Maryellen Brunson McClain ·
Jeffrey D. Shahidullah ·
Katherine R. Mezher
Editors

Interprofessional Care Coordination for Pediatric Autism Spectrum Disorder

Translating Research into Practice

Springer

Editors
Maryellen Brunson McClain
Department of Psychology
Utah State University
Logan, UT, USA

Jeffrey D. Shahidullah
Department of Psychiatry
University of Texas at Austin
Dell Medical School
Austin, TX, USA

Katherine R. Mezher
Department of Educational Psychology
Miami University
Oxford, OH, USA

ISBN 978-3-030-46294-9 ISBN 978-3-030-46295-6 (eBook)
https://doi.org/10.1007/978-3-030-46295-6

This Springer imprint is published by the registered company Springer Nature Switzerland AG
The registered company address is: Gewerbestrasse 11, 6330 Cham, Switzerland

Maryellen Brunson McClain:

For my husband, Abraham Verdoes, for his continued love and support throughout my graduate training and academic career. And for my parents, Edwin and Leana McClain, who instilled in me a passion for learning and education.

Jeffrey D. Shahidullah:

I am forever grateful to my wife (Ashley) and children (Jalen, Jazlene, and Benjamin) for their love, support, and patience during the writing of this book.

Katherine R. Mezher:

To my husband and children—Mike, Eleanor, Michael, and George—for your unwavering support.

Acknowledgments

We would like to acknowledge Megan E. Golson for her hard work and editorial assistance during the writing of this book.

Contents

Editors and Contributors

About the Editors

Maryellen Brunson McClain, Ph.D., is an Assistant Professor of Psychology at Utah State University. She is also core faculty with the Utah Regional Leadership Education in Neurodevelopmental and related Disabilities (URLEND) program. Dr. McClain's research, clinical, and teaching interests are related to autism spectrum disorder and related neurodevelopmental disorders. She is particularly interested in assessment considerations, interprofessional coordinated care, measure development, and appropriate assessment and identification of culturally and linguistically diverse children. Dr. McClain earned a BA in Psychology from the College of Wooster and a Ph.D. in School Psychology from Indiana University. Dr. McClain completed her APA-accredited predoctoral internship at the University of Tennessee Professional Psychology Internship Consortium at the University of Tennessee Health Science Center (UTHSC). She completed a postdoctoral fellowship in developmental disabilities at the Boling Center for Developmental Disabilities (BCDD) at UTHSC. Dr. McClain is a licensed psychologist in the state of Utah. She was a LEND trainee as a graduate student (Riley Hospital for Children), a predoctoral intern (UTHSC), and a postdoctoral fellow (BCDD).

Jeffrey D. Shahidullah, Ph.D., is an Assistant Professor of psychiatry at The University of Texas at Austin Dell Medical School. He is a Co-director of research for Developmental and Behavioral Pediatrics. Dr. Shahidullah holds the Health Service Psychologist (HSP) and Nationally Certified School Psychologist (NCSP) credentials. He is a Pediatric Psychologist within a Developmental and Behavioral Pediatrics clinic at Dell Children's Medical Center of Central Texas and UT Health Austin. He also provides consultative telephonic support for mental/behavioral health concerns to rural primary care practices and schools as part of state-funded telemedicine initiatives, Texas Child Psychiatry Access Network (CPAN) and Texas Child Health Access through Telemedicine Program (TCHAT). Dr. Shahidullah earned a BA in psychology and EdS in school psychology from

Baylor University. He then earned a Ph.D. in school psychology at Michigan State University. He completed his APA-accredited predoctoral internship at The Children's Hospital of Philadelphia (CHOP) and postdoctoral fellowship at Geisinger Health System, both in pediatric psychology. While at CHOP, he was a Leadership Education in Neurodevelopmental Disabilities (LEND) fellow. Previously, he was an Assistant Professor within the Graduate School of Applied and Professional Psychology (GSAPP) at Rutgers University—New Brunswick, where he also held an adjunct appointment as an Assistant Professor of pediatrics at Rutgers Robert Wood Johnson Medical School. Dr. Shahidullah's clinical, research, and training interests pertain to integrating behavioral health services within schools and primary care settings. He is also interested in models of interprofessional training and collaboration among healthcare providers. He is the Author of the *Handbook of Pediatric Behavioral Healthcare: An Interdisciplinary Collaborative Approach*, which is also published by Springer Publishing Company.

Katherine R. Mezher, Ph.D., is an Assistant Clinical Professor and the School Psychology Program Coordinator, in the Department of Educational Psychology at Miami University (Oxford, Ohio). She received her Ph.D. in School Psychology from the University of Tennessee, Knoxville. Dr. Mezher completed a postdoctoral fellowship in the Kelly O'Leary Center for Autism Spectrum Disorder at Cincinnati Children's Hospital Medical Center and is a licensed Psychologist in the state of Ohio. While at Cincinnati Children's Hospital, she was also a fellow in the Leadership Education in Neurodevelopment and Related Disabilities (LEND) interdisciplinary training program. Dr. Mezher's interests include early intervention, autism spectrum disorder and developmental disabilities, service coordination, and individual academic and behavior interventions in school settings. She has taught 10 courses at Miami, including but not limited to behavior intervention, psychoeducational assessment, education of individuals with exceptionalities, autism trends and research, and educational research. She currently also serves as the School Psychology Internship Coordinator.

Contributors

Jessica S. Akers Department of Educational Psychology, Baylor University, Waco, TX, USA

Amanda Austin Department of School Psychology, Graduate School of Applied and Professional Psychology, Rutgers University, New Brunswick, NJ, USA

Gazi F. Azad Division of Child and Adolescent Psychiatry, New York State Psychiatric Institute and Columbia University, New York, NY, USA

Rebecca A. Baum Clinical Associate Professor of Pediatrics, Division of Developmental Behavioral Pediatrics, Nationwide Children's Hospital, The Ohio State University College of Medicine, Columbus, OH, USA

Kristen E. Beck Clinical Assistant Professor of Pediatrics, Nationwide Children's Hospital, The Ohio State University College of Medicine, Columbus, OH, USA

Paul J. Bellino Department of Pediatrics, Geisinger Health System, Danville, PA, USA

Jan Blacher Graduate School of Education, University of California, Riverside, Riverside, CA, USA

Yasamin Bolourian Graduate School of Education, University of California, Riverside, Riverside, CA, USA

Briana Brukilacchio Department of Educational Psychology, The University of Texas at Austin, Austin, TX, USA

Kaitlin Bundock Department of Special Education and Rehabilitation Counseling, Utah State University, Logan, UT, USA

Jonathan M. Campbell Department of Psychology, Western Carolina University, Cullowhee, NC, USA

Atilla T. Ceranoglu Department of Psychiatry, Bressler Clinical and Research Program for Autism Spectrum Disorders, Harvard Medical School, Massachusetts General Hospital, Boston, MA, USA

Susan Copeland Department of Special Education, University of New Mexico, Albuquerque, NM, USA

Benjamin Covington Department of Psychology, Utah State University, Logan, UT, USA

Geraldine Dawson Department of Psychiatry and Behavioral Sciences, Duke Center for Autism and Brain Development, Duke University School of Medicine, Durham, NC, USA

John-Joe Dawson-Squibb Center for Autism Research in Africa, Division of Child and Adolescent Psychiatry, University of Cape Town, Cape Town, South Africa

Kathryn A. DeHart Department of Pediatrics, Geisinger Health System, Danville, PA, USA

Amie Duncan Department of Pediatrics, Cincinnati Children's Hospital Medical Center, Cincinnati, OH, USA

Morgan Engelmann Department of Educational Psychology, The University of Texas at Austin, Austin, TX, USA

Autumn Fikki Department of Educational Psychology, The University of Texas at Austin, Austin, TX, USA

Susan G. Forman Department of School Psychology, Rutgers University, New Brunswick, NJ, USA

Samantha Fuld School of Social Work, University of Maryland, Baltimore, MD, USA

Terisa P. Gabrielsen Counseling, Psychology and Special Education, Brigham Young University, Provo, UT, USA

Megan E. Golson Department of Psychology, Utah State University, Logan, UT, USA

Brigid K. Groves Department of Pharmacy, Columbus, OH, USA

Christina Harkins Department of Human Services, Curry School of Education and Human Development, University of Virginia, Charlottesville, VA, USA

Bryn Harris School of Education and Human Development, Department of Pediatrics, University of Colorado Denver, Denver, CO, USA

Jill H. Harris Children's Specialized Hospital, New Brunswick, NJ, USA

Ashley J. Harrison Educational Psychology Department, University of Georgia, Athens, GA, USA

Cassity R. Haverkamp Department of Psychology, Utah State University, Logan, UT, USA

Michelle Heyman Graduate School of Education, University of California, Riverside, Riverside, CA, USA

Trenesha Hill Pediatric Mental Health Institute, Children's Hospital Colorado, Aurora, CO, USA

Meredith I. Holley Department of Psychiatry, The University of Texas at Austin, Austin, TX, USA

Judith Holt Utah State University, Logan, UT, USA

Cody A. Hostutler Pediatric Psychology and Neuropsychology, Columbus, OH, USA;
Department of Pediatrics, The Ohio State University College of Medicine, Columbus, OH, USA

Jill Howard Department of Psychiatry and Behavioral Sciences, Duke Center for Autism and Brain Development, Duke University School of Medicine, Durham, NC, USA

Gagan Joshi Department of Psychiatry, Bressler Clinical and Research Program for Autism Spectrum Disorders, Harvard Medical School, Massachusetts General Hospital, Boston, MA, USA

Christopher J. Keary Department of Psychiatry, Harvard Medical School, Lurie Center for Autism, Massachusetts General Hospital, Boston, MA, USA

Paul W. Kettlewell Department of Psychiatry, Geisinger Health System, Danville, PA, USA

Marie Kirkpatrick Department of Educational Psychology, Baylor University, Waco, TX, USA

Sharon L. Larson Center for Population Health Research, Main Line Health System, Thomas Jefferson University, Philadelphia, PA, USA

David S. Mandell Center for Mental Health, Perelman School of Medicine, University of Pennsylvania, Philadelphia, PA, USA

Stacy Shumway Manwaring Communication Sciences and Disorders, University of Utah, Salt Lake City, UT, USA

Micah O. Mazurek Department of Human Services, Curry School of Education and Human Development, University of Virginia, Charlottesville, VA, USA

Maryellen Brunson McClain Department of Psychology, Utah State University, Logan, UT, USA

Christopher J. McDougle Department of Psychiatry, Harvard Medical School, Lurie Center for Autism, Massachusetts General Hospital, Boston, MA, USA

Laura Lee McIntyre College of Education, University of Oregon, Eugene, OR, USA

Michelle Menezes Department of Human Services, Curry School of Education and Human Development, University of Virginia, Charlottesville, VA, USA

Katherine R. Mezher Department of Educational Psychology, Miami University, Oxford, OH, USA

Kyla E. Minton Center for Autism and Related Disorders, Kennedy Krieger Institute, Baltimore, MD, USA

Amy Norton Autism Department, Children's Specialized Hospital, New Brunswick, NJ, USA

Bill Ogletree Department of Communication Sciences and Disorders, Western Carolina University, Cullowhee, NC, USA

Tiffany Otero Department of Special Education, University of New Mexico, Albuquerque, NM, USA

Sirin Ozdemir Department of Psychiatry, Harvard Medical School, Massachusetts General Hospital, Boston, MA, USA

Kristen Padilla Department of Educational Psychology, Baylor University, Waco, TX, USA

Gretchen Gimpel Peacock Department of Psychology, Utah State University, Logan, UT, USA

Sarah E. Pinkelman Department of Special Education and Rehabilitation, Utah State University, Logan, UT, USA

Johanna Price Department of Communication Sciences and Disorders, Western Carolina University, Cullowhee, NC, USA

Sheri Ravenscroft Developmental-Behavioral Pediatrics, Dell Children's Medical Group, Austin, TX, USA

Nuri Reyes Departments of Pediatrics and Psychiatry, University of Colorado School of Medicine, Anschutz Medical Campus, Aurora, CO, USA

Jessie Richard Nationwide Children's Hospital, Center for Autism Spectrum Disorders, Columbus, OH, USA

Kristen Rolf Department of Special Education and Rehabilitation, Utah State University, Logan, UT, USA

Amy Rose Department of Communication Sciences and Disorders, Western Carolina University, Cullowhee, NC, USA

Jeffrey D. Shahidullah Department of Psychiatry, University of Texas at Austin Dell Medical School, Austin, TX, USA

Susan M. Sheridan College of Education and Human Sciences, University of Nebraska Lincoln, Lincoln, NE, USA

Stephanie Y. Shire College of Education, University of Oregon, Eugene, OR, USA

Vicki Simonsmeier Sorenson Legacy Foundation Center for Clinical Excellence, Utah State University, Logan, UT, USA

Tyanna C. Snider Division of Pediatric Psychology and Neuropsychology, Nationwide Children's Hospital, Columbus, OH, USA

Neelkamal Soares Pediatric and Adolescent Medicine, Western Michigan University Homer Stryker M.D. School of Medicine, Kalamazoo, MI, USA

Kristin Sohl Department of Child Health, University of Missouri, Columbia, MO, USA

Dasha Solomon Boston Children's Hospital, Harvard Medical School, Boston, MA, USA

Ashley L. Stuart Pediatrics, University of Utah, Salt Lake City, UT, USA

Brianna J. Williams Department of Counseling, Educational Psychology, and Special Education, Michigan State University, East Lansing, MI, USA

Sarah Winter Department of Pediatrics, University of Utah, Salt Lake City, UT, USA

Lisa Wisman Weil Department of Communication Sciences and Disorders, Emerson College, Boston, MA, USA

Luodi Yu Autism Research Center, School of Psychology, South China Normal University, Guangzhou, China;
Department of Speech-Language-Hearing Sciences, University of Minnesota Twin Cities, Minneapolis, MN, USA

Introduction to Interprofessional Care Coordination for Pediatric Autism Spectrum Disorder

Maryellen Brunson McClain, Jeffrey D. Shahidullah, and Katherine R. Mezher

Abstract This chapter introduces this book and its central purpose. Autism spectrum disorder, its associated symptoms, and rising prevalence warrant service provision from several disciplines and professions. The rationale and benefits of interprofessional care coordination are discussed. The following chapters in this book are written by professionals from diverse fields to encourage and improve readers' interprofessional care coordination.

Autism spectrum disorder (ASD) is a lifelong neurodevelopmental disorder characterized by deficits in social communication and interaction and is accompanied by restricted, repetitive patterns of behavior (American Psychiatric Association, 2013). The prevalence rates of ASD have dramatically increased in recent years with current estimates suggesting that 1 in 54 children (approximately 1.9%) in the United States have ASD (Maenner et al., 2020). The lifetime cost of education, healthcare, and other service needs for an individual with ASD can range from $1.4 to $2.4 million dollars (Buescher, Cidav, Knapp, & Mandell, 2014).

ASD is complex and can impact several areas of functioning, including social, behavioral, mental health, and academic. Moreover, many children with ASD experience high rates of co-occurring medical and mental health problems. As a result of the complex nature of the disorder and the co-occurring problems, many children with ASD receive care from a variety of providers. Providers represent numerous disciplines (e.g., psychology, speech-language pathology, medicine), work in several settings (e.g., hospitals, community clinics, schools, primary care), and are involved at all stages of care from screening and evaluation/identification to service provision and management. Because children with ASD have a wide range of symptom manifestations and needs that change over time, service management can present

M. B. McClain (✉)
Department of Psychology, Utah State University, Logan, UT, USA
e-mail: maryellen.mcclainverdoes@usu.edu

J. D. Shahidullah
Department of Psychiatry, University of Texas at Austin Dell Medical School, Austin, TX, USA

K. R. Mezher
Department of Educational Psychology, Miami University, Oxford, OH, USA

M. B. McClain et al. (eds.), *Interprofessional Care Coordination for Pediatric Autism Spectrum Disorder*, https://doi.org/10.1007/978-3-030-46295-6_1

particular challenges for clinicians. The multiple medical, developmental, educational, and behavioral outcomes associated with ASD necessitate interprofessional care coordination (ICC) of services, advocacy, and engagement in care on behalf of children with ASD and their families.

ICC consists of streamlining services across professionals and disciplines both within and across settings (Shahidullah, Azad, Mezher, McClain, & McIntyre, 2018). ICC may reduce unmet healthcare needs, gaps in care across settings, and duplication of services for children with ASD and their families (McClain et al., 2019). Engagement in ICC requires interprofessional collaboration, which occurs when "multiple health workers from different professional backgrounds provide comprehensive services by working with patients, their families, careers and communities to deliver the highest quality of care across settings" (Gilbert, Yan, & Hoffman, 2010; p. 13). Working as part of successful interprofessional teams is pivotal in addressing unmet healthcare needs. Characteristics of strong interprofessional teams include providing clarity of roles and responsibilities, optimizing individual professional skills, and improving the provision and coordination of care through team-work and camaraderie (Bridges, Davidson, Odegard, Maki, & Tomkowiak, 2011).

The purpose of this book is to present how professionals across various disciplines and settings can collaborate in an interprofessional manner in working with children who have ASD and their families with an emphasis on both identification and service provision. There lacks consensus in the literature regarding the terminology to describe the ways in which professionals across disciplines interact in providing clinical care (Chamberlain-Salaun, Mills, & Usher, 2013). However, in general, interprofessional and interdisciplinary refer to professionals from various disciplines collaborating and working together to provide services. In this book, authors use both interdisciplinary and interprofessional to refer to this overarching definition. Chapters emphasize broad (e.g., screening and surveillance, identification, service provision) as well as specialized (e.g., ASD and trauma, international perspectives, social skills) considerations. Chapters also highlight the importance of interprofessional care across various settings (e.g., primary care, schools) and during specific services (e.g., speech-language therapy, applied behavior analysis, school-based interventions, psychopharmacology).

This book is designed for professionals across a range of disciplines that provide services to children with ASD and their families. It is our hope that this book will provide an easy reference guide for clinicians across pediatric healthcare settings, schools, and community clinics including primary care physicians, developmental–behavioral pediatricians, child and adolescent psychiatrists, pediatric medical specialists, nurses, medical geneticists, pharmacists, school and clinical psychologists, social workers, speech and language pathologists, occupational therapists, physical therapists, audiologists, counselors, behavior therapists and analysts, psychometricians, and educators. We hope these chapters will provide professionals who have ICC experience with new and innovative ideas to strengthen current and develop new collaborative interprofessional relationships. We also strive to encourage clinicians who do not yet engage in ICC to consider developing such interprofessional relationships.

References

American Psychiatric Association. (2013). Diagnostic and statistical manual of mental disorders (5th ed.). Washington DC: American Psychiatric Association.

Bridges, D. R., Davidson, R. A., Odegard, P. S., Maki, I. V., & Tomkowiak, J. (2011). Interprofessional collaboration: Three best practice models of interprofessional education. *Medical Education Online, 16,* 1.

Buescher, Ariane V. S., Cidav, Z., Knapp, M., Mandell, D. S. (2014). Costs of autism spectrum disorders in the United Kingdom and the United States. *JAMA Pediatrics, 168*(8), 721

Chamberlain-Salaun, J., Mills, J., & Usher, K. (2013). Terminology used to describe health care teams: An integrative review of the literature. *J. Multidisciplinary Healthcare, 6,* 65–74.

Gilbert, J. H., Yan, J., & Hoffman, S. J. (2010). A WHO report: Framework for action on interprofessional education and collaborative practice. *Journal of Allied Health, 39,* 196–197. https://scholar.harvard.edu/hoffman/publications/who-report-framework-action-interprofessionaleducation-and-collaborative-pract.

Maenner, M. J., Shaw, K. A., Baio, J., Washington, A., Patrick, M & Dietz, P. M. (2020). Prevalence of autism spectrum disorder among children aged 8 years—autism and developmental disabilities monitoring network, 11 Sites, United States, 2016. *MMWR Surveillance Summaries, 69*(4), 1–12.

McClain, M. B., Shahidullah, J. D., Mezher, K., Olson, K., Haverkamp, C., & Schwartz, S. (2019). School-clinic care coordination for youth with ASD: A national survey of school psychologists. *Journal of Autism and Developmental Disorders.*

Shahidullah, J. D., Azad, G. F., Mezher, K., McClain, M. B., & McIntyre, L. L. (2018). Linking the medical and educational home to support children with autism spectrum disorder: Practice recommendations. *Clinical Pediatrics, 57,* 1496–1505.

Medical Comorbidities in Pediatric Autism Spectrum Disorder

Amanda Austin and Jeffrey D. Shahidullah

Abstract Youth with autism spectrum disorder (ASD) have many and varied social, emotional, behavioral, and academic needs. In many cases, these children also have medical needs, adding to the level of care they require. Medical conditions commonly co-occur in children with ASD; some of the most common include epilepsy, gastrointestinal issues, sleep problems, and feeding disorders. The diagnosis and treatment of these conditions is often complicated by their ASD symptoms. The care and collaboration of professionals from multiple disciplines is needed to effectively conceptualize and treat these conditions. This chapter provides a review of common co-occurring medical conditions in children with ASD and highlights the need for interprofessional collaboration.

Medical conditions commonly co-occur in children with autism spectrum disorder (ASD) (Coury, 2010; Levy et al., 2010; Vargason, Frye, McGuinness, & Hahn, 2019). Some of the most common include epilepsy, gastrointestinal issues, sleep problems, and feeding disorders (Kohane et al., 2012). Children with ASD are also significantly more likely than children without ASD to have a variety of psychiatric conditions, non-emergency and hospital emergency care, and high medication usage (Gurney, McPheeters, & Davis, 2006). These medical conditions can be a challenge to manage clinically and can have a dramatic impact on the quality of child and family life (Devnani & Hegde, 2015; Kohane et al., 2012). This chapter provides an overview of commonly co-occurring medical conditions in youth with ASD and highlights the need for interprofessional care for this population.

A. Austin
Department of School Psychology, Graduate School of Applied and Professional Psychology, Rutgers University, New Brunswick, NJ, USA
e-mail: afa72@gsapp.rutgers.edu

J. D. Shahidullah (✉)
Department of Psychiatry, Dell Medical School, University of Texas at Austin, Austin, TX, USA
e-mail: Jeff.Shahidullah@austin.utexas.edu

M. B. McClain et al. (eds.), *Interprofessional Care Coordination for Pediatric Autism Spectrum Disorder*, https://doi.org/10.1007/978-3-030-46295-6_2

Epilepsy

Epilepsy and seizure disorders are common co-occurring medical conditions in children with ASD. Epilepsy is a brain disease characterized by: (1) at least two unprovoked seizures that occur more than 24 h apart, (2) one unprovoked seizure and a probability of 60% or greater of further seizures after two unprovoked seizures, occurring over the next 10 years, or (3) diagnosis of an epilepsy syndrome (Fisher et al., 2014). An epileptic seizure is caused by abnormal electrical activity in the brain and can manifest differently across both individuals and occurrences, varying in topography and severity. The three primary types of seizures include focal, generalized, and unclassified seizures, and individuals may experience one or more of these types. Focal seizures occur in one or more localized brain regions, while generalized seizures affect both sides of the brain. Unclassified seizures have unknown or unclear onsets. Generally, seizures may involve staring spells; sudden jerking of the extremities, face, or neck; and/or loss of consciousness. Individuals may also experience symptoms, or auras, such as sensations or mood changes, prior to the onset of a seizure that signal that they will soon experience one (Follansbee-Junger, Smith, Guilfoyle, & Modi, 2018).

Epilepsy affects between 8–30% of children with ASD (Tuchman & Cuccaro, 2011), compared to 1–2% of the general population (Spence & Schneider, 2009). This overrepresentation is consistent across many studies of epilepsy in children with and without ASD. Additionally, it appears that heredity is unable to explain these increased rates, as a study that examined parent and sibling prevalence rates of epilepsy found that compared to the 12.2% of children with ASD in the study who experienced seizures, only 4.1% of their parents and 2.7% of their siblings also experienced seizures (Aldinger, Lane, Veenstra-VanderWeele, & Levitt, 2015). This suggests that the prevalence of epilepsy and seizures among youth with ASD is likely more attributable to the fact that they have ASD and not because they may have inherited it from family members. Conclusively, it has been reported that having epilepsy increases the risk for ASD, and that having ASD increases the risk of epilepsy (Amiet et al., 2008).

A high rate of epilepsy is found in children with both ASD and an intellectual disability. Having an intellectual disability is considered a risk factor for epilepsy, with more severe intellectual disabilities leading to a greater risk for developing epilepsy. A meta-analysis found that the pooled prevalence of epilepsy in individuals with ASD and an intellectual disability was 21.4% compared to 8% of children with epilepsy and ASD without an intellectual disability (Amiet et al., 2008). There is a particular risk for developing both ASD and intellectual disabilities among infants demonstrating epileptic encephalopathies and infantile spasms (Tuchman, Alessandri, & Cuccaro, 2010; Tuchman & Cuccaro, 2011). One study found that 14% of infants with the onset of epilepsy within their first year of life developed ASD.

Epilepsy diagnoses are typically made based on several factors, among them patient history, description of seizures, and tests that detect abnormal electrographic activity in the brain (i.e., EEGs and MRIs; Follansbee-Junger et al., 2018). This diagnostic process can become complicated by ASD symptoms and/or diagnoses. Significant abnormal EEGs are found in as many as 60% of individuals with ASD without any clinical seizure activity (Chez, Chang, Krasne, Coughlan, Kominsky, & Schwartz, 2006; Spence & Schneider, 2009). Additionally, some seizure symptoms may be difficult to differentiate from typical ASD behaviors (e.g., not responding to name, repetitive movements; Tye, Rinicles, & Whitehouse, 2019). Given the elevated rates of epilepsy and seizures among children with ASD, it is important to be aware of subtle symptoms that can be the result of either ASD or epilepsy (Kagan-Kushnir, Roberts, & Snead, 2005). Collaboration between professionals in the areas of epilepsy and ASD is needed to ensure proper diagnosis and to discriminate between symptoms of ASD and symptoms of epilepsy. Parent or caregiver input is also necessary in determining a proper diagnosis, as they will be most familiar with how their child's symptoms manifest.

For individuals with both epilepsy and ASD, the most common treatment option is the use of anti-epileptic drugs, which works for approximately two-thirds of individuals. Additional treatment options for the one-third of children who are treatment-resistant include surgery, vagal nerve stimulation, and dietary changes (Follansbee-Junger et al., 2018). Psychosocial interventions can also help supplement these treatments in countering the developmental delays that can accompany epilepsy and ASD but do not typically change as a result of traditional treatments (Spence & Schneider, 2009; Tuchman et al., 2010). Monitoring the effects of treatments will require collaboration between a child's parent or caregiver, the prescriber of any medication, implementers of other treatments, and those with whom the child works within any other capacity (e.g., teachers, therapists).

Having diagnoses of both ASD and epilepsy can be indicative of a variety of poorer outcomes than those with ASD without epilepsy. Areas of greater risk include cognitive, adaptive, behavioral, social, and medical domains (Hara, 2007; Turk et al., 2009; Viscidi et al. 2014). Overall, individuals with ASD and epilepsy report a lower quality of life (Tye et al., 2019). Specifically, regarding behavioral outcomes, these children tend to exhibit more maladaptive behaviors associated with ASD, including self-injurious, compulsive, and ritualistic behaviors (Viscidi et al., 2014). Socially, they may have impaired facial recognition and theory of mind (Richard & Scheffer, 2017), lower social maturity (Tye et al., 2019), increased staring behavior (i.e., staring too hard and too long), and overall increased difficulties with social interactions (Turk et al., 2009). Also elevated in this population are rates of earlier mortality (Gillberg, Billstedt, Sundh, & Gillberg, 2010) and the use of psychotropic medications (Hara, 2007).

Gastrointestinal Issues

Gastrointestinal (GI) issues are among common medical conditions associated with ASD. GI symptoms and conditions that exist at elevated rates in this population include abdominal pain, chronic constipation with or without diarrhea (Buie et al.,

2010), gastroesophageal reflux disease (GERD), Crohn's disease, inflammatory bowel disease (IBD), and colitis (Bauman, 2010). While the most common symptom is not universally agreed upon, it is suggested that the most common symptoms include chronic constipation (Holingue, Newill, Lee, Pasricha, & Fallin, 2018) and diarrhea (Coury, 2010).

While prevalence rates vary among studies, numerous studies have found significantly higher rates of GI issues among children with ASD than children without ASD. A meta-analysis found that GI issues occur four times as frequently in children with ASD than in children without ASD (McElhanon, McCracken, Karpen, & Sharp, 2014). Other studies examining specific GI symptoms have determined a prevalence rate for constipation of 33.9%, which occurs in 17.6% of those without ASD (Ibrahim, Voigt, Katusic, Weaver, & Barbaresi, 2009), 0.83% for IBD (0.54% non-ASD; Kohane et al., 2012), and 11.74% for bowel disorders not including IBD (4.5% non-ASD; Kohane et al., 2012). As with epilepsy, it appears that heredity is unable to explain these increased rates; Aldinger et al. (2015) found that compared to the 42.2% of children with GID and ASD in their sample, 26.5% of their parents and 12.2% of their siblings had GID.

GI issues often lead to or are accompanied by issues with incontinence, including nocturnal enuresis, daytime enuresis, and encopresis. A systematic review found that prevalence rates for all three issues are higher in children with ASD than in typical peers (2–41%, 4.3–25%, 2–12.5%, respectively; Niemcyzk, Wagner & von Gontard, 2018). These issues, specifically encopresis, commonly stem from both medical and behavioral difficulties, causing the integration of care from several providers to be of particular importance.

Diagnosing GI issues in this population is often more difficult than it is in the general population. Due to impairments in communication, frequently the only indicator of GI issues in children with ASD is the exacerbation of problem behavior (Bauman, 2010); thus, it is important for multiple providers to collaboratively assess and determine whether behaviors are being exhibited due to pain or another cause. Treatment of GI issues in ASD may include dietary interventions and behavioral interventions focused on feeding and diet, nutritional supplements, and medication. Treatment of enuresis and encopresis is largely behavioral, as medical interventions alone are typically designed to treat isolated episodes (Furuta et al., 2012); however, when integrated with behavioral interventions, medical treatment can be beneficial in promoting continence. As medical approaches are implemented to relieve instances of constipation, sitting on the toilet prior to a bowel movement can be prompted and reinforced (Call, Mevers, McElhanon, & Scheithauer, 2017). Such interventions require extensive collaboration between professionals (e.g., behavior analysts, pediatric gastroenterologists, nursing staff), as they often deviate from and are more intensive than treatments used in typically developing children. Treatment packages and the extent of collaboration needed will vary depending on the child and any barriers to typical treatment the child experiences (e.g., medication intolerance, feeding issues, behavioral issues).

Sleep Problems

Issues with sleep are commonly experienced by children with ASD. Sleep problems include delayed sleep onset, night waking, early awakening, a reduced need for sleep or shorter duration of sleep, parasomnias such as nightmares, and sleep-related breathing and movement disorders (Bauman, 2010). The most commonly reported concern is insomnia, which includes problems surrounding sleep onset and night waking. The prevalence of sleep problems in children with ASD vary, but range from 40–80% (Cortesi, Giannotti, Ivanenko, & Johnson, 2010), while the prevalence in children without ASD is approximately 30% (Krakowiak, Goodlin-Jones, Hertz-Picciotto, Croen, & Hansen, 2008).

Sleep problems affect daytime behavior and can cause neurocognitive dysfunction and behavioral disruptions (Mazurek, Dovgan, Neumeyer, & Malow, 2019). They have been found to be predictive of ASD symptom severity (Schreck, Mulick, & Smith, 2004), and lead to attention difficulties, hyperactivity, and anxiety (Mazurek et al., 2019). Not only do they have an impact on child quality of life, but they also affect the functioning and quality of life of the family (Devnani & Hegde, 2015). Because sleep problems often have behavioral components (Johnson & Malow, 2008), treatment typically involves improving sleep hygiene, behavioral interventions, and may also include pharmacological treatments (e.g., melatonin). Improving sleep hygiene includes establishing environmental cues and bedtime routines that can make it more likely a child will fall asleep quicker and stay asleep longer. These can include keeping bedtime and wake times the same each day, putting away electronics at least 30 min before bed, and keeping a cool temperature in the bedroom.

For a child who has established any maladaptive sleep associations (e.g., parent in room while falling asleep), parents can work to break the association by gradually distancing themselves from the child's bed each night to foster independent sleep onset (Maxwell-Horn & Malow, 2017). For children who frequently leave their bed during the night ("curtain calls"), the "bedtime pass" intervention may be used (Friman, Hoff, Schnoes, Freeman, Woods, & Blum, 1999). This involves giving the child a card, or "bedtime pass," that she can redeem once per night to get out of bed for any reason. Any problem behaviors that occur after the card is traded in are ignored and any attempts to escape from the bedroom are redirected with minimal attention. If a bedtime pass is left unused, then it can be redeemed the next morning for a special reward that the child ordinarily does not get outside of this program. Collaboration between caregivers and behavior specialists is needed to select appropriate interventions and ensure proper implementation, and prescribers of any medications must be involved in treatment to monitor its effects on sleep disturbances.

Feeding Disorders

Feeding problems represent a substantial concern among children with ASD, impacting not only those with ASD, but also their families and teachers (Ledford & Gast, 2006). Children with ASD are five times more likely than children without ASD to develop a feeding issue (Sharp et al., 2013). A review found that 46–89% of children with ASD are present with feeding issues (Ledford & Gast, 2006). The most common feeding problem among this population is food selectivity, which can include narrow food preferences, refusal of certain textures, or requiring specific food presentations (Schreck, Williams, & Smith, 2004). Such concerns can greatly impact the daily lives of affected families, as their children with ASD may not eat the same meals that the rest of the family eats, they may have to shop for specific foods, and their ability to eat at restaurants may be impeded. Children with feeding issues, if untreated, are also at an elevated risk of developing psychiatric disorders (Zucker et al., 2015), nutritional deficits (Cornish, 1998), and having impaired growth (Schwarz, 2003).

Feeding issues in children with ASD often have behavioral components (Ledford & Gast, 2006). Feeding issues can occur due to difficulties with compliance, cognitive rigidity, and/or sensory-based aversions, and can be maintained through caregiver reinforcement and lack of contingency management. Treatment of feeding issues typically includes a behavioral intervention(s), such as simultaneous presentation, sequential presentation, differential reinforcement, stimulus fading, escape extinction, and appetite manipulation. Behavior therapists specializing in feeding disorders must work closely with caregivers to implement and monitor interventions and ensure interventions are being implemented with fidelity by caregivers. It is important for medical professionals to rule out any medical origins for feeding problems. Feeding disorders should be treated as early as possible to lessen the risk of nutritional deficits and other health issues that can arise (Ledford & Gast, 2006).

Conclusion

The overrepresentation of co-occurring medical conditions in children with ASD leads to an increased need for enhanced interprofessional collaboration among care providers for this population. In addition to the most common co-occurring conditions described above, children with ASD are at an increased risk of many others including obesity, hypotonia, allergic diseases, and immune dysfunction (Bauman, 2010). As comorbid medical conditions often lead to higher risks of negative social, behavioral, medical, educational, and/or psychiatric outcomes (Neuhaus, Bernier, Tham, & Webb, 2018), multiple providers are needed to provide the most comprehensive treatment and increase the likelihood of a better quality of life for both children and their families. Currently, ensuring collaborative and interprofessional services is made challenging by each provider's distinct setting and approach to care, lack of communication between providers, and gaps in services (Shahidullah et al., 2018).

While many medical conditions occur at increased rates in children with ASD and have been shown to share underlying mechanisms, there is much uncertainty surrounding what causes these enhanced rates, making it difficult to take preventive measures. The exacerbation of ASD symptoms by some medical conditions, difficulty with identification as a result of ASD, and treatment of ASD and comorbid medical conditions make it necessary for a higher quality of care and screening. Due to complications in the diagnostic and treatment processes of medical conditions in children with ASD, it is important for professionals to engage in collaborative service management.

References

Aldinger, K. A., Lane, C. J., Veenstra-VanderWeele, J., & Levitt, P. (2015). Patterns of risk for multiple co-occurring medical conditions replicate across distinct cohorts of children with autism spectrum disorder. *Autism Research, 8,* 771–781.

Amiet, C., Gourfinkel-An, I., Bouzamondo, A., Tordjman, S., Baulac, M., Lechat, P., … Cohen, D. (2008). Epilepsy in autism is associated with intellectual disability and gender: Evidence from a meta-analysis. *Biological Psychiatry, 64,* 577–582.

Bauman, M. L. (2010). Medical comorbidities in autism: Challenges to diagnosis and treatment. *Neurotherapeutics: The Journal of the American Society for Experimental NeuroTherapeutics, 7,* 320–327.

Buie, T., Campbell, D. B., Fuchs, G. J., Furuta, G. T., Levy, J., Van de Water, J., … Winter, H. (2010). Evaluation, diagnosis, and treatment of gastrointestinal disorders in individuals with ASDs: A consensus report. *Pediatrics, 125,* S1–S18.

Call, N., Mevers, J. L., McElhanon, B. O., & Scheithauer, M. C. (2017). A multidisciplinary treatment for encopresis in children with developmental disabilities. *Journal of Applied Behavior Analysis, 50,* 332–344.

Chez, M. G., Chang, M., Krasne, V., Coughlan, C., Kominsky, M., & Schwartz, A. (2006). Frequency of epileptiform EEG abnormalities in a sequential screening of autistic patients with no known clinical epilepsy from 1996 to 2005. *Epilepsy & Behavior, 8,* 267–271.

Cornish, E. (1998). A balanced approach towards healthy eating in autism. *Journal of Human Nutrition & Dietetics, 11,* 501–509.

Cortesi, F., Giannotti, F., Ivanenko, A., & Johnson, K. (2010). Sleep in children with autistic spectrum disorder. *Sleep Medicine, 11,* 659–664.

Coury, D. (2010). Medical treatment of autism spectrum disorders. *Current Opinion in Neurology, 23,* 131–136.

Devnani, P. A., & Hegde, A. U. (2015). Autism and sleep disorders. *Journal of Pediatric Neurosciences, 10,* 304–307.

Fisher, R. S., Acevedo, C., Arzimanoglou, A., Bogacz, A., Cross, H., Elger, C. E., … Wiebe, S. (2014). A practical clinical definition of epilepsy. *Epilepsia, 55,* 475–482.

Follansbee-Junger, K., Smith, A. W., Guilfoyle, S., & Modi, A. C. (2018). Epilepsy. In S. G. Forman & J. D. Shahidullah (Eds.), *Handbook of pediatric behavioral healthcare: An interdisciplinary collaborative approach* (pp. 85–98). Switzerland: Springer.

Friman, P. C., Hoff, K. E., Schnoes, C., Freeman, K. A., Woods, D. W., & Blum, N. (1999). The bedtime pass. *Archives of Pediatric and Adolescent Medicine, 153*(10), 1027–1029.

Furuta, G. T., Williams, K., Kooros, K., Kaul, A., Panzer, R., Coury, D. L., Fuchs, G. (2012). Management of constipation in children and adolescents with autism spectrum disorders. *Pediatrics, 130,* S98–S105.

Gillberg, C., Billstedt, E., Sundh, V., & Gillberg, I. C. (2010). Mortality in autism: A prospective longitudinal community-based study. *Journal of Autism and Developmental Disorders, 40,* 352–357.

Gurney, J. G., McPheeters, M. L., & Davis, M. M. (2006). Parental report of health conditions and health care use among children with and without autism. *Archives of Pediatric and Adolescent Medicine, 160,* 825–830.

Hara, H. (2007). Autism and epilepsy: A retrospective follow-up study. *Brain and Development, 29,* 486–490.

Holingue, C., Newill, C., Lee, L., Pasricha, P., & Fallin, M. D. (2018). Gastrointestinal symptoms in autism spectrum disorder: A review of the literature on ascertainment and prevalence. *Autism Research, 11,* 24–36.

Ibrahim, S. H., Voigt, R. G., Katusic, S. K., Weaver, A. L., & Barbaresi, W. J. (2009). Incidence of gastrointestinal symptoms in children with autism: A population-based study. *Pediatrics, 124,* 680–686.

Johnson, K. P., & Malow, B. A. (2008). Sleep in children with autism spectrum disorders. *Current Treatment Options in Neurology, 10,* 350–359.

Kagan-Kushnir, T., Roberts, S. W., & Snead, O. C. (2005). Screening electroencephalograms in autism spectrum disorders: Evidence-based guideline. *Journal of Child Neurology, 20,* 197–206.

Kohane, I. S., McMurry, A., Weber, G., MacFadden, D., Rappaport, L., Kunkel, L., et al. (2012). The co-morbidity burden of children and young adults with autism spectrum disorders. *PLoS ONE, 7,* 1–7.

Krakowiak, P., Goodlin-Jones, B., Hertz-Picciotto, I., Croen, L. A., & Hansen, R. L. (2008). Sleep problems in children with autism spectrum disorders, developmental delays, and typical development: A population-based study. *Journal of Sleep Research, 17,* 197–206.

Ledford, J. R., & Gast, D. L. (2006). Feeding problems in children with autism spectrum disorders: A review. *Focus on Autism and Other Developmental Disabilities, 21,* 153–166.

Levy, S. E., Giarelli, E., Lee, L., Schieve, L., Kirby, R. S., Cunniff, C., … Rice, C. E. (2010). Autism spectrum disorder and co-occurring developmental, psychiatric, and medical conditions among children in multiple populations of the United States. *Journal of Developmental & Behavioral Pediatrics, 31,* 267–274.

Maxwell-Horn, A., & Malow, B. A. (2017). Sleep in autism. *Seminars in Neurology, 37,* 413–418.

Mazurek, M. O., Dovgan, K., Neumeyer, A. M., & Malow, B. A. (2019). Course and predictors of sleep and co-occurring problems in children with autism spectrum disorder. *Journal of Autism and Developmental Disorders, 49,* 2101–2115.

McElhanon, B. O., McCracken, C., Karpen, S., & Sharp, W. G. (2014). Gastrointestinal symptoms in autism spectrum disorder: A meta-analysis. *Pediatrics, 133,* 872–883.

Neuhaus, E., Bernier, R. A., Tham, S. W., & Webb, S. J. (2018). Gastrointestinal and psychiatric symptoms among children and adolescents with autism spectrum disorder. *Frontiers in Psychiatry, 9,* 515.

Niemczyk, J., Wagner, C., & von Gontard, A. (2018). Incontinence in autism spectrum disorder: A systematic review. *European Child and Adolescent Psychiatry, 27,* 1523–1537.

Richard, A. E., Scheffer, I. E., & Wilson, S. J. (2017). Features of the broader autism phenotype in people with epilepsy support shared mechanisms between epilepsy and autism spectrum disorder. *Neuroscience and Biobehavioral Reviews, 75,* 203–233.

Schreck, K. A., Mulick, J. A., & Smith, A. F. (2004). Sleep problems as predictors of intensified symptoms of autism. *Research in Developmental Disabilities, 25,* 57–66.

Schreck, K. A., Williams, K., & Smith, A. F. (2004). A comparison of eating behaviors between children with and without autism. *Journal of Autism and Developmental Disorders, 34,* 433–438.

Schwarz, S. M. (2003). Feeding disorders in children with developmental disabilities. *Infants and Young Children, 16,* 317–330.

Shahidullah, J. D., Azad, G., Mezher, K. R., McClain, M. B., & McIntyre, L. L. (2018). Linking the medical and educational home to support children with autism spectrum disorder: Practice recommendations. *Clinical Pediatrics, 57,* 1496–1505.

Sharp, W. G., Berry, R. C., McCracken, C., Nuhu, N. N., Marvel, E., Saulnier, C.A., … Jaquess, D. L. (2013). Feeding problems and nutrient intake in children with autism spectrum disorders: A meta-analysis and comprehensive review of the literature. *Journal of Autism and Developmental Disorders, 43,* 2159–2173.

Spence, S., & Schneider, M. T. (2009). The role of epilepsy and epileptiform EEGs in autism spectrum disorders. *Pediatric Research, 65,* 599–606.

Tuchman, R., Alessandri, M., & Cuccaro, M. (2010). Autism spectrum disorders and epilepsy: Moving towards a comprehensive approach to treatment. *Brain and Development, 32,* 719–730.

Tuchman, R., & Cuccaro, M. (2011). Epilepsy and autism: Neurodevelopmental perspective. *Current Neurology and Neuroscience Reports, 11,* 428–434.

Turk, J., Bax, M., Williams, C., Amin, P., Eriksson, M., & Gillberg, C. (2009). Autism spectrum disorder in children with and without epilepsy: Impact on social functioning and communication. *Acta Paediatrica,* 675–681.

Tye, C., Runicles, A. K., Whitehouse, A. J. O., & Alvares, G. A. (2019). Characterizing the interplay between autism spectrum disorder and comorbid medical conditions: An integrative review. *Frontiers in Psychology, 9,* 1–21.

Vargason, T., Frye, R. E., McGuinness, D. L., & Hahn, J. (2019). Clustering of co-occurring conditions in autism spectrum disorder during early childhood: A retrospective analysis of medical claims data. *Autism Research, 12,* 1275–1285.

Viscidi, E. W., Johnson, A. L., Spence, S. J., Buka, S. L., Morrow, E. M., & Triche, E. W. (2014). The association between epilepsy and autism symptoms and maladaptive behaviors in children with autism spectrum disorder. *Autism, 18,* 996–1006.

Zucker, N., Copeland, W., Franz, L., Carpenter, K., Keeling, L., Angold, A., Egger, H. (2015). Psychological and psychosocial impairment in preschoolers with selective eating. *Pediatrics, 136,* e582–e590.

Screening and Surveillance

Terisa P. Gabrielsen, Stacy Shumway Manwaring, and Ashley L. Stuart

Abstract Within the context of typical development, it is not unusual for a child to show a slight delay in reaching a developmental milestone. Healthcare providers and parents may adopt a wait-and-see approach for some delays with little consequence to the child's outcome. In the case of early signs of autism spectrum disorder (ASD) that often manifest as developmental delays, however, acting early to evaluate the child's development and provide early intervention is key to better outcomes. Early identification is defined as having a comprehensive developmental evaluation of possible ASD symptoms no later than age 3, but a growing body of research has shown identification can be accurate and stable at younger ages. Navigating the differences between minor delays and signs of ASD is best conducted by combining forces between parents and health or other early childhood care providers using both ASD screening and developmental surveillance. This chapter outlines guidelines and resources for both screening and surveillance from professional organizations, ASD researchers, and healthcare agencies.

Early Identification of Autism Spectrum Disorder

The first 3 years of life are characterized by tremendous brain growth and skill development. These are also the years in which symptoms of autism spectrum disorder (ASD) become apparent (Guthrie, Swineford, Nottke, & Wetherby, 2013; Zwaigenbaum et al., 2013). Developmental theorists and scientists have provided ample evidence for typical developmental trajectories and timeframes within early childhood development (Centers for Disease Control [CDC], 2019), allowing both parents and providers to monitor development. In addition to gains in height, weight, and head

T. P. Gabrielsen (✉)
Counseling, Psychology and Special Education, Brigham Young University, Provo, UT, USA
e-mail: Terisa_gabrielsen@byu.edu

S. S. Manwaring
Communication Sciences and Disorders, University of Utah, Salt Lake City, UT, USA

A. L. Stuart
Pediatrics, University of Utah, Salt Lake City, UT, USA

M. B. McClain et al. (eds.), *Interprofessional Care Coordination for Pediatric Autism Spectrum Disorder*, https://doi.org/10.1007/978-3-030-46295-6_3

circumference, development in cognitive, motor, social–emotional, language, and adaptive skill domains may be tracked and noted in personal and medical records. Collaboration across healthcare disciplines, early childhood care, and education is key to early identification of ASD. While primary care providers (PCPs) have consistent access and play a substantial role in early identification (Baio et al., 2018), parents and other providers can join with PCPs as a team to recognize early signs and act on delays or differences at the earliest opportunity (Glascoe, 1999).

As will be discussed below, over the last 20 years, researchers have focused efforts on identifying the earliest signs of ASD. Prospective studies examining the development of infants and toddlers at risk for ASD have led to an increased understanding of the social communication, language, and motor delays that may be observed in this population. Further, research has shown that screening for ASD can result in earlier diagnosis (Chlebowski, Robins, Barton, & Fein, 2013; Miller et al., 2011; Robins et al., 2014).

Social and Communication Development

First smiles, cooing, and eye contact are among the earliest social milestones expected in typical development (CDC, 2019). If vision and hearing are intact, and a child does not achieve these social milestones, parents and providers can begin to work on identifying possible delays through early intervention referrals and increasing interventions aimed at developing social interaction skills (Fein, Holt, Brennan, & Barton, 2015). Communication entails verbal and/or nonverbal interactive exchanges between people. Deficits in communication are a core feature of ASD and include impairments in both verbal and nonverbal communication forms (DSM-5; American Psychiatric Association [APA], 2013). Infants and toddlers later diagnosed with ASD have been found to show decreased use of a range of prelinguistic communication skills including eye gaze, facial expressions, sharing attention and enjoyment, communicative vocalizations, and gestures (e.g., Shumway & Wetherby, 2009; Veness et al., 2012; Wetherby et al., 2004; Wetherby, Watt, Morgan, & Shumway, 2007). In relation to gesture, studies of infants at increased genetic risk for ASD (due to having an older sibling diagnosed with the disorder) indicate that reduced gesture use is present in infancy (Mitchell et al., 2006) and persists over time (Iverson et al., 2018). Parents and providers can be watching for these social communication skills to develop, paying special attention to the frequency of use as well as the purpose for which the communication is used. For example, how clear is the communicative intent? Does the child integrate different forms of communication, such as pairing a gesture with eye gaze? Is the communication directed to another person? Does the child communicate for a variety of purposes—to request, comment, etc.? Reduced frequency of communication as well as the variety of communicative intent may point to an important area for targeted intervention.

Language Delays

While communication deficits are a core feature of ASD, a delay in language is not specific to ASD. Even so, language delay is among the first concerns most commonly reported by parents of children later diagnosed with ASD (Matheis et al., 2017) and language impairment is common enough to warrant status as a specifier of ASD in the *Diagnostic and Statistical Manual of Mental Disorders, Fifth Edition* (APA, 2013). In addition to expressive language delays, early delays in receptive language are also often present in infants and toddlers later diagnosed with ASD, and these delays have a substantial impact on social communication development and learning opportunities (Camarata, 2014). The American Academy of Pediatrics (AAP) recommends hearing evaluation as a first step when communication delays are observed in order to rule out the presence of hearing loss, even temporary hearing loss, which can impact language development (Johnson & Myers, 2007).

Motor Development

Esther Thelen's work in early development focused on the underlying brain capability for motor movement requiring dynamic sub-systems of interplay between body systems, tasks, and environment (Thelen, 1995). While not diagnostic of ASD, early deficits in motor skills have been found in young children later diagnosed with ASD. For example, an association has been identified between low muscle tone, or hypotonia, in infancy and later symptoms of ASD (Serdarevic et al., 2017). Head lag has been shown to be another early indicator of deviation from typical development in children later diagnosed with ASD (Flanagan, Landa, Bhat, & Bauman; 2012). Differences in gait symmetry have also been found in toddlers with ASD (Esposito, Venuti, Apicella, & Muratori, 2011). Emerging research points to prolonged retainment of primary reflexes (e.g., grasping, rooting, and sucking) beyond the normal developmental period as impacting motor development in children later diagnosed with ASD (Chinello, Di Gangi, & Valenza, 2018). Importantly, early motor delays have been linked with subsequent social communication, expressive language, and adaptive developmental delays in children with ASD (Bhat, Galloway, Landa, 2012; LeBarton & Iverson, 2013; Provost, Lopez, & Heimerl, 2007).

Age of Identification of ASD

The first few years of life are a sensitive developmental period (Uylings, 2006), so researchers continue efforts to identify ASD at earlier ages (Jones & Klin, 2013; Ozonoff et al., 2010). The majority of ASD diagnoses made by 2 years of age are stable over time (Chawarska, Klin, Paul, Macari, & Volkmar, 2009, Guthrie et al.,

2013; Zwaigenbaum et al., 2013), and the target for early identification of ASD is before 3 years of age (Baio et al., 2018; Johnson & Myers, 2007). Other factors involved in determining this target include United States federal law, the Individuals with Disabilities Education Improvement Act (IDEA, 2004), whose Part C specifies a mandate for Child Find activities for children with disabilities from birth to three years for the express purpose of providing early intervention services, primarily in home settings. Part C or Early Intervention (EI) services are generally provided at low or no cost to families with the intention of equalizing access to care regardless of socioeconomic status.

Although 3 years or younger has been identified as the target age for early identification of ASD, according to data collected over the past decade or more in the United States, the average age of diagnosis ranges from 3 years, 11 months for children with severe symptomatology to 4 years, 9 months for children with ASD who have milder symptoms including age-appropriate cognitive and language abilities (Maenner et al., 2020). Although developmental concerns are often documented by 3 years of age in the majority (85%) of children with ASD, only 42% have been reported to have completed a comprehensive evaluation (including measures of cognitive, adaptive, language, and behavioral development) by age 3 years. Recent studies of 4-year-olds with ASD show 84% have evaluations before 36 months, however (Shaw et al., 2020). While a formal medical diagnosis of ASD is not required to receive EI services, a comprehensive developmental evaluation is typically performed as part of EI eligibility determination. A study of enrollment in EI services for all disabilities found a wide disparity across states between the estimated number of eligible infants and toddlers and those that are enrolled in EI services (Rosenberg, Robinson, Shaw, & Ellison, 2013). Improving the implementation of best practices in surveillance and screening could help to close this gap, providing earlier entry into EI services and additional therapies as needed. For more information regarding EI and transition services, please see the chapter "Transition to Early Schooling for Children with ASD".

Conversations About Developmental Concerns

Although pediatric care providers, including family practice providers, have the most consistent professional access to children in the first 3 years of life, any professional who works with this population should be aware of early signs of developmental delays, including those specific to ASD, to ensure early identification. Extensive specialty training is not required for the wide range of early childhood professionals to identify possible signs of delays. However, awareness of the importance of developmental monitoring and understanding what to do if signs of ASD or other delays are present are needed to connect parents with resources for assessment (including experts with specialty training) and early intervention options. One example of reaching out to the broader range of early childhood professionals is the research that has been done to integrate surveillance and ASD screening into the Special Supplemental Nutrition Program for Women, Infants, and Children (WIC) in some areas

(First5LA, 2011; Guerrero, Inkelas, Whaley, & Kuo, 2013; Zuckerman, Chavez, & Reeder, 2017).

Trajectories Versus Timeframes

Developmental trajectories are stable and consistent in humans, but the exact timeframes for developmental milestones may vary slightly. Parents may be concerned about potentially minor delays in reaching developmental milestones, which could be indicative of the variability seen in typical development. In contrast, parents may be unaware of more significant delays if similar age infants or toddlers are not consistently available for comparison. Either way, professionals need to take action if they or the parents have concerns. Parent concerns can be the most valuable source of early detection of ASD risk, as the brief observation available during a pediatric visit may not be a reliable sample of behavior (Gabrielsen et al., 2015). Conversations about development are an established part of well-child visits with the child's pediatric care provider (AAP, 2019), although less is known about how these conversations occur and how best to assess parent concerns. Recognizing that diversity of culture, language, education, and family circumstances can all affect the reporting of parent concerns is critical (Donohue, Childs, Richards, & Robins, 2019). While a wait-and-see approach may seem like a logical response to parent concerns given the variation within typical development, in the case of developmental concerns related to ASD risk, early action is strongly recommended over wait-and-see approaches (CDC, 2019; Hyman, Levy, Myers, & Council and Children with Disabilities, 2020; Johnson & Myers, 2007).

Gender Differences

Differences in symptom presentation between females and males are important to note both in surveillance and screening. In the past, females identified with ASD were usually severely affected, with intellectual disability and language disorder profiles. In contrast, current research suggests that females with ASD may have better social communication skills than males with ASD, may imitate social behavior better (Ormond, Brownlow, Garnett, Rynkiewicz, & Attwood, 2017), and may have restricted or repetitive interests that are more focused on animals or people than objects (Lai, Lombardo, Auyeung, Chakrabarti, & Baron Cohen, 2015). Thus, it is critical to consider that concerns may be reported less often or interpreted as less urgent when the child is female. However, research has yet to provide specific information to guide parents and providers when considering early developmental profiles specific to females with ASD. Some screening research suggests that a focus on social communication and interaction deficits or differences may be useful (Evans, Boan, Bradley, & Carpenter, 2019).

Cultural Differences

ASD is generally thought to be equally present across cultures and genetic groups globally, but prevalence rates (and therefore identification rates) vary widely (Norbury & Sparks, 2013). Given the longstanding delays in the identification of children from ethnic or racial minority groups (Maenner et al., 2020; Baio et al., 2018), provider outreach and communication with culturally diverse families is critical to early identification. Latino families have reported that the stress of the diagnostic process, lack of parent knowledge about ASD, and lack of understanding the medical system are the leading barriers to receiving a timely diagnosis and appropriate intervention (Zuckerman et al., 2017). Other studies suggest that cultural influences on the way caregivers discuss behaviors with a provider might obscure ASD symptoms for a provider who is listening for typically White, Western cultural behavior descriptions (Norbury & Sparks, 2013). Both screening and surveillance can help to mitigate these barriers (Begeer, El Bouk, Boussaid, Terwogt, & Koot, 2009; Dawson, 2016). Please see the chapters "Clinical and School Identification and Intervention for Youth with ASD: Culturally and Linguistically Responsive Interdisciplinary Considerations" and "International Perspectives in Coordinated Care for Individuals with ASD" for more information regarding culture and ASD.

Education About Developmental Milestones

Each state in the United States (U.S.) has a federally funded *Learn the Signs, Act Early* Ambassador to coordinate early identification efforts within their state. For more information and to find your state's ambassador, see: https://www.cdc.gov/ncbddd/actearly/ambassadors-list.html. Supporting local efforts are the nationally accessible training modules and resources for both parents and providers available from the Centers for Disease Control (see Table 1). Although these efforts are aimed at identifying ASD in the early years, developmental milestone monitoring is useful for all developmental delays or other conditions affecting development. Resources range from developmental milestone handouts to milestone tracker apps for parents. Provider resources include training, most notably the *Autism Case Training (ACT)* and *Watch Me!* online training modules with continuing education credit available. Materials are adapted for various professional settings (e.g., healthcare, WIC, home visitors, Head Start). All are free downloads, with options to order hard copies (e.g., books, pamphlets, charts, magnets).

ASD-specific educational resources can also be accessed through the extensive resource, *Autism Navigator®* (Autism Navigator, LLC, 2019), listed in Table 2. Among the many resources available through the *Autism Navigator®*, perhaps the most illustrative is the Video Glossary, which shows side-by-side video examples of typical development and delays that may be seen in ASD in the toddler years. Intervention options are also shown in the Video Glossary, making it a rich source of information for both parents and providers.

For professionals across disciplines, the *Birth to 5 Watch Me Thrive!* website from the U.S. Department of Health and Human Services (2017) contains extensive data

Table 1 Learn the signs act early resources for early identification of ASD. All available from https://www.cdc.gov/ncbddd/actearly/index.html, free, and available in English and Spanish unless otherwise noted

Audience	Online training/educational awareness resources	Developmental milestones
Parents	• Milestones in action: photos and videos • If you're concerned (steps to take) • How to get help for your child	• Milestones tracker app • Milestones checklist *(Arabic, Brazilian Portuguese, Haitian Creole, Chinese, Somali, Vietnamese)* • Milestones moments booklet *(Chinese, Korean)* • Baby's busy day: Being one is so much fun! (Book) • Where is bear? A terrific tale for 2-year-olds (Book) • Amazing me: It's busy being 3 (Book) • How to help your child tipsheets and how to talk to your doctor tipsheets (Vietnamese, Korean, Haitian Creole) • Milestone brochure (Spanish, Vietnamese, Korean, Haitian Creole) • Flyers (first tooth, almost walking, watch me) • Growth charts (grow up healthy and milestones) • Developmental monitoring and screening fact sheet
Providers or educators	• Health care providers primer • Early childhood educators primer • WIC program staff primer • Early head start and head start program primer • Home visiting program primer • Child find program primer • Narrated PowerPoint presentation for health care providers (English only) • Narrated PowerPoint presentation of parents of young children • Watch me! celebrating milestones and sharing concerns (1-hr training with credit available) • Autism Case Training (ACT) online (English Only) • ACT in-classroom curriculum (English only)	• Milestone tracker app, milestones matter posters • Web button (English only) • Videos to share on website (English)

Table 2 Autism Navigator® early identification resources available in English, Spanish, and Creole, all available through https://autismnavigator.com/

Audience	Free educational resources	Fee-based resources
Parents	A seamless path for families • 16 by 16™ LookBooks • Social communication growth charts About autism in toddlers • 3-hr course for anyone ASD video glossary (English only)	A seamless path for families • Social communication video growth charts How-to guide for families (8-hr course) *Some fee-based resources could be free for families if providers or families are enrolled in research or have a group rate*
Professionals	What is ASD? (Handout) Early red flags of autism (poster)	Autism Navigator® for primary care (8-hr course)

Table 3 Birth to Five, Watch Me Thrive! https://www.acf.hhs.gov/ecd/child-health-development/watch-me-thrive (available in English and Spanish unless otherwise indicated)

Developmental and behavioral screening practices	Screening measures
• Early child care and educator guide • Early intervention service and early special education provider's guide • Primary Care Provider's Guide • Community guide (English only) • Child welfare caseworker's guide (English only) • Home visitor's guide • Behavioral Health Provider's Guide (English only) • Housing and homeless shelter provider's guide (English only) • Developmental screening passport	Compendium of screening measures (2014) reviews of commonly used measures. • Ages and Stages Questionnaire (ASQ) • Brigance • Developmental Assessment of Young Children (DAY-C) • Learning Accomplishment Profile-Diagnostic Screens (LAP-D) • Early Screening Profiles • Parents' Evaluation of Developmental Status (PEDS) • FirstSTEP • Infant developmental inventory • Survey of Well-Being of Young Children (SWYC)

for developmental surveillance, including a *Compendium of Screening Measures* (See Table 3). The website also offers links to resources in each state for early identification and intervention.

Ongoing Professional Surveillance

In the 2020 AAP Clinical Report aimed at offering guidance to clinicians providing pediatric care to individuals with ASD, developmental surveillance for ASD is defined as talking with caregivers about concerns about their child's development or behavior, making informal observations, and monitoring of symptoms in the context of routine health supervision (Hyman et al., 2020). This Clinical Guide is an excellent resource for all care providers, as it provides excellent care information from early identification through treatment, and is freely available online at https://pediatrics.aappublications.org/content/145/1/e20193447.

The Bright Futures National Center has been developing guidelines over several decades by and for multidisciplinary pediatric care professionals, currently involving the AAP, the Maternal Child Health Bureau, Health Resources and Service Administration, and the Centers for Medicare & Medicaid Services. Although overall health is the focus of Bright Futures, some of their resources include guidelines for ongoing surveillance of development (Table 4). A brief summary of the timing of surveillance activities is provided in the Bright Futures/AAP Periodicity Schedule within the Guidelines. The Schedule indicates ages for surveillance and screening of developmental and behavioral health, beginning with Newborn visits through age 21 years. Developmental screening is indicated at 9, 18, and 30 months, and ASD-specific screening at 18 and 24 months, consistent with the AAP recommendations (Hyman et al., 2020; Johnson & Myers, 2007; Lipkin, Macias, & Council for Children with Disabilities, 2020).

Surveillance begins with a family history of developmental delays, including ASD. Asking open-ended questions about concerns as well as age-specific questions about developmental milestones constitute ongoing surveillance. General developmental screening tools, such as those described in the Compendium of Screening Resources (see Table 3) are an important part of surveillance, but the conversations between providers and parents about development and concerns are critical for

Table 4 American Academy of Pediatrics and Bright Futures guidelines and resources https://brightfutures.aap.org/materials-and-tools/Pages/default.aspx

Audience	Free resources	Fee-based or subscription resources
Parents		Patient education handouts for ASD (AAP) (in English and Spanish) *Many handouts are available for care across the lifespan, only surveillance handouts are listed here* • What is your one-year old telling you? • Is your toddler communicating with you?
Providers	• Bright futures guidelines • Periodicity table • Pocket guidebook • Developmental, behavioral, psychosocial, screening, and assessment forms (links) • Presentation templates for education • Clinical practice tools	• Bright futures: guidelines for health supervision of infants, children and adolescents, 4th edition (print and e-book) • Bright futures toolkit (AAP) • AAP autism toolkit (English only) https://shop.aap.org/autismtoolkit/

early identification of ASD, as provider observation alone is not likely to provide a comprehensive picture of development (Gabrielsen et al., 2015).

The AAP surveillance and screening algorithm specific to ASD outlined in the 2007 guidelines (Johnson & Myers, 2007) has recently been expanded to include a broader range of neurodevelopmental disorders and behavioral and emotional problems, titled "Promoting optimal development: Identifying infants and young children with developmental disorders through developmental surveillance and screening." (Lipkin et al., 2020). The new algorithms are freely available online through the *Pediatrics* portal (https://pediatrics.aappublications.org/content/pediatrics/145/1/e20193449.full.pdf). At health supervision visits, Bright Futures' developmental and ASD-specific screening previously described are supplemented by specific actions to take if screens are positive and/or surveillance reveals concern for motor development specifically, for developmental concerns, or for any unaddressed concerns. The algorithm indicates that surveillance should continue throughout childhood, and extends from early concerns through the initiation of chronic conditions management (Lipkin et al., 2020).

The AAP Policy Statement and Technical Report regarding identification and evaluation of ASD first published in 2007 describes surveillance as a ". . . 'moving picture' of the child's unfolding development, [and] screening represents 'snapshots' of the child's development at specific times." (p. 1195, Johnson & Myers, 2007). Although developmental screening is important, general screeners may not be sensitive to social symptoms associated with ASD, requiring ASD-specific screening tools to maximize the chances of identifying ASD early (Hyman et al., 2020).

Universal Screening for ASD

The AAP recommendations for ASD screening are for universal screening of children for ASD at their 18- and 24-month well-child visits, *or at any time there is a parent or provider concern* (Hyman et al., 2020; Johnson & Myers, 2007; Lipkin et al., 2020). Universal screening is slowly being adopted in the U.S., with recent surveys indicating that 17% (Self, Parham, & Rajagopalan, 2015) to 65% of pediatricians report using a formal screener to screen for ASD (Coury et al., 2017). While this is encouraging, universal screening is not without controversy (Al-Qabandi, Gorter, & Rosenbaum, 2011; Charman & Gotham, 2013). In 2016, the United States Preventative Services Task Force (USPSTF) finalized their report on universal screening for ASD, stating there is currently insufficient evidence to directly connect better outcomes to universal screening. The report clearly states that screening is not harmful, and that screeners with satisfactory performance data do exist, but that without more research on outcomes from universal screening, they could not endorse screening on a universal basis (Siu et al., 2016). Similar recommendations were published in Canada and the United Kingdom (Allaby & Sharma, 2011; Canadian Task Force on Preventative Health, 2016).

One of the flaws in the standard methodology employed by recommendation bodies, such as the AAP or the USPSTF, is that treatment outcomes are the only outcome of interest, whereas many would argue that age of identification could be justified as an outcome (Coury, 2015: Pierce, Courchesne, & Bacon, 2016). There is a well-established body of research tying early intervention to favorable outcomes, as well as some large studies showing that screening results in earlier identification (Chlebowski, Robins, Barton, & Fein, 2013; Robins et al., 2014). However, because these two bodies of literature are not connected, the gap in the literature between screening and treatment outcomes has become a barrier to the endorsement of universal screening. Although many have been concerned about excessive false positive results based on screening research to date (Charman & Gotham, 2013), newer research with longitudinal follow-up is documenting risk for false negative results as well (Beacham et al., 2018; Carbone et al., 2020; Guthrie et al., 2019). The USPSTF judged that adequate evidence exists that screening tests can detect ASD in children aged 18–30 months (Siu et al., 2016), and prominent ASD researchers urge continuation of universal screening as the benefits (including earlier detection of ASD in underserved populations) outweigh the concerns raised (Dawson, 2016).

In 2015, a large group of ASD researchers published a report titled *Early Screening of Autism Spectrum Disorder : Recommendations for Practice and Research* (Zwaigenbaum et al., 2015). The report is publicly available in *Pediatrics* and may be found at: https://pediatrics.aappublications.org/content/136/Supplement_1/S41. A selection of screening measures discussed in the report for universal screening of toddlers (Level 1) and more targeted at-risk screening measures (Level 2) are listed in Table 5. Other screening measures commonly used in the U.S. and available to the public are also provided.

Not included in the table are screeners often used in research, but not readily available except through contacting the authors, e.g., the First Year Inventory (FYI: Baranek, Watson, Crais & Reznick, 2003; Lee et al., 2019) for 12-month-olds, from the Program for Early Autism Research, Leadership and Service (PEARLS), at the University of North Carolina School of Medicine. In addition, some measures with additional screening options, such as the Autism Spectrum Rating Scales (ASRS: Simek & Wahlberg, 2011; Goldstein & Naglieri, 2009), were not included because the short form of the ASRS (derived from the long form's 15 most highly predictive items) has extremely limited psychometric data available regarding its performance as a screener. Broad developmental measures with limited research on effectiveness for ASD screening (Dolata, Sanford-Keller, & Squires, 2019) were also not included as ASD screeners, e.g., Ages and Stages Questionnaires: Social–Emotional, Second Edition (ASQ:SE; Squires et al., 2015) and the Brief Infant-Toddler Social and Emotional Assessment (BITSEA: Briggs-Gowan & Carter, 2006; Giserman Kiss, Feldman, Sheldrick, & Carter, 2017). (See Table 3 for general developmental screeners.) Finally, measures commonly used in diagnostic or educational classification decision-making (Level 3 evaluation measures) were not included in the table as screeners. See the chapter "Interdisciplinary Evaluation of Autism Spectrum Disorder" for interdisciplinary evaluation measures.

Table 5 Commonly used ASD-specific screening and broadband developmental measures by age range

Age range	Measure copyright	Availability	Psychometrics	Level 1—Universal or Level 2—At Risk
*9–24 months	*Infant Toddler Checklist (ITC)—Part of the Communication and Symbolic Behavior Scales Developmental Profile* (Wetherby & Prizant, 2002, Brookes Publishing)	Parent Questionnaire Free download https://brookespublishing.com/product/csbs-dp-itc/ Scoring information https://firstwords.fsu.edu/pdf/Checklist_Scoring_Cutoffs.pdf Spanish available https://firstwords.fsu.edu/pdf/infant-toddler_Spanish.pdf	*Not recommended for < 9 months. PPV (for all delays, not specifically ASD) PPV = 0.42 – 0.79; NPV = 0.87 – 0.99[1]	Level 1 Broadband needs ASD follow-up measure for Level 2
9–24 months	*Early Screening for Autism and Communication Disorders (ESAC) and SmartESAC* (Autism Navigator, LLC)	Autism Navigator® product https://firstwordsproject.com/screen-my-child/ Parent questionnaires online—can connect with providers, fees for providers	Extremely limited evidence available publicly. Preliminary field-testing indicated sensitivity from 0.84 to 0.86 and specificity from 0.83 to 0.85 for a total of 47 items[2]	Level 1 or Level 2
16–30 months	*Modified Checklist for Autism in Toddlers™—Revised with follow up (M-CHAT-R/F)* (Robins, Fein, & Barton, 2009)	Parent Questionnaire Free https://mchatscreen.com/mchat-rf/ Multiple languages and a picture version	Strong evidence for use PPV 0.475 for ASD, but if all developmental disorders are included PPV = 0.946[1]	Level 1 (Questionnaire) and Level 2 (follow-up interview)

(continued)

Table 5 (continued)

Age range	Measure copyright	Availability	Psychometrics	Level 1—Universal or Level 2—At Risk
18–35 months	*Parents' Observations of Social Interactions (POSI)* (Perrin, et al., 2016)	Parent questionnaire Free Part of the Survey of Well-being of Children www.TheSWYC.org Multiple languages	Very limited evidence in referred populations only—early comparisons with MCHAT are favorable, but PPV has not been provided.[3,4]	Level 1
24–36 months	*Screening Tool for Autism in Toddlers and Young Children (STAT™)* (Stone Coonrod, & Ousely, 2000, Vanderbilt Univ.)	In-person interactive observation measure Kit, protocols, and online training (required)[5] available through https://stat.vueinnovations.com/	Strong evidence for use, 24–35 mos. Promising for 14–23 mo. [1]	Level 2 in-person measure
Ages 4 + years ASD Lower cutoff for ages 2–4	*Social Communication Questionnaire (SCQ)—Current version Lifetime version* (Rutter, Bailey & Lord, 2003, WPS)	Parent Questionnaire (can be completed by others) Purchase from WPS Multiple languages Available in hard copy and online versions Lifetime Version is phrased for children older than 5 years, but some have advocated it for children younger than age 4 (consider the last 12 months) because of more stable psychometric properties than the Current Version.[6]	Metanalysis shows acceptable accuracy AUC = 0.827–0.885, sensitivities 0.47–0.96, specificities 0.52–0.99.[6] Cutoff of 12 (rather than 15) overall showed high sensitivity of 0.82, but lower specificity of 0.56.[7] A lower cutoff score of 11 has better psychometrics for children 2–4.[8,9]	Level 2

(continued)

Table 5 (continued)

Age range	Measure copyright	Availability	Psychometrics	Level 1—Universal or Level 2—At Risk
2.5 years and up ASD	*Social Responsiveness Scales-Second Edition (SRS-2)* (Constantino & Gruber, 2012, WPS)	Parent/Teacher Questionnaire Purchase from WPS Available in hard copy and online versions Spanish available	Norms separated by gender (in school age version only). Sensitivity 0.45–1.00 Specificity 0.73–0.83 PPV = 0.33–0.60 NPV = 0.71–1.00 AUC = 0.59–0.93[10]	Level 2

PPV = Positive Predictive Value. NPV = Negative Predictive Value. WPS = Western Psychological Services. MHS = Multi-health Systems Assessments, Inc.
[1]Evaluation of adequacy and psychometric data are quoted from Zwaigenbaum et al., 2015
[2]Wetherby et al., 2009
[3]Salisbury, Nyce, Hannum, Sheldrick & Perring, 2018
[4]Smith, Shledrick, & Perrin, 2013
[5]Requires formal training on administration and coding
[6] Chesnut, Wei, Barnard-Brak & Richman, 2017
[7] Corsello et al., 2007
[8] Wiggins, Bakeman, Adamson & Robins, 2007
[9] Allen, Silove, Williams & Hutchins, 2007
[10] Dovekot, van der Ende, Verhulst & Greaves-Lord (2015), Dutch version of SRS, deemed equivalent in raw scores to SRS-2 because questions were the same. The addition of a Teacher Report to the Parent Report increased the psychometric properties of the SRS. Results were similar to previous studies by the authors, Constantino & Gruber, 2012, and other external validation studies (Boltë et al., 2011 and Charman et al., 2007)

Next Steps for Referral

When screening and surveillance efforts result in a decision to pursue evaluation, there are several options to consider, and all can be pursued simultaneously to find the option that will result in the earliest evaluation. Comprehensive evaluations for ASD are time-consuming and may take place over multiple days and/or multiple visits. As early intervention efforts are symptom dependent rather than diagnosis dependent, for children under 3 years of age, the first and typically fastest path to an evaluation is to refer to the local Early Intervention agency (https://ectacenter.org/contact/ptccoord.asp). For children over age 3, contact the local school for an evaluation. These evaluations are low or no cost and may result in access to intervention if the child meets eligibility criteria for services (which vary by state). These evaluations typically cover multiple domains of development; however, they may not include ASD-specific assessment measures.

In some cases, access to therapies at the level of intensity desired by families, or access to specialist assessment may be beyond the school system capabilities (Irvin, McBee, Boyd, Hume, & Odom, 2012). Families may wish to supplement school-based services with private assessment and/or therapies. Health insurance mandates for ASD services are now in place throughout the U.S., providing many families with insurance coverage for Applied Behavior Analysis (ABA) services, which along with speech-language and occupational therapy services, are the most commonly prescribed intensive treatments for ASD in the early years (Bitterman, Daley, Misra, Carlson, & Markowitz, 2008). Medical diagnoses are required for insurance coverage, so evaluations outside of the education system may be necessary to access the intensity of treatment services desired. Medical diagnoses for ASD are generally given by physicians or PhD-level psychologists. In cases where neither of these professionals with appropriate ASD expertise are available, and/or there is a speech-language pathologist (SLP) with significant ASD training and experience available, an SLP may diagnose ASD. Note, however, that not all insurance companies accept an SLP diagnosis for ASD-specific services, such as ABA therapy.

In the 2020 Clinical Report Guidance, the primary care provider is charged with both discussing the importance of assessment and assisting the family in navigating the assessment process, including connecting families with community resources, with extra support required for families with low income or language barriers (Hyman et al., 2020). This charge applies to other community providers as well, given that pediatricians may not always be the first point of contact when a concern is discussed.

Waitlists for medical diagnoses from specialists can be long, but ASD specialty clinics in many states have been trying novel approaches to reduce the wait in order to provide diagnoses earlier (Austin et al., 2016; Gordon-Lipkin, Foster, & Peacock, 2016; Rotholz, Kinsman, Lacy, & Charles, 2017). Most states have ASD specialty clinics associated with a university medical center or large healthcare system or hospital, and specialty clinics exist independently as well. See the chapter "Interdisciplinary Evaluation of Autism Spectrum Disorder" for more details. When specialist waitlists are long, and if general pediatricians and child psychologists are experienced and comfortable with the application of the DSM-5 criteria, they can make an initial clinical diagnosis to begin eligibility for services (Hyman et al., 2020).

Case Examples

There are many pathways and approaches to screening, early identification, and early intervention for very young children with ASD. The following case examples illustrate the benefits of screening and surveillance used together to improve outcomes.

Case 1 male: Surveillance by the pediatrician identified significant ASD concerns at age 12 months, including possible seizures and speech delay. The parents were unaware of ASD symptoms or anything about ASD but sought community-based gross motor play therapy. Physical therapists discussed multiple developmental concerns with parents, leading to follow-up with the pediatrician. ASD-specific screening was failed at age 27 months, which prompted parents to seek evaluation and more intensive intervention. Evaluation resulted in an ASD diagnosis, followed by enrollment in EI services, special education preschool, and a specialized preschool for ASD. Other family members, including extended family, have subsequently received ASD diagnoses.

Case 2 female: Although parents were not concerned, the pediatrician identified concerns with weight at 18 months. Some severely restricted feeding behaviors were initially attributed to reflux. At 23 months, pediatrician concerns about low weight resulted in a referral to EI services for feeding difficulties. ASD screening was also failed at 23 months, with subsequent evaluation confirming ASD. She was able to enroll in EI services for speech/language, feeding, and ASD, then an ASD specialty preschool with Medicaid funding. Parents report she is doing very well.

Case 3 male: Parents were concerned about speech development, which was monitored by the pediatrician from 18 months to 24 months. Recommendations at that time were to do at-home speech enrichment activities. The child's extended family had no concerns, commenting that he had some well-developed routines that were enjoyable for all every day and they thought he was fine. His mother had been taking courses in child development, which raised her level of concern about ASD specifically. At his 24-month well-child visit, an ASD screen result was borderline failed by parent report, but the pediatrician urged further action because of the mother's concerns. Subsequent evaluation confirmed significant ASD symptoms. He enrolled in EI services, his mother attended seminars on various treatment options to help with decision-making, and he transitioned into an intensive special education preschool in his school district.

Summary

There is no single perfect approach to identifying ASD, so multiple efforts are required. Parents and providers across disciplines (healthcare, speech and language, education, early childhood care, and early intervention), working together to coordinate surveillance and screening can result in earlier identification of ASD, which is the key to early intervention access. For example, concerns regarding social interaction or play skills may first be noted by early education and/or childcare providers, while differences in nonverbal communication may be more apparent to speech therapists. Communication with parents and among providers about concerns is key to taking earlier action. Improved outcomes for ASD rely on early intervention, so the importance of combining ASD screening with surveillance cannot be understated. Given the importance of early identification, redundant systems and methods are required for the best outcome (e.g., screening in healthcare, early intervention, and early childhood care centers). Surveillance of development requires that all early childhood care providers have conversations with parents, and that both professionals and parents are educated about development. Fortunately, many resources are available for no or low cost to improve education about developmental milestones and red flags for ASD. Considerations of culture, language, and gender differences within these conversations are important to avoid missing identification of ASD at the earliest opportunities. Screening measures are available at low or no cost and in multiple languages, improving identification across cultures and languages. Finally, although universal screening for toddlers has not yet been fully adopted in the U.S., use of ASD-specific screening measures for children with and without significant concerns has been shown to improve early identification of ASD (Baio et al., 2018; Chelbowski et al., 2013; Oosterling et al., 2010; Robins et al., 2014), giving families options for earlier treatment and better outcomes.

References

Allaby, M., & Sharma, M. (2011). *Screening for autism spectrum disorders in children below the age of 5 years*. United Kingdom: UK National Screening Committee.

Allen, C. W., Silove, N., Williams, K., & Hutchins, P. (2007). Validity of the social communication questionnaire in assessing risk of autism in preschool children with developmental problems. *Journal of Autism and Developmental Disorders, 37*(7), 1272–1278.

Al-Qabandi, M., Gorter, J. W., & Rosenbaum, P. (2011). Early autism detection: Are we ready for routine screening? *Pediatrics, 128*(1), e211–e217.

American Academy of Pediatrics. (2019). Bright futures/AAP recommendations for preventive pediatric health care (periodicity schedule). Retrieved from https://www.aap.org/en-us/Documents/periodicity_schedule.pdf.

American Psychiatric Association (2013). Diagnostic and statistical manual of mental disorders, Fifth edition. Author.

Austin, J., Manning-Courtney, P., Johnson, M., Weber, R., Johnson, H., Murray, D., et al. (2016). Improving access to care at autism treatment centers: A system analysis approach. *Pediatrics, 137*(Supplement 2), S149–S157.

Autism Navigator, LLC. (2019) *Autism Navigator®*. Retrieved from https://autismnavigator.com/

Baio, J., Wiggins, L., Christensen, D. L., Maenner, M. J., Daniels, J., Warren, Z., … Dowling, N. F. (2018). Prevalence of autism spectrum disorder among children aged 8 years—Autism and developmental disabilities monitoring network, 11 sites, United States, 2014. *MMWR Surveillance Summaries, 67*(No. SS-6), 1–23.

Baranek, G. T., Watson, L. R., Crais, E., & Reznick, S. (2003). *First-year inventory (FYI) 2.0.* Chapel Hill, NC: University of North Carolina at Chapel Hill

Beacham, C., Reid, M., Bradshaw, J., Lambha, M., Evans, L., Gillespie, S., et al. (2018). Screening for autism spectrum disorder: Profiles of children who are missed. *Journal of Developmental and Behavioral Pediatrics, 39*(9), 673–682.

Begeer, S., El Bouk, S., Boussaid, W., Terwogt, M. M., & Koot, H. M. (2009). Underdiagnosis and referral bias of autism in ethnic minorities. *Journal of Autism and Developmental Disorders, 39*(1), 142–148.

Bhat, A. N., Galloway, J. C., Landa, R. J. (2012). Relationship between early motor delay and later communication delay in infants at risk for autism. *Infant Behavior Development, 35*(4), 838–846.

Bitterman, A., Daley, T. C., Misra, S., Carlson, E., & Markowitz, J. (2008). A national sample of preschoolers with autism spectrum disorders: Special education services and parent satisfaction. *Journal of Autism and Developmental Disorders, 38*(8), 1509–1517.

Bölte, S., Westerwald, E., Holtmann, M., Freitag, C., & Poustka, F. (2011). Autistic traits and autism spectrum disorders: The clinical validity of two measures presuming a continuum of social communication skills. *Journal of Autism and Developmental Disorders, 41*(1), 66–72.

Briggs-Gowan, M. J., & Carter, A. S. (2006). *Examiner's manual for the Brief Infant-Toddler Social and Emotional Assessment (BITSEA)*. San Antonio, Texas: Psychological Corporation, Harcourt Press.

Camarata, S. (2014). Early identification and early intervention in autism spectrum disorders: Accurate and effective? *International Journal of Speech-Language Pathology, 16,* 1–10.

Canadian Task Force on Preventative Health Care. (2016). Recommendations on screening for developmental delay. *Canadian Medical Association Journal, 188*(8), 1–9.

Carbone, P., Campbell, C., Wilkes, J., Stoddard, G., Huynh, K., Young, P. C. & Gabrielsen, T.P. (2020). Primary care autism screening and later autism diagnosis. Pediatrics [doi TBA, accepted March 16, 2020]

Centers for Disease Control. (2019). CDC's Developmental Milestones. Retrieved from https://www.cdc.gov/ncbddd/actearly/milestones/index.html

Charman, T., Baird, G., Simonoff, E., Loucas, T., Chandler, S., Meldrum, D., et al. (2007). Efficacy of three screening instruments in the identification of autistic-spectrum disorders. *British Journal of Psychiatry, 191,* 554–559.

Charman, T., & Gotham, K. (2013). Measurement issues: Screening and diagnostic instruments for autism spectrum disorders—lessons from research and practice. *Child and Adolescent Mental Health, 18*(1), 52–64.

Chawarska, K., Klin, A., Paul, R., Macari, S., & Volkmar, F. (2009). A prospective study of toddlers with ASD: Short-term diagnostic and cognitive outcomes. *Journal of Child Psychology and Psychiatry, 50*(10), 1235–1245.

Chesnut, S. R., Wei, T., Barnard-Brak, L., & Richman, D. M. (2017). A meta-analysis of the social communication questionnaire: Screening for autism spectrum disorder. *Autism, 21*(8), 920–928.

Chinello, A., Di Gangi, V., & Valenza, E. (2018). Persistent primary reflexes affect motor acts: Potential implications for autism spectrum disorder. *Research in Developmental Disabilities, 83,* 287–295.

Chlebowski, C., Robins, D., Barton, M., & Fein, D. (2013). Large-scale use of the modified checklist for autism in low-risk toddlers. *Pediatrics, 131*(4), e1121–e1127.

Constantino, J., & Gruber, C. P. (2012). *Social responsiveness scale* (2nd ed.). Torrance, CA: Western Psychological Services.

Corsello, C., Hus, V., Pickles, A., Risi, S., Cook, E. H., Leventhal, B., et al. (2007). Between a ROC and a hard place: Decision making and making decisions about using the SCQ. *Journal of Child Psychology and Psychiatry, 48*(9), 932–940.

Coury, D. L. (2015). Babies, bathwater, and screening for autism spectrum disorder: Comments on the USPSTF recommendations for autism spectrum disorder screening. *Journal of Developmental and Behavioral Pediatrics, 36*(9), 661–663.

Coury, D., Wolfe, A., Lipkin, P.H., Baer, B., Hyman, S., Levy, S., ... Sisk, B. (2017). Screening of young children for autism spectrum disorders: Results from a national survey of pediatricians. Presented at the Pediatric Academic Societies Annual Meeting, 2017, San Francisco, CA

Dawson, G. (2016). Why it's important to continue universal autism screening while research fully examines its impact. *JAMA Pediatrics, 170*(6), 527–528.

Department of Health and Human Services. (2017). *Birth to 5, Watch Me Thrive!* Retrieved from https://www.acf.hhs.gov/ecd/child-health-development/watch-me-thrive.

Dolata, J. K., Sanford-Keller, H., & Squires, J. (2019). Modifying a general social-emotional measure for early autism screening. *International Journal of Developmental Disabilities*, 1–8.

Donohue, M. R., Childs, A. W., Richards, M., & Robins, D. L. (2019). Race influences parent report of concerns about symptoms of autism spectrum disorder. *Autism, 23*(1), 100–111.

Duvekot, J., van der Ende, J., Verhulst, F., & Greaves-Lord, K. (2015). The screening accuracy of the parent and teacher-reported Social Responsiveness Scale (SRS): Comparison with the 3Di and ADOS. *Journal of Autism and Developmental Disorders, 45*(6), 1658–1672.

Esposito, G., Venuti, P., Apicella, F., & Muratori, F. (2011). Analysis of unsupported gait in toddlers with autism. *Brain and Development, 33*(5), 367–373.

Evans, S. C., Boan, A. D., Bradley, C., & Carpenter, L. A. (2019). Sex/gender differences in screening for autism spectrum disorder: Implications for evidence-based assessment. *Journal of Clinical Child & Adolescent Psychology, 48*(6), 840–854.

Fein, D., Holt, M., Brennan, L., & Barton, M. (2015). *The activity kit for babies and toddlers at risk*. New York, NY: Guilford Press.

First5LA. (2011). *Research report: Early Developmental Screening and Intervention Initiative (EDSI): Lessons learned 2005–2010.* Retrieved from https://www.first5la.org/files/EDSI_Report_final_10092012.pdf.

Flanagan, J. E., Landa, R., Bhat, A., & Bauman, M. (2012). Head lag in infants at risk for autism: A preliminary study. *American Journal of Occupational Therapy, 66*(5), 577–585.

Gabrielsen, T. P., Farley, M., Speer, L., Villalobos, M. Baker, C. & Miller, J. (2015). Identifying autism in a brief observation. *Pediatrics, 135*(2), e330–e338. https://doi.org/10.1542/peds.2014-1428

Giserman Kiss, I., Feldman, M. S., Sheldrick, R. C., & Carter, A. S. (2017). Developing autism screening criteria for the Brief Infant Toddler Social Emotional Assessment (BITSEA). *Journal of Autism and Developmental Disorders, 47*(5), 1269–1277.

Glascoe, F. P. (1999). Using parents' concerns to detect and address developmental and behavioral problems. *Journal of the Society of Pediatric Nurses, 4*(1), 24–35.

Goldstein, S., & Naglieri, J. (2009). *Autism spectrum rating scales*. Toronto, Canada: Multi-Health Systems Inc.

Gordon-Lipkin, E., Foster, J., & Peacock, G. (2016). Whittling down the wait time: Exploring models to minimize the delay from initial concern to diagnosis and treatment of autism spectrum disorder. *Pediatric Clinic North America, 63*(5), 851–859.

Guerrero, A. D., Inkelas, M., Whaley, S. E., & Kuo, A. (2013). A WIC-based curriculum to enhance parent communication with healthcare providers. *Journal of Community Health, 38,* 958–964.

Guthrie, W., Swineford, L., Nottke, C., & Wetherby, A. (2013). Early diagnosis of autism spectrum disorder: Stability and change in clinical diagnosis and symptom presentation. *Journal of Child Psychology and Psychiatry, 54*(5), 582–590.

Guthrie, W., Wallis, K., Bennett, A., Brooks, E., Dudley, J., Gerdes, M., et al. (2019). Accuracy of pediatric screening in a large pediatric network. *Pediatrics, 144*(4), e20183963.

Hyman, S. L., Levy S. E., Myers, S. M., AAP Council on Children with Disabilities, Section on Developmental and Behavioral Pediatrics. (2020). Identification, evaluation, and management of children with autism spectrum disorder. *Pediatrics, 145*(1), e20193447

Individuals with Disabilities Education Act, 20 U.S.C. § 1400 (2004).

Irvin, D. W., McBee, M., Boyd, B. A., Hume, K., & Odom, S. L. (2012). Child and family factors associated with the use of services for preschoolers with autism spectrum disorder. *Research in Autism Spectrum Disorders, 6*(1), 565–572.

Iverson, J. M., Northrup, J. B., Leezenbaum, N. B., Parlade, M. V., Koterba, E. A., & West, K. L. (2018). Early gesture and vocabulary development in infant siblings of children with autism spectrum disorder. *Journal of Autism and Developmental Disorders, 48*(1), 55–71.

Johnson, C. P., & Myers, S. M. (2007). Identification and evaluation of children with autism spectrum disorders. *Pediatrics, 120*(5), 1183–1215.

Jones, W., & Klin, A. (2013). Attention to eyes is present but in decline in 2-6-month-old infants later diagnosed with autism. *Nature, 504*(7480), 427–431.

Lai, M. C., Lombardo, M. V., Auyeung, B., Chakrabarti, B., & Baron Cohen, S. (2015). Sex/gender differences and autism: Setting the scene for future research. *Journal of the American Academy of Child and Adolescent Psychiatry, 54*(1), 11–24.

LeBarton, E. S., & Iverson, J. M. (2013). Fine motor skill predicts expressive language in infant siblings of children with autism. *Developmental Science, 16,* 815–827.

Lee, H. Y., Vigen, C., Zwaigenbaum, L., Bryson, S., Smith, I., Brian, J., et al. (2019). The performance of the First Year Inventory (FYI) Screening on a sample of high-risk 12-month-olds diagnosed with Autism Spectrum Disorder (ASD) at 36 months. *Journal of Autism and Developmental Disorders, 49*(12), 4957–4973.

Lipkin, P. H., Macias, M. M., & Council on Children with Disabilities, Section on Developmental and Behavioral Pediatrics. (2020). Promoting optimal development: Identifying infants and young children with developmental disorders through developmental surveillance and screening. *Pediatrics, 145*(1), e20193440.

Maenner, M.J., Shaw, K.A., Baio, J., Washington, A., Patrick, M., DiRienzo, M., Christensen, D.L., Wiggins, L.D., Pettygrove, S. Andrews, J.G., Lopez, M., Hudson, A., Baroud, T., Schwenk, Y., White, T., Rosenberg, C.R., Lee, L-C., Harrington, R.A., Huston, M., Hewitt, A., . . . Patricia M. Dietz, (2020). Prevalence of autism spectrum disorder among children aged 8 years—autism and developmental disabilities monitoring network, 11 Sites, United States, 2016. *MMWR. Surveillance Summaries, 69*(4), 1–12.

Matheis, M., Matson, J. L., Burns, C. O., Jiang, X., Peters, W. J., Moore, M., et al. (2017). Factors related to parental age of first concern in toddlers with autism spectrum disorder. *Developmental Neurorehabilitiation, 20,* 228–235.

Miller, J., Gabrielsen, T., Villalobos, M., Alleman, R., Wahmhoff, N., & Segura, B. (2011). The each child study: Systematic screening for autism spectrum disorders in a pediatric setting. *Pediatrics, 127,* 866–871.

Mitchell, S., Brian, J., Zwaigenbaum, L., Roberts, W., Szatmari, P., Smith, I., et al. (2006). Early language and communication development of infants later diagnosed with autism spectrum disorder. *Journal of Developmental and Behavioral Pediatrics, 27*(2 Suppl), S69–78.

Norbury, C. F., & Sparks, A. (2013). Difference or disorder? Cultural issues in understanding neurodevelopmental disorders. *Developmental Psychology, 49*(1), 45–58.

Oosterling, I. J., Wensing, M., Swinkels, S. H., van der Gaag, R. J., Visser, J. C., Woudenberg, T., et al. (2010). Advancing early detection of autism spectrum disorder by applying an integrated two-stage screening approach. *Journal of Child Psychology and Psychiatry, 51,* 250–258.

Ormond, S., Brownlow, C., Garnett, M. S., Rynkiewicz, A., & Attwood, T. (2017). Profiling autism symptomatology: An exploration of the Q-ASC parental report scale in capturing sex differences in autism. *Journal of Autism and Developmental Disorders, 48,* 389–403.

Perrin, E. C., Sheldrick, C., Visco, Z., & Mattern, K. (2016). The survey of well-being of young children user's manual. *Tufts Medical Center.* https://www.floatinghospital.org/-/media/

Brochures/Floating-Hospital/SWYC/SWYC-Manual-v101-Web-Format-33016.ashx?la=en&hash=E0C2802F003ED312E9D5268374C540A112151FB3
Pierce, K., Courchesne, E., & Bacon, E. (2016). To screen or not to screen for ASD universally is not the question: Why the task force got it wrong. *Journal of Pediatrics, 176,* 182–194.
Provost, B., Lopez, B. R., & Heimerl, S. (2007). A comparison of motor delays in young children: autism spectrum disorder, developmental delay, and developmental concerns. *Journal of Autism and Developmental Disorders, 37*(2), 321–328.
Robins, D. L., Casagrande, K., Barton, M., Chen, C.-M. A., Dumont-Mathieu, T., & Fein, D. (2014). Validation of the Modified Checklist for Autism in Toddlers, Revised With Follow-up (M-CHAT-R/F). *Pediatrics, 133*(1), 37–45.
Robins, D. L., Fein, D. & Barton, M. (2009). The modified checklist for autism in toddlers, revised with follow up. https://mchatscreen.com/mchat-rf/
Rosenberg, S. A., Robinson, C. C., Shaw, E. F., & Ellison, M. C. (2013). Part C early intervention for infants and toddlers: Percentage eligible versus served. *Pediatrics, 131*(1), 38–46.
Rotholz, D., Kinsman, A., Lacy, K., & Charles, J. (2017). Improving early identification and intervention for children at risk for autism spectrum disorder. *Pediatrics, 139*(2), e20161061.
Rutter, M., Bailey, A., & Lord, C. (2003). *Social communication questionnaire.* Los Angeles, CA: Western Psychological Services.
Ozonoff, S. Iosif, A., Baguio, F., Cook, I., Hill, M. M., Hutman, T., … Young, G. S. (2010). A prospective study of the emergence of early behavioral signs of autism. *Journal of the American Academy of Child & Adolescent Psychiatry, 49*(3), 256–266. e1–2.
Salisbury, L. A., Nyce, J. D., Hannum, C. D., Sheldrick, R. C., & Perrin, E. C. (2018). Sensitivity and specificity of 2 autism screeners among referred children between 16 and 48 months of age. *Journal of Developmental and Behavioral Pediatrics, 39*(3), 254–258.
Self, T. L., Parham, D. F., & Rajagopalan, J. (2015). Autism spectrum disorder early screening practices: A survey of physicians. *Communication Disorders Quarterly, 36*(4), 195–207.
Serdarevic, F., Ghassabian, A., van Batenburg-Eddes, T., White, T., Blanken, L., Jaddoe, V., et al. (2017). Infant muscle tone and childhood autistic traits: A longitudinal study in the general population. *Autism Research, 10*(5), 757–768.
Shaw, K.A., Maenner, M.J., Baio, J., Washington, A., Christensen, D.L., Wiggins, L.D., Pettygrove, S., Andrews, J.D., White, T., Rosenberg, C.R., Constantino, J.N., Fitzgerald, R.T., Zahorodny, W., Shenouda, J., Daniels, J.L., Salinas, A., Durkin, M.S., & Dietz, P.M. (2020). Early identification of autism spectrum disorder among children aged 4 years—early autism and developmental disabilities monitoring network, Six Sites, United States, 2016. *MMWR Surveill Summ, 69*(SS-3), 1–11. https://doi.org/10.15585/mmwr.ss6903a1
Shumway, S., & Wetherby, A. (2009). Communicative acts of children with autism spectrum disorders in the second year of life. *Journal of Speech, Language and Hearing Research, 52,* 1139–1152.
Simek, A. N., & Wahlberg, A. C. (2011). Test review: Autism spectrum rating scales. *Journal of Psychoeducational Assessment, 29*(2), 191–195.
Smith, N. J., Sheldrick, R. C., & Perrin, E. C. (2013). An abbreviated screening instrument for autism spectrum disorders. *Infant Mental Health Journal, 34*(2), 149–155.
Stone, W. L., Coonrod, E. E., & Ousley, O. Y. (2000). Screening Tool for Autism in Two-year-olds (STAT): Development and preliminary data. *Journal of Autism and Developmental Disorders, 30*(6), 607–612.
Thelen, E. (1995). Motor development: A new synthesis. *American Psychologist, 50,* 79–95.
Uylings, H. B. M. (2006). Development of the human cortex and the concept of "critical" or "sensitive" periods. *Language Learning, 56*(Suppl 1), 59–90.
Veness, C., Prior, M., Bavin, E., Eadie, P., Cini, E., & Reilly, S. (2012). Early indicators of autism spectrum disorders at 12 and 24 months of age: A prospective, longitudinal comparative study. *Autism, 16*(2), 163–177.
Wetherby, A., Lord, C., Woods, J., Guthrie, W., Pierce, K., Shumway, S., et al. (2009). *The Early Screening for Autism and Communication Disorders (ESAC): Preliminary field-testing of an*

autism-specific screening tool for children 12 to 36 months of age. Chicago, IL: Oral presentation at the International Meeting for Autism Research.

Wetherby, A., & Prizant, B. (2002). *Communication and symbolic behavior scales developmental profile—First* (normed ed.). Baltimore, MD: Brookes.

Wetherby, A. M., Watt, N., Morgan, L., & Shumway, S. (2007). Social communication profiles of children with autism spectrum disorders late in the second year of life. *Journal of Autism and Developmental Disorders, 37*(5), 960–975.

Wetherby, A., Woods, J., Allen, L., Cleary, J., Dickinson, H., & Lord, C. (2004). Early indicators of autism spectrum disorders in the second year of life. *Journal of Autism and Developmental Disorders, 34,* 473–493.

Wiggins, L. D., Bakeman, R., Adamson, L. B., & Robins, D. L. (2007). The utility of the social communication questionnaire in screening for autism in children referred for early intervention. *Focus on Autism and Other Developmental Disabilities, 22*(1), 33–38.

Zuckerman, K. E., Chavez, A. E., & Reeder, J. A. (2017a). Decreasing disparities in child development assessment: Identifying and discussing possible delays in the Special Supplemental Nutrition Program for Women, Infants, and Children (WIC). *Journal of Developmental and Behavioral Pediatrics, 38*(5), 301–309.

Zuckerman, K. E., Lindly, O. J., Reyes, N. M., Chavez, A. E., Macias, K., Smith, K. N., et al. (2017b). Disparities in diagnosis and treatment of autism in Latino and non-Latino white families. *Pediatrics, 139*(5), e20163010.

Zwaigenbaum, L., et al. (2013). Early identification of autism spectrum disorders. *Behavioral Brain Research, 251*, 133–146.

Zwaigenbaum, L., Bauman, M. L., Fein, D., Pierce, K., Buie, T., Davis, P. A., Newschaffer, C., Robins, D. L., Wetherby, A., Choueiri, R., Kasari, C., Stone, W. L. Yirmiya, N., Estes, A., Hansen, R. L., McPartland, J. C., Natowicz, M. R., Carter, A., Granpeesheh, D., Mailloux, Z., Smith Roley, S., Wagner, S. (2015). Early screening of autism spectrum disorder: Recommendations for Practice and Research. *PEDIATRICS, 136*(Supplement), S41–S59. https://doi.org/10.1542/peds.2014-3667D

Developmental Screening in Community-Based Settings

Jeffrey D. Shahidullah, Susan G. Forman, Jill H. Harris, and Amy Norton

Abstract Autism spectrum disorder (ASD) is a neurodevelopmental disorder affecting 1 in 59 children in the United States. The benefits of early detection and intervention for ASD have been clearly documented. However, significant delays exist in access to early screening, diagnosis, and service provision. Despite the American Academy of Pediatrics' guidelines recommending developmental screening for ASD at 18 and 24 months, less than 20% of children with ASD receive their diagnosis before age 3. For many, this diagnosis comes several years later, which further delays entry into support services. There are documented barriers to appropriate developmental screening occurring in primary care, largely due to the lack of time that primary care clinicians have to conduct this screening. Thus, there is a need to expand developmental screening to also occur in accessible community-based settings, such as the home, preschool, child care, and other community programs. This chapter provides the rationale for developmental screening to occur in community settings and describes several existing models that may be positioned to offer innovative solutions to overcome the limitations with families solely relying on the primary care clinic as a developmental screening source.

Autism spectrum disorder (ASD) is a neurodevelopmental disorder affecting 1 in 59 children in the United States (Baio et al., 2018). The benefits of early detection and intervention for ASD have been clearly documented (Helt et al., 2008; Reichow & Wolery, 2009; Zwaigenbaum et al., 2015). However, significant delays exist in access to early screening, diagnosis, and service provision (Bishop-Fitzpatrick & Kind,

J. D. Shahidullah (✉)
Department of Psychiatry, Dell Medical School, University of Texas at Austin, Austin, TX, USA
e-mail: Jeff.Shahidullah@austin.utexas.edu

S. G. Forman
Department of School Psychology, Rutgers University, New Brunswick, NJ, USA

J. H. Harris
Children's Specialized Hospital, New Brunswick, NJ, USA

A. Norton
Autism Department, Children's Specialized Hospital, New Brunswick, NJ, USA

M. B. McClain et al. (eds.), *Interprofessional Care Coordination for Pediatric Autism Spectrum Disorder*, https://doi.org/10.1007/978-3-030-46295-6_4

2017). Despite the American Academy of Pediatrics' guidelines (AAP; Johnson & Myers, 2007) recommending developmental screening for ASD at 18 and 24 months, less than 20% of children with ASD receive their diagnosis before age 3 (Zablotsky et al., 2017). For many, this diagnosis comes several years later, which further delays entry into support services (Baio et al., 2018). There are documented barriers to appropriate developmental screening occurring in primary care, largely due to the lack of time that primary care clinicians have to conduct this screening (Morelli et al., 2014). Thus, there is a need to expand developmental screening to also occur in accessible community-based settings, such as the home, preschool, child care, and other community programs. This chapter provides a rationale for developmental screening to occur in community settings and describes several existing models that may be positioned to offer innovative solutions to overcome the limitations with families solely relying on the primary care clinic as a developmental screening source.

Current Status of Developmental Screening and Referral

Primary care clinicians (i.e., nurses, pediatricians, and family medicine physicians) are uniquely positioned to promote children's developmental health within the medical home. Primary care clinicians have regular and longitudinal contact with children and families through routine well-visits, as well as sick-visits. Many children with developmental delays/disorders and behavioral concerns/disorders have subtle symptoms that are not easily detectable in the absence of measurement using validated screening tools and approaches. The AAP has recommended that ASD screening occurs at the 18- and 24-month primary care well-visit (Johnson & Myers, 2007). This early screening is important as research has shown that an ASD diagnosis at the age of two can be considered very reliable (Lord et al., 2006). However, pediatricians cite lack of time, training, and resources as barriers to conduct screening often needed for later diagnosis (Morelli et al., 2014).

In part due to the lack of uptake of developmental and ASD screening in the primary care medical home, there are noteworthy delays between the onset of parental concerns and comprehensive evaluation and diagnosis of ASD. For children with ASD, symptoms are often present by 12 months of age, but the typical age of diagnosis is 4–5 years (Baio et al., 2018), and those with low SES or racial and ethnic minorities, including African–American, Hispanic–American, and Asian–American children, have been found to be identified later (Durkin et al., 2010). The majority of children are identified after age 3 (when eligibility for Early Intervention services may end), and one third to one half are identified after school age (Sheldrick, Maye, & Carter, 2017). In a large, multi-site ASD surveillance study (Baio et al., 2018), despite the parents of 85% of children with ASD expressing concerns to a provider about their child's development by 36 months of age, the median age of diagnosis was 52 months, and ranged from 46 to 67 months depending on symptom severity. In a survey in the United Kingdom of over 1,000 parents of children with an ASD diagnosis, there was an average delay of around 3.5 years from when they first approached a provider with their concerns to actually receiving an ASD diagnosis (Crane, Chester, Goddard, Henry, & Hill, 2016).

Comparison of the age at which parents or caregivers are first aware of potential problems, and when children are typically diagnosed as having ASD, and when children diagnosed as having ASD receive services underscores the need for expanded and innovative screening and referral processes. Parents may first notice that their child is behaving or learning differently than other children, or a friend or relative may express to the parent that they are concerned about the child's development. Child care providers or preschool teachers may note that the child's language development, social interactions, and other behaviors are different than their peers. Clinicians who become aware of child symptoms that may result in an ASD diagnosis often take a "wait and see" approach, citing concerns about unnecessarily alarming parents, and/or lack of knowledge of appropriate community resources (Earls, Andrews, & Hay, 2009).

Equally concerning are data indicating that when children are screened and problems are identified, they may not be referred for appropriate services. For example, King et al. (2010) found that when a child failed a developmental screening instrument administered in a medical practice, physicians referred them for services only 61% of the time. However, another study found that when pediatricians did talk with parents about developmental concerns, it was found that 90% of children who would be eligible for intervention services did not access the necessary services (Jimenez, Barg, Guevara, Gerdes, & Fiks, 2012). Branson and Bingham (2017) found that child care providers were able to identify children who were at risk for developmental delays, but did not indicate that they would refer these children for further evaluation. Concerns about parent reactions, feelings of not being qualified to make referrals, lack of knowledge about referral agencies, and child care center policies and procedures were cited by the child care providers as reasons for not making referrals. Parents not understanding how to contact the referral agency or the importance of the intervention were factors that were found to influence parent follow-through.

Early identification and intervention are practices that can improve child development and reduce the negative outcomes often associated with disabilities (Brown & Guralnick, 2012), and screening is the first step to diagnosis and provision of early intervention services. Although children with ASD will likely need continued support into their adult years, early identification and intervention can improve their outcomes in areas such as communication skills, social interaction, social relatedness, cognitive ability, independence, quality of life, and ASD symptomology (Braddock & Twyman, 2014; Dawson et al., 2010, 2012; Robins, 2008; Sallows & Graupner, 2005). Early identification and intervention may also reduce parent stress related to the child's diagnosis (Earhart & Zamora, 2015), and improve the interaction between the child and caregivers (Paschall & Mastergeorge, 2016). Failure to screen and refer early negates the potential for reducing the burden of ASD on individuals, families, and society.

Models of Community-Based Screening and Referral

Child Care Setting Models

There are several advantages of conducting developmental screening within child care (i.e., day care) settings. For example, many young children (although certainly not all) spend a considerable part of their day in child care, thus allowing ample opportunities for child care staff to observe the child across a variety of activities and skill areas (Larsen et al., 2018). These skills include social interaction, emotion regulation, language development, and motor development. Child care staff may also be well-suited to detect individual differences by virtue of exposure to large groups of same-age student peers. Staff also have frequent and ongoing access to check-in with parents regarding follow-up (e.g., daily drop-off/pick-up). However, there are few published studies that examine actual child care developmental screening practices.

Branson and Bingham (2017) noted child care staff were able to identify concerns regarding children in their classrooms; however, they typically express discomfort sharing those concerns with parents (e.g., worries about alarming parents regarding their child's development). In another study, Shahidullah and colleagues (2020) surveyed childcare staff from all counties in New Jersey who attended a developmental screening workshop to determine their views on conducting developmental screening in their classrooms. While most respondents viewed screening as beneficial, many were not conducting developmental screening for all children in their centers. Identified barriers included funding to purchase screening materials, need for more training on discussing screening results with parents, and information about referral resources. The Quality Rating Improvement System (QRIS Resource Guide, 2018) attempts to address these concerns by establishing standards of care that include developmental screening. The QRIS is offered to states and includes provider supports, such as training, mentoring, and technical assistance to help programs achieve higher levels of quality. Programs are financially incentivized for implementation of standards which include universal screening.

When implementing screening programs within child care centers, considerations include selection of a screening tool (e.g., access, training availability, ease of use, cost, administration time), determination of respondents (e.g., parent, staff, or both), frequency of screening, establishing buy-in by promoting the benefits of universal screening over referral-based screening, methods for sharing results with parents, identification of referral resources, and follow-up processes.

Researchers have demonstrated that child care providers are good identifiers of developmental or ASD-specific concerns with or without the use of a standardized screening tool (Branson and Bingham, 2017; Janvier et al., 2015). However, we did not find published examples of studies that quantify actual referral for, and successful linkage to, services. For example, in a universal ASD screening study (Janvier et al., 2016) conducted in Head Start settings, both child care workers and parents independently completed several ASD screening questionnaires. In this study, child care providers were not asked to make referrals as study staff offered diagnostic evaluations within the Head Start setting to children who scored at-risk on any of the tools (parent or teacher). In the Branson and Bingham (2017) study, while child care providers accurately identified children at risk for developmental delay, they did not always report that they would make referrals for those identified.

Home-Based Models

Major advantages of home-based screening programs are privacy and comfort for parents/families, accessibility, and likelihood of increased parent engagement. Home-based models remove barriers such as transportation, cost, and impact on the parent work schedule. Home models include telephone programs (Bogin, 2006; Dworkin, 2006; Nelson et al., 2019; Roux et al., 2012), screening through web-based/phone apps (Bardhan et al., 2016; Thabtah, 2018), and home visiting programs (Michalopoulos et al., 2017, 2019).

The disadvantages of home-based models include reliance on parent initiative. For example, if the parent does not have a concern, they are unlikely to initiate or participate in screening. Indeed, parents who are a racial minority, low income, and/or low parental education may be less likely to report developmental or ASD concerns (Zuckerman et al, 2014). A disadvantage specific to online screening models is that there typically is no one to ask if the parent has any questions about a screening item. Access to a computer or smartphone may be a barrier for some families.

An example of a phone-based model of developmental and ASD screening used a 2-1-1 program within an area serving a large population of low-income and racial and ethnic minority children (Nelson et al., 2019; Roux et al., 2012). In the Roux et al. (2012) study, a portion of parents of children aged 0–5 years old who called a 2-1-1 information center serving Los Angeles County were offered phone screening by a trained care coordinator using the Parents' Evaluation of Developmental Status (PEDS Online, Glascoe, 2010). The Modified Checklist of Autism in Toddlers (M-CHAT, Robins, 1999) was also given to parents of those children aged 16–48 months. Results were immediately shared with the parent, and local referrals for evaluation and intervention were provided with the parent on the phone to demonstrate how to advocate for child needs. Phone follow-up to ensure service linkage was also provided. Of children screened, over half were considered at developmental risk and almost all of those were given at least one new referral. At follow-up, a high percentage of children were either receiving recommended services or had services pending. The authors note that replication would require adequately trained staff, established referral relationships, as well as technologic infrastructure and funding. Nelson et al. (2019) varied this approach by randomly assigning families seen at a health clinic to treatment as usual in the clinic (control) or treatment as usual plus connection with 2-1-1 for phone-based developmental screening, resource information, and follow-up to determine service initiation. Those children in the intervention group had greater rates of referrals and linkage to services.

The *Help Me Grow* program includes healthcare provider training, phone access to screening, and resource linkage (Bogin, 2006; Dworkin, 2006). Phone-based care coordinators may either conduct developmental screening during the call or tell parents how they can access online developmental screening (typically using the Ages and Stages Questionnaire, Third Edition; ASQ-3). For those completing online screening, the completed screen is linked to staff at a central intake system who then calls the parent to discuss results and offer resources. Successful linkage to referral services may not be guaranteed as McKay and colleagues (2006) reported that almost half of families in their study were either lost to follow-up or had not followed through with resource recommendations despite an average of seven contacts after the initial call. There are several examples of ASD screening phone apps or mobile access for home or office use (Bardhan et al., 2016; Thabtah, 2018). These apps may use pictorial examples or video snippets with which parents can compare their child's behavior. Easter Seals offers free online ASQ screening (see http://www.easterseals.com/mtffc/asq/).

Birth to Five: Help Me Thrive! (2014) provides a manual available online for home visiting programs that includes information about screening tools, how to discuss concerns with families, and information about locating referral resources. In 2018, 74% of children participating in Maternal, Infant, and Early Childhood Home Visiting Programs had received timely developmental screening (MCHI, 2019). Long-term impact of home visiting programs suggests long-term cost effectiveness based on reduced spending on government programs and increased individual parent earnings (Michalopoulos et al., 2017) although different areas of focus within the model resulted in different types and levels of impact (Michalopoulos et al., 2019).

Community-Focused Models

Advantages of community-based screening models include the opportunity to promote collaboration to support integration of care and effective communication (Roux et al., 2012) and awareness of developmental screening across community programs and providers. Community-based programs are typically located in easily accessible and family-oriented agencies, such as family success centers and public libraries. Another advantage is that when community-based programs are offered, staff involved are trained in the use of screening tools, sharing of results with families is part of the process, staff is knowledgeable of referral sources, and in some models, follow-up is a built-in component. Disadvantages include limitation in the number of children served, cost, staffing, need for outreach to inform families of the program, and family buy-in. For example, parents who do not have a concern may be unlikely to participate unless they are aware of/buy-into the importance of screening for young children. How the family learns of the program is important. Parents may be more likely to participate when someone they trust tells them about the program versus learning about a program in a flyer or advertisement.

The *Quick Peek* model is one example of community-based developmental screening (Harris & Norton, 2016). Free, interactive screening using the ASQ-3 (Squires, Twomby, Bricker & Potter, 2009) is offered for children aged 1–5 years, in both English and Spanish by trained child development experts. The Modified Checklist for Autism in Toddlers-Revised (MCHAT-R, Robins et al., 2009) is administered for children aged 16–30 months. Clinics are primarily located in low-income cities, in easily accessible community programs such as public libraries, family success centers, and child care resource and referral agencies. All families receive anticipatory guidance resources and a summary letter of results to share with their healthcare provider. Families of children determined to be at risk receive referral information for evaluation and intervention and are called one month later for follow-up. In this model, more than 50% of children screened were deemed at developmental risk. A clear majority of those reached at one-month follow-up had arranged recommended evaluations and services (Harris & Norton, 2016).

Books, Balls, & Blocks (2017) is a scalable community-based model that may be offered as part of the larger Help Me Grow program. It consists of an interactive parent event to provide information about child development, offer developmental screenings, and provide community resources. It differs from some other models in its focus on fun activities that parents can do with their child. Joining with community partners may make the event more successful by providing a location, marketing and encouraging families to attend. This program is relatively new and research on impact is currently unavailable.

Discussion

Universal developmental screening in accordance with AAP guidelines should ideally occur in all pediatric primary care settings. This is due to the frequent and continuous contact that primary care clinicians have with young children and their families and the unique rapport and trust that families have with these clinicians. However, the current standard of screening in primary care practice does not align with AAP guidelines, and many children "fall through the cracks" with missed or delayed diagnoses leading to delays to treatment. Fortunately, several innovative models exist for developmental screening to occur in community settings that may be positioned to overcome the limitations with families solely relying on the primary care clinic as a developmental screening source. These models make access to early childhood screening accessible to families by positioning screening services in common community touchpoints, such as child care settings and public libraries. In many settings, such as child care centers, individuals are well positioned to provide input around screening in the context of their ability to compare a child to a sample of same-age peer comparisons who also function in a structured social setting.

Given the importance of family buy-into recognize the importance of early screening and referral initiation, these models may provide families with the support needed through partnerships around working with the family to problem-solve around barriers to follow-through and access to referrals. These models often provide follow-up support to determine successful linkage and/or the need for further assistance. Given difficulties with making referrals after a young child has been screened (e.g., not knowing where to refer, not following up), more research should look at innovative models of engagement with families around following-through with referrals so that barriers with referral follow-through do not negate the impact of developmental or ASD screening programs.

Developing feasible and scalable methods to train a non-healthcare clinician workforce to conduct brief developmental screening with young children, discuss and engage the family around the importance of developmental screening, and empower the individual to discuss screening results in a family-centered way will be important. The value-add of providing this training to non-healthcare clinicians in community settings (e.g., child care centers, community centers) should be articulated and framed in the context of the financial and societal return-on-investment. This return-on-investment perspective will be important for securing funding structures to continue to support training and program development in this area to ensure long-term viability and sustainability of programming.

References

Baio, J., Wiggins, L., Christensen, D. L., Maenner, M., Daniels, J., Warren, Z., & Dowling, N. F. (2018). Prevalence of autism spectrum disorder among children aged 8 years-Autism and Developmental Disabilities Monitoring Network, 11 sites, United States, 2014. *Morbidity and Mortality Weekly Report, 67*, 1–23.

Bardhan, S., Mridha, G. M., Ahmed, E., Ullah, A., Ahmed, H. U., Rabbani M. G., … Al Mamun, A. (2016). Autism BARTA–A smart device based automated autism screening tool for Bangladesh. In *Fifth International Conference on Informatics*. Retrieved form https://ieeexplore.ieee.org/document/7760073.

Birth to Five: Watch me Thrive. Available from https://www.acf.hhs.gov/ecd/child-health-development/watch-me-thrive.

Bishop-Fitzpatrick, L., & Kind, A., J., H. (2017). A scoping review of health disparities in autism spectrum disorder. *Journal of Autism and Developmental Disorders, 47*, 3380–3391.

Bogin, J. (2006). Enhancing developmental services in primary care: The Help Me Grow experience. *Journal of Developmental and Behavioral Pediatrics, 27,* S8–S12.

Books, Blocks and Balls program manual. Available from Help Me Grow- Utah, Provo, UT. March, 2017. Retrieved from https://helpmegrownational.org/resources/books-balls-and-blocks-manual/.

Braddock, B., & Twyman, K. (2014). Access to treatment for toddlers with autism spectrum disorders. *Clinical Pediatrics, 53*, 225–229.

Branson, D., & Bingham, A. (2017). Child care providers' competence and confidence in referring children at risk for developmental delays. *Infants & Young Children, 30,* 41–57.

Brown, S. E., & Guralnick, M. J. (2012). International human rights to early intervention for infants and young children with disabilities. *Infants and Young Children, 25*, 270–285.

Crane, L., Chester, J. W., Goddard, L., Henry, L. A., & Hill, E. (2016). Experiences of autism diagnosis: A survey of over 1000 parents in the United Kingdom. *Autism, 20*, 153–162.

Dawson, G., Jones, E. J., Merkle, K., Venema, K., Lowy, R., Faja, S., Kamara, K., & Webb, S. J. (2012). Early behavioral intervention is associated with normalized brain activity in young children with autism. *Journal of the American Academy of Child and Adolescent Psychiatry, 51*, 1150–1159.
Dawson, G., Rogers, S., Munson, J., Smith, M., Winter, J., Greenson, J., Donaldson, A., & Varley, J. (2010). Randomized, controlled trial of an intervention for toddlers with autism: The Early Start Denver Model. *Pediatrics, 125*, 17–23.
Durkin, M. S., Maenner, M. J., Meaney, F., J., Levy, S. E., DiGuiseppi, C., Nicholas, J. S., & Schieve, L. A. (2010). Socioeconomic inequility in the prevalence of autism spectrum disorder: Evidence from a U. S. cross-sectional study. *PLoS One, 12*, e11551.
Dworkin, P. (2006). Historical overview: From ChildServ to Help Me Grow. *Journal of Developmental and Behavioral Pediatrics, 27*, S5–S7.
Easter Seals: Make the first five count. Retrieved from https://www.easterseals.com/mtffc/asq/ July2019.
Earhart, J., & Zamora, I. (2015). Achievement together: The development of an intervention using relationship-based strategies to promote positive learning habits. *Infants and Young Children, 28*, 32–45.
Earls, M. F., Andrews, J. E., & Hay, S. S. (2009). A longitudinal study of developmental and behavioral screening and referral in North Carolina's assuring better health and development participating practices. *Clinical Pediatrics, 48*, 824–833.
Glascoe, F. P. (2010). *Parents' evaluation of developmental status: Online (PEDS online)*. Nashville, TN: Ellsworth and Vandermeer Press LLC.
Harris, J., & Norton, A. (2016). The Quick Peek program: A model for developmental screening within underserved communities. *Infants & Young Children, 29*, 290–298.
Helt, M., Kelley, E., Kinsbourne, M., Pandey, J., Boorstein, H., Herbert, M., & Fein, D. (2008). Can children with autism recover? If so, how? *Neuropsychological Review, 18*, 339–366.
Janvier, Y. M., Harris, J. F., Coffield, C. N., Louis, B., Xie, M., Cidav, Z., et al. (2015). Screening for autism spectrum disorder in underserved communities: Early childcare providers as reporters. *Autism, 20*, 364–373.
Janvier, Y. M., Harris, J. F., Coffield, C. N., Louis, B., Xie, M., Cidav, Z., et al. (2016). Screening for autism spectrum disorder in underserved communities: Early childcare providers as reporters. *Autism, 20*, 364–373.
Jimenez, M. E., Barg, F. K., Guevara, J. P., Gerdes, M., & Fiks, A. G. (2012). Barriers to evaluation for early intervention services: Parent and early intervention employee perspectives. *Academic Pediatrics, 12*, 551–557.
Johnson, C. P., Myers, S. M., & American Academy of Pediatrics Council on Children with Disabilities. (2007). *Pediatrics, 120*, 1183–215.
King, T. M., Tandon, S. D., Macias, M. M., Healy, J. A., Duncan, P. M., Swignoski, N. L., & Lipkin, P. H. (2010). Implementing developmental screening and referrals: Lessons learned from a national project. *Pediatrics, 125*, 350–360.
Larsen, K., Aasland, A., & Diseth, T. H. (2018). Identification of symptoms of autism spectrum disorders in the second year of life at day-care centers by day-care staff: Step one in the development of a short observation list. *Journal of Autism and Developmental Disorders, 48*, 2267–2277.
Lord, C., Risi, S., DiLavore, P. S., Shulman, C., Thurm, A., & Pickles, A. (2006). Autism from 2 to 9 years of age. *Archives of General Psychiatry, 63*, 694–701.
Maternal Child Health Initiatives (MCHI). Retrieved from https://mchb.hrsa.gov/maternal-child-health-initiatives/home-visiting-overview.
McKay, K., Shannon, A., Vater, S., & Dworkin, P. H. (2006). ChildServ: Lessons learned from the design and implementation of a community-based developmental surveillance program. *Infants & Young Children, 19*, 371–377.
Michalopoulos, C., Faucetta, K., Hill, C. J., Portilla, X, A., Burrell, L., Lee, H., Duggan, A., & Knox, V. (2019). *Impacts on family outcomes of evidence-based early childhood home visiting: Results from the Mother and Infant Home Visiting Program Evaluation* (OPRE Report 2019-07).

Washington, DC: Office of Planning, Research, and Evaluation, Administration for Children and Families, U.S. Department of Health and Human Services. Retrieved from https://www.acf.hhs.gov/sites/default/files/opre/mihope_impact_report_final20_508.pdf.

Michalopoulos, C., Faucetta, K., Warren, A., & Mitchell, R. (2017). *Evidence on the long-term effects of home visiting programs: Laying the groundwork for long-term follow-up in the Mother and Infant Home Visiting Program Evaluation (MIHOPE)* (OPRE Report 2017-73). Washington, DC: Office of Planning, Research and Evaluation, Administration for Children and Families, U.S. Department of Health and Human Services. Retrieved from https://www.acf.hhs.gov/sites/default/files/opre/mihope_lt_long_term_evidence_brief_508_compliant_corrected.pdf.

Morelli, S. A., Rameson, L. T., Lieberman, M. D. (2014). The neural components of empathy: Predicting daily prosocial behavior. *Scane, 9*, 39–47.

National Center on Early Childhood Quality Assurance. (2018). QRIS Resource Guide. US. Retrieved from https://ecquality.acf.hhs.gov/resource-guide.

Nelson, B. B., Thompson, L. R., Herrera, P., Biely, C., Zarate, D. A., Aceves, I., et al. (2019). Telephone-based developmental screening and care coordination through 2-1-1: A randomized trial. *Pediatrics, 143,* e20181064.

Paschall, K. W., & Mastergeorge, A. M. (2016). A review of 25 years of research in bidirectionality in parent-child relationships: An examination of methodological approaches. *International Journal of Behavioral Development*, *40*, 442–451.

Reichow, B., & Wolery, M. (2009). Comprehensive synthesis of early intensive behavioral interventions for young children with autism based on teh UCLA young autism project model. *Journal of Autism and Developmental Disorders, 39*, 23–41.

Robins, D. L. (1999). The modified checklist for Autism in toddlers (M-CHAT). Storrs, CT: self-published.

Robins, D. L. (2008). Screening for autism spectrum disorders in primary care settings. *Autism, 12*, 537–556.

Robins, D. L., Fein, D., & Barton, M. (2009). *The modified checklist for autism in toddlers*. Revised with Follow-Up (M-CHAT-R/F): Self-published.

Roux, A. M., Herrera, P., Wold, C. M., Dunkle, M. C., Glascoe, F. P., & Shattuck, P. T. (2012). Developmental and autism screening through 2-1-1: Reaching underserved families. *American Journal of Preventive Medicine, 43,* S457–S463.

Sallows, G. O., & Graupner, T. D. (2005). Intensive behavioral treatment for children with autism: Four-year outcome and predictors. *American Journal of Mental Retardation, 110*, 417–438.

Shahidullah, J. D., Forman, S. G., Norton, A., Harris, J., Palejwala, M. H., & Chaudhuri, A. (2020). Implementation of developmental screening by childcare providers. *Infants & Young Children, 33,* 21–34.

Sheldrick, R. C., Maye, M. P., & Carter, A. S. (2017). Age at first identification of autism spectrum disorder: An analysis of two US surveys. *Journal of the American Academy of Child and Adolescent Psychiatry, 56*, 313–320.

Squires, J., Twomby, E., Bricker, D. D., & Potter, L. (2009). Ages and stages Questionnaire-3 User's guide. Paul H Brookes Publishing.

Thabtah, F. (2018). An accessible and efficient autism screening method for behavioural data and predictive analyses. *Health Informatics Journal.* Retrieved from https://journals.sagepub.com/doi/pdf/10.1177/1460458218796636.

Zablotsky, B., Black, L. I., Blumberg, S. J. (2017). Estimated prevalence of children with diagnosed developmental disabilities in the United States, 2014–2016. U.S. Department of Health and Human Services, National Center for Health Statistics Data Brief, 291.

Zuckerman, K. E., Sinche, B., Cobian, M., Cervantes, M., Meija, A., Becker, T., et al. (2014). Conceptualization of autism in the Latino community and its relationship with early diagnosis. *Journal of Developmental and Behavioral Pediatrics, 35,* 522–532.

Zwaigenbaum, L., Bauman, M., L., Stone, W., L., Yirmiya, N., Estes, A., Hansen, R., L., & Wetherby, A. (2015). Early identification of autism spectrum disorder: Recommendations for practice and research. *Pediatrics, 136*, S10–S40.

Interdisciplinary Evaluation of Autism Spectrum Disorder

Jonathan M. Campbell, Bill Ogletree, Amy Rose, and Johanna Price

Abstract Authors introduce key features of interdisciplinary evaluation of autism spectrum disorder. The Comprehensive-Developmental Approach (CDA) is identified as a useful framework for conducting interdisciplinary evaluation. The CDA emphasizes the role of cohesive team functioning as critical for assessment work with families. Principles of evidence-based assessment and diagnostic instruments that meet evidence-based guidelines are identified. Links between interdisciplinary evaluation and intervention planning are described, including possibilities for "co-treatment" by interdisciplinary teams after the evaluation is complete. Strengths and limitations of interdisciplinary evaluation and intervention are introduced and authors conclude that interdisciplinary collaboration is worthwhile. The chapter concludes with a case study that illustrates interdisciplinary evaluation within a school setting.

Evaluation of children and youth with Autism Spectrum Disorder (ASD) may focus on initial diagnostic evaluation or ongoing assessment for individuals with a confirmed diagnosis. A range of social-communicative, behavioral, and language symptoms may be present for individuals with ASD, such as individuals who have limited speech to those with well-developed verbal language. Children with ASD also show various co-occurring difficulties beyond social-communicative and restrictive behavior or interests that characterize core symptoms of ASD. Co-occurring challenges may include other neurodevelopmental disorders (e.g., attention-deficit hyperactivity disorder; intellectual disability), medical conditions (e.g., seizure disorder), psychological and behavioral disorders (e.g., depression; disruptive behavior disorders), among others. Please refer to chapter "Medical Comorbidities in Pediatric Autism Spectrum Disorder" regarding medical comorbidities for more information. Given

J. M. Campbell (✉)
Department of Psychology, Western Carolina University, Cullowhee, NC, USA
e-mail: jmcampbell@wcu.edu

B. Ogletree · A. Rose · J. Price
Department of Communication Sciences and Disorders, Western Carolina University, Cullowhee, NC, USA

M. B. McClain et al. (eds.), *Interprofessional Care Coordination for Pediatric Autism Spectrum Disorder*, https://doi.org/10.1007/978-3-030-46295-6_5

the range of presenting core symptoms and the breadth of possible co-morbid conditions associated with ASD, an interdisciplinary or interprofessional assessment approach is warranted and recommended.

In this chapter, authors introduce interdisciplinary principles for assessment of ASD and identify and describe evidence-based assessment guidelines to inform diagnostic evaluation and special education eligibility decision-making. Authors provide a brief and selective introduction to diagnostic measures that meet evidence-based assessment guidelines. Next, authors describe strategies and approaches to use assessment results to inform intervention and educational programming. This section is followed by recommendations for synthesizing and communicating findings derived from an interdisciplinary assessment. The chapter concludes with a case example illustrating principles of interdisciplinary evaluation.

Evidence-Based Assessment Guidelines for Diagnostic Evaluation and Special Education Eligibility

Children and youth with ASD will likely interface with multiple service delivery systems, such as schools, outpatient mental health providers, and other professionals. Schools serve as the "de facto" service delivery settings and school professionals the "de facto" service providers for many children and youth with ASD. Given the frequent and necessary intersection between school and non-school professional providers, it is important for professionals to understand the similarity and difference between (a) medical/psychiatric diagnosis and (b) educational classification of ASD. Medical and psychiatric diagnosis of ASD is most commonly based on the diagnostic definition provided by the Diagnostic and Statistical Manual of Mental Disorders–Fifth Edition (DSM-5; American Psychiatric Association (APA), 2013). DSM-5 defines ASD as a neurodevelopmental disorder characterized by deficits in social communication and the presence of restrictive/repetitive behavior, interests, or activities (APA, 2013). Further, symptoms must be present in early development and yield significant impairment in social, occupational, or other areas of functioning.

Children and youth with ASD may also be eligible for special education services through meeting ASD eligibility criteria presented in the Individuals with Disabilities Education Improvement Act (2004). Many aspects of the educational definition of ASD match well with the medical definition; for example, social, communication, and behavioral components are included in the educational definition of ASD as in the psychiatric definition. In contrast to the medical definition of ASD, however, educational impact must be present for students with ASD to qualify for special education services. It is also important to note that there is variability in ASD identification and eligibility criteria requirements across states (Barton et al., 2016).

Comprehensive-Developmental Approach to Assessment

The Comprehensive-Developmental Approach (CDA; Klin, Saulnier, Tsatsanis, & Volkmar, 2005) articulates a valuable interdisciplinary model for assessing children and youth with ASD. The CDA provides a useful framework to incorporate assessment findings from various domains of functioning across disciplines, i.e., the comprehensive aspect of the model, that are interpreted from a developmental perspective. As noted, children and youth with ASD demonstrate difficulties and strengths across various domains that warrant comprehensive assessment. For example, cognitive functioning may be well-developed in the presence of significant limitations in social-communicative abilities, expressive language, academic achievement, and adaptive functioning.

Several principles of the CDA inform interdisciplinary assessment. First, cohesive team functioning is important for optimal assessment as this encourages discussion, allows for reconciliation of disparate findings, and, ultimately, yields a complete picture of the individual's strengths and limitations (e.g., Klin et al., 2005). Second, parent or caregiver involvement is crucial to the assessment process. Parents and caregivers directly observe individuals and provide important details needed for diagnosis, such as the onset of symptom presentation, and adaptive functioning, such as exhibited in the home context. Finally, the CDA emphasizes assessment of functional adjustment for individuals with ASD. For example, an adolescent with ASD may have well-developed cognitive and language abilities (e.g., superior-range measured intelligence), but not demonstrate everyday adaptive skills (e.g., independent dressing, telling time, purchasing items). Given these discrepancies, functional adjustment is critical to assess (Klin et al., 2005).

Introduction to Evidence-Based Assessment for Autism Spectrum Disorder

Evidence-based Assessment (EBA) principles should inform assessment for individuals with suspected or confirmed ASD. The basic tenet of EBA is that assessment instruments and practices should be grounded in evidentiary support, particularly psychometric evidence (e.g., standardization, norming, reliability, validity) that is replicated by multiple investigators or investigative groups. Ozonoff, Goodlin-Jones, and Solomon (2005) identified an initial set of instruments that met EBA guidelines for ASD. Roughly a decade later, Campbell, Ruble, and Hammond (2014) updated a review of measures meeting EBA guidelines for assessment of ASD, including several diagnostic instruments introduced in the next section.

A brief overview of diagnostic instruments that meet EBA guidelines. From EBA standards, three measures demonstrate strong psychometric support for diagnosis of ASD. The measures elicit diagnostic information through behavior observation, interview, or combination of both sources. Despite differences between the measures, each satisfies EBA criteria.

Autism Diagnostic Observation Schedule—Second Edition (ADOS-2; Lord, Rutter, DiLavore, Risi, Gotham, & Bishop, 2012*)*. The ADOS-2 is considered a "gold standard" diagnostic instrument for identification of ASD. The ADOS-2 consists of various activities, including play and interviews, that are administered in a semi-structured format to elicit social-communicative and behavioral symptoms indicative of ASD (Lord et al., 2012). As such, the ADOS-2 presents an opportunity to collect behavioral observation data, typically within the context of a clinical setting. The ADOS-2 features five modules that are administered based upon an individual's age and expressive language ability, ranging from activities that are appropriate for toddlers (e.g., simple routine-based play) to adults (e.g., interview questions related to social difficulties). Behavioral observations are coded to reflect the presence and degree of social-communicative and behavioral indicators of ASD to inform diagnostic decision-making. Codes are tallied within a diagnostic algorithm which produces an ADOS-2 diagnostic decision regarding the presence of an ASD. The ADOS-2 requires extensive training for reliable administration and scoring. The ADOS-2 features strong psychometric support and is consistently identified as an evidence-based diagnostic assessment for ASD (Campbell et al., 2014).

Autism Diagnostic Interview–Revised (ADI-R; Rutter, LeCouteur, & Lord, 2003*)*. The ADI-R is also considered a "gold standard" diagnostic instrument for ASD. The ADI-R is a comprehensive diagnostic interview completed with a caregiver that assesses the presence and onset of core social-communicative and behavioral indicators of ASD. Interview responses are coded and produce a diagnostic algorithm score that yields a diagnostic decision regarding the presence of ASD. Like its counterpart, the ADOS-2, the ADI-R requires extensive training for reliable and valid administration and scoring. The ADI-R features strong psychometric support and is consistently identified as an evidence-based diagnostic assessment for ASD (Campbell et al., 2014).

Childhood Autism Rating Scale–Second Edition (CARS-2; Schopler, Reichler, & Renner, 2010*)*. The CARS-2 is a rating scale completed by a trained evaluator to summarize the presence and severity of symptoms indicative of ASD. The CARS-2 features two forms, the Standard Version (CARS-2-ST), appropriate for children below the age of 6 and individuals with limited cognitive or language ability, and the High Functioning Version (CARS-2-HFA), appropriate for children six years or older with average or greater intellectual ability. Both forms sample 15 domains of functioning. CARS-2 ratings are informed by various sources of information, such as direct behavioral observation, parent report, and record review. Ratings are summed to produce an overall CARS-2 score, which falls within one of three categories representing the degree of ASD symptomatology. The CARS-2 is a useful tool for organizing and summarizing information about ASD-related symptoms from various sources and should be used in tandem with other "gold standard" diagnostic instruments.

Outside of autism-specific diagnostic instruments, several domains of functioning should be assessed to describe an individual with ASD. Core areas of assessment include cognitive functioning, language abilities, social–emotional adjustment, and adaptive behavior. Depending on the individual's age, abilities, and other presenting concerns, other domains of functioning should be assessed, such as academic achievement. Given the range of domains that should be assessed, interdisciplinary assessment is warranted.

Incorporating and Communicating Findings from Interdisciplinary Assessment

After all assessment data are collected, members of the interdisciplinary team meet to discuss results, draw conclusions regarding the diagnosis of ASD, and develop recommendations for the child (Prelock, Beatson, Bitner, Broder, & Ducker, 2003). In some settings, the team immediately meets with the family to discuss their diagnostic impressions and recommendations (Self, Mitchell, Hess, Marble, & Swails, 2017; Volkmar, Booth, McPartland, & Wiesner, 2014). In other settings, a single team member, such as a social worker (Koushik, Bacon, Stancin, 2015), psychologist (Koushik et al., 2015), or assessment coordinator (Prelock et al., 2003), coordinates the assessment findings of all team members and meets with the family to discuss findings and recommendations.

Written Report

The team's written report should present a comprehensive, holistic representation of the child and his or her strengths and needs, rather than disjointed results and impressions from each professional (Klin et al., 2005; Volkmar et al., 2014). An effectively organized and integrated report may begin with an integrated case history, followed by findings of individual professionals, and conclude with an integrated summary (Volkmar et al., 2014). Reports may also be entirely integrated, with individual professionals' results combined into a single, cohesive section.

Assessment reports generally include the child's developmental history, quantitative and qualitative descriptions of the child's performance on standardized tools, and descriptions of the child's behavior in naturalistic contexts, both as observed by professionals and reported by family members. Reports should profile the child's strengths and needs, and specific and meaningful recommendations to address the child's needs should be included (Huerta & Lord, 2012; Scottish Intercollegiate Guidelines Network [SIGN], 2016). These recommendations specify important targets for treatment, identify community and educational resources that should be utilized to support the child's development, and describe strategies for parents, teachers, and others that address their specific concerns and equip them to optimize their interactions with the child. In the case of diagnostic evaluations, reports should clearly state whether a diagnosis of ASD was made, explain why this conclusion was reached, and include the diagnostic criteria used (Huerta & Lord, 2012; SIGN, 2016).

An initial draft of the assessment report may be reviewed by the family and school personnel (Prelock et al., 2003; Self et al., 2017). Of particular importance is their perspectives regarding whether the behaviors demonstrated by the child during the assessment process are consistent with behaviors observed on a daily basis at home and at school (Prelock et al., 2003). Once family input has been incorporated, the report is finalized and distributed to the family as well as to relevant agencies and service providers with appropriate consent (Prelock et al., 2003; Self et al., 2017).

When drafting the report, teams may also consider using language that reflects a "strengths perspective" (Braun, Dunn, & Tomchek, 2017). Recently, Braun and colleagues (2017) found that interdisciplinary teams' diagnostic evaluation reports for children with suspected ASD contained significantly more language associated with a deficits perspective than a strengths perspective. A strengths perspective requires language that is descriptive, neutral, and/or positive, focusing on a child's abilities rather than disabilities. For example, the statements "Social interactions were difficult [for Bob]" and "Daisy had a great deal of difficulty sitting during the evaluation" maintain a deficit perspective, while "Bob responded to questions and comments. He did not make comments or ask the examiner questions" and "Throughout the evaluation, Daisy frequently got up from her seat" are descriptive and neutral, thus supporting a strengths perspective (Braun et al., 2017, p. 979). Because diagnostic reports are often a family's first source of information specific to their child's diagnosis and may be shared with many service providers, maintaining a strengths perspective in the report is an important part of encouraging the family and school personnel to view the child and his or her abilities positively (Braun et al., 2017).

Reporting Assessment Information to Caregivers and Educational Professionals

The initial assessment of a child with ASD includes sharing a diagnosis of ASD with the child and caregivers. This is a challenging task for professionals and a significant experience for families. Professionals identified the most difficult aspects of delivering the diagnosis as follows: (a) making certain that caregivers comprehend the diagnosis and reasons it was given, (b) delivering information at an appropriate level of complexity, and (c) handling caregivers' emotional reactions (Rogers, Goddard, Hill, Henry, & Crane, 2016). For parents, their perceptions of this experience influence their reaction to their child's diagnosis, with positive perceptions associated with greater acceptance and less anxiety regarding the child's diagnosis of ASD (Chua, 2012). Given both the inherent difficulty and lasting effects of sharing the diagnosis, it is important for professionals to be well-prepared to implement evidence-based practices during this task.

To foster a more positive experience, professionals' communication with parents is paramount (SIGN, 2016). Strongly recommended practices include providing both oral and written information that is clear, accurate, accessible, and understandable to families (SIGN, 2016). Ensuring opportunities for caregivers and the child (as appropriate) to ask questions at the time diagnostic information is shared is also strongly recommended (SIGN, 2016). Other recommended practices include providing child care, as feasible, for younger children at the time diagnostic information is shared; considering sharing information with adolescents separately from their parents; and providing opportunities for families to ask further questions at a later time (SIGN, 2016). Professionals' behavior has been correlated with parents' satisfaction of the diagnostic process for ASD, with empathy, understanding of the family's concerns, direct communication, being approachable, and open to questions associated with greater parent satisfaction (Brogan & Knussen, 2003). Therefore, professionals should be aware of their interpersonal skills during the diagnostic process, showing empathy to stress and anxiety that families will likely feel (SIGN, 2016; Marcus, Kunce, & Schopler, 2005). Additionally, the use of language aligned with a strengths perspective may encourage families to view their child and the ASD diagnosis in a positive light.

Cases of Diagnostic Uncertainty

In some cases, professionals may not be able to definitively diagnose ASD. Diagnostic uncertainty is more likely for (a) very young children who may not comply with testing protocols and are developing rapidly; (b) mildly affected children whose difficulties may not be readily detected or characterized; and (c) children with severe behavioral difficulties who are difficult to assess (Huerta & Lord, 2012; Volkmar et al., 2014). In these instances, professionals should clearly communicate to families why ASD could not be either diagnosed or ruled out, as well as recommendations for future action (Huerta & Lord; SIGN, 2016; Volkmar et al., 2014). Appropriate recommendations may include monitoring and re-evaluating the child within a specified time frame, such as 6 to 12 months (Huerta & Lord, 2012), and referring to other specialists (SIGN, 2016).

Sharing Information at Later Assessments

After the initial diagnosis of ASD is determined, the child should periodically participate in additional assessments. These assessments may be part of routine re-evaluations required by local education agencies, such as end of year or triennial special education re-evaluations. Results from these assessments are important for shaping appropriate intervention goals, as the child develops and his or her strengths and needs change, and as the child transitions to different systems of care, such as from early intervention to school-based services. During these assessments, clear oral and written communication with parents, the child, and other stakeholders continues to be important. Professionals should provide opportunities for all involved individuals to ask questions. Interpersonal aspects of communication are also important, and professionals should demonstrate empathy and understanding. Use of oral and written language that reflects a strength perspective of the child continues to be an important aspect of oral and written communication with families, educators, and other service providers.

Using Assessment Results to Inform Intervention and Educational Programming

When serving any student with ASD, optimal therapeutic management and educational programming, hereafter referred to collectively as "treatment," should be driven by the assessment findings of a collaborative team (Wilkinson, 2017). Assessment teams, often comprised of the student with ASD, family members, educators, psychologists, occupational and physical therapists, speech-language pathologists, and medical professionals, should conduct assessments in a manner that informs treatment goal-setting, ongoing management, and treatment evaluation (Riccio & Prickett, 2019). As initial team-based assessments targeting diagnoses or developmental/educational status are completed, data should be in place to make effective treatment decisions. Ongoing assessment should be dynamic in nature, and employ test-treat-test formats and utilize a variety of trial instructional methods (Budoff, 1987).

The Team's Role in Effective Treatment Planning and Implementation

The decision to treat from a team perspective has benefits and costs. Benefits include the multiple perspectives of varied team members, opportunities for cross disciplinary work, and the potential for a broader systems-based approach that promotes a holistic intervention environment. Costs of team-based intervention can include the time and effort required to create a truly integrated treatment effort; however, a recent pilot documented reduced amount of wait-time and financial costs of evaluation when interdisciplinary assessment teams were created (Williams-Arya et al., 2019). There are also risks specific to violating perceived territorial practice boundaries established by educational and health disciplines since their inception. In sum, releasing professional roles, even in small degrees, can be challenging.

Is it worth the effort to treat in teams? Sylvester, Ogletree, and Lunnen (2017) respond with a resounding "yes" in their description of co-treatment as a vehicle for children with more significant disabilities. These authors highlight a variety of ways professionals can co-treat effectively ranging from more casual collaborations to integrated hands-on interventions. What follows is a review of a few ways professionals may treat together in the pursuit of developmental, behavioral, social, and educational gains for students with ASD.

Teams can set goals. Collaborative teams often work together to select treatment goals that are strength-based; address developmental, behavioral, educational, and social needs; and promote socially valid outcomes (Wilkinson, 2017). Goals emerge from data generated throughout the comprehensive assessment process. As team-based assessment discussions move to treatment, team members should work together to create a broad-based treatment plan. Collaborative treatment planning and goal generation assures that team members are knowledgeable specific to all student goals. Team awareness of goals across developmental, behavioral, educational, and social domains creates fertile ground for integrated disciplinary work supporting all student needs. Finally, student goals should be measurable, with clear expectations and criteria for advancement or termination stated.

Teams can choose methodologies. Recently, Ogletree, Rose, and Hambrecht (2019) reviewed effective methods for promoting skill acquisition in children with ASD. Although these authors targeted communication skill growth, the ideas and treatment approaches they presented have broader applications. Ogletree et al. (2019) suggest that treatment methods must be both scientifically supported and practitioner-friendly. Scientifically supported treatments were described as those reported in reliable journals with critical peer review. Robey (2004) reports five levels of evidence for scientifically supported treatments based upon the strength and integrity of research processes. These include, in declining order as to rigor, meta-analyses, randomized controlled studies, quasi-experimental studies without randomization, observational efforts with controls, and observations without controls. Fortunately, when choosing treatment methods, collaborative teams have several options that meet rigorous standards of scientific support. These evidenced-based treatments have been described in several sources (National Autism Center, 2015; Prior, Rogers, Roberts, Williams, & Sutherland, 2011; Simpson, 2004, 2005; Wong et al., 2013).

Ogletree et al. (2019) suggest that practitioner-friendly approaches are easy to apply with respect to resources and effort. The authors also note that "friendly" methods are learnable, efficient, and effective. The concept of practitioner-friendliness is reasonably new and will necessitate clinical judgment from the intervention team. This said, team-based decisions regarding method friendliness may require trial and error applications and discussions.

Teams can treat together. As mentioned earlier, team members can treat together (Sylvester et al., 2017). This can take a more passive form such as consultation or observation or it can be active as in integrated co-treatment efforts. It is likely that some disciplines may work together due to natural affinities. For example, psychologists and speech-language pathologists both have interest in the potential communicative value of behavior and may find that active co-treatment promotes broader gains than siloed intervention and works to help others understand behavioral outbursts. Likewise, physical therapists may seek out speech-language pathologists for co-treatment after observing increased vocal behaviors during movement. While it may be unlikely for all members of the team to co-treat a given child, opportunities for team-based treatments abound.

Teams can evaluate the treatment progress. Throughout treatment, teams encounter the need to alter or even end intervention efforts based on student progress. Therefore, one element of effective team-based intervention is ongoing evaluation. Prior to evaluating and potentially modifying any treatment effort, practitioners must assure that intervention procedures have been implemented with fidelity, i.e., conducted as planned and in a comparable manner over time (Mandell, Stahmer, Shin, Xie, Reisinger, & Marcus, 2013). Procedures used in research studies, such as ongoing external data-keeping on treatment sequences use, would seem appropriate to monitor fidelity in team-based intervention contexts. For example, team monitoring of fidelity of a reinforcement based intervention is important to ensure that reinforcement is delivered reliably when the appropriate behavior is demonstrated. If reinforcement is not reliably delivered, intervention may be ineffective due to reinforcing other behavior or resulting in reinforcement schedule that is too thin. In fact, fidelity data-keeping during treatment would seem to be a valuable use of team member time, assuming data collectors are not actively engaged in the treatment itself.

If treatments have been conducted with fidelity, there is still the need to assess progress against criterion established in initial goals statements. Performance criterion can be written in ways that make goals easily measurable through the collection of frequency, percentage, or event descriptive data. Once again, treatments emanating from teams typically involve more interventionists allowing for assistance with data collection. Team-based interventions also allow unique windows into performance on all student goals across intervention contexts and providers. Of course, this requires considerable planning, collaboration, and time.

Teams can modify methodologies. Team members should always be open to modifying treatments based upon the process described above. If methods are not successful, they must be altered or terminated in favor of other treatment options. For example, if a student has participated in a communication intervention employing Milieu Training (i.e., a routine-based, more natural application of Applied Behavioral Analysis (Fey et al., 2006)) to promote verbal requesting, yet there is no appreciable change after three months of intervention conducted with fidelity, modifying treatment would be warranted. A new approach may be needed, or simple adjustments to training may work such as new activities, procedures, or reinforcement contingencies. Team staffing meetings provide excellent venues for processing and problem-solving methodological changes during treatment.

Teams can assist with dismissal decisions. One of the more challenging actions taken by therapists is treatment dismissal. While students will ASD predictably progress through various graduated school grades and settings, the need may arise for the termination of non-educational therapy services. These dismissal decisions typically occur when students have closed need gaps, be they developmental, psychological, behavioral, or social. Clearly, the thoughts of a collaborative team can be helpful with treatment dismissal decisions. Team members other than the individual directing a specific intervention effort may have useful insights specific to dismissal that prevent the early disruption or protracted unnecessary prolongation of treatment efforts.

Infusing Intervention and Educational Programing

For school-aged students with ASD, all developmental, behavioral, psychological, and social treatments should be conducted with educational needs of the child in mind. Simply put, interventions should be implemented seamlessly across a child's educational day and support, whenever possible, access to the general education curriculum (Karger, 2005). This requires significant collaboration between general/special education teachers and other members of the intervention team. Please refer to chapter "Promoting Academic Success" regarding promoting academic success for additional information.

Fortunately, team staffing meetings and more casual team interactions provide excellent formats for holistic discussions of educational and other needs presented by children with ASD. One can certainly imagine how an Individualized Educational Program (IEP) meeting would provide critical educational information to psychologists, physical therapists, occupational therapists, speech-language pathologists, and others who, in turn, could use classroom priorities in co-treatment efforts. For example, knowledge of a general or special education focus on addition and subtraction, may provide the impetus the co-treating speech-language pathologist and occupational therapist to focus on expressive vocabulary and fine motor activities related to arithmetic. The collaboration described above can cost teams time but intuitively contribute to more integrated and effective treatment efforts.

Case Example for Interdisciplinary Evaluation

Josiah

Josiah is a 10-year-old boy currently receiving special education services at a local public elementary school. He was initially evaluated at age seven, in the second grade, due to academic and behavioral concerns expressed by his classroom teacher. He met criteria for special education eligibility under the category of Specific Learning Disability with significant delays in basic reading skills, reading comprehension skills, and written expression. At his initial Individualized Education Program (IEP) meeting, the team made the decision to provide Josiah with specialized instruction for three hours each day in a resource classroom along with classroom accommodations and modifications.

The three years from initial placement in second grade until his current fifth-grade placement in a self-contained classroom for children with emotional disabilities have been considerably arduous for Josiah, his teachers, and parents. In resource and general education classes, Josiah was noted to be aggressive toward his peers and displayed some differences in communication skills. Classroom teachers frequently called Josiah's parents to come to pick him up from school due to his behavior and increasing anxiety. Josiah's parents were simultaneously struggling with his behavior at home and sought ideas and help from close family members and friends. He was seen by numerous physicians who each had a different perspective of what might be the cause of Josiah's challenging behavior. He was ultimately diagnosed with ADHD and bipolar disorder and placed on several medications, including lithium, Depakote, and Ritalin.

Josiah is now due for his three-year reevaluation. A reevaluation occurs at least every three years with the purpose of helping the IEP team determine if a child still qualifies for special education services. It also helps the IEP team with planning for current and future educational needs. Due to some of Josiah's repetitive and aggressive behaviors and communication differences, a referral has been made to the local school districts "Autism Support Team" to assist with his upcoming reevaluation.

Evaluation Approach

In this case, an interdisciplinary assessment team model or "Autism Support Team" was chosen due to the nature and complexity of Josiah's academic and behavioral needs and question of an ASD diagnosis. Autism Support Teams are becoming more prevalent in public schools to build capacity in the provision of services to students with ASD. They often work in collaboration with other teams, such as Assistive Technology and/or Behavioral Support Teams, to improve the implementation of evidence-based practices.

As there are required screenings and formal evaluations to determine eligibility under the category of ASD in the public-school system, members of the team are often prescriptive and include a school psychologist, a special education teacher, a speech-language pathologist, a behavioral specialist, and parents/caregivers. General education teachers, occupational therapists, and social workers may also be involved depending on school district or student needs.

Case Illustration

Referral

A referral for the Autism Support Team's involvement in Josiah's reevaluation was received by the case coordinator for consideration and action. A meeting was subsequently scheduled to obtain parent consent for evaluation and to establish assessment goals and plans for team collaboration. The team identified five critical priorities: (a) focused assessment on obtaining the most appropriate primary and secondary special education eligibility categories for Josiah; (b) a thorough behavioral assessment that will lead to successful intervention strategies in both home and school environments; (c) significant parent and physician input and collaboration due to medications and current medical diagnoses; (d) coordination and collaboration on type and timing of assessments to ensure an adequate representation of strengths and needs; and (e) incorporation of social and friendship skills assessments.

Evaluation

Due to Josiah's current eligibility category of Specific Learning Disability, placement in a classroom for children with emotional disabilities, and a question of possible ASD diagnosis, the evaluation protocol included assessments/measures required for several possible areas of primary and secondary eligibility categories. Through collaborative discussion, the team felt that Autism Spectrum Disorder should be ruled in or out as a priority. Therefore, ADOS-2 administration was prioritized. Additional testing included a psychological evaluation, an educational evaluation, a functional behavior assessment, classroom/school observations, hearing and vision screenings, and completion of parent/teacher questionnaires.

Josiah's parents were integral members of the team and relayed information from and to the physician. They were also interviewed in-depth and provided the team with significant developmental, family, adaptive, and social history, giving context and a more complete picture of Josiah's strengths and needs.

Findings and Results

After all evaluations were completed, members of the team met to share and discuss results openly to generate the most accurate picture of Josiah's abilities and needs. Josiah's strengths were numerous and included good progress with basic reading skills since his initial evaluation. He excels at math and exhibits age-appropriate voice, fluency, and articulation skills. Josiah's language skills are a relative strength, especially his single word receptive and expressive vocabulary. Josiah's non-verbal intelligence is within the average range, with strengths in perceptual organization and visual-motor proficiency. Teachers and parents report that Josiah is sensitive, caring, and has specific interests (i.e., animals, being outside, and video games). Josiah functions well in the home and classroom settings when he is on routine.

Josiah's parents and teachers report that he does get upset during times of transition or when something or someone new is introduced into the home or classroom. He prefers to talk about things he is interested in and struggles with making and/or keeping friends. Josiah's classroom teacher reported that he struggles with written expression and this is an area of significant frustration for him as he likes to get things "right." Of particular concern is that Josiah does not get along well with his peers. During group activities, he will often go off on his own or cause a disruption within the group. The classroom teacher also reported that Josiah does not seem to ask questions in class and will not ask for help when needed.

Formal testing by the school psychologist, speech-language pathologist, behavioral specialist, and occupation therapist revealed a Total Score on the ADOS-2 of 10 which exceeds the Autism Cutoff Score of 9, suggesting a diagnosis of autistic disorder. Formal intelligence testing revealed scores ranging from borderline to average with higher non-verbal reasoning abilities when compared to verbal reasoning. Educational testing revealed significant difficulties in the academic areas of written expression and reading comprehension. Sensory integration, aggressive behavior during times of transition or presentation of new tasks or people, and social language skills were additional areas of need.

Summary and Treatment Plan

The Case coordinator with input from the family integrated the above findings into a summary and treatment plan. Josiah was deemed eligible for special education services under the Autism category. Intervention services were provided based on the assessment data collected by the interdisciplinary team.

Chapter Conclusions

Interdisciplinary evaluation constitutes best practice for assessment and intervention planning for children and youth with suspected or confirmed ASD. The Comprehensive-Developmental Approach is a useful framework for guiding and informing interdisciplinary evaluation for ASD by capitalizing on complementary expertise of evaluation teams. For interdisciplinary teams to function maximally, cohesion is critical. Team cohesion elicits interdisciplinary discussion, allows for a thorough understanding of an individual's strengths and weaknesses, and produces a coherent diagnostic picture for parents and caregivers. Interdisciplinary evaluation should feature evidence-based assessment instruments and processes. Interdisciplinary evaluation should also inform interdisciplinary intervention, which may include treatment by team members simultaneously or involve consultation. Ongoing interdisciplinary evaluation is recommended to assess the effectiveness of the intervention and modify treatment as needed. Although interdisciplinary evaluation may require front-end investment of planning and coordination, there is evidence that interdisciplinary evaluation reduces time to diagnosis and client costs (Williams-Arya et al., 2019).

References

American Psychiatric Association. (2013). *Diagnostic and statistical manual of mental disorders* (5th ed.). Washington, DC: Author.

Barton, E. E., Harris, B., Leech, N., Stiff, L., Choi, G., & Joel, T. (2016). An analysis of state autism educational assessment practices and requirements. *Journal of Autism and Developmental Disorders, 46,* 737–748.

Braun, M. J., Dunn, W., & Tomchek, S. D. (2017). A pilot study on professional documentation: Do we write from a strengths perspective? *American Journal of Speech-Language Pathology, 26,* 972–981.

Brogan, C. A., & Knussen, C. (2003). The disclosure of a diagnosis of an autistic spectrum disorder: Determinants of satisfaction in a sample of Scottish parents. *Autism: The International Journal of Research & Practice, 7,* 31–46.

Budoff, M. (1987). Measures for assessing learning potential. In C. S. Lidz (Ed.), *Dynamic assessment: An interactional approach to evaluating learning potential* (pp. 173–195). New York: Guilford.

Campbell, J. M., Ruble, L. A., & Hammond, R. K. (2014). Evidence-based assessment of autism spectrum disorders. In L. A. Wilkinson (Ed.), *Autism spectrum disorders in children and adolescents: Evidence-based assessment and intervention* (pp. 51–73). Washington, DC: American Psychological Association.

Chua, A. K. (2012). Parental experience of having a child diagnosed with Autistic Spectrum Disorder: An integrative literature review. *Singapore Nursing Journal, 39,* 8–18.

Fey, M. E., Warren, S. F., Brady, N., Finestack, L. H., Bredin-Oja, S., Fairchild, M., … Yoder, P. J. (2006). Early effects of responsivity education/prelinguistic milieu teaching for children with developmental delays and their parents. *Journal of Speech, Language and Hearing Research, 49,* 526–547.

Huerta, M., & Lord, C. (2012). Diagnostic evaluation of autism spectrum disorders. *Pediatric Clinics of North America, 59,* 103–111.

Individuals with Disabilities Education Improvement Act of 2004. Pub L. No. 108–446, 118 Stat. 2647. (2004).

Karger, J. (2005). *Access to the General Education Curriculum for Students with Disabilities: A Discussion of the Interrelationship between IDEA '04 and NCLB.* Wakefield, MA: National Center on Accessing the General Curriculum. Retrieved August 27, 2019, from http://aem.cast.org/about/publications/2005/ncac-curriculum-access-idea04-nclb.html.

Klin, A., Saulnier, C., Tsatsanis, K., & Volkmar, F. R. (2005). Clinical evaluation in autism spectrum disorders: Psychological assessment within a transdisciplinary framework. In F. R. Volkmar, R. Paul, A. Klin, & D. Cohen (Eds.), *Handbook of autism and pervasive developmental disorders* (3rd ed., pp. 772–798). Hoboken, NJ: Wiley.

Koushik, N. S., Bacon, B., & Stancin, T. (2015). An interprofessional care model for evaluating autism spectrum disorders (ASDs) among low-income children. *Clinical Practice in Pediatric Psychology, 3,* 108–119. https://doi.org/10.1037/cpp0000093.

Lord, C., Rutter, M., DiLavore, P., Risi, S., Gotham, K., & Bishop, S. (2012). *Autism Diagnostic Observation Schedule, Second Edition (ADOS-2) Manual.* Torrance, CA: Western Psychological Services.

Mandell, D. S., Stahmer, A. C., Shin, S., Xie, M., Reisinger, E., & Marcus, S. C. (2013). The role of treatment fidelity on outcomes during a randomized field trial of an autism intervention. *Autism, 17,* 281–295.

Marcus, L. M., Kunce, L. J., & Schopler, E. (2005). Working with families. In F. R. Volkmar, R. Paul, A. Klin, & D. Cohen (Eds.), *Handbook of autism and pervasive developmental disorders: Assessment, interventions, and policy* (3rd ed., Vol. 2, pp. 1055–1086). Hoboken, NJ: John Wiley & Sons.

National Autism Center (NAC). (2015). *Findings and conclusions: National standards project Phase 2*. Randolph, MA: Author.

Ogletree, B. T., Rose, A., & Hambrecht, G. (2019). Evidence-based methods for teaching school-aged children and youth with autism spectrum disorder and complex communication needs. In J. B. Ganz & R. L. Simpson (Eds.), *Interventions for individuals with autism spectrum disorders and complex communication needs* (pp. 193–223). Baltimore, MD: Paul H. Brookes.

Ozonoff, S., Goodlin-Jones, B. L., & Solomon, M. (2005). Evidence-based assessment of autism spectrum disorders in children and adolescents. *Journal of Clinical Child and Adolescent Psychology, 34,* 523–540.

Prelock, P. A., Beatson, J., Bitner, B., Broder, C., & Ducker, A. (2003). Interdisciplinary assessment of young children with autism spectrum disorder. *Language, Speech, and Hearing Services in Schools, 34,* 194–202.

Prior, M., Roberts, J. M. A., Rodger, S., Williams, K., & Sutherland, R. (2011). *A review of the research to identify the most effective models of practice in early intervention of children with autism spectrum disorders*. Australia: Australian Government Department of Families, Housing, Community Services and Indigenous Affairs.

Riccio, C. A., & Prickett, C. S. (2019). Autism-focused assessment and program planning. In J. B. Ganz & R. L. Simpson (Eds.), *Interventions for individuals with autism spectrum disorder and complex communication needs* (pp. 21–46). Baltimore, MD: Paul H. Brookes.

Robey, R. R. (2004). A five-phase model for clinical-outcome research. *Journal of Communication Disorders, 37,* 401–411.

Rogers, C. L., Goddard, L., Hill, E. L., Henry, L. A., & Crane, L. (2016). Experiences of diagnosing autism spectrum disorder: A survey of professionals in the United Kingdom. *Autism: The International Journal of Research & Practice, 20,* 820–831.

Rutter, M., LeCouteur, A., & Lord, C. (2003). *Autism diagnostic interview-revised.* Los Angeles: Western Psychological Services.

Schopler, E., Reichler, R. J., & Renner, B. R. (2010). *Childhood Autism Rating Scale, Second Edition (CARS-2).* Los Angeles: Western Psychological Services.

Scottish Intercollegiate Guidelines Network (SIGN). (2016). *Assessment, diagnosis and interventions for autism spectrum disorders.* SIGN publication no. 145. Edinburgh: SIGN. Retrieved from http://www.sign.ac.uk.

Self, T. L., Mitchell, L. M., Hess, S., Marble, K. J., & Swails, J. (2017). Developing a university-based interprofessional education diagnostic team to identify children with possible autism spectrum disorder. *Communication Disorders Quarterly, 38,* 185–192.

Simpson, R. L. (2004). Finding effective intervention and personnel preparation practices for students with autism spectrum disorders. *Exceptional Children, 70,* 125–144.

Simpson, R. L. (2005). Evidence-based practices and students with autism spectrum disorders. *Focus on Autism and Other Developmental Disabilities, 20,* 140–149.

Sylvester, L., Ogletree, B. T., & Lunnen, K. (2017). Cotreatment as a vehicle for interprofessional collaborative practice: Physical therapists and speech-language pathologists collaborating in the care of children with severe disabilities. *American Journal of Speech-Language Pathology, 26,* 206–216.

Volkmar, F. R., Booth, L. L., McPartland, J. C., & Wiesner, L. A. (2014). Clinical evaluation in multidisciplinary settings. In F. R. Volkmar, S. J. Rogers, R. Paul, & K. A. Pelphrey (Eds.), *Handbook of autism and pervasive developmental disorders: Assessment, interventions, and policy* (4th ed., Vol. 2, pp. 661–672). Hoboken, NJ: John Wiley & Sons.

Wilkinson, L. A. (2017). *A best practice guide to assessment and intervention for autism spectrum disorders in schools* (2nd ed.). Philadelphia, PA: Jessica Kingsley Publishers.

Williams-Arya, P., Anixt, J., Kuan, L., Johnson, H., Kent, B., Bing, N., … Manning-Courtney, P. (2019). Improving access to diagnostic assessments for autism spectrum disorder using an arena model. *Journal of Developmental and Behavioral Pediatrics, 26.*

Wong, C., Odom, S. L., Hume, K., Cox, A. W., Fettig, A., Kucharczyk, S, … Schultz, T. R. (2013). *Evidence-based practices for children, youth, and young adults with autism spectrum disorder.* Chapel, Hill, NC: The University of North Carolina, Frank Porter Graham Child Development Institute, Autism Evidenced-Based Practice Review Group.

Dell Children's (S)TAAR Model of Early Autism Assessment

Meredith I. Holley, Sheri Ravenscroft, Briana Brukilacchio, Morgan Engelmann, and Autumn Fikki

Abstract Here, we describe a transdisciplinary effort to efficiently and equitably improve access to comprehensive evaluations for young children at-risk for autism and related neurodevelopmental disorders in the Austin, Texas community. What emerged from this collaboration between Dell Children's Medical Group and The University of Texas at Austin is a flexible clinical approach that emphasizes patient-centered care, community partnerships, best practices, and provider satisfaction. This chapter outlines integral components of our (Sin Exclusión) Transdisciplinary Autism Assessment & Resources (S)TAAR model, with the hope of providing an example of early autism assessment that can be implemented in medically underserved communities through pediatric specialty clinics. Future iterations of the model are aimed at increasing professional training opportunities for students and early career clinicians and further increasing post-diagnostic family supports. The benefits and limitations of the current model are discussed and avenues for expansion are considered in greater detail.

Introduction

Current practice parameters recommend that all children be screened for autism spectrum disorder (ASD) (hereafter, autism) at age 18 and 24 months, along with regular developmental surveillance (Zwaigenbaum et al., 2015). It is an integral function of developmental-behavioral pediatricians (DBPs) and psychologists to address concerns related to children who screen positive for the risk of autism (Hansen et al., 2016). DBPs and psychologists working with this population are trained to provide

M. I. Holley (✉)
Department of Psychiatry, The University of Texas at Austin, Austin, TX, USA
e-mail: meredith.brinster@ascension.org

S. Ravenscroft
Developmental-Behavioral Pediatrics, Dell Children's Medical Group, Austin, TX, USA

B. Brukilacchio · M. Engelmann · A. Fikki
Department of Educational Psychology, The University of Texas at Austin, Austin, TX, USA

M. B. McClain et al. (eds.), *Interprofessional Care Coordination for Pediatric Autism Spectrum Disorder*, https://doi.org/10.1007/978-3-030-46295-6_6

complex developmental evaluations, including history of present illness, developmental testing, and assistance in the coordination of a treatment plan. DBPs also provide medical expertise in response to a variety of concerns expressed by the patient and referring physician. For example, DBPs routinely assess the impact of pre-existing health conditions (e.g., prematurity) and the presence of related disorders (e.g., seizure activity). They prescribe medications, order tests as needed, and frequently direct patients to relevant subspecialties for more extensive workups (e.g., genetics for whole-exome sequencing). Psychologists with specialized training in autism assessment provide complementary expertise to thoroughly address psychosocial and behavioral concerns, cognitive abilities, academic skills, and family functioning. Additionally, psychologists serving this population are extensively trained in the administration and interpretation of standardized cognitive and academic measures, gold-standard autism diagnostic instruments (e.g., ADOS-2) and are prepared to rule-out or diagnose comorbid psychological disorders.

For both DBPs and psychologists alike, autism assessment is often a time-intensive process that is minimally reimbursable by insurance, produces an arduous amount of documentation (e.g., electronic medical records, report-writing), and limits the number of patients who can receive comprehensive care in a reasonable timeframe. Barriers include (1) time and resources needed to address complex patients, (2) burnout incurred from the time required to document complex concerns, and (3) resultant long waitlists that plague the profession and the community at large. Accordingly, there is a burgeoning movement in the field to update existing diagnostic pathways through evaluation models that increase collaboration across systems and providers (Gerdts et al., 2018; Gordon-Lipkin, Foster, & Peacock, 2016; Williams-Arya et al., 2019).

To address this challenge in the Austin, Texas community, a transdisciplinary team was formed through the Developmental-Behavioral Pediatrics Program within Ascension/Seton Dell Children's Medical Group and Pediatric Psychology within Dell Medical School/The University of Texas at Austin. This collaboration formed the Comprehensive Autism Program (CAP) housed at Dell Children's Developmental-Behavioral Pediatrics Program (hereafter, CAP). Through a comprehensive needs assessment, barriers to quality care were identified and used to inform program objectives. In the pursuit of these objectives, the *(Sin Exclusión) Transdisciplinary Autism Assessment and Resources Model ((S)TAAR)* was developed to address challenges through innovative transdisciplinary procedures. Here we discuss the results of our local needs assessment, introduce our approach to addressing each barrier, describe programmatic activities and objectives, present an example patient case, and describe future avenues for improvement and expansion.

Barriers to Quality Care in Autism Assessment

A multi-method needs assessment was conducted by the CAP team to guide program development. Goals of the assessment were to (1) determine the expressed level of need within the community through analyzing the clinic waitlist; (2) explore qualitative accounts of family experiences with autism assessment in the literature; (3) determine community characteristics and expected number of children with autism in the region; (4) collate a list of local agencies, service providers, and resources serving families of children with autism in the region; (5) determine areas of overlapping expertise and clinical capacity within clinic staff; (6) identify possible gaps in clinic expertise to inform hiring; (7) review the criteria for autism assessment provided by each major insurance provider billed by the clinic; (8) monitor clinicians' adherence to best practices in autism assessment; and (9) review the literature on healthcare disparities and unmet needs in autism assessment related to patient sex, race, ethnicity, language, and socioeconomic status.

Sources of information included a review of relevant literature, census data, national surveys, analysis of the clinic waitlists, caregiver report, live observation monitoring fidelity of best practices in usual care, and an investigation of community resources. Four primary barriers to quality care were identified through this process, including: (1) accessibility to diagnostic services (e.g., length of time from initial parent concern to receiving a diagnosis; excluding medically underserved communities), (2) efficiency of assessment procedures (e.g., patients lost-to-follow-up due to multiple diagnostic appointments), (3) threats to diagnostic accuracy in autism assessment (e.g., under-identification of racial minorities), and (4) negative caregiver experiences (e.g., high frustration and parental stress during diagnostic odyssey).

Strengths were also identified, which provided CAP with a roadmap to address challenges by leveraging existing capacities within the clinic and community. These included (1) multilingualism within clinic staff and access to in-person interpreting services, (2) clear areas of overlapping and complementary expertise across clinic staff; (3) high level of adherence to best practices in usual care; and (4) enthusiasm from community organizations to partner with the clinic. Each aspect of the (S)TAAR model directly corresponds with an identified barrier and addresses it through an existing clinic/community strength. First, accessibility issues are addressed through a staff commitment to inclusivity, community outreach, and language access (S). Next, inefficiency and redundancy are targeted using a transdisciplinary team approach (T). Diagnostic accuracy is prioritized by continuing to use gold-standard assessment procedures (AA). Finally, social work and community partnerships were leveraged to improve caregivers' experiences and connections to local resources (R). In the next section, the results of our needs assessment are described and contextualized to provide background for CAP's objectives and activities.

Accessibility

Access to care is arguably the largest obstacle faced by patients and developmental-behavioral health providers alike (Mansell & Morris, 2004; Miller et al., 2008). Although valid ASD diagnoses can increasingly be made in infants and toddlers (Mandell, Novak, & Zubritsky, 2005), the median age of identification in the United

States is 5.7 years (Shattuck et al., 2009). This gap is due, in large part, to a nationwide shortage of clinicians specializing in the diagnosis of pediatric behavioral and developmental disorders (Mayer & Skinner, 2009). The primary consequence of this bottleneck is a delay in access to appropriate interventions, which causes many children who have already been identified and referred for an evaluation, to miss out on opportunities for early intervention (Zwaigenbaum et al., 2015). This pattern differentially impacts families who are unable to afford out-of-pocket fees for private evaluation services (Bisgaier, Levinson, Cutts, & Rhodes, 2011; Chiri & Warfield, 2012). Additionally, it is well-documented that later age of ASD diagnosis is associated with race and lower socioeconomic status (SES) (Jo et al., 2015; Mandell, Listerud, Levy, & Pinto-Martin, 2002).

Although diagnostic bottlenecks have been reported across the country, the 2005-2006 National Survey of Children with Special Healthcare Needs further revealed large variations between states in terms of difficulty accessing ASD services (Thomas, Parish, Rose, & Kilany, 2012). In Texas, 53% of families of children with ASD experienced problems getting referrals, 13% had delayed or forgone care, 47% had unmet care coordination needs, and 24% experienced difficulty utilizing services (Thomas, Parish, Rose, & Kilany, 2012). Presently, Dell Children's Medical Group (DCMG) employs one of the only medical providers (DBP) specializing in autism assessment that accepts insurance, including Medicaid, in the greater Austin area. Therefore, CAP operates within the national, state, and local systems that perpetuate well-documented inefficiencies and obstacles to adequate care for families of children with ASD.

Texas is also one of five majority-minority states in the U.S. whose population is composed of less than 50% Non-Hispanic White residents (U.S. Census Bureau, 2018). Further, over 35% of Texans speak a language other than English. Consistent with these statistics, many patients referred to Developmental-Behavioral Pediatrics at Dell Children's are demographically, culturally, and/or linguistically diverse. Given that healthcare disparities differentially impact children with ASD from minority backgrounds, and minority families experience additional delays in the age of initial diagnosis (Fountain, King, & Bearman, 2011; Magaña, Parish, Rose, Timberlake, & Swaine, 2012; Mandell et al., 2002), CAP is committed to creating a diagnostic model that is responsive to the needs and barriers impacting the local community.

Efficiency

As of June 2018, the waitlist for new patients at Dell Children's Developmental-Behavioral Pediatrics clinic was upwards of 18 months. Therefore, a child exhibiting for a comprehensive evaluation by a general pediatrician during their 18-month well-child visit could spend an additional 18 months awaiting their first appointment. Once evaluated by the clinic, families were typically scheduled for multiple appointments prior to receiving the final diagnosis. Therefore, a child exhibiting atypical development in infancy would likely experience a lag of nearly 2 years before receiving an autism diagnosis that qualified them for intervention services. On average, caregivers report lags between 2 and 3.5 years between their initial developmental concerns and the date of diagnosis (Chamak, Bonniau, Oudaya, & Ehrenberg, 2011; Crane, Chester, Goddard, Henry, & Hill, 2016; Siklos & Kerns, 2007), with long wait times cited as a key cause of parental stress (Crane et al., 2016). Early access to a streamlined diagnostic service is crucial in lessening the impact of stress on families and improving overall satisfaction.

In addition to lengthy new patient waitlists, inefficiencies in the diagnostic process prolong the time between referral and diagnosis. By design, existing interdisciplinary diagnostic models require 2–3 visits prior to diagnosis (Gerdts et al., 2018). Multiple clinic visits disproportionately impact families with limited resources because transportation, childcare, and time off from work pose substantial limitations. Given the clinic's location within Central Texas, families from rural areas often travel for hours to attend visits. For these reasons, the clinic has made a concerted effort to limit the amount of face-to-face assessment time required by patients and families, without sacrificing quality or diagnostic accuracy.

Diagnostic Accuracy

Given that ASD remains a behavioral diagnosis, it is inherently subject to potential limitations including gender bias, linguistic, and cultural norms that vary across individual patients, and an individual provider's subjective lens (Chapman, Kaatz, & Carnes, 2013; Peris, Teachman, & Nosek, 2008). Racial and ethnic disparities in quality healthcare plague the process of autism diagnosis (Blair et al., 2013; Ennis-Cole, Durodoye, & Harris, 2013; Magaña et al., 2012). For example, African-American children were diagnosed an average of 1.4 years later than White children (Mandell et al., 2002) and are much more likely to have received a previous diagnosis of conduct or adjustment disorder (Mandell, Ittenbach, Levy, & Pinto-Martin, 2007). Hispanic children are diagnosed almost one year later than White children, receive fewer specialty services, and have higher unmet service needs (Magaña, Lopez, Aguinaga, & Morton, 2013). Additionally, girls with autism continue to be more likely to be missed or misdiagnosed (Bargiela, Steward, & Mandy, 2016; Fuss, Briken, & Klein, 2018; Gould & Ashton-Smith, 2011; Werling & Geschwind, 2013).

In addition to these known sources of bias that have the potential to skew the perception of any provider, patients frequently present to this clinic with complex histories that further complicate behavioral diagnostics. For example, pre/perinatal complications (e.g., in utero toxic exposure), trauma histories (e.g., fleeing danger in a home country), interruptions to caregiver support (e.g., foster care), and forms of ongoing instability (e.g., housing) commonly surface during our evaluations. The transdisciplinary aspect of this model has evolved to deliver culturally-sensitive and truly comprehensive evaluations to a highly heterogeneous patient population and, in doing so, hopefully, increase diagnostic accuracy. A primary component of this approach involves diagnostic consensus between providers, each of whom represents diverse backgrounds and clinical orientations. This safeguard against accidental bias has been built into the (S)TAAR model to address the potential for diagnostic inaccuracy and increase accountability across providers.

Negative Caregiver Experiences

Caregivers of children with autism typically engage in intensive self-education, beginning when they first develop concerns about their child's growth and behavior (Stoner et al., 2005). Time spent looking for information and services reportedly detracts from other activities and leads to feelings of burnout (Weiss, Wingsiong, & Lunsky, 2014). This information-seeking process continues after the child's initial diagnosis because parents report that information about ASD is typically only delivered during one visit in an overwhelming fashion (Carlsson, Miniscalco, Kadesjö, & Laakso, 2016), and during a time when they are also experiencing emotional turmoil around their child's prognosis (Stoner et al., 2005).

Caregivers of children with autism consistently report high levels of stress in response to parenting demands, even beyond those endorsed by caregivers of children with chronic illnesses or other developmental disabilities (Blacher & McIntyre, 2006; Mungo, Ruta, Arrigo & Mazzona, 2007; Olsson & Hwang, 2001). These feelings of stress have been linked to low awareness about autism, inadequate service provision, difficulty accessing existing services, and difficulty understanding the disorder (Divan, Vajaratkar, Desai, Strik-Lievers, & Patel, 2012; Keen, Couzens, Muspratt, & Rodger, 2010). Families of children with autism who have access to fewer financial resources are particularly affected (Pickard & Ingersoll, 2016; Stuart & McGrew, 2009), as are single parents (Meadan, Halle, & Ebata, 2010), and those responsible for multiple children (Harper, Dyches, Harper, Roper, & South, 2013). Although clinicians set out to serve families, clinical and educational programs have been implicated as an additional source of stress for caregivers of children with autism (Altiere & von Kluge, 2009).

Caregivers whose children are diagnosed with special healthcare needs, such as autism, further report that their first step following the appointment is to search for information and practical advice (Jackson et al., 2008). They typically seek information regarding associated symptoms, the course and prognosis of the disorder, and available treatments (Hodgetts, Zwaigenbaum, & Nicholas, 2015). Other common questions are related to the causes of autism, whether there are blood tests to diagnose the disorder, whether a cure exists, and how to plan for having another child (Gona et al., 2015). When parents encounter difficulty acquiring or accessing this information, they tend to develop increased levels of anxiety (Kai, 1996), further compounding the degree of stress they experience related to their child's special educational and healthcare needs. Therefore, given the amount of information parents must learn about autism, and the number of systems they are tasked with navigating for their child, these families may require more family-centered care and extensive case management throughout the diagnostic process. In response to the evident need for family-centered practices in autism assessment, this model incorporates aspects of family navigation, therapeutic assessment, and post-diagnostic support.

Program Objectives and Activities

(Sin Exclusión)

(S)TAAR was developed to be inclusively responsive to the needs and goals of a specific patient population: children under the age of four with a chief complaint of delayed or disordered development, including primary concerns related to language development, behavior, and/or specific concerns for autism. The Developmental-Behavioral Pediatrics Department at Dell Children's Medical Group provides more than 500 new patient visits per year. Of those, at least 50% are diagnosed with autism. About 50% of all DBP new patients are seen in the CAP clinic.

The (S)TAAR model of autism assessment does not exclude patients based on language spoken, insurance provider, or other sociocultural factors. As described above, a majority of Texas residents are Non-White (U.S. Census Bureau, 2018). In addition, the Hispanic population is projected to be the largest demographic group in Texas by 2020. Given that approximately 1 in every 10 children in the United States lives in Texas (7.3 million; State of Texas Children, 2016), addressing state-specific barriers to autism diagnosis through culturally and linguistically-inclusive practice is an essential component of public health. Over 35% of Texans speak a language other than English, with approximately 30% comprised of Spanish speakers (U.S. Census Bureau, 2018). To ensure language access for non-English speakers in our clinic, bilingual providers were utilized and the hospital system frequently arranged for in-person interpreter services. In the past year, bilingual services have been provided in Spanish and Mandarin. Live interpreting services have been arranged for a variety of languages, for example, including Spanish, Farsi, Nepalese, Amharic, Kurdish, and American Sign Language.

Insurance type has also been implicated as an important predictor for time to diagnosis, access to services, and an overall financial burden (Wang, Mandell, Lawer, Cidav, & Leslie, 2013). In our current healthcare system, availability and quality of services is largely dependent on insurance coverage. However, insurance reimbursement rates vary significantly, and therefore, the number of qualified providers accepting all major insurance plans presents another barrier to equitable care and early diagnosis. In Texas, 44% of children are covered by employer-provided insurance, and 43% receive care through federally- or state-funded public insurance programs. Dell Children's Developmental-Behavioral Pediatrics clinic accepts all major insurance, including Medicaid and other state-contracted managed care health plans (e.g., STAR, STAR+Plus, CHIP). Importantly, these statistics are reflected in the patient demographics of those seen in Dell Children's DBP clinic where 40% of patients are insured through Medicaid. Clinic staff is available to assist with insurance support and case management prior to the appointment, and insurance limitations are taken into consideration when providing resources and referrals.

Transdisciplinary

The terms multidisciplinary, interdisciplinary, and transdisciplinary are increasingly used in the literature, but often ambiguously and interchangeably. While each term implies a team approach that draws upon the knowledge and expertise from different disciplines, multi and interdisciplinary approaches typically dictate that professionals from each discipline stay within their boundaries of expertise. In contrast, transdisciplinary work suggests an integration of expertise that transcends traditional professional boundaries. The (S)TAAR model is intentionally transdisciplinary in nature, creating a whole developmental assessment team that is greater than the sum of its parts.

(S)TAAR clinical assessment team, as defined by the subset of staff involved in direct patient care during the diagnostic appointment, is composed of a developmental-behavioral pediatrician (MD/DBP), nurse practitioner (FNP-C), licensed pediatric psychologist (Ph.D./Psych), and a licensed clinical social worker (LCSW) with support from medical assistants. Each team member provides a unique clinical contribution; however, the synchronous model allows overlap between skill sets of each provider, ensuring flexibility in the delivery of services. Medical providers (e.g., FNP-C and DBP) can flexibly deliver diagnostic interview and medical examination procedures. Diagnostic providers (e.g., DBP, Psych) flexibly administer developmental and diagnostic assessment procedures. Behavioral health providers (e.g., Psych/Social Work) flexibly provide counseling and provision of resources.

Through a transdisciplinary approach involving each specialty listed above, the amount of direct provider care within a single appointment always exceeds the length of the visit itself, providing the patient and family with the most value for their time in clinic. For example, during a 90-min visit, a family may have 45 min of face-to-face time with the DBP, 60 min with the psychologist, 80 min with a nurse practitioner, and 15 min with a social worker because providers work alongside one another, moving in and out of the exam and adjoining observation rooms as needed (see Fig. 1). Essential to the overall evaluation procedure is the additional role of nurse coordinator who serves to manage referrals, waitlists, patient communication, triage, scheduling, and gathering of pre-existing records. It is through this role that much of the evaluation process is initiated prior to the new patient assessment appointment, including documentation of past medical history and previous test results.

Documentation time is an issue that plagues comprehensive assessments in that there is a large amount of pre- and post-visit workflow. Care that occurs after the visit, or post-visit workflow, largely refers to time spent completing reports and documenting procedures, which can average three to five pages according to the

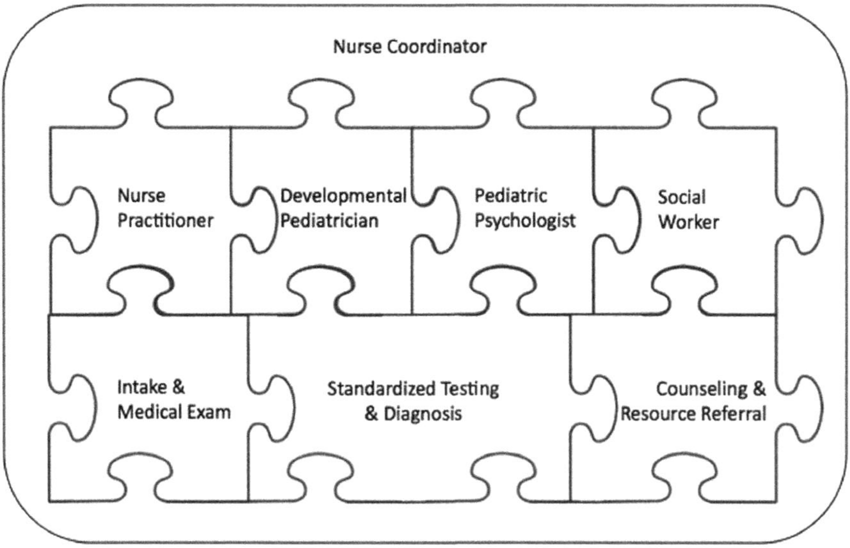

Fig. 1 Interconnection and overlap of (S)TAAR transdisciplinary providers

DBP workflow paper (Soares, Baum, & Frick, 2015). The (S)TARR model addresses this challenge by delegating the pre-visit workload to the nurse practitioner who is responsible for reviewing and documenting the visit prior to the appointment. The post-visit medical decision-making and plan of care is documented by the physician or nurse practitioner after the visit. Testing results and interpretations are delegated to psychology during and after the visit. In this way, charting is shared among providers and highlights unique clinical skills from each discipline. In practice, this has allowed for minimization of computer use in the room while increasing provider engagement with family members and patients. The nurse practitioner actively charts during the visit while the psychologist and physician are freed from the electronic medical record (EMR) to perform assessments and orient themselves more responsively to the patient and their family members. This is especially valuable when some EMRs do not allow for multiple people documenting in the chart at the same time and represents an area for medical residents to integrate into future iterations of the model.

Autism Assessment

At the time of referral, patients meeting inclusion criteria for the (S)TAAR program are identified by the nurse coordinator. This includes patients under the age of four with a chief complaint of developmental delay, behavior, speech, or autism.

Chief concerns are typically expressed in referral paperwork as physician and/or parent concern and may include failed developmental screeners from well-child visits, school districts, or community programs. A minority of patients in the (S)TAAR program also present with provisional diagnoses of autism seeking second opinions and require more comprehensive evaluations and case management to qualify for and access appropriate services.

Prior to scheduling, (S)TAAR patients are categorized into one of two referral groups. Patients with existing developmental testing or behavioral screening measures (e.g., Battelle Developmental Inventory, Second Edition Newborg, 2005; Modified Checklist for Autism in Toddlers (M-CHAT-R/F; Robins, Fein, & Barton, 1999; Robins et al., 2014)) are assigned to the DATA group. Appointments for this group typically include more extensive record review and supplementary direct assessment in clinic. Patients with minimal previous developmental or clinical data (e.g., physician reported concern for autism without administration of screening instruments) are assigned to the NADA group. Appointments for this group typically include less extensive record review and more extensive direct assessment in clinic. The primary purposes of this categorization process are to (1) provide structure and balance to the demands and workflow within the clinic, (2) allow sufficient time for documentation, and (3) tentatively plan specific duties each member of the interdisciplinary team will need to complete during each patient's visit. For example, administration of developmental assessments (e.g., Mullen Scales of Early Learning (MSEL; Mullen, 1989, 1995; Akshoomoff, 2006) is typically administered during NADA visits and those materials are inventoried and placed in the room in advance of the visit. Second opinion visits typically require an ADOS-2 and those materials are prepared in advance as well.

Presently, the (S)TAAR model is implemented during one clinic day per week. These days begin with a team huddle, at which point the DBP, nurse practitioner, psychologist, nurse coordinator, and social worker discuss the day's patients. Providers review existing patient records, including referral questions, chief concerns, medical history, any prior developmental testing or screening instruments, and new patient paperwork. This information is used to determine which assessments are necessary to inform the diagnosis and treatment plan, identify families who will utilize an interpreter, and screen for families that may require unique support from social work (e.g., those who have disclosed housing or food insecurity on new patient paperwork). During these discussions, the nurse practitioner begins the documentation of history and previous assessment results.

(S)TAAR currently provides five new patient appointments per clinic day. While data collection and the evaluation process begins much prior to the appointment, families participate in 90-min, face-to-face consultation/assessment with the transdisciplinary team. Appointment duration varies slightly based on the breadth of previously acquired background information and the complexity of information needed to make a diagnostic determination. Consistent with a transdisciplinary approach, providers work together from start to finish, fluidly blending clinical skills and perspectives from DBP and psychology. For example, developmental testing is conducted with the child while thorough clinical background information is collected via a caregiver interview. Each provider observes the child from their lens of expertise while also working together to form a well-rounded conceptualization of the patient. This assessment approach reduces redundancy that can often occur in interdisciplinary assessment, requires less time from the patient and family, less repetition from parents interacting with different team members at separate times, and improves communication between specialists.

After direct testing, providers inform the family that they will briefly conference in another room. At this point, the team conducts a brief case conference to reach consensus regarding diagnosis, referrals, treatment recommendations, and follow-up plans. Same-day feedback is typically provided by the DBP unless further diagnostic information is required. Feedback is delivered empathically and collaboratively such that the family's initial questions are reiterated and addressed one by one. Diagnoses are provided clearly and an emphasis is placed on avenues for intervention and support. Feedback is delivered with 1–2 staff in the room to allow the family greater privacy. One staff member is primarily oriented towards the parent(s) while another staff member is available to entertain the patient and start showing parents examples of how they can build therapeutic supports into their daily interactions (e.g., show parents how to elicit speech or eye contact by withholding the desired object, improving social reciprocity by engaging in peek-a-boo or tickling, etc.). An emphasis is placed on strengths, introducing parents to recommended intervention services, and helping families prioritize their treatment goals and balance their time/resources according to their child's needs and the family's values. Families that receive a same-day diagnosis are immediately introduced to the clinic's social worker who helps them process the diagnostic experience, provides resources, and explains the role of social work in ongoing case management. If further testing is needed or the parents express a lack of receptiveness to an autism diagnosis, families are referred to the pediatric psychologist for an additional workup. If the referral is due to a lack of diagnostic consensus among staff, the family will return for additional testing and is provided with autism rating scales for teachers, and/or other caregivers to complete. This is often the case for more mild cases of autism particularly those involving co-occurring medical disorders such as a child with epilepsy presenting with social communication deficits. If the referral is due to a lack of buy-in from the parents regarding a potential developmental disability, the psychologist will follow-up about parental concerns which sometimes include cultural norms, stigma, or highly elevated parental stress/depression. The clinic prioritizes efficiency in delivering an accurate diagnosis, but not at the expense of family autonomy or buy-in. Therefore, these rare cases involving significant push-back from parents are treated with particular care and curiosity on the part of CAP providers (Fig. 2).

A typical new patient appointment may include the following procedures:

1. Transdisciplinary morning rounds focused on initial case conceptualization, visit plan, and coordination with social work.
2. The patient is checked in for the appointment and their caregiver is asked to complete a standardized developmental rating scale.

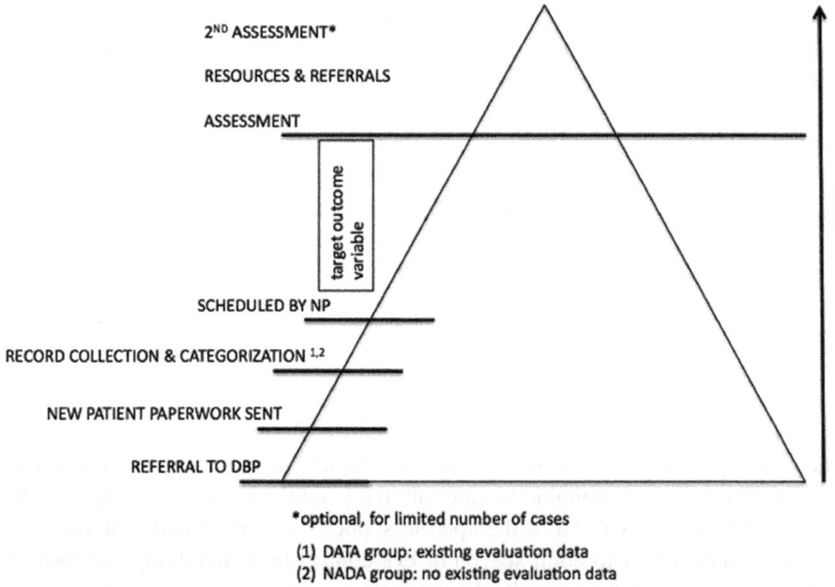

Fig. 2 Timeline of (S)TAAR evaluation, highlighting pre-appointment process and efficiency of assessment procedures

3. Assessment team members enter the room, introduce themselves, and provide an overview of visit procedures.
4. Caregivers are asked to identify chief concerns and their goals for the appointment.
5. Simultaneous delivery of the following clinical services:
    a. Diagnostic interview with the caregiver, derived from The Diagnostic and Statistical Manual of Mental Disorders (5th edition; American Psychiatric Association, 2013) and Autism Diagnostic Interview-Revised (Rutter, Le Couteur, & Lord, 2003)
    b. Standardized developmental assessment with patient
    c. Gathering information from the parent interview and direct observation of the patient to complete a standardized observation rating scale used to determine the existence and severity of autistic symptoms.
6. Medical provider performs a physical exam and discusses co-occurring or differential medical conditions.
7. Providers exit the room to privately conference about the patient. Diagnostic impressions are discussed, standardized assessments are scored, data are reviewed, and the treatment plan is formulated.
8. Feedback is provided to the patient:
    a. Psychologist shares assessment results, including strengths and weaknesses
    b. DBP delivers relevant diagnostic information and explains the treatment plan

   c. Nurse practitioner begins to visit documentation and referrals process
   d. Social worker joins team members to provide support and answer questions.
9. Each patient is scheduled for a one-month follow-up visit to check on the status of referrals and provide an additional opportunity for questions and support.

Resources

Essential to the (S)TAAR model's success is collaborative partnerships with community providers in the areas of early childhood intervention services, general pediatrics, private therapy providers, and connections with high-risk developmental follow-up clinics through local hospital services. Referrals *from* such providers significantly increase the amount of clinically useful information received prior to the assessment appointment. Referrals *to* these providers and other community resources aim to bridge the gap between diagnosis and intervention. Early detection often assumes early intervention, however, parents often report confusion regarding immediate next steps, difficulty accessing services, and general difficulties navigating autism service delivery (Kogan et al., 2008; Moodie-Dyer, Joyce, Anderson-Butcher, & Hoffman, 2014). Despite being well-documented, the process of accessing intervention services post-diagnosis has not improved much over time (Kohler, 1999; Sperry, Whaley, Shawn, & Brame, 1999). In contrast, parents who reported positive experiences emphasize the importance of increased collaboration and social support (Moodie-Dyer et al., 2014).

To provide this level of social support, the (S)TAAR model includes the role of social work as a vital part of the diagnostic process. After receiving the diagnosis and having individual questions answered by the diagnostic team, the clinic social worker is introduced to families through a "warm handoff" procedure. Warm handoffs are a common and often recommended feature of programs that integrate behavioral health services into medical care. Typically, this transitional procedure is designed to facilitate engagement and further appointment attendance with behavioral health providers within the clinic. However, the role of social work in the (S)TAAR model is to provide empowerment and support in helping families access outside community supports in a timely fashion that minimizes feelings of isolation and confusion. The social worker provides an informational packet of vetted, evidence-based informational resources and ongoing assistance to connect with community agencies and quickly enroll in appropriate interventions. Parents are also connected with educational and support services available in-house through clinic psychologists or in the community through nonprofit agencies (e.g., pro bono educational advocacy services for parents of children with autism). Conversations regarding existing and available social and financial supports take place, questions are answered, and families are provided with the social worker's direct phone number to be contacted with additional questions and concerns.

Case Example

We present an example case from spring 2019 to illustrate the flexibility of the (S)TAAR model in meeting individual needs through efficient and comprehensive evidence-based evaluations. This example highlights the experience of Sonia (pseudonym), a 32-month-old female referred for an evaluation by her pediatric otolaryngologist due to significant speech delays and global developmental concerns. Her parents are Middle Eastern refugees that resettled in the greater Austin, Texas area. She was born in the United States and experienced a complicated and premature birth due to a congenital infectious disease affecting the central nervous system. Sonia's disease caused her to develop vision impairments and bilateral sensorineural hearing loss (for which she received cochlear implants). Sonia resides with her parents and extended family in a suburb of Austin, Texas. English and Pashto were spoken in the home.

Sonia was seen in Developmental-Behavioral Pediatrics within 3 months of her referral date. Prior to the appointment, records from otolaryngology, audiology, neuropsychology, speech therapy, physical therapy, occupational therapy, and the local school district's early intervention program were obtained and extensively reviewed during the team huddle and documented by the nurse practitioner. The previous testing included a failed M-CHAT-R, and severely delayed development based on the Mullen Scales of Early Learning and Bayley Scales of Infant and Toddler Development, Third Edition. New patient paperwork including symptom checklists and parental concerns were reviewed prior to the appointment. A full summary of her developmental and medical history, previous test results, and parental concerns was summarized by the nurse coordinator and reviewed by the full assessment team during the team huddle. The assessment team spent approximately 10 min discussing Sonia's case and determined that the Childhood Autism Rating Scale, Second Edition, Standard Version (CARS2-ST; Schopler, Van Bourgondien, Wellman, & Love, 2010), the Developmental Profile 3 (DP-3; Alpern, 2007), a semi-structured parent interview, and physical exam were appropriate to provide additional information regarding developmental and behavioral functioning and evaluate concerns for autism spectrum disorder.

Results of the full evaluation indicated that Sonia was not communicating with any spoken language, used limited eye contact, pointing, and gestures, did not seek comfort from familiar caregivers or engage with others, did not engage in play, repetitively threw or mouthed objects on a regular basis, engaged in hand-flapping, hand-posturing, and repetitive pacing, occasionally sought physical play with adults but did not engage with peers, and did not spontaneously imitate others' speech or actions. The CARS2-ST was completed based on direct observation of Sonia's behavior and parent-report during a semi-structured interview. Scores indicated severe symptoms of autism spectrum disorder. Sonia's parents reported severely impaired adaptive, social-emotional, cognitive, and communication abilities on a norm-referenced measure.

The assessment team met for approximately 10 min and reached a consensus that autism spectrum disorder, speech impairment, and global developmental delay were appropriate diagnoses. Appropriate referrals and resources were discussed during the brief case conference and a plan was developed to deliver feedback and connect the family with ongoing support.

The patient's family was immediately provided with feedback regarding Sonia's developmental delays, lack of progress in speech therapy, and behavioral symptoms consistent with an autism diagnosis. Applied behavior analysis (ABA) was discussed as an appropriate intervention option with her parents, including a specific referral to a local agency accepting Medicaid. Parents were counseled regarding eventual placement in a public school or school for the Deaf. The team made referrals to ophthalmology for a second opinion regarding vision impairment, ABA therapy to support developmental, communicative, and behavioral gains, and ongoing speech, occupation, and physical therapies to continue addressing additional areas of Sonia's delayed development. Genetic testing and an electroencephalogram (EEG) were ordered, the family was introduced to the social worker for ongoing case management, and a medical follow-up visit was scheduled for 6 months.

This family was highly vulnerable to barriers outlined in our needs assessment. They were recently resettled asylum-seekers with public insurance whose primary language is Pashto. Additionally, Sonia presented with a complex medical history (prematurity, disease affecting the central nervous system) and multiple disabilities (vision impairment, hearing impairment), which complicated the diagnostic process. Despite these factors, Sonia was seen within 3 months of referral date and required only one 90-min office visit. She was provided with a comprehensive, evidence-based, transdisciplinary evaluation resulting in same-day feedback regarding multiple diagnoses, referrals back into the community, and post-diagnostic social and medical support.

Discussion

The (S)TAAR model has positively impacted our community's access to care via significant reductions in waitlist time (approximately 77% reduction) and significantly increased the number of new patients seen per month (approximately 190% growth). It is our hope that reductions in time to diagnosis, partnered with a high quality transdisciplinary assessment, ultimately reduce caregiver stress and translate to efficient access to early intervention. As such, we believe that our assessment process targets many of the issues in autism care that plague caregivers and providers alike. Qualitatively, our team reports high provider satisfaction in terms of quality and efficiency with the assessment process. Additional benefits of the (S)TAAR model include an infrastructure that lends itself well to training. The team-based approach offers the possibility of live supervision and observation of assessment techniques.

(S)TAAR is unique from other published models involving collaboration across multiple specialties in that it does not utilize a speech-language pathologist (SLP).

Much discussion occurred surrounding the cost/benefit of including an SLP in the assessment team. Most insurance providers only reimburse two speech evaluations per year and SLPs in the community reported to CAP that they conduct their own speech assessment as part of the process of initiating therapy and developing individualized treatment goals. Therefore, while our team evaluates broad receptive and expressive language using developmental assessments (e.g., MSEL) and notes unusual or aberrant vocalizations and patterns of communication, we chose to leave more comprehensive speech evaluations to SLPs in the community who provide the service when speech therapy is initiated. This minimizes the threat of test-retest effects that occur when patients are redundantly evaluated within a short time period and reduces the amount billed to insurance for the patient's appointment at CAP.

Though (S)TAAR is limited in its age range, improvements that emerge through this model have secondary impacts on patients of all ages. Because high-risk infants and toddlers constitute a significant portion of overall referrals, activities implemented for this group of new patients were anticipated to indirectly benefit the broader clinic population as well. In addition, as children age, other community providers (e.g., public school systems) often capture those who demonstrate developmental or behavioral differences. As the model continues to improve access to care for the youngest members of our community, it is our plan to expand the age range to include 4- and 5-year-olds in order to capture all children who are not yet eligible for enrollment in public kindergarten programs. In future iterations, older patients might benefit from more extensive evaluation, including speech/language (e.g., pragmatics, semantics), academic skills, adaptive and social-emotional behavior.

Program evaluation for the (S)TAAR model is ongoing and outcome data have not yet been published. The team hypothesizes that quality and cost-effectiveness metrics will increase in relation to the single-provider multi-visit model that was previously in place. In terms of quality (determined through fidelity checks and quality monitoring), the team is actively collecting data regarding the timeline from referral to diagnosis, patient satisfaction, and provider satisfaction. In terms of cost-effectiveness, billable hours, no-shows, and rate of follow-up will be compared between baseline and the initial implementation phases of the (S)TAAR model. Future program goals include expanding the model with fidelity to further increase the number of new patient appointments, with particular emphasis on increasing training opportunities for graduate students and medical residents.

Finally, the nature of transdisciplinary work poses unique, and often subtle implementation challenges. Through our execution of the (S)TAAR model, we have experienced a team synchrony that appears integral to the success of the model. This synchrony requires hidden parameters related to leadership, communication, coordination, and an emergent "flow." In positive psychology, flow is a mental state in which a person performing an activity is fully engaged in a feeling of high focus, complete involvement, and enjoyment in the process. It has been our experience that effective leadership from the CAP team, individual responsibility for components of the assessment process, clear communication, and genuine enjoyment of working as a group to support families has helped to foster a flow that appears to have a significantly positive impact on the providers' and patients' experience. Future research may help to elucidate the key components to our model's successes that go beyond fiscal or productivity goals, but also speak to the heart involved in being the beginning of a family's lifelong journey with autism.

References

Akshoomoff, N. (2006). Use of the mullen scales of Early Learning for the assessment of young children with autism spectrum disorders. *Child Neuropsychology, 12*(4–5), 269–277.

Alpern, G. D. (2007). *Developmental profile 3 (DP-3)*. Los Angeles, CA: Western Psychological Services.

Altiere, M. J., & von Kluge, S. (2009). Family functioning and coping behaviors in parents of children with autism. *Journal of Child and Family Studies, 18*(1), 83.

American Psychiatric Association (2013) *Diagnostic and statistical manual of mental disorders: diagnostic and statistical manual of mental disorders* (5th ed.). Arlington, VA: American Psychiatric Association, 2013.

Bargiela, S., Steward, R., & Mandy, W. (2016). The experiences of late-diagnosed women with autism spectrum conditions: An investigation of the female autism phenotype. *Journal of Autism and Developmental Disorders, 46*(10), 3281–3294.

Bisgaier, J., Levinson, D., Cutts, D. B., & Rhodes, K. V. (2011). Access to autism evaluation appointments with developmental-behavioral and neurodevelopmental subspecialists. *Archives of Pediatrics and Adolescent Medicine, 165,* 673–674.

Blacher, J., & McIntyre, L. L. (2006). Syndrome specificity and behavioural disorders in young adults with intellectual disability: Cultural differences in family impact. *Journal of Intellectual Disability Research, 50*(3), 184–198.

Blair, I. V., Steiner, J. F., Fairclough, D. L., Hanratty, R., Price, D. W., Hirsh, H. K., et al. (2013). Clinicians' implicit ethnic/racial bias and perceptions of care among Black and Latino patients. *The Annals of Family Medicine, 11*(1), 43–52.

Carlsson, E., Miniscalco, C., Kadesjö, B., & Laakso, K. (2016). Negotiating knowledge: Parents' experience of the neuropsychiatric diagnostic process for children with autism: Negotiating knowledge. *International Journal of Language & Communication Disorders, 3*, 328–338.

Chamak, B., Bonniau, B., Oudaya, L., & Ehrenberg, A. (2011). The autism diagnostic experiences of French parents. *Autism, 15*(1), 83–97.

Chapman, E. N., Kaatz, A., & Carnes, M. (2013). Physicians and implicit bias: How doctors may unwittingly perpetuate health care disparities. *Journal of General Internal Medicine, 28*(11), 1504–1510.

Chiri, G., & Warfield, M. E. (2012). Unmet need and problems accessing core health care services for children with autism spectrum disorder. *Maternal and Child Health Journal, 16*(5), 1081–1091.

Crane, L., Chester, J. W., Goddard, L., Henry, L. A., & Hill, E. (2016). Experiences of autism diagnosis: A survey of over 1000 parents in the United Kingdom. *Autism, 20*(2), 153–162.

Divan, G., Vajaratkar, V., Desai, M. U., Strik-Lievers, L., & Patel, V. (2012). Challenges, coping strategies, and unmet needs of families with a child with autism spectrum disorder in Goa, India. *Autism Research, 5,* 190–200.

Ennis-Cole, D., Durodoye, B. A., & Harris, H. L. (2013). The impact of culture on autism diagnosis and treatment: Considerations for counselors and other professionals. *The Family Journal, 21*(3), 279–287.

Fountain, C., King, M. D., & Bearman, P. S. (2011). Age of diagnosis for autism: individual and community factors across 10 birth cohorts. *Journal of Epidemiology and Community Health, 65*(6), 503–510.

Fuss, J., Briken, P., & Klein, V. (2018). Gender bias in clinicians' pathologization of atypical sexuality: A randomized controlled trial with mental health professionals. *Scientific Reports, 8*(1), 3715–3719.

Gerdts, J., Mancini, J., Fox, E., Rhoads, C., Ward, T., Easley, E., et al. (2018). Interdisciplinary team evaluation: An effective method for the diagnostic assessment of autism spectrum disorder. *Journal of Developmental and Behavioral Pediatrics, 39*(4), 271–281.

Gona, J. K., Newton, C. R., Rimba, K., Mapenzi, R., Kihara, M., van de Vijver, F., & Ali, A. (2015). Parents' and professionals' perceptions on causes and treatment options for autism spectrum disorders (ASD) in a multicultural context on the Kenyan coast. *PLoS One, 10*(8), e0132729.

Gordon-Lipkin, E., Foster, J., & Peacock, G. (2016). Whittling down the wait time: exploring models to minimize the delay from initial concern to diagnosis and treatment of autism spectrum disorder. *Pediatric Clinics, 63*(5), 851–859.

Gould, J., & Ashton-Smith, J. (2011). Missed diagnosis or misdiagnosis? Girls and women on the autism spectrum. *Good Autism Practice (GAP), 12*(1), 34–41.

Hansen, R. L., Blum, N. J., Gaham, A., Shults, J., & DBPNet Steering Committee. (2016). Diagnosis of autism spectrum disorder by developmental-behavioral pediatricians in academic centers: a DBPNet study. *Pediatrics*, *137*(Supplement 2), S79–S89.

Harper, A., Dyches, T. T., Harper, J., Roper, S. O., & South, M. (2013). Respite care, marital quality, and stress in parents of children with autism spectrum disorders. *Journal of autism and developmental disorders*, *43*(11), 2604–2616.

Hodgetts, S., Zwaigenbaum, L., & Nicholas, D. (2015). Profile and predictors of service needs for families of children with autism spectrum disorders. *Autism, 19*(6), 673–683.

Jackson, R., Baird, W., Davis-Reynolds, L., Smith, C., Blackburn, S., & Allsebrook, J. (2008). Qualitative analysis of parents' information needs and psychosocial experiences when supporting children with health care needs. *Health Information & Libraries Journal,* (1), 31–37.

Jo, H., Schieve, L. A., Rice, C. E., Yeargin-Allsopp, M., Tian, L. H., Blumberg, S. J., Boyle, C. A. (2015). Age at Autism Spectrum Disorder (ASD) diagnosis by race, ethnicity, and primary household language among children with special health care needs, United States, 2009/2010. *Maternal and Child Health Journal*, 1687–1697.

Kai, J. (1996). Parents' difficulties and information needs in coping with acute illness in preschool children: A qualitative study. *BMJ, 313*(7063), 987–990.

Keen, D., Couzens, D., Muspratt, S., & Rodger, S. (2010). The effects of a parent-focused intervention for children with a recent diagnosis of autism spectrum disorder on parenting stress and competence. *Research in Autism Spectrum Disorders, 4*(2), 229–241.

Kogan, M. D., Strickland, B. B., Blumberg, S. J., Singh, G. K., Perrin, J. M., & van Dyck, P. C. (2008). A national profile of the health care experiences and family impact of autism spectrum disorder among children in the United States, 2005–2006. *Pediatrics, 122*(6), e1149–e1158.

Kohler, F. W. (1999). Examining the services received by young children with autism and their families: A survey of parent responses. *Focus on autism and other developmental disabilities, 14*(3), 150–158.

Magaña, S., Parish, S., Rose, R., Timberlake, M., & Swaine, J. (2012). Racial and ethnic disparities in quality of health care among children with autism and other developmental disabilities. *Intellectual and Developmental Disabilities, 50*(4), 287–299.

Magaña, S., Lopez, K., Aguinaga, A., & Morton, H. (2013). Access to diagnosis and treatment services among Latino children with autism spectrum disorders. *Intellectual and Developmental Disabilities, 51*(3), 141–153.

Mandell, D. S., Listerud, J., Levy, S. E., & Pinto-Martin, J. A. (2002). Race differences in the age at diagnosis among Medicaid-eligible children with autism. *Journal of the American Academy of Child and Adolescent Psychiatry, 41*(12), 1447–1453.

Mandell, D. S., Novak, M. M., & Zubritsky, C. D. (2005). Factors associated with age of diagnosis among children with autism spectrum disorders. *Pediatrics, 116*(6), 1480–1486.

Mandell, D. S., Ittenbach, R. F., Levy, S. E., & Pinto-Martin, J. A. (2007). Disparities in diagnoses received prior to a diagnosis of autism spectrum disorder. *Journal of Autism and Developmental Disorders, 37*(9), 1795–1802.
Mansell, W., & Morris, K. (2004). A survey of parents' reactions to the diagnosis of an autistic spectrum disorder by a local service: Access to information and use of services. *Autism, 4*, 387–407.
Mayer, M. L., & Skinner, A. C. (2009). Influence of changes in supply on the distribution of pediatric subspecialty care. *Archives of Pediatrics and Adolescent Medicine, 163*(12), 1087–1091.
Meadan, H., Halle, J. W., & Ebata, A. T. (2010). Families with children who have autism spectrum disorders: Stress and support. *Exceptional children, 77*(1), 7–36.
Miller, A. R., Armstrong, R. W., Mâsse, L. C., Klassen, A. F., Shen, J., & O'Donnell, M. E. (2008). Waiting for child developmental and rehabilitation services: An overview of issues and needs. *Developmental Medicine and Child Neurology, 50*(11), 815–821.
Moodie-Dyer, A., Joyce, H. D., Anderson-Butcher, D., & Hoffman, J. (2014). Parent–caregiver experiences with the autism spectrum disorder service delivery system. *Journal of Family Social Work, 17*(4), 344–362.
Mullen, E. (1989). Mullen scales of early learning. Cranston, RI: TOTAL Child.
Mullen, E. M. (1995). *Mullen scales of early learning* (pp. 58–64). Circle Pines, MN: AGS.
Mungo, D., Ruta, L., Arrigo, V., & Mazzona, L. (2007). Impairment of quality of life in parents of children and adolescents with pervasive developmental disorder. *Health and Quality of Life Outcomes, 5*(22), 1–9.
Olsson, M. B., & Hwang, C. P. (2001). Depression in mothers and fathers of children with intellectual disability. *Journal of Intellectual Disability Research, 45*(6), 535–543.
Peris, T. S., Teachman, B. A., & Nosek, B. A. (2008). Implicit and explicit stigma of mental illness: Links to clinical care. *The Journal of Nervous and Mental Disease, 196*(10), 752–760.
Pickard, K. E., & Ingersoll, B. R. (2016). The role of socioeconomic status on parent-reported service knowledge, service use, unmet service needs, and barriers to service use. *Autism, 20*(1), 106–115.
Robins, D. L., Fein, D., & Barton, M. L. (1999). *Modified checklist for autism in toddlers (M-CHAT) follow-up interview*. Author: Publisher.
Robins, D. L., Casagrande, K., Barton, M., Chen, C. M. A., Dumont-Mathieu, T., & Fein, D. (2014). Validation of the modified checklist for autism in toddlers, revised with follow-up (M-CHAT-R/F). *Pediatrics, 133*(1), 37–45.
Rutter, M., Le Couteur, A., & Lord, C. (2003). Autism diagnostic interview-revised. *Los Angeles, CA: Western Psychological Services, 29*(2003), 30.
Schopler, E., Van Bourgondien, M. E., Wellman, G. J., & Love, S. R. (2010). *Childhood Autism rating scale* (2nd ed.). Los Angeles: Western Psychological Services.
Shattuck, P. T., Durkin, M., Maenner, M., Newschaffer, C., Mandell, D. S., Wiggins, L., ... & Baio, J. (2009). Timing of identification among children with an autism spectrum disorder: findings from a population-based surveillance study. *Journal of the American Academy of Child & Adolescent Psychiatry, 48*(5), 474–483.
Siklos, S., & Kerns, K. A. (2007). Assessing the diagnostic experiences of a small sample of parents of children with autism spectrum disorders. *Research in Developmental Disabilities, 28*(1), 9–22.
Soares, N. S., Baum, R. A., & Frick, K. D. (2015). Improving developmental-behavioral pediatric care workflow. *Journal of Developmental and Behavioral Pediatrics, 36*(1), 45–52.
Sperry, L. A., Whaley, K. T., Shawn, E., & Brame, K. (1999). Services for young children with autism spectrum disorders: Voices of parents/caregivers and providers. *Infants and Young Children, 11*(4), 17–33.
Stoner, J. B., Bock, S. J., Thompson, J. R., Angell, M. E., Heyl, B. S., & Crowley, E. P. (2005). Welcome to our world: Parent perceptions of interactions between parents of young children with ASD and education professionals. *Focus on Autism and Other Developmental Disabilities, 20*(1), 39–51.

Stuart, M., & McGrew, J. H. (2009). Caregiver burden after receiving a diagnosis of an autism spectrum disorder. *Research in Autism Spectrum Disorders*, *3*(1), 86–97.
Thomas, K. C., Parish, S. L., Rose, R. A., & Kilany, M. (2012). Access to care for children with autism in the context of state Medicaid reimbursement. *Maternal and Child Health Journal, 16*(8), 1636–1644.
U.S. Census Bureau. (2018). 2013–2017 ACS 5-year estimates. Retrieved from https://www.census.gov/quickfacts/TX.
Wang, L., Mandell, D. S., Lawer, L., Cidav, Z., & Leslie, D. L. (2013). Healthcare service use and costs for autism spectrum disorder: a comparison between Medicaid and private insurance. *Journal of Autism and Developmental Disorders, 43*(5), 1057–1064.
Weiss, J. A., Wingsiong, A., & Lunsky, Y. (2014). Defining crisis in families of individuals with autism spectrum disorders. *Autism, 18*(8), 985–995.
Werling, D. M., & Geschwind, D. H. (2013). Sex differences in autism spectrum disorders. *Current Opinion in Neurology, 26*(2), 146.
Williams-Arya, P., Anixt, J., Kuan, L., Johnson, H., Kent, B., Bing, N., et al. (2019). Improving access to diagnostic assessments for Autism spectrum disorder using an arena model. *Journal of Developmental and Behavioral Pediatrics, 40*(3), 161–169.
Zwaigenbaum, L., Bauman, M. L., Fein, D., Pierce, K., Buie, T., Davis, P. A., et al. (2015). Early screening of autism spectrum disorder: Recommendations for practice and research. *Pediatrics, 136*(Supplement 1), S41–S59.

Management

Laura Lee McIntyre and Stephanie Y. Shire

Abstract Autism spectrum disorder (ASD) is a lifelong neurodevelopmental disorder that requires ongoing coordinated care and management across caregivers and professionals. A variety of interventions are used in the management of ASD, and it is important to evaluate the effectiveness and implementation of interventions and programs. First, this chapter discusses ASD core challenges for young children such as social engagement, play skills, and social communication, to set the stage for intervention and management strategies. Then, family navigation approaches are described given their relevance for coordinated care in management strategies. The chapter concludes with a case example of an interdisciplinary management approach.

Introduction

Autism spectrum disorder (ASD) is a lifelong neurodevelopmental disorder that requires ongoing coordinated care and management across caregivers and professionals to improve outcomes and improve overall functioning and quality of life (Hyman et al., 2020). Core symptoms of ASD include difficulties with social communication and the presence of restricted interests and repetitive behaviors (American Psychiatric Association, 2013). People with ASD commonly have co-occurring medical or behavioral health disorders which underscore the need for interdisciplinary care coordination to ensure comprehensive care and seamless integration of treatment across providers and disciplines (Shahidullah, Azad, Mezher, McClain, & McIntyre, 2018). These comorbid conditions may range from seizures to sleep disorders to anxiety (e.g., Hyman et al., 2020) and significantly impact the family and caregivers (Blacher & McIntyre, 2006).

The purpose of this chapter is to discuss the evidence supporting a variety of interventions in the management of ASD. Interdisciplinary coordinated care will be discussed within the context of these management approaches. Coordinated care

L. L. McIntyre (✉) · S. Y. Shire
College of Education, University of Oregon, Eugene, OR, USA
e-mail: llmcinty@uoregon.edu

M. B. McClain et al. (eds.), *Interprofessional Care Coordination for Pediatric Autism Spectrum Disorder*, https://doi.org/10.1007/978-3-030-46295-6_7

involves teaming with a range of providers in the evaluation, treatment, and management of core symptoms and related conditions. Coordinated care also includes consultation and planning with the family in order to best understand and support the goals and priorities of the family and child (Shahidullah, McClain, Azad, Mezher, & McIntyre, in press). ASD core challenges will be discussed first to set the stage for intervention and management strategies. Then, family navigation approaches will be described given their relevance for coordinated care in management strategies. We conclude with a case example of an interdisciplinary management approach.

Core Challenges

Over the first two to three years of life, children demonstrate rapid growth in their social engagement with people and objects during daily interactions (Tomasello et al., 2005). Children can practice communicating their ideas and needs and practice actions with objects through routine interactions with their caregivers. These moments allow caregivers the opportunity to scaffold their children's bids into increasingly more clear and sophisticated communication and play skills (Adamson et al., 2012). Seminal early childhood research has demonstrated the link between access to these early learning opportunities and children's growing language and cognitive skills (e.g., Risley & Hart, 2006). However, many young children with autism spectrum disorder (ASD) may miss out on a number of these early learning opportunities due to differences in early social engagement (e.g., Adamson, Bakeman, Deckner, & Romski, 2009) leading to a cascading impact on development in other core early childhood skill domains including play and social communication.

Social Engagement

While typically developing young children will master the ability to sustain long periods of coordination between people and shared activities, known as joint engagement (Adamson, Bakeman, & Deckner, 2004) by about 18 months, this can be an ongoing challenge for young children with ASD. Research has demonstrated that children with ASD spend significantly more time focused exclusively and intensely on objects or not engaged with either objects or people (unengaged) than typically developing children and children with other developmental disorders (e.g., Adamson et al., 2009). When children are exclusively object engaged or unengaged, they are not noticing the input of adults who provide a critical mapping of spoken language and gestures to the materials in the environment. Further, children may also miss out on the actions that the adult may demonstrate with the materials, key opportunities to learn to develop the skills to appropriately use these items. Joint engagement creates a critical foundation for early learning contributing to children's cognitive and communicative development (Adamson, Bakeman, Suma, & Robbins, 2019).

Play Skills

When children are not noticing an adult's actions on objects, children lose information on how to functionally use these objects. A child's actions on objects can be categorized as functional or symbolic play acts (Sigman & Ungerer, 1984). Functional play emerges first between approximately 12 and 24 months followed by symbolic play (Sigman and Ungerer, 1981). The development of play skills is associated with gains in social, cognitive, and communicative skills (e.g., Pierucci, Barber, Gilpin, Crisler, & Klinger, 2015; Toth, Munson, Meltzoff, & Dawson, 2006). Yet, for young children with ASD, the emergence of this hierarchy of skills may take more time (Jarrold, Boucher, & Smith, 1996; Rutherford, Young, Hepburn, & Rogers, 2007). In particular, additional support may be required to advance symbolic level play skills (e.g., Kasari & Chang, 2014). Further, the diversity or number of different ways that children can flexibly play with an object may be more limited whereby play is often rote and repetitive than the play of their typically developing peers (Jarrold et al., 1996). This insistence to use an object, in the same way, each time, or intense interest in a play topic, character, physical feature of a toy, or specific action may range in intensity where some children show little repetition and others may experience significant distress if change occurs. This can pose a substantial barrier to dynamic social play with peers who may not want to engage in the same topic or action as often as the child with ASD. These social demands are significant and require children to flexibly play with the objects appropriately in the context of reciprocal, dynamic interactions. Peer play interactions require negotiation and navigation of the social context with other children, such that intervention is often required in order for children with ASD to participate in common early childhood and preschool activities such as free play and outside playtime.

Social Communication

The symbolism and abstraction required for higher level social play is also required for children's use of words as communication symbols. As such, it is logical that the development of joint engagement and play skills are intertwined with the development of children's nonverbal and spoken communication skills (e.g., Adamson & Bakeman, 2006; Tomasello, Carpenter, & Liszkowski, 2007). Children's spontaneous nonverbal communication both to request (e.g., pointing to ask for an item that is out of reach) and for the purpose of social sharing (joint attention, for example, holding up a toy to show it to another person) are key skills that are often missing for young children with ASD. Initiations of joint attention (IJA), in particular, (e.g., pointing to share an airplane in the sky with another person) are unique challenges that are used to differentially diagnose ASD from other developmental disorders. Developing children's IJA skills can bolster children's expressive language skills (e.g., Kasari et al., 2008; Mundy, Sigman, & Kasari, 1990).

It is estimated that approximately 30–50% of children with ASD will not have word combinations and may have few or no spontaneous, functional words to request or comment by school entry (e.g., Tager-Flusberg & Kasari, 2013). Reducing social communication challenges in early childhood is one of the best predictors of later developmental outcomes (Anderson, Liang, & Lord, 2014). Therefore, core challenges that present during early childhood including joint engagement, play skills, and initiations of joint attention are key targets for care management.

Management Approaches

Given the complexity of ASD and the range of symptoms associated with core features and co-occurring conditions, a number of approaches have been used in the management and care of people with ASD. The lion share of the research on interventions for people with ASD focuses on early behavioral intervention given some of the seminal studies demonstrating that early, intensive interventions may significantly improve intellectual and adaptive functioning and special education outcomes (e.g., Lovass, 1987). Beyond strict behavioral approaches, interventions have been developed that are based on naturalistic and developmental approaches that are intended to address core symptoms.

Applied Behavior Analysis (ABA)

The overwhelming majority of evidence-based intervention models in ASD are based on the principles of ABA (National Autism Center, 2015; Rogers & Vismara, 2008). ABA approaches involve using behavioral theory to systematically teach skills and/or reduce challenging behavior by modifying the environment and manipulating the antecedents and consequences surrounding a target behavior. Discrete trial training is one of the most well-known and well-researched forms of intervention based on ABA (Bogin, 2008; National Autism Center, 2015). In discrete trial training, specific skills are taught systematically through structured, one-on-one teaching sessions. In each adult directed teaching trial, the task is clearly presented to the learner and a programmed consequence is provided after each learner's response (e.g., verbal praise following a correct response) to increase the occurrence of desired behavior or decrease the occurrence of undesired behavior (Bogin, Sullivan, Rogers, & Stabel, 2010). Discrete trial training and other forms of ABA approaches have been demonstrated to be effective in producing gains in adaptive and intellectual functioning in comparison to eclectic treatment approaches (Howard, Sparkman, Cohen, Green, & Stanislaw, 2005). Although there are numerous studies demonstrating the efficacy of ABA-based approaches in preschool and early elementary school (e.g., Cohen, Amerine-Dickens, & Smith, 2006; Eikeseth, Smith, Jahr, & Eldevik, 2002; Howard et al., 2005; Remington et al., 2007), there remain challenges with using strict ABA approaches to symptom management. For example, some studies use small sample sizes and nonexperimental research designs (for a review see Reichow, Hume, Barton, & Boyd, 2018), which make the evidence less compelling. Although discrete trial training programs are effective in teaching discrete skills, the skills may not generalize to other settings, teachers, or materials. Further, children may become overly reliant on adult prompts, and therefore, reduce their spontaneous interactions or initiations with adults and peers (Schreibman et al., 2015). Most notably, ABA approaches may not comprehensively address core symptoms in young children with ASD. For these reasons, there have been a number of recent advances in naturalistic developmental approaches in an effort to address some of these limitations.

Naturalistic developmental behavioral interventions (NDBIs). NDBIs were developed in part, to address some of the concerns with strict ABA and discrete trial training approaches. NDBIs, although behaviorally based, focus on a range of naturalistic approaches to teach early developmental and prerequisite skills such as joint attention, play skills, and initiating requests (Schreibman et al., 2015). Some specific NDBIs include Pivotal Response Training (PRT; Koegel & Koegel, 2006), Early Start Denver Model (ESDM; Dawson et al., 2010), and Joint Attention Symbolic Play Engagement and Regulation (JASPER; Kasari, Freeman, & Paparella, 2006). JASPER, in particular, has quite a few randomized controlled trials that support its efficacy in enhancing early social communication skills in children with ASD (Kasari et al., 2006, 2008, 2010, 2014). JASPER is a targeted social communication intervention that has been shown to improve joint attention, language, play skills, and engagement in toddlers, preschoolers, and minimally verbal children with ASD (Kasari et al., 2014).

Care Management in the Community: Intervention Effectiveness Trials

A number of behavioral interventions have been developed in university research settings to address the core challenges children with ASD can experience in social engagement, play, and communication (Smith & Iadarola, 2015). Although significant advances in intervention development and testing have been accomplished, leading to gains for children and their families who are able to reach university clinics in large urban centers, fewer interventions have been tested when delivered by community clinicians to diverse samples of children in the community who demonstrate great heterogeneity in their profiles of strengths and needs.

Understanding where to start: Setting service targets. Although children with ASD are unified as a group by challenges in social engagement, play, and communication skills, there is significant variability in the rate of acquisition of these skills and thus, individualization of care is necessary. Tools have been developed for use by community practitioners and educators to identify individualized targets matched to our understanding of the developmental emergence of these skills in early childhood. For example, the Short Play and Communication Evaluation (SPACE: Shire, Shih, Chang, & Kasari, 2018) is a tool that was developed and tested with preschool teachers. The brief, play-based assessment is designed to help the practitioner identify which play and social communication skills the child has mastered and then to identify a developmentally appropriate target for intervention. The tool has been validated with gold standard tools to assess play and social communication which are used in research settings, demonstrating that the intervention targets identified through the brief SPACE administered by teachers are not significantly different than those identified by researchers using the longer, more complex protocols (Shire et al., 2018). Such freely available tools are examples of resources available to community clinicians to help identify the unique needs of a child experiencing some delays in the core developmental domains and to set personalized and developmentally appropriate targets for service. Communication between parents, community clinicians, and early childhood educators is critical to identify the most relevant developmental targets for psychoeducational management approaches.

Transitioning efficacious interventions into the community. Interventions that have an established base demonstrating the efficacy of the intervention under highly controlled conditions with research staff delivering the intervention, must also be tested when transported and potentially adapted to fit the community care context. Considerations in the community for adoption of an intervention service include those related to the implementation of the intervention (e.g., training for clinicians to reach and maintain implementation fidelity, clinical supervision, etc.), as well as the sustainability of the intervention within the local service context, a challenge which is not presented in short term clinical research (Proctor, Powell, & McMillen, 2013). Therefore, a partnership between the community service team and the research team is needed to bring together an understanding of the facilitators and barriers to service adoption and implementation and then select the implementation strategies to best support success. This partnership model is demonstrated in Community Partnered Participatory Research (CPPR: Jones & Wells, 2007). While *community-based* research takes place in community settings, CPPR emphasizes joint leadership and shared decision-making power amongst the team of community and research members (Jones & Wells, 2007). CPPR sets the context to understand how interventions may be adapted to best fit the needs of the community.

Testing effectiveness in the community. Several empirically supported efficacious interventions that target the development of social engagement, communication and/or play skills have been tested when delivered by community clinicians or educators under real-world conditions. NDBIs utilize natural contingencies and behavioral strategies in natural settings to teach developmentally appropriate targets have the greatest number of examples of programs that have been tested in randomized controlled trial designs. To best understand how the intervention is being delivered by those who will use it in the community and whether or not children are making significant gains, it is important to examine both the effectiveness (e.g., outcomes for children and caregivers) and implementation (e.g., fidelity) of the program. Effectiveness trials have included various community stakeholders who learn the intervention strategies and deliver the program with the child including caregivers, educators, and community clinicians. These trials differ from when research staff deliver the intervention in the context of a natural setting such as a school or a family's home. Comprehensive reviews of efficacy and effectiveness trials are available (e.g., Green & Garg, 2018; Smith & Iadarola, 2015), as well as interventions targeting core early childhood skills (e.g., joint attention interventions: Murza, Schwartz, Hahs-Vaughn, & Nye, 2016).

As highlighted by Green and Garg (2018), caregiver mediated interventions, in particular, have demonstrated consistent effects to increase children's time jointly engaged and children's dyadic social interaction. Interventions focused on creating this foundation in order to advance children's social communication skills have been demonstrated by models including the Preschool Autism Communication Trial (PACT: Green et al., 2010), a developmental intervention developed in the United Kingdom and JASPER (Kasari, Gulsrud, Paparella, Hellemann, & Berry, 2015), an NDBI developed in the United States. Both the PACT and JASPER caregiver mediated interventions have been adapted and then tested in community settings. The PACT intervention has been adapted for delivery by community providers working in India and Pakistan (Rahman et al., 2016). Further, JASPER has been tested when delivered in families' home focusing on families who are underserved and under-resourced in five centers across the United States (Kasari et al., 2014) leading to increases in children's initiations of joint attention, as well as their play skills. The JASPER intervention has also been mediated by paraprofessional and head teachers in preschool and toddler classroom settings, similarly leading to gains in children's joint engagement, initiations of joint attention, and language (Chang et al., 2016; Shire et al., 2017).

Service Navigation and Care Coordination for Families

Families report finding timely access to high quality care is a significant topic of concern and stress (Brookman-Frazee, Baker-Ericzen, Stadnick, & Taylor, 2012). With multiple intervention models at various stages of development, efficacy, and effectiveness, existing within a fragmented service systems and often no single point of entry within a community, significant supports are required to help families understand which services may be available in one's community, let alone match the possible options to best fit the unique needs of the children and their families. Family Navigation (FN, also referred to as Patient Navigation in the medical literature) has emerged as a strategy to support timely access to both diagnostic and intervention services by integrating the disconnected parts of the system for the benefit of the user (Broder-Fingert et al., 2019). FN is a case management framework that has been applied to support an individual or family's ability to quickly and efficiently find their way to assessment and service which has been studied in medical interventions (e.g., cancer treatment), as well as mental health and substance abuse. However, the application of

FN to families' navigation of the autism assessment and intervention service system has emerged more recently.

The navigator is an individual who is trained to provide information that is communicated in an accessible form to the family. Through qualitative studies including navigators and families who have accessed FN services, several core features of FN have been reported. Specific to FN services for mental health and addiction services, successful navigation services were defined first by the navigator's abilities including the ability to understand the needs of the child and their family, to build strong rapport without judgment, be reliable, demonstrate strong communication skills, demonstrate expertise and knowledge, as well as flexibility, and provide family centered support (Markoulakis, Chan, & Levitt, 2019). Second, the actions of the family also contributed to successful navigation, including involvement in the creation and implementation of the navigation plan and engaging in open communication (Markoulakis et al., 2019). Findings from this study also emphasize how the bidirectional relationship between the navigator and the family access the service is key to perceptions of a successful fit for the match of navigator to family. The combination of responsive services that connect with the child, knowledgeable and supportive service providers, as well as both the child and family, demonstrating a willingness to engage with the recommendations and services provided by the navigator and clinicians led to the highest perceptions of successful FN. In addition to these characteristics, recent examination of care components of FN specific to serving children with ASD and their families emphasize additional considerations. For example, considering the need for care over time, ongoing navigator training and supervision including fidelity monitoring is recommended through regular check-ins to continue to support challenging cases (Broder-Fingert et al., 2019).

FN has been piloted to target a reduction in disparities in the time to diagnosis for families of 40 young children referred for ASD diagnostic evaluation (Feinberg et al., 2016). The study focused on families who are traditionally underserved (e.g., from racial/ethnic minority groups, born outside the United States, speak a language other than English) and under-resourced (e.g., with income less than 200% of the federal poverty level). Three targeted in-person visits and three phone contacts were provided to families randomized to FN. Significantly more families who received FN completed the diagnostic assessment (19 of 20) than those who received community access as usual (11 of 19). This is one of the first examples of FN case management as a strategy to support families of young children with ASD. FN is also highly applicable to support families' access to timely and appropriate intervention services with a trial exploring the application to service access underway (Broder-Fingert et al., 2018).

Care Coordination

Given the breadth and scope of management approaches to support people with ASD in early childhood and across the lifespan, care coordination is critical. A number of professionals may be working with a child with ASD and their family. For example, special educators, psychologists, speech and language pathologists, and a variety of medical specialists may be involved in the child's care. Progress on IEP goals and objectives, data on speech and language targets, and sleep, diet, and behavioral data can all be shared across the team for more seamless planning.

Case Example

Barry is 30-month old who received an autism specific screening tool during a routine well-child visit with his primary care physician. Barry's mother reported concerns with sleep, intense tantrums, and speech. Barry used about 10 words to communicate and had few functional play skills. Barry's primary care physician referred Barry to receive a comprehensive developmental evaluation to assess for autism spectrum disorder. Barry also was assigned to a Family Navigator (FN) who met with Barry's caregivers at home and in the primary care physician's office. The FN helped Barry's caregivers the early intervention referral process while Barry was on a waiting list for a comprehensive developmental evaluation. Barry was determined to be eligible for early intervention services under federal special education law (Individuals with Disabilities Education Improvement Act, 2004). Barry received specialized instruction delivered for an early childhood special educator in a community preschool. The early childhood educators at the preschool received training and implementation guidance of the JASPER intervention and the multidisciplinary team, comprised of Barry's caregivers, a special educator, paraeducator, speech-language pathologist, and occupational therapist conducted an assessment of Barry's social, communication, and play skills to develop intervention targets. Progress on Barry's individualized education plan was shared with the medical team conducting the comprehensive developmental evaluation. Medical management and follow-up was provided to Barry by a developmental pediatrician and nurse practitioner on an annual basis. During the medical management visits, Barry's caregivers shared the progress on Barry's educational and behavioral goals that were being tracked by Barry's early childhood special education team. Barry's team noted that on days in which Barry had significant sleep disruptions, his maladaptive behavior intensified. Barry's caregivers, in conjunction with the school team, were able to chart these co-occurrences and share with Barry's developmental pediatrician. Although no medical treatment was initially recommended to address the sleep and disruptive behavior issues, the developmental pediatrician recommended that the educational team consult with a pediatric school psychologist who was well versed in behavioral approaches to improving sleep problems and behavior problems. Barry's caregivers continued to work with the FN who assisted with care coordination and psychoeducation to Barry's family.

References

Adamson, L. B., & Bakeman, R. (2006). The development of displaced speech in early mother-child conversations. *Child Development, 77,* 186–200.

Adamson, L. B., Bakeman, R., & Deckner, D. F. (2004). The development of symbol-infused joint engagement. *Child Development, 75*(4), 1171–1187.

Adamson, L. B., Bakeman, R., Deckner, D. F., & Romski, M. (2009). Joint engagement and the emergence of language in children with autism and Down syndrome. *Journal of Autism and Developmental Disorders, 39*(1), 84.

Adamson, L. B., Bakeman, R., Deckner, D. F., & Nelson, P. B. (2012). Rating parent–child interactions: Joint engagement, communication dynamics, and shared topics in autism, down syndrome, and typical development. *Journal of Autism and Developmental Disorders, 42*(12), 2622–2635.

Adamson, L. B., Bakeman, R., Suma, K., & Robins, D. L. (2019). An expanded view of joint attention: Skill, engagement, and language in typical development and autism. *Child Development, 90*(1), e1–e18.

American Psychiatric Association. (2013). *Diagnostic and statistical manual of mental disorders (DSM 5),* 5th Edn. Washington, D.C.: American Psychiatric Association.

Anderson, D. K., Liang, J. W., & Lord, C. (2014). Predicting young adult outcome among more and less cognitively able individuals with autism spectrum disorders. *Journal of Child Psychology and Psychiatry, 55*(5), 485–494.

Blacher, J., & McIntyre, L. L. (2006). Syndrome specificity and behavioural disorders in young adults with intellectual disability: Cultural differences in family impact. *Journal of Intellectual Disability Research, 50,* 184–198.

Bogin, J. (2008). *Overview of discrete trial training*. Sacramento, CA: National Professional Development Center on Autism Spectrum Disorders, M.I.N.D. Institute, The University of California at Davis Medical School.

Bogin, J., Sullivan, L., Rogers, S., & Stabel. A. (2010). *Steps for implementation: Discrete trial training*. Sacramento, CA: The National Professional Development Center on Autism Spectrum Disorders, The M.I.N.D. Institute, The University of California at Davis School of Medicine.

Broder-Fingert, S., Walls, M., Augustyn, M., Beidas, R., Mandell, D., Wiltsey-Stirman, S., et al. (2018). A hybrid type I randomized effectiveness-implementation trial of patient navigation to improve access to services for children with autism spectrum disorder. *BMC Psychiatry, 18*(1), 79.

Broder-Fingert, S., Qin, S., Goupil, J., Rosenberg, J., Augustyn, M., Blum, N., … & Silverstein, M. (2019). A mixed-methods process evaluation of Family Navigation implementation for autism spectrum disorder. *Autism, 23*(5), 1288–1299.

Brookman-Frazee, L., Baker-Ericzén, M., Stadnick, N., & Taylor, R. (2012). Parent perspectives on community mental health services for children with autism spectrum disorders. *Journal of Child and Family Studies, 21*(4), 533–544.

Chang, Y. C., Shire, S. Y., Shih, W., Gelfand, C., & Kasari, C. (2016). Preschool deployment of evidence-based social communication intervention: JASPER in the classroom. *Journal of Autism and Developmental Disorders, 46*(6), 2211–2223.

Cohen, H., Amerine-Dickens, M., & Smith, T. (2006). Early intensive behavioral treatment: Replication of the UCLA model in a community setting. *Journal of Developmental and Behavioral Pediatrics, 27*(2), 145–155.

Dawson, G., Rogers, S., Munson, J., Smith, M., Winter, J., Greenson, J., et al. (2010). Randomized, controlled trial of an intervention for toddlers with autism: the Early Start Denver Model. *Pediatrics, 125*(1), 17–23.

Eikeseth, S., Smith, T., Jahr, E., & Eldevik, S. (2002). Intensive behavioral treatment at school for 4–7 year-old children with autism. *Behavior Modification, 26*(1), 49–68.

Feinberg, E., Abufhele, M., Sandler, J., Augustyn, M., Cabral, H., Chen, N., et al. (2016). Reducing disparities in timely autism diagnosis through family navigation: results from a randomized pilot trial. *Psychiatric Services, 67*(8), 912–915.

Green, J., Charman, T., McConachie, H., Aldred, C., Slonims, V., Howlin, P., et al. (2010). Parent-mediated communication-focused treatment in children with autism (PACT): a randomised controlled trial. *The Lancet, 375*(9732), 2152–2160.

Green, J., & Garg, S. (2018). Annual research review: the state of autism intervention science: progress, target psychological and biological mechanisms and future prospects. *Journal of Child Psychology and Psychiatry, 59*(4), 424–443.

Howard, J. S., Sparkman, C. R., Cohen, H. G., Green, G., & Stanislaw, H. (2005). A comparison of intensive behavior analytic and eclectic treatments for young children with autism. *Research in Developmental Disabilities, 26*(4), 359–383.

Hyman, S. L., Levy, S. E., Myers, S. M., & AAP Council on Children with Disabilities, Section on Developmental and Behavioral Pediatrics. (2020). Identification, evaluation, and management of children with autism spectrum disorder. *Pediatrics, 145*(1), e20193447.

Jarrold, C., Boucher, J., & Smith, P. K. (1996). Generativity deficits in pretend play in autism. *British Journal of Developmental Psychology, 14*(3), 275–300.

Jones, L., & Wells, K. (2007). Strategies for academic and clinician engagement in community-participatory partnered research. *JAMA, 297*(4), 407–410.

Kasari, C., & Chang, Y. C. (2014). *Play development in children with autism spectrum disorders: Skills, object play, and interventions. Handbook of Autism and Pervasive Developmental Disorders*, 4th Edn.

Kasari, C., Freeman, S., & Paparella, T. (2006). Joint attention and symbolic play in young children with autism: a randomized controlled intervention study. *Journal of Child Psychology and Psychiatry, 47*(6), 611–620.

Kasari, C., Gulsrud, A., Paparella, T., Hellemann, G., & Berry, K. (2015). Randomized comparative efficacy study of parent-mediated interventions for toddlers with autism. *Journal of consulting and clinical psychology, 83*(3), 554.

Kasari, C., Paparella, T., Freeman, S., & Jahromi, L. B. (2008). Language outcome in autism: Randomized comparison of joint attention and play interventions. *Journal of Consulting and Clinical Psychology, 76*(1), 125–137.

Kasari, C., Gulsrud, A. C., Wong, C., Kwon, S., & Locke, J. (2010). Randomized controlled caregiver mediated joint engagement intervention for toddlers with autism. *Journal of Autism and Developmental Disorders, 40*(9), 1045–1056.

Kasari, C., Kaiser, A., Goods, K., Nietfeld, J., Mathy, P., Landa, R., et al. (2014). Communication interventions for minimally verbal children with autism: a sequential multiple assignment randomized trial. *Journal of the American Academy of Child and Adolescent Psychiatry, 53*(6), 635–646.

Koegel, R. L., & Koegel, L. K. (2006). *Pivotal response treatments for autism: Communication, social, & academic development*. Baltimore, MD: Paul H. Brookes Publishing.

Lovaas, O. I. (1987). Behavioral treatment and normal educational and intellectual functioning in young autistic children. *Journal of Consulting and Clinical Psychology, 55*(1), 3–9.

Markoulakis, R., Chan, S., & Levitt, A. (2019). Identifying the key features and outcomes of family navigation services for mental health and/or addictions concerns: a Delphi study. *BMC health services research, 19*(1), 137.

Mundy, P., Sigman, M., & Kasari, C. (1990). A longitudinal study of joint attention and language development in autistic children. *Journal of Autism and Developmental Disorders, 20*(1), 115–128.

Murza, K. A., Schwartz, J. B., Hahs-Vaughn, D. L., & Nye, C. (2016). Joint attention interventions for children with autism spectrum disorder: a systematic review and meta-analysis. *International journal of language & communication disorders, 51*(3), 236–251.

National Autism Center. (2015). *Findings and conclusions: National standards project, phase 2*. Randolph, MA: Author.

Pierucci, J. M., Barber, A. B., Gilpin, A. T., Crisler, M. E., & Klinger, L. G. (2015). Play assessments and developmental skills in young children with autism spectrum disorders. *Focus on Autism and Other Developmental Disabilities, 30*(1), 35–43.

Proctor, E. K., Powell, B. J., & McMillen, J. C. (2013). Implementation strategies: Recommendations for specifying and reporting. *Implementation Science, 8*(1), 139.

Rahman, A., Divan, G., Hamdani, S. U., Vajaratkar, V., Taylor, C., Leadbitter, K., … & Patel, V. (2016). Effectiveness of the parent-mediated intervention for children with autism spectrum disorder in south Asia in India and Pakistan (PASS): a randomised controlled trial. *The Lancet Psychiatry, 3*(2), 128–136.

Reichow, B., Hume, K., Barton, E. E., & Boyd, B. A. (2018). Early intensive behavioral intervention (EIBI) for young children with autism spectrum disorders (ASD*). Cochrane Database of Systematic Reviews, 5,* CD009260.

Remington, B., Hastings, R. P., Kovshoff, H., degli Espinosa, F., Jahr, E., Brown T., … Ward, N. (2007). Early intensive behavioral intervention: Outcomes for children with autism and their parents after two years. *American Journal on Mental Retardation, 112*(6), 418–438.

Risley, T. R., & Hart, B. (2006). promoting early language development. In N. F. Watt, C. Ayoub, R. H. Bradley, J. E. Puma, & W. A. LeBoeuf (Eds.), *Child psychology and mental health. The crisis in youth mental health: Critical issues and effective programs, vol. 4. Early intervention programs and policies* (pp. 83–88). Praeger Publishers/Greenwood Publishing Group.

Rogers, S. J., & Vismara, L. A. (2008). Evidence-based comprehensive treatments for early autism. *Journal of Clinical Child and Adolescent Psychology, 37,* 8–38.

Rutherford, M. D., Young, G. S., Hepburn, S., & Rogers, S. J. (2007). A longitudinal study of pretend play in autism. *Journal of Autism and Developmental Disorders, 37*(6), 1024–1039.

Schreibman, L., Dawson, G., Stahmer, A. C., Landa, R., Rogers, S. J., McGee, G. G., et al. (2015). Naturalistic developmental behavioral interventions: Empirically validated treatments for autism spectrum disorder. *Journal of Autism and Developmental Disorders, 45*(8), 2411–2428.

Shahidullah, J. D., Azad, G. F., Mezher, K., McClain, M. B., & McIntyre, L. L. (2018). Linking the medical and educational home to support children with autism spectrum disorder: Practice recommendations. *Clinical Pediatrics, 57,* 1496–1505.

Shahidullah, J. D., McClain, M. B., Azad, G., Mezher, K. R., & McIntyre, L. L. (in press). Coordinating autism care across schools and medical settings: Considerations for school psychologists. *Intervention in School and Clinic.*

Shire, S. Y., Chang, Y. C., Shih, W., Bracaglia, S., Kodjoe, M., & Kasari, C. (2017). Hybrid implementation model of community-partnered early intervention for toddlers with autism: A randomized trial. *Journal of Child Psychology and Psychiatry, 58*(5), 612–622.

Shire, S. Y., Shih, W., Chang, Y. C., & Kasari, C. (2018). Short Play and Communication Evaluation: Teachers' assessment of core social communication and play skills with young children with autism. *Autism, 22*(3), 299–310.

Sigman, M., & Ungerer, J. (1981). Sensorimotor skills and language comprehension in autistic children. *Journal of Abnormal Child Psychology, 9*(2), 149–165.

Sigman, M., & Ungerer, J. A. (1984). Cognitive and language skills in autistic, mentally retarded, and normal children. *Developmental Psychology, 20*(2), 293.

Smith, T., & Iadarola, S. (2015). Evidence base update for autism spectrum disorder. *Journal of Clinical Child & Adolescent Psychology, 44*(6), 897–922.

Tager-Flusberg, H., & Kasari, C. (2013). Minimally verbal school-aged children with autism spectrum disorder: The neglected end of the spectrum. *Autism research, 6*(6), 468–478.

Tomasello, M., Carpenter, M., Call, J., Behne, T., & Moll, H. (2005). Understanding and sharing intentions: The origins of cultural cognition. *Behavioral and Brain Sciences, 28*(5), 675–691.

Tomasello, M., Carpenter, M., & Liszkowski, U. (2007). A new look at infant pointing. *Child Development, 78*(3), 705–722.

Toth, K., Munson, J., Meltzoff, A. N., & Dawson, G. (2006). Early predictors of communication development in young children with autism spectrum disorder: Joint attention, imitation, and toy play. *Journal of Autism and Developmental Disorders, 36*(8), 993–1005.

Transition to Early Schooling for Children with ASD

Michelle Heyman, Yasamin Bolourian, and Jan Blacher

Abstract The transition to school can be difficult for any child, but children with autism spectrum disorder (ASD) encounter additional problems and obstacles during this time. ASD is a lifelong disorder. Yet, the earlier a child with ASD receives intervention, the more promising the long-term outcomes. One way for children to be identified with ASD before entering school is through yearly appointments with their primary care doctor. Under federal legislation of IDEA, children from birth to age three with, or at risk of having, developmental delays have a legal right to early intervention. However, not everyone has equal access to services. Geographical location, race, and socioeconomic status are a few factors that contribute to uneven access to interventions for families. Culturally sensitive providers should be aware of early signs of ASD and be knowledgeable about referring families to appropriate education and treatment. Ultimately, to close the service gap, parents who have children with ASD should be aware of their rights and how to navigate the system to receive treatment.

Introduction

All children experience a transition to early schooling, although the point of transition may vary. Some children remain at home with their caregiver until mandatory kindergarten, some attend preschool prior to kindergarten, and some may experience daycare from infancy onward. Regardless, it is not uncommon for many children to find the demands of kindergarten rather rigorous—to listen, to get along with others, and to exert a fair degree of self-regulation (McIntyre, Blacher, & Baker, 2006; Rimm-Kaufman, Curby, Grimm, Nathanson, & Brock, 2009; Rosanbalm & Murray, 2017).

Transitioning for children with autism spectrum disorder (ASD) may be a more challenging time for parents and children. Most of the skills that require "fine-tuning" upon school entry, including social skills and self-regulation, are likely to be far less

M. Heyman (✉) · Y. Bolourian · J. Blacher
Graduate School of Education, University of California, Riverside, Riverside, CA, USA
e-mail: mheym001@ucr.edu

M. B. McClain et al. (eds.), *Interprofessional Care Coordination for Pediatric Autism Spectrum Disorder*, https://doi.org/10.1007/978-3-030-46295-6_8

well developed in children with ASD (Larcombe, Joosten, Cordier, & Vaz, 2019). Some studies indicate that children with ASD may be less emotionally ready to engage with their peers upon school entry, while others may have difficulty with on-task and direction-following behaviors (Kemp & Carter, 2005; Marsh, Spagnol, Grove, & Eapen, 2017). What is absolutely critical is that teachers, parents, and other professionals (e.g., speech therapists, behavior therapists, psychologists, the kindergarten teacher, preschool teacher) work harmoniously to prepare children with ASD for this transition, and all this is largely dependent on *when* the child was first diagnosed with ASD.

The Role of Autism Identification and Early Schooling

In considering how ASD may affect the transition to early schooling, it is important to understand what constitutes the diagnosis and how the timing of diagnosis may impact the process. ASD is a lifelong condition characterized by pervasive impairments in social communication and interaction, along with restricted patterns of behaviors and interests (American Psychiatric Association [APA], 2013). Symptoms of ASD that are most prominent in early development are social and communication deficits (Martínez-Pedraza & Carter, 2009; Woods & Wetherby, 2003). Although many parents report autistic-like concerns in children as young as 18 months, professionals often delay giving a diagnosis and take a "wait and see" approach until the child is older. A delay in initial diagnosis can be attributed to the array of behaviors demonstrated by each child with ASD, uninformed professionals, or inappropriate referrals provided to the family (Woods & Wetherby, 2003).

Current diagnostic assessments are reliable when administered by appropriately trained professionals to children from about 18 to 24 months, and these children are more than likely to retain their diagnosis as they age (Lord & Luyster, 2006; National Research Council, 2001; Woods & Wetherby, 2003). Factors that may influence the time of diagnosis during early childhood include the family's socioeconomic background, race/ethnicity, and child gender (Rosenberg, Kaufmann, Law, & Law, 2011). For example, research has consistently shown that age at diagnosis is delayed for racially/ethnically diverse children and females (Hyman, Levy, & Myers, 2020; Mandell, Listerud, Levy, & Pinto-Martin, 2002; Rosenberg et al., 2011). It is also important to note the cultural context of ASD, as some parents (e.g., White versus Latinx) may report different symptoms (see chapter "Clinical and School Identification and Intervention for Youth with ASD: Culturally and Linguistically Responsive Interdisciplinary Considerations"; Blacher, Stavropoulos, & Bolourian, 2019).

Importantly, a delay in the detection of ASD affects *when* families and children can start receiving intervention services. Children diagnosed at an earlier age have more promising trajectories, largely due to earlier access to appropriate interventions. Specifically, these children often show more improved cognitive and language outcomes compared to children diagnosed later in life (Hyman et al., 2020; Turner & Stone, 2007; Warren et al., 2011). Access to early intervention can also help reduce familial stress, as well as future financial burden for the community in terms of education costs (Järbrink, 2007; Koegel, Koegel, Ashaugh, & Brahshaw, 2014; Rosenberg et al., 2011). Thus, as the growing body of evidence suggests, early identification and treatment of ASD is crucial to the wellbeing of individuals with ASD, their families, and, arguably, the public.

With that being said, in 2020, the Association of American Physicians (AAP) published a historic update to their clinical recommendations on ASD. In their report (Hyman et al., 2020), the authors endorsed providing early intervention or school-based services to children who have documented delays even before an official diagnosis of ASD is given. This shift among pediatricians shows support for the body of evidence for the early treatment of ASD symptoms and attempts to break barriers to service access in early childhood years.

One way to improve the identification of ASD is to increase awareness and knowledge of expected developmental milestones among medical and school-based service providers. It is critical for professionals to understand behaviors that indicate early signs of ASD versus behaviors that are part of a child's normative development (Martínez-Pedraza & Carter, 2009; National Research Council, 2001). In an effort to improve early identification of ASD, the CDC launched a health education campaign to help families, healthcare providers, and early childhood educators identify and monitor developmental milestones called "Learn the signs. Act Early." Their program includes free and simple online checklists, training videos, and tracking tools (Center for Disease Control and Prevention, 2019). For example, an early sign of ASD is echolalia, which is the repetition of heard words or phrases. While first learning a language, it may be normative for a child to repeat another's spoken words. However, if the child mimics the precise intonation and inflection of heard words, it may be an indicative symptom of ASD (Martínez-Pedraza & Carter, 2009). In order to recognize the spectrum of symptoms in the early years, ASD-specific training needs to be provided to medical and school-based professionals. Collaborations with trained professionals across fields of medicine, behavioral health, and education can assist with making earlier, more accurate diagnoses and improving health outcomes for families and young children with ASD (National Research Council, 2001). This chapter will discuss interdisciplinary issues pertaining to early schooling for children with ASD, and will conclude with recommendations for how to promote interdisciplinary care among relevant providers during the time of transition, thus reducing overall transition challenges.

Legal Mandates Guiding the Process of Early Schooling

In the United States, the Individuals with Disabilities Education Act (IDEA, 2004) is the nation's education mandate for providing free, appropriate public education to all children with disabilities. There are two parts of IDEA that support families of children transitioning into the school aged years, with the intention of providing continuity of supports and services in the community and school settings.

Infants and Toddlers

Part C of IDEA (2004) is intended for children from birth to 3 years of age and mandates that early intervention (EI) be provided to families of children who are considered at risk, who have a developmental delay, or who have a physical or psychological/mental condition associated with developmental delay (Scarborough, Hebbeler, & Spiker, 2006). EI has been shown to improve long-term child emotional, cognitive, and social development. Examples of EI services include screenings and assessments, therapy (e.g., physical, occupational, and speech/language therapy), and transportation (National Research Council, 2001). If the child qualifies for these services, a written Individualized Family Service Plan, or IFSP, will be developed by a team of providers, depending on the child and family's needs, to legally document which services the state will provide. The IFSP is a document indicating goals as specified jointly by the parent(s) and service providers (Lipkin & Okamoto, 2015).

Research has demonstrated that variability exists with regards to the Part C eligibility criteria used to identify children with developmental delays (Adams & Tapia, 2013; Stahmer & Mandell, 2007). For example, some states define developmental delays quantitively (e.g., the number of standard deviations the child is away from the normative development) or it is defined in more vague terms (e.g., not demonstrating expected behaviors based on chronological age). States also range on the type of professional who can determine if the child meets the state's eligibility of developmentally delayed (e.g., licensed health care provider, "qualified personal") (Shackelford, 2006, p. 12). Such inconsistencies in what populations are served make it difficult to evaluate and compare the effectiveness of EI programs. However, findings from a meta-analysis of studies on early intervention for children with ASD (mean age of 37.4 months) revealed stronger cognitive and adaptive behavior outcomes for programs associated with universities, hospitals, and research, compared to community-based settings (Nahmias, Pellecchia, Stahmer, & Mandell, 2019).

It is highly recommended that children with ASD be immediately referred for EI. Referrals are most commonly made by family members or healthcare professionals and less frequently by professionals within the education system, although, this situation will likely change with the more widespread awareness of ASD (Stahmer & Mandell, 2007). It is also less common for infants and toddlers to be in formal school settings, and thus, pediatricians and primary care physicians have an obligation as one of the first providers to observe atypical developmental behaviors and implement a screening assessment.

The services and supports that families are given through EI assist the child with long-term development (e.g., emotional, cognitive, and social; National Research Council, 2001). Research has shown that children with ASD who are minimally verbal are more likely to improve language skills if they receive intervention before entering the school system (at about 5 years of age) in comparison to children who start services after the age of five. Additionally, EI can help prevent the development of secondary symptoms associated with ASD (e.g., behavioral issues).

Preschool-Aged Children and the Transition to Kindergarten

Under IDEA Part B, children with disabilities between the ages of 3 to 22 years old have access to a free and appropriate public education (FAPE) within the least restrictive environment (LRE) through the school district (Lipkin & Okamoto, 2015; Trohanis, 2008, p. 143). FAPE is not plainly described within the IDEA legislation, but it refers to equal educational opportunity, at no cost, to every child (Lipkin & Okamoto, 2015). Another component of IDEA, Part B, is LRE. The aim of LRE is to integrate children with disabilities into the regular education environment "to the maximum extent possible" (Lipkin & Okamoto, 2015, p. e1651). Ideally, the child should spend a full school day in general education, but sometimes the child spends 50% or more in Special Education. An Individualized Education Program (IEP) is developed based on the child's needs, as determined by appropriate assessments. Similar to the IFSP, an IEP is a legal document that specifies the services that the school district will provide. However, the IEP document is more specific, it involves a range of interdisciplinary professionals and evolves as the child goes through school. School-based support and intervention may be deemed necessary to ensure the educational success of the child. As described by IDEA, states are in control of defining the eligibility criteria for such services (Lipkin & Okamoto, 2015).

The transition to early schooling is a crucial time for determining the portion of the school day that the child will have access to typically developing peers (LRE). It is critical for children with disabilities to have access to typically developing peers to assist with further development of the child's language and social skills. Finally, the IEP document helps to ensure some continuity of care, by hopefully continuing the types of services provided in early intervention, e.g., behavioral intervention, speech within the school system. One longitudinal study with a positive outcome followed children from preschool into kindergarten. In kindergarten, it was demonstrated that the child's classroom placement and services provided were consistent with those received prior to entry to early schooling (Towle, Vacanti-Shova, Higgins D'Alessandro, Ausikaitis & Reynolds, 2018).

Continuity of Care

ASD is a disorder that involves two main systems of care. The earliest is the medical system because physicians are most likely to see children prior to school age and are often involved in either diagnosing or referring the child for a more comprehensive evaluation. Once early intervention ensues, however, treatment is primarily educational. To maximize success for children with ASD, children need to be first identified and found.

Screening and Evaluation

Under IDEA, Child Find is an obligation for state agencies to identify children at risk of developmental delay in order to refer them for further evaluations and supports (Dosreis, Weiner, Johnson, & Newschaffer, 2006). For children under 3 years of age who are demonstrating behaviors of concern or are not meeting developmental milestones, parents have two options. Parents may request a free evaluation from their local EI provider or schedule a well-child visit with the child's pediatrician. At well-child visits, parents have the opportunity to voice their concerns about their child's development and discuss behavioral concerns. For primary care physicians, it is vital to educate parents about typical developmental milestones versus atypical development, and to provide a universal screening questionnaire or checklist to determine whether existing developmental or behavioral concerns may require formal supports. For first time parents, well-child visits may be even more important because they may not be as familiar with or informed about behaviors that require developmental monitoring (Barton, Dumont-Mathieu, & Fein, 2012). Despite how critical these visits are for children and parents, data from the Child and Adolescent Health Measurement Initiative (2016/2017) indicate that the national prevalence of developmental screenings by healthcare providers is low, with only about 35% of parents of children (ages 0–5) indicating that their doctor asked about developmental or behavioral concerns, and 31% of parents of infants and very young children (ages 9–35 months) indicating that they had completed a developmental screening tool. Reported barriers to pediatric screenings include increased physician time needed to implement testing and staffing needed to address potential issues or questions that may arise from the screening (Barton et al., 2012).

After the completion of a developmental screening, the primary care physician may make a referral for a comprehensive diagnostic evaluation in order to receive a medical diagnosis; this can be done by a screening clinic, specialist, or an EI team. A medical diagnosis is often considered the first step toward obtaining services for ASD, though it is not always required. The diagnostic evaluation should be done by a licensed physician, trained psychologist, or an educator who has experience or training in conducting developmental evaluations and assessing developmental disabilities. The evaluation should involve a review of developmental history and records, a parent interview, play-based observations, and assessments of cognitive and adaptive functioning. A neurological assessment or genetic consultation may be recommended to rule out biological or medical diagnoses. Based on the assessment results, a comprehensive report is developed for families to submit to the child's insurance company and to begin the provision of any needed family-based services (National Research Council, 2001). Figure 1 shows the steps families can take if their child is under 3 years old.

For children between the ages of 3 and 5 years, the screening and assessment process may differ depending on when parents initiate evaluation and services with the public schools. First, parents should discuss any behavioral observations and developmental concerns with a pediatrician or, if the child attends daycare or preschool,

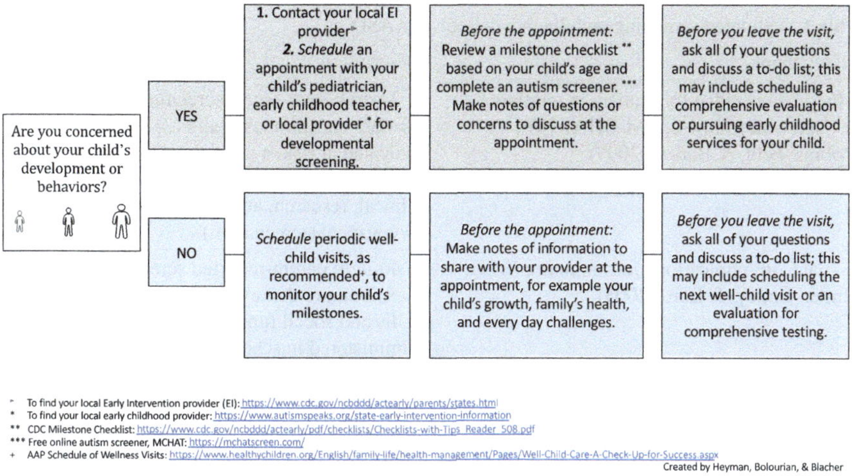

Fig. 1 Flowchart of the Early Developmental Screening Process for Families

a teacher. Depending on the pediatrician, a screening for ASD may be conducted, or a referral may be provided to the specialist (National Research Council, 2001). Alternatively, parents may submit a written letter to the school district detailing specific concerns and request an evaluation. The school district has the right to deny the parent's evaluation request, so it is important to include any previous records that support the parents' concerns. If the request is accepted and the evaluation indicates that there is a disability or delay, special education services will be provided to address issues before the start of kindergarten (Lipkin & Okamoto, 2015).

The selection of ASD-specific screening and diagnostic instruments is dependent on the diagnostic provider. Table 1 summarizes some validated screeners that can be used by healthcare and school-based professionals to identify behaviors indicating child risk for ASD. The Table also indicates gold-standard ASD assessments that should be administered by a trained provider if the child is deemed to be at risk. Such screening and diagnostic tools are described in detail in chapters "Screening and Surveillance" and "Interdisciplinary Evaluation of Autism Spectrum Disorder".

Utilization of Services

Medical Care

Children with ASD are at increased risk for co-occurring medical conditions (see chapter "Medical Comorbidities in Pediatric Autism Spectrum Disorder") and, thus, have higher costs of healthcare services, including hospitalizations, clinic visits, and prescription medication (Croen, Najjar, Ray, Lotspeich, & Bernal, 2006). Such

Table 1 Validated screening and diagnostic tools for ASD

Assessment	Description
Modified checklist for Autism in toddlers, revised with follow-up (M-CHAT-R/F; Robins, Fein, & Barton, 2009)	A 2-part parent-report screening tool: (1) a 20-item questionnaire, and (2) if the child is indicated at risk, a more detailed interview with the parent. Available for download for clinical, research, and educational purposes (www.mchatscreen.com)
Social Communication Questionnaire (SCQ; Rutter, Bailey, & Lord, 2003)	A 40-item parent-reported screening questionnaire that evaluates communication skills and social functioning. Can be administered in school and clinic settings
Childhood Autism rating scale, Second Edition (CARS2; Schopler, Van Bourgondien, Wellman, & Love, 2010)	A 15-item parent-completed rating scale that considers child behaviors (e.g., frequency, intensity, peculiarity, and duration) when formulating a potential diagnosis. Can be administered in school and clinic settings
Autism behavior checklist (ABC; Krug, Arick, & Almond, 1980)	A 57-item checklist, completed by a parent or teacher, often used in schools to help identify ASD among children with severe disabilities
Gilliam Autism rating scale-Third Edition (Gilliam, 2014)	A 58-item test, completed by parents or teachers. Used to screen for ASD in individuals, from 3 to 22 years of age with behavioral concerns
Autism diagnostic observation schedule, Second Edition (ADOS-2; Lord et al., 2012)	Gold-standard diagnostic tool, used by a trained professional, to determine if individuals meet diagnostic criteria for ASD. Semi-structured, play-based set of observations
Autism diagnostic interview-revised (ADI-R; Rutter, Le Couteur, & Lord, 2003)	A semi-structured interview (93 items), administered by a trained professional, with parents of children suspected of having ASD

expenditures for families of children with ASD are significantly greater than for families of children without ASD (Shimabukuro, Grosse, & Rice, 2007). Prior studies also reported that children with ASD have higher utilization of acute care, such as emergency department visits, than the general population (Deavenport-Saman, Lu, Smith, & Yin, 2015). This remains to be true when controlling for demographic characteristics and comorbid physical and mental conditions (Cummings et al., 2016).

Health care provided through an emergency or urgent-care facilities is often costlier and less effective. In ASD research, factors associated with fewer, non-urgent emergency visits include being older (six years of age and above) and individuals identifying as non-Hispanic. A great majority of visits by children with ASD also classified as primary care treatable, indicating that the use of emergency care was not required (Deavenport-Saman et al., 2015). Such findings may indicate that families of children with ASD need better, earlier access to effective healthcare services that may decrease the need to seek emergency care. In addition, in a sample of 396 adolescents and adults with ASD, Lunsky and colleagues (2015) found that one of the strongest predictors of emergency service use was previous emergency visits. Thus, improving healthcare access and utilization in early childhood years may divert the course of frequent and sometimes preventable emergency department visits.

Psychiatric Care

Children with ASD also experience significant co-occurring mental health conditions (see chapters "Interprofessional Roles to Support Psychotropic Medication Prescribing for ASD" and "Psychopharmacology of Autism Spectrum Disorder"). Previous research has shown that children with ASD utilize primary and specialty care (e.g., psychiatric visits, neurology visits) at higher rates than children without ASD (Croen et al., 2006; Gurney, McPheeters, & Davis, 2006; Kalb, Stuart, Freedman, Zablotsky, & Vasa, 2012; Lavelle et al., 2014; Liptak, Stuart, & Auinger, 2006). In a comparison of more than 30,000 children with or without ASD (ages 2–18) enrolled in the Kaiser Permanente Medical Care Program, Croen and colleagues (2006) found that children with ASD were significantly more likely to have a comorbid psychiatric diagnosis, such as a mood or impulse disorders. Specifically, for 2 to 4 year old children with ASD, psychiatric outpatient visits were 13 times more frequent than for children without ASD; for all other ages, psychiatric visits were 7 times more frequent in the ASD group. These findings point to the need for improving pediatric psychiatric services within networks of care for children with ASD. In addition, the mental health needs of the child with ASD affect families as well (Blacher & Baker, 2017), and thus, treatment should wrap around the needs of parents. Finally, the school professionals also need to be made aware of comorbid disorders in children with ASD. Notably, internalizing disorders may be under-reported by teachers (Llanes, Blacher, Stavropoulos, & Eisenhower, 2018). Additionally, children with ASD, with or without concomitant intellectual disability, have high rates of comorbid psychiatric disorders (Baker & Blacher, 2019), although more research on this topic relevant to young and school-age children with ASD is needed.

Coordinated Care

In contrast to care provided through emergency departments, the medical home model concentrates on primary inter-coordinated care. The medical home model, originated by the AAP, defines this mode of primary care as accessible, family-centered, continuous, comprehensive, coordinated, compassionate, and culturally effective (Medical Home Initiatives for Children with Special Needs Project Advisory Committee, 2002). Importantly, the most recent statement from the AAP indicates that the medical home system should allow parents to be able to develop a relationship with their child's physician that is characterized by mutual responsibility and trust. These perspectives on healthcare have the potential for substantial changes within the lives of families who have children with special needs. For example, Cheak-Zamora and Farmer (2015) found that access to family-centered care and care coordination was associated with lower unmet healthcare needs of children with ASD. A recent national survey supported by the Health Resources and Services Administration indicated that about 43% of children (ages 0–17) with special health care needs received care within a medical model, although some state-by-state variability exists (60.9% in Nebraska versus 24.6% in Nevada; Child and Adolescent Health Measurement Initiative, 2017).

Despite the comprehensive conceptualization of the medical home model, significant barriers to its implementation have been reported, including inadequate reimbursement for office and follow-up visits (Golnik, Ireland, & Borowsky, 2009; Medical Home Initiatives for Children with Special Needs Project Advisory Committee, 2002). Moreover, in a national survey of pediatricians and family physicians, respondents indicated a need for additional training and education about ASD, beyond training on overall special health care needs (Golnik et al., 2009). Families of children with ASD have also reported a lack of coordinated family-centered care, poor access to medical home, delayed referrals, lack of clinician knowledge about available community services, and limited confidence in the provided level of care (Brachlow, Ness, McPheeters, & Gurney, 2007; Carbone, Behl, Azor, & Murphy, 2010; Carbone et al., 2013).

Telehealth has been identified as a new, possible solution to certain barriers within systems of care (Todorow, Connell, & Turchi, 2018), such as long waitlists, transportation issues, and inadequate service access. As such, the focus of telehealth among families of children with ASD has primarily been on improving access to services among rural, underserved areas. In 2018, the Health Resources and Service Administration (HRSA) funded the Washington State Department of Health to improve access to statewide coordinated care for children with ASD through telehealth practices. Findings from the initial capacity assessment revealed that there is support among service providers and families. However, implementation issues with telehealth include technology knowledge, equipment, maintenance, billing, and reimbursement (Washington State Department of Health, 2017). In addition, telehealth has been touted as a model that can support the goals of early intervention, specifically through parent education and training. There is accumulating evidence to suggest that families can effectively help their children learn new skills in their natural environment (Boisvert & Hall, 2014). Interestingly, few studies have examined school-based telehealth services for children with ASD (Langkamp, McManus, & Blakemore, 2015).

Issues Impeding Access to Services

Effective interventions and services should be accessible across socioeconomic levels and among diverse groups. However, families of children with ASD experience substantial disparities in health care access and health promotion for several reasons. One factor associated with such disparities is geography, or location of residence. For example, families living in non-metropolitan areas report fewer service options and access, which may lead to increased use of emergency departments to address healthcare needs (Thomas, Ellis, McLaurin, Daniels, & Morrissey, 2007; Zhang, Mason, Boyd, Sikich, & Baranek, 2017). Notably, these families likely have less access to university or research-based services, which are often shown to be more effective than community-based service programs (Nahmias et al., 2019)

In a recent review of service disparities, race and socioeconomic status (SES) were identified as the prominent disadvantaging factors for children with ASD (Bishop-Fitzpatrick & Kind, 2017). Race, and to some extent culture, have consistently been found to predict disparities in service access and receipt (Blacher, Cohen, & Azad, 2014; Blacher et al., 2019; Broder-Fingert, Shui, Pulcini, Kurowski, & Perrin, 2013; Doshi, Tilford, Ounpraseuth, Kuo, & Payakachat, 2017; Liptak et al., 2008; Magaña, Parish, Rose, Timerblake & Swaine, 2012; Magaña, Parish, & Son, 2015; Parish, Magaña, Rose, Timberlake, & Swaine, 2012). Overall, studies have indicated differences in the quantity and quality of care. Qualitatively, parents of non-White children with ASD, compared to parents of White children with ASD, are more likely to report the following: having limited access to physicians who listen; receiving less timely care; experiencing less time with child's physician; experiencing less attention to cultural and familial values; needing more information about ASD (Liptak et al., 2008; Magaña et al., 2012, 2015; Parish et al., 2012). In addition, non-White families of children with ASD, when compared to White families, are also less likely to receive specialized care (e.g., neurology, gastroenterology, psychiatry) or coordinated, family-centered care (Broder-Fingert et al., 2013; Doshi et al., 2017). In a follow-up study of trends in healthcare service access for families of children with ASD, Magaña and colleagues (2015) found that low-quality care persisted over a 5-year period, suggesting that disparities tend not to improve.

Belonging to a family with low socioeconomic status (SES) has been associated with poorer quality of care and being uninsured (Liptak et al., 2008). High SES families have been shown to have greater access to care within a medical home model (Sobtoka, Francis, Vander, & Booth, 2016). However, the relationship between SES and healthcare may be mediated or partially explained by parent knowledge of service systems, such that higher SES is associated with greater knowledge about ASD-related services, which is associated with a higher number of services used (Pickard & Ingersoll, 2015).

Conclusion: Making the Transition to Early Schooling Less Challenging

During early childhood development, families of young children with ASD experience stressful situations, often before the diagnostic process begins. Even highly resourced parents face roadblocks in obtaining a diagnostic evaluation for ASD and subsequently advocating for appropriate treatments, so it is often the case that under-resourced families face even greater obstacles. The number of reported barriers to accessing and receiving quality inter-coordinated services suggests that there is room for improvement. This section contains key areas that address some of these barriers.

Parent and Community Outreach

First, it is important to equip parents with the knowledge needed to navigate service systems during preschool or early intervention in order for them to later advocate for ASD-related services and become better able to secure necessary supports on behalf of their children and families. This is vitally important when all parents do not have equal access to such service systems. In the U.S., national trends indicate an increase in racial diversity, with Latinx populations increasing by almost 20 million between 2000 and 2014 (Colby & Ortman, 2015). Recognizing service disparities related to race and the nation's diversity, there is clearly a need to train professionals to work effectively with underserved families of children with ASD using a culturally responsive approach (e.g., learning cultural beliefs about child development and disability). Moreover, as most evidence-based ASD interventions have been validated with White families, research should seek to adapt interventions for culturally and racially diverse children with ASD, and address gaps in the research related to the effectiveness of early intervention programs in the community versus academic settings (Cohen, 2013).

As described previously, families who have insufficient access to services are also likely to be from underserved communities that are often difficult to reach, perhaps due to geographic location or lack of transportation. It is crucial, then, to find ways to reach these families—through the dissemination of information on systems of care, especially to families who are disconnected from service providers. Culturally relevant programs and practices need to be developed to help these families to increase access to screening, intervention services, and advocacy. For example, Zuckerman et al. (2014) conducted focus groups targeting Latinx families whose children were diagnosed with ASD at 2.8 years, on average. Family members reported that they had limited access to information with regards to ASD within their community and received little support from their community when they wanted to discuss their child's behaviors and symptoms related to ASD. Additionally, the parents experienced difficulty when finding the care their child with ASD needed; when they found professionals to assist with their initial diagnosis, the appointments were described as being confusing, long, and tedious for the child.

An example of successful outreach to under-resourced families exists in the Inland Empire of Southern California (i.e., the counties of Riverside and San Bernardino, as well as the desert communities of Palm Springs and Coachella Valley), a population of about four million. Under the auspices of the University of California, Riverside, the SEARCH Center is an organization that is dedicated to providing Support, Education, Advocacy, Resources, Community, and Hope to families who have children with ASD. With a focus on screening and educational access for underrepresented groups, SEARCH reaches about 100 children a year at no financial cost to families. To date, slightly over 50% of children screened have been Latinx and 20% have been Spanish-speaking, and research has indicated that there are cultural differences in the concerns that parents bring to the screening clinic (Blacher et al., 2019). Through educational consultations and parent education programs, SEARCH helps affected families understand ASD, and to learn how to select appropriate programs and services designed to meet their children's developmental, behavioral, and academic needs. SEARCH is supported by institutional and research funding and has partnered with ASD-related and disability agencies in the area to promote equity and reduce disparities in the services for youth with ASD or developmental disabilities. The net result is an effort to disseminate information on ASD to regions in need in a culturally sensitive manner—to inform, educate, and link families to existing services. The more readily parents expand their networks while their children with ASD are very young, and the more they use their skills to advocate for their child, the smoother the transition to kindergarten and early schooling will be.

Here is a case brought to the SEARCH Center:

V. is the Latina mother of a 3 ½ -year old son, Ivan. V. spoke English, but not well. When his mother first contacted SEARCH, her specific concerns were conveyed to staff in Spanish, and included Ivan's difficulty with even the slightest changes in routine—for example, moving from play to lunch. Ivan also did not speak more than 20 words, and did not engage in any conversations or back-and-forth interactions with his siblings, parents or children in his preschool class. V. consulted her non-Spanish-speaking pediatrician when her son was 2 ½ years old. The pediatrician said that these types of delays were common, but she administered a brief developmental checklist anyway. The pediatrician admitted that she was not sure but thought the parent should be referred to the SEARCH Center, a local autism screening center, to rule out the possibility of ASD. V. waited another year before calling SEARCH. The importance of pursuing further assessment as soon as possible was not conveyed to V., and she and her immediate friends and family were not aware of red flags for ASD. The pediatrician also did not mention that the services at SEARCH were free.

During the phone-call with the SEARCH team member, V. completed the *Social Communication Questionnaire* (SCQ; Rutter, Bailey, & Lord, 2003). Based on the SCQ, Ivan appeared to be in the risk range for ASD, and a full assessment was scheduled. At the assessment appointment, the team administered the ADOS-2 (Lord et al., 2012) and a cognitive assessment to Ivan. V. completed an interview about Ivan's development, an adaptive behavior interview (*Vineland Adaptive Behavior*

Scales; Sparrow, Ciccetti, & Saulnier, 2016). Several parent-completed questionnaires focused on possible child behavior problems and autism symptomatology. Ivan did meet criteria for ASD, and also appeared to have meet criteria for a developmental delay, based on his adaptive and cognitive development. V. was shown how to contact her local regional center to request services, additional evaluations (i.e., speech), and behavioral intervention services for Ivan. Since V. was employed full-time, a behaviorally-oriented intensive early intervention center-based preschool program was recommended. Notably, Ivan missed the opportunity to enter the early intervention system at age 2 ½, and valuable time for speech and cognitive development had been lost.

Professional Training

There is still a reported need for inter-disciplinary trainings related to ASD-specific knowledge (e.g., Golnik et al., 2009), as well as to positive relationship development between professionals and family members of children with ASD. The production of ASD-specific training programs should begin in graduate school (e.g., education and psychology doctoral/master's programs, teacher credential programs, medical school). While the foundation of these programs should be content-based, courses may be enhanced by using practitioner-based research or case-based learning in order to support reflective thinking about one's own practice. By investing in training programs that increase expertise in ASD, we can help meet the service and treatment challenges these families face.

Developed by the CDC and the Health Resources and Services Administration's Maternal Child Health Bureau in 2011, the Autism Case Training (ACT) curriculum targets developmental-behavioral pediatrics and is designed to train future clinicians on the identification, diagnosis, and management of ASD through real-life scenarios. ACT has been peer-reviewed and endorsed by the American Academy of Pediatrics (Major, 2015). Pilot studies indicate that the program is found to be useful by pediatric residents and is associated with positive short-term changes in overall knowledge and perceived competence (Major, Peacock, Ruben, Thomas, & Weitzman, 2013). The ACT modules and resources (e.g., facilitator guide, discussion questions, handouts, video library) are downloadable at no cost through the CDC website (http://www.cdc.gov/AutismCaseTraining) to ensure that autism education is accessible for all practicing pediatric clinicians (see chapter "Interprofessional Education and Training").

Removing the Disconnect from Early Intervention to Public Schools

Lastly, greater communication among service providers across disciplines is needed. Engaging in a collaborative exchange with professionals across disciplines will help generate and synthesize knowledge of individual families in order to provide more appropriate supports, and these are desperately needed at the transition from preschool to "big school," or kindergarten. This will require a collaborative effort on the part of families, insurers, government, medical educators, and other systems of care who support families through early intervention. Collaborative partnerships will help to assure smooth sailing for these families.

Acknowledgments We appreciate the support from the SEARCH Family Autism Resource Center, Graduate School of Education at UC Riverside, and from the Vernon Eady Endowment.

References

Adams, R. C., & Tapia, C. (2013). Early intervention, IDEA part C services, and the medical home: Collaboration for best practice and best outcomes. *Pediatrics, 132,* e1073–e1088.
American Psychiatric Association. (2013). *Diagnostic and statistical manual of mental disorders* (5th ed.). Washington, DC: Author.
Baker, B. L., & Blacher, J. (2019). Brief report. Behavior disorders and social skills in adolescents with autism spectrum disorder: Does IQ matter? *Journal of Autism and Developmental Disorders.*
Barton, M. L., Dumont-Mathieu, T., & Fein, D. (2012). Screening young children for autism spectrum disorders in primary practice. *Journal of Autism and Developmental Disorders, 42,* 1165–1174.
Bishop-Fitzpatrick, L., & Kind, A. J. H. (2017). A scoping review of health disparities in autism spectrum disorder. *Journal of Autism and Developmental Disorders, 47,* 3380–3391.
Blacher, J., & Baker, B. L. (2017). Collateral effects of youth disruptive behavior disorders on mothers' psychological distress: Adolescents with autism spectrum disorder, intellectual disability, or typical development. *Journal of Autism and Developmental Disorders, 49,* 2810–2821.
Blacher, J., Cohen, S. R., & Azad, G. F. (2014). In the eye of the beholder: Reports of autism symptoms by Anglo and Latino parents. *Research in Autism Spectrum Disorders, 8*(12), 1648–1656.
Blacher, J., Stavropoulos, K. K. M., & Bolourian, Y. (2019). Anglo-Latino differences in parental concerns and service inequities for children at risk of ASD. *Autism: International Journal of Research and Practice, 23,* 1554–1562.
Boisvert, M., & Hall, N. (2014). The use of telehealth in early autism training for parents: A scoping review. *Smart Homecare Technology and Telehealth, 2,* 19–27.
Brachlow, A. E., Ness, K. K., McPheeters, M. L., & Gurney, J. G. (2007). Comparison of indicators for a primary care medical home between children with autism or asthma and other special health care needs. *Archives of Pediatrics and Adolescent Medicine, 161*(4), 399–405.
Broder-Fingert, S., Shui, A., Pulcini, C. D., Kurowski, D., & Perrin, J. M. (2013). Racial and ethnic differences in subspecialty service use by children with autism. *Pediatrics, 132,* 94–100.
Carbone, P. S., Behl, D. D., Azor, V., & Murphy, N. A. (2010). The medical home for children with autism spectrum disorders: Parent and pediatrician perspectives. *Journal of Autism and Developmental Disorders, 40,* 317–324.

Carbone, P. S., Murphy, N. A., Norlin, C., Azor, V., Sheng, X., & Young, P. C. (2013). Parent and pediatrician perspectives regarding the primary care of children with autism spectrum disorders. *Journal of Autism and Developmental Disorders, 43,* 964–972.

Center for Disease Control and Prevention. (2019). learn the signs. Act early. https://www.cdc.gov/ncbddd/actearly/index.html.

Cheak-Zamora, N. C., & Farmer, J. E. (2015). The impact of the medical home on access to care for children with autism spectrum disorders. *Journal of Autism and Developmental Disorders, 45,* 636–644.

Child and Adolescent Health Measurement Initiative. (2016/2017). National survey of children's health (NSCH) data query. Data resource center for child and adolescent health supported by cooperative agreement U59MC27866 from the U.S. Department of Health and Human Services, Health Resources and Services Administration's Maternal and Child Health Bureau (HRSA MCHB). Retrieved from https://www.childhealthdata.org.

Cohen, S. R. (2013). Advocacy for the "Abandonados": Harnessing cultural beliefs for Latino families and their children with intellectual disabilities. *Journal of Policy and Practice in Intellectual Disabilities, 10,* 71–78.

Colby, S. L., & Ortman, J. M. (2015). *Projections of the size and composition of the US population: 2014 to 2060. Current population reports.* Washington, DC: U.S. Census Bureau. Retrieved from https://www.census.gov/content/dam/Census/library/publications/2015/demo/p25-1143.pdf.

Croen, L. A., Najjar, D. V., Ray, G. T., Lotspeich, L., & Bernal, P. (2006). A comparison of health care utilization and costs of children with and without autism spectrum disorders in a large group-model health plan. *Pediatrics, 118*(4), e1203–e1211.

Cummings, J. R., Lynch, F. L., Rust, K. C., Coleman, K. J., Madden, J. M., & Croen, L. A. (2016). Health services utilization among children with and without autism spectrum disorders. *Journal of Autism and Developmental Disorders, 46,* 910–920.

Deavenport-Saman, A., Lu, Y., Smith, K., & Yin, L. (2015). Do children with autism overutilize the emergency department? Examining visit urgency and subsequent hospital admissions. *Maternal and Child Health Journal, 20*(2), 306–314.

Doshi, P., Tilford, J., Ounpraseuth, S., Kuo, D., & Payakachat, N. (2017). Do insurance mandates affect racial disparities in outcomes for children with autism? *Maternal and Child Health Journal, 21*(2), 351–366.

Dosreis, S., Weiner, C. L., Johnson, L., & Newschaffer, C. J. (2006). Autism spectrum disorder screening and management practices among general pediatric providers. *Journal of Developmental and Behavioral Pediatrics, 27,* S88–S94.

Gilliam, J. E. (2014). *Gilliam Autism Rating Scale* (3rd ed.). Austin, TX: PRO-ED.

Golnik, A., Ireland, M., & Borowsky, I. W. (2009). Medical homes for children with autism: A physician survey. *Pediatrics, 123*(3), 966–971.

Gurney, J. G., McPheeters, M. L., & Davis, M. M. (2006). Parental report of health conditions and health care use among children with and without autism: National survey of children's health. *Archives of Pediatrics and Adolescent Medicine, 160*(8), 825–830.

Hyman, S. L., Levy, S. E., & Myers, S. M. (2020). Identification, evaluation, and management of children with autism spectrum disorder. *Pediatrics, 145,* 1–64.

Individuals with Disabilities Education Act, 20 U.S.C. § 1400. (2004).

Järbrink, J. (2007). The economic consequences of autistic spectrum disorder among children in a Swedish municipality. *Autism, 11,* 452–463.

Kalb, L. G., Stuart, E. A., Freedman, B., Zablotsky, B., & Vasa, R. (2012). Psychiatric-related emergency department visits among children with an autism spectrum disorder. *Pediatric Emergency Care, 28,* 1269–1276.

Kemp, C., & Carter, M. (2005). Identifying skills for promoting successful inclusion in kindergarten. *Journal of Intellectual and Developmental Disability, 30,* 31–44.

Koegel, L. K., Koegel, R. L., Ashbaugh, K., & Bradshaw, J. (2014). The importance of early identification and intervention for children with or at risk for autism spectrum disorders. *International Journal of Speech-Language Pathology, 16,* 50–56.

Krug, D. A., Arick, J., & Almond, P. (1980). Behavior checklist for identifying severely handicapped individuals with high levels of autistic behavior. *Journal of Child Psychology and Psychiatry, 21,* 221–229.

Langkamp, D. L., McManus, M. D., & Blakemore, S. D. (2015). Telemedicine for children with developmental disabilities: A more effective clinical process than office-based care. *Telemedicine and e-Health, 21,* 110–114.

Larcombe, T. J., Joosten, A. V., Cordier, R., & Vaz, S. (2019). Preparing children with autism for transition to mainstream school and perspectives on supporting positive school experiences. *Journal of Autism and Developmental Disorders, 49,* 3073–3088.

Lavelle, T. A., Weinstein, M. C., Newhouse, J. P., Munir, K., Kuhlthau, K. A., & Prosser, L. A. (2014). Economic burden of childhood autism spectrum disorders. *Pediatrics, 133,* e520–e529.

Lipkin, P. H., & Okamoto, J. (2015). The Individuals with Disabilities Education Act (IDEA) for children with special educational needs. *Pediatrics, 136,* e1650–e1662.

Liptak, G. S., Stuart, T., & Auinger, P. (2006). Health care utilization and expenditures for children with autism: Data from U.S. National Samples. *Journal of Autism and Developmental Disorders, 36,* 871–879.

Liptak, G. S., Benzoni, L. B., Mruzek, D. W., Nolan, K. W., Thingvoll, M. A., Wade, C. M., & Fryer, G. E. (2008). Disparities in diagnosis and access to health services for children with autism: Data from the national survey of children's health. *Journal of Developmental and Behavioral Pediatrics, 29,* 152–160.

Llanes, E., Blacher, J., Stavropoulos, K. K. M., & Eisenhower, A. (2018). Parent and teacher reports of comorbid anxiety and ADHD symptoms in children with ASD. *Journal of Autism and Developmental Disorders,* 1–12. https://doi.org/10.1007/s10803-018-3701-z.

Lord, C., & Luyster, R. (2006). Early diagnosis of children with autism spectrum disorders. *Clinical Neuroscience Research, 6*(3–4), 189-194.

Lord, C., Rutter, M., DiLavore, P., Risi, S., Gotham, K., & Bishop, S. (2012). *Autism Diagnostic Observation Schedule–2nd Edition (ADOS-2).* Los Angeles, CA: Western Psychological Corporation.

Lunsky, Y., Paquette-Smith, M., Weiss, J. A., & Lee, J. (2015). Predictors of emergency service use in adolescents and adults with autism spectrum disorder living with family. *Emergency Medical Journal, 32*(10), 787–792.

Magaña, S., Parish, S. L., Rose, R. A., Timberlake, M., & Swaine, J. G. (2012). Racial and ethnic disparities in quality of health care among children with autism and other developmental disabilities. *Intellectual and Developmental Disabilities, 50*(4), 287–299.

Magaña, S., Parish, S. L., & Son, E. (2015). Have racial and ethnic disparities in the quality of health care relationships changed for children with developmental disabilities and ASD? *American Journal of Intellectual and Developmental Disabilities, 120,* 504–513.

Major, N. E. (2015). Autism education in residency training programs. *AMA Journal of Ethics, 17*(4), 318–322.

Major, N. E., Peacock, G., Ruben, W., Thomas, J., & Weitzman, C. C. (2013). Autism training in pediatric residency: Evaluation of a case-based curriculum. *Journal of Autism and Developmental Disorders, 43,* 1171–1177.

Mandell, D. S., Listerud, J., Levy, S. E., & Pinto-Martin, J. A. (2002). Race differences in the age at diagnosis among medicaid-eligible children with autism. *Journal of the American Academy of Child and Adolescent Psychiatry, 41*(12), 1447–1453.

Marsh, A., Spagnol, V., Grove, R., & Eapen, V. (2017). Transition to school for children with autism spectrum disorder: A systematic review. *World Journal of Psychiatry, 7,* 184.

Martínez-Pedraza, F. D. L., & Carter, A. S. (2009). Autism spectrum disorders in young children. *Child and Adolescent Psychiatric Clinics, 18*(3), 645–663.

McIntyre, L. L., Blacher, J., & Baker, B. L. (2006). The transition to school: Adaptation in young children with and without developmental disability. *The Journal of Intellectual Disability Research, 50,* 349–361.

Medical Home Initiatives for Children with Special Needs Project Advisory Committee. (2002). The medical home. *Pediatrics, 110,* 184–186.

Nahmias, A. S., Pellecchia, M., Stahmer, A. C., & Mandell, D. S. (2019). Effectiveness of community-based early intervention for children with autism spectrum disorder: A meta-analysis. *Journal of Child Psychology and Psychiatry, 60,* 1200–1209.

National Research Council. (2001). Educating children with autism. Committee on educational interventions for children with autism. In C. Lord and J. P. McGee (Eds.), *Division of behavioral and social sciences and education.* Washington, DC: National Academy Press. Accessed 11 Dec 2011.

Parish, S., Magaña, S., Rose, R., Timberlake, M., & Swaine, J. G. (2012). Health care of Latino children with autism and other developmental disabilities: Quality of provider interaction mediates utilization. *American Journal on Intellectual and Developmental Disabilities, 117,* 304–315.

Pickard, K. E., & Ingersoll, B. R. (2015). From research settings to parents: The role of parent social networks in the choices parents make about services for their child with autism spectrum disorder. *Clinical Psychological Science, 3,* 256–269.

Rimm-Kaufman, S. E., Curby, T. W., Grimm, K. J., Nathanson, L., & Brock, L. L. (2009). The contribution of children's self-regulation and classroom and classroom quality to children's adaptive behaviors in the kindergarten classroom. *Developmental Psychology, 45*(4), 958–972.

Robins, D. L., Fein, D., & Barton, M. L. (2009). *Modified Checklist for Autism in Toddlers, Revised with Follow-Up (M-CHAT-R/F).* Self-published.

Rosanbalm, K. D., & Murray, D. W. (2017). *Promoting self-regulation in early childhood: A practice brief. OPRE Brief#2017–79.* Washington, DC: Office of Planning, Research, and Evaluation, Administration for Children and Families, US. Department of Health and Human Services.

Rosenberg, R. E., Kaufmann, W. E., Law, J. K., & Law, P. A. (2011). Parent report of community psychiatric comorbid diagnoses in autism spectrum disorders. *Autism Research and Treatment, 2011,* 1–10.

Rutter, M., Bailey, A., & Lord, C. (2003). *The Social Communication Questionnaire: Manual.* Western Psychological Services.

Rutter, M., Le Couteur, A., & Lord, C. (2003). *Autism diagnostic interview-revised.* Los Angeles, CA: Western Psychological Services.

Rutter, M., Bailey, A., & Lord, C. (2003). *Manual for the social communication questionnaire.* Los Angeles, CA: Western Psychological Services.

Scarborough, A. A., Hebbeler, K. M., & Spiker, D. (2006). Eligibility characteristics of infants and toddlers entering early intervention services in the United States. *Journal of Policy and Practice in Intellectual Disabilities, 3,* 57–64.

Schopler, E., Van Bourgondien, M., Wellman, J., & Love, S. (2010). *Childhood Autism Rating Scale—Second Edition (CARS2): Manual.* Los Angeles: Western Psychological Services.

Shackelford, J. (2006). *State and Jurisdictional eligibility definitions for infants and toddlers with disabilities under IDEA. NECTAC notes,* Issue No. 21. National Early Childhood Technical Assistance Center (NECTAC).

Shimabukuro, T. T., Grosse, S. D., & Rice, C. (2007). Medical expenditures for children with an autism spectrum disorder in a privately insure population. *Journal of Autism and Developmental Disorders, 38,* 546–552.

Sobotka, S. A., Francis, A., Vander, P., & Booth, K. (2016). Associations of family characteristics with perceptions of care among parents of children with autism. *Child: Care, Health and Development, 42,* 135–140.

Sparrow, S. S., Cicchetti, D. V., & Saulnier, C. A. (2016). *Vineland Adaptive Behavior Scales, (Vineland-3)* (3rd ed.). San Antonio, TX: Pearson.

Stahmer, A. C., & Mandell, D. S. (2007). State infant/toddler program policies for eligibility and services provision for young children with autism. *Administration and Policy in Mental Health and Mental Health Services Research, 34,* 29–37.

Thomas, K. C., Ellis, A. R., McLaurin, C., Daniels, J., & Morrissey, J. P. (2007). Access to care for autism-related services. *Journal of Autism and Developmental Disorders, 37,* 1902–1912.

Todorow, C., Connell, J., & Turchi, R. M. (2018). The medical home for children with autism spectrum disorder: An essential element whose time has come. *Current Opinions in Pediatrics, 30,* 311–317.

Towle, P. O., Vacanti-Shova, K., Higgins-D'Alessaddro, A., Ausikaitis, A., & Reynolds, C. (2018). A longitudinal study of children diagnosed with autism spectrum disorder before age three: School services at three points time for three levels of outcome disability. *Journal of Autism and Developmental Disorders, 49,* 3747–3760.

Trohanis, P. L. (2008). Progress in providing services to young children with special needs and their families: An overview to and update on the implementation of the Individuals with Disabilities Education Act (IDEA). *Journal of Early Intervention, 30,* 140–151.

Turner, L. M., & Stone, W. L. (2007). Variability in outcome for children with an ASD diagnosis at age 2. *Journal of Child Psychology and Psychiatry, 48,* 793–802.

Warren, Z., McPheeters, M. L., Sathe, N., Foss-Feig, J. H., Glasser, A., & Veenstra-VanderWeele, J. (2011). A systematic review of early intensive intervention for autism spectrum disorders. *Pediatrics, 127,* e1303–e1311.

Washington State Department of Health. (2017). 2017 AS3D telehealth capacity assessment. Retrieved from https://www.doh.wa.gov/Portals/1/Documents/Pubs/970-225-AS3D2017THCapacityAssessmentExecutiveSummary.pdf.

Woods, J. J., & Wetherby, A. M. (2003). Early identification of and intervention for infants and toddlers who are at risk for autism spectrum disorder. *Language, Speech, and Hearing Services in Schools, 34,* 180–193.

Zhang, W., Mason, A. E., Boyd, B., Sikich, L., & Baranek, G. (2017). A rural–urban comparison in emergency department visits for U.S. children with autism spectrum disorder. *Journal of Autism and Developmental Disorders, 47,* 590–598.

Zuckerman, K. E., Sinche, B., Mejia, A., Cobian, M., Becker, T., & Nicolaidis, C. (2014). Latino parents' perspectives on barriers to autism diagnosis. *Academic Pediatrics, 14*(3), 301–308.

Promoting Academic Success

Kaitlin Bundock, Vicki Simonsmeier, Megan E. Golson, Benjamin Covington, and Maryellen Brunson McClain

Abstract Students with Autism Spectrum Disorder (ASD) comprise a large percentage of students receiving special education services in schools. Students with ASD have particular areas of need that may influence their academic and school success. In this chapter, we describe some of the reading, mathematics, and communication difficulties students with ASD may have in schools and provide an overview of effective strategies and interventions. Using an applied fictional case example, we highlight how interdisciplinary collaboration can be used within schools to maximize the success of all students with ASD.

One in 59 children have Autism Spectrum Disorder (ASD) and an average of 65–70% of these children receive special education services (Baio et al., 2018).[1] Autism is the largest growing special education eligibility category for students under the Individuals with Disabilities Education Act (IDEA, 2004; Kim, Bal, & Lord, 2018; McDonald et al., 2019). Students with ASD have a wide range of academic skills and abilities and are served in a variety of educational placements, from specialized

[1]Autism refers the special education eligibility category whereas autism spectrum disorder (ASD) refers to the Diagnostic and Statistical Manual of Mental Disorders, 5th edition (DSM-5; American Psychiatric Association, 2013) disorder. Autism is used to describe students who receive special education services under this eligibility category whereas ASD describes individuals with a medical diagnosis of ASD. It should be noted that a child may have both a medical diagnosis of ASD AND receive special education services or one or the other. In this chapter, although we are focusing on the school setting, we are referring to children with ASD who are students in schools, including those who do and do not receive special education services.

K. Bundock (✉)
Department of Special Education and Rehabilitation Counseling, Utah State University, Logan, UT, USA
e-mail: kaitlin.bundock@usu.edu

V. Simonsmeier
Sorenson Legacy Foundation Center for Clinical Excellence, Utah State University, Logan, UT, USA

M. E. Golson · B. Covington · M. B. McClain
Department of Psychology, Utah State University, Logan, UT, USA

M. B. McClain et al. (eds.), *Interprofessional Care Coordination for Pediatric Autism Spectrum Disorder*, https://doi.org/10.1007/978-3-030-46295-6_9

schools and self-contained classrooms, to fully inclusive general education settings (McDonald et al., 2019). Most students with ASD in public schools are included in general education settings for at least some of the school day (McDonald et al., 2019).

Students with ASD may require services at different times throughout their lives. This chapter focuses on services and supports for K-12 students with ASD under IDEA Part B by (a) describing broadly what students with ASD need to be successful in school, (b) providing an overview of the strengths and needs of students with ASD in reading, mathematics, and communication, (c) describing the associated research-based interventions that address these needs, (d) highlighting how interdisciplinary collaboration between school service providers can best meet the needs of students with ASD in academic settings, and (e) illustrating a case example of a successful interdisciplinary collaboration within multi-tiered systems of support.

What Supports Do Students with ASD Need to Be Successful in School?

Students with ASD experience a wide range of educational outcomes, in part due to the broad range of skills and abilities of individuals with ASD. Even though approximately half of the students diagnosed with ASD have average to above average cognitive skills (White et al., 2016) they have lower rates of college enrollment compared to other students with and without disabilities (Wei, Yu, Shattuck, & Blackorby, 2017). These indicators, combined with the increasing prevalence rates of ASD (McDonald et al., 2019), necessitate that school and community professionals work collaboratively to improve the academic success of students with ASD (Guldberg et al., 2011).

When working with students who have ASD, it is important to avoid focusing solely on academic deficits. Instead, practitioners should assess and recognize the strengths of students with ASD and use them when designing proactive and responsive instructional supports and interventions. Additionally, practitioners should recognize that the presence of ASD does not automatically mean that students will face academic deficits. In fact, many students with ASD are gifted in a variety of content areas (Kim et al., 2018). As a result, instructional planning for students with ASD should also include opportunities for extension and enrichment to allow gifted students with ASD opportunities to meet their academic potential and incorporate their personal preferences (Bianco et al., 2009).

Students with ASD may have specific areas of need related to school success. Multiple authors (e.g., Kasari & Patterson, 2012; Prelock & McCauley, 2012) have also identified difficulties in joint attention as a core difficulty for students with ASD, a skill which is typically developed during early childhood (before age 2). In a review of cognitive training technologies used to treat emotion, language-literacy, and social skills, Wass and Porayska-Pomsta (2014) found that while students made some improvement when using technologies, there was a little carry over into other settings. Based on these results, they conclude that the difficulties students with ASD may have in transferring and generalizing knowledge may in part be due to difficulties applying new knowledge and skills in noisy, distracting, real-world settings. Therefore, when working with students with ASD, it is important to attend not only to their needs related to skills and knowledge, but also to consider how to support generalization of these skills to novel environments. With these needs in mind, we turn to patterns of academic performance of students with ASD.

School Functioning and Students with ASD

The achievement needs and supports of students with ASD vary within and across individuals. When students with ASD receive services in inclusive environments, priority should be placed on providing them access to the general education environment and curriculum. Within these settings, it is essential that professionals within and outside of schools collaborate to meet the needs of students with ASD. Similar to all individuals, people with ASD can have varying cognitive abilities and achievement across academic domains (Bianco et al., 2009; Kim et al., 2018). Practitioners should rely primarily on individual student assessment when determining specific profiles of academic and functional performance and only use the information below for general guidance.

Reading

Students with ASD exhibit variable reading skills and predictive factors (i.e., decoding abilities, vocabulary, social communication skills, attention, eye-tracking, language abilities, cognitive abilities) of reading skills within this population are also wide-ranging (e.g., Brown, Oram-Cardy, & Johnson, 2013; Micai, Holly, Vulchanova, & Saldana, 2017; Nation, Clarke, Wright, & Williams, 2016; Norbury & Nation, 2011). In comparison to neurotypical peers, many students with ASD demonstrate comparable reading fluency skills, but significantly poorer reading comprehension skills (McIntyre et al., 2017). Subsequently, many students with ASD may appear to be strong readers when they read text fluently (reading fluency), but they may not be understanding what they read (reading comprehension). Text that is high in social content or requires inferential skills may be even more challenging for students with ASD (e.g., Davidson, Kaushanskaya, & Weismer, 2018; Tirado & Saldaña, 2016). The development of reading comprehension skills is important as students begin to use these skills to learn content from and demonstrate mastery of other academic areas (e.g., science). The assessment of both reading fluency and comprehension skills for students with ASD is critical to adequately determine needs and educational planning surrounding literacy.

Mathematics

Several studies indicate that the mathematical abilities of autistic children are also highly variable. Within-group research suggests that there may be multiple profiles of ASD and math performance, ranging from very low to very high while controlling for intellectual quotient (IQ) and other competencies (Chen et al., 2019; Jones et al., 2009; Wei et al., 2015). For example, Jones et al. (2009) found three distinct math/IQ profiles for 14- to 16-year-olds diagnosed with ASD, including groups whose numerical operations abilities exceeded, fell short of, or matched their full-scale IQ . Similarly, Chen et al. (2019) found that while typically developing 7- to 12-year-olds exhibited homogeneous math and reading abilities, age-matched children with an ASD could be distinctly divided into two groups: those with lower math than reading skills and those with higher math than reading skills.

When students with ASD reach higher levels of academic mathematics, their performance may be largely affected by their verbal comprehension, perceptual reasoning (e.g., the ability to abstract and comprehend conceptual relationships), and anxiety (Oswald et al., 2016). In other words, inferior mathematics performance may not be the result of an auxiliary deficit, but rather may be a consequence of hallmark social and communication deficits at the core of ASD. Given that mathematics instruction is inextricably linked to language comprehension, as well as social interaction between the teacher and the student, deficits may relate more to instructional method than to subject matter.

Communication

Communication skills are tied to student performance in all content areas and are integral to navigating the academic and social context of schools (White et al., 2016). In 1943, when Kanner described students with what we now call ASD, he noted "if language developed" it was marked by echolalia, pronoun reversals, and concreteness (Volkmar et al., 2014). As we have improved and changed the diagnostic criteria for ASD, we now understand that students may have these difficulties, but their difficulties in speech, language, and communication are varied. Difficulties in communication, particularly in social-pragmatic communication, are now considered one of the defining characteristics of individuals who are identified as having ASD. The DSM-5 (APA, 2013) describes the social-pragmatic difficulties in greeting, sharing, using verbal and non-verbal communication, and difficulties in understanding idioms, humor, metaphors, and multiple meaning in varied contexts. Consequently, most research in the communication of individuals with ASD has focused on the pre-linguistic and developing language skills of students with ASD (see chapter 'Coordinating Speech-Language Pathology Services for Youth with Autism Spectrum Disorder' for additional information) rather than on the academic language needs of these same students as they age and progress through the educational system.

The heterogeneity of symptoms in students with ASD is also evidenced in their communication skills. Difficulties in communication are found in non-verbal, as well as verbal skills. Students with ASD often do not point to express interest (DSM-5, 2013; Volkmar et al., 2014). For those who are non-verbal or deaf or hard of hearing, difficulties in use and understanding of gestures may mean that sign language will not be an appropriate alternative communication modality. Other students may have superior receptive and expressive language skills and yet lack understanding of social norms within their classroom or school. Some individuals with ASD are also noted to use restricted or stereotyped communication (they may be an expert on the solar system), or repetitive phrases (e.g., "hmmm, let me think a minute" becomes an automatic response each time the student is asked a question). Many students with ASD have difficulties in the use of correct prosody or intonational patterns in speech. This makes it difficult for the listener to know if the student is excited or distraught without looking for more information. This difference in understanding the prosody of others, sometimes referred to as a supralinguistic aspect of communication also makes it difficult for them to understand the subtle difference in the utterances (e.g., Is this yours? vs. Is THIS yours? vs. Is this YOURS?). Difficulties in supralinguistic skills may mean that these students may have difficulty understanding things not explicitly stated, understanding figurative language or jokes that their peers laugh at, problem-solving, and identifying the main idea and supporting arguments. These difficulties may occur in the classroom when information is presented verbally, when students read information, and when students are presented with higher level math word problems (Knight & Sartini, 2015).

While communication difficulties are a hallmark of ASD, they are also one of the best predictors of outcomes. A child's overall cognitive ability and communication at the sentence level at 5 years of age is the best predictor of long-term prognosis (Volkmar et al., 2014). Kim and colleagues (2018) also found that students with IQ scores below 85 showed consistently lower academic achievement and that students who displayed a significant difference between their cognitive and academic scores on standardized assessments also had a discrepancy in at least one academic area. Even for those with average cognitive abilities, 22% of 9-year-old and 32% of 18-year-old students in the study were below or low average in at least one academic domain (Kim et al., 2018).

Speech in ASD

There is little consistent information available regarding the speech sound production, speech fluency, nor speech prosody of students with ASD. A systematic review by Broome, McCabe, Docking, and Doble (2017) was inconclusive in identifying specific characteristics of the speech (articulation, voice problems, prosody, fluency) of students with ASD. As discussed above, while difficulties in prosody can be heard in the communication of some students with ASD, this is not a universal characteristic. There is currently no standardized assessment tool to evaluate and measure difficulties in prosody. It may be that prosody is affected by speech fluency, word finding difficulties, or sensory system feedback. Currently, Holbrook (in preparation) has a tool in development entitled The Brief Prosody Rating Scale for ASD which may prove helpful to clinicians and researchers alike in classifying and identifying the underlying difficulties in speech-language prosody.

Specific Interventions to Support Academic Success of Students with ASD

In the next section, we describe specific interventions that have been demonstrated through research to provide positive results for students with ASD. We recommend that practitioners select research-based interventions when working with students with ASD.

Reading Interventions for Students with ASD

The current research on reading interventions is still emerging for students with ASD but several interventions have been determined to be effective. The majority of research has focused on interventions for reading comprehension skills, although some studies have explicitly addressed reading fluency skills. Several interventions and strategies are effective for reading fluency, such as listening passage preview, repeated readings, reread-adapt and answer-comprehend (RAAC), error correction, fluency training, discrete trial instruction, and Reading Mastery curriculum (Guthrie, 2017; Hua et al., 2012; Kamps et al., 2016; Nopprapun & Holloway, 2014; Reisener, Lancaster, McMullin, & Ho, 2014). Specific to reading comprehension, the use of several techniques, such as peer-based strategies, cooperative learning groups, reading aloud, direct instruction, video modeling, priming, self-management, graphic organizers, computer-assisted technology, story mapping, and reciprocal questioning, have been shown to be effective (Chiang & Lin, 2007; El Zein, Solis, Vaughn, & McCulley, 2014; Fleury et al., 2014; Finnegan & Mazin, 2016; Randi, Newman, & Grigorenko, 2010; Schatz, 2017; Senokossoff, 2016). Determining the effectiveness of reading interventions for students with ASD who have cognitive delays is also warranted as most of the aforementioned studies focus on students with ASD who have at least average cognitive abilities.

Mathematics Interventions for Students with ASD

A primary recommendation from recent research reviews on mathematics interventions for students with ASD is the use of explicit instruction with prompts and consequences incorporated, both for teaching mathematics topics, as well as for teaching content-vocabulary (King, Lemons, & Davidson, 2016; Spooner, Root, Saunders, & Browder, 2019). Explicit instruction (with connected prompting strategies and positive reinforcement) should form the foundation of mathematics instruction and intervention for students with ASD.

Spooner et al. (2019) recommend using systematic and explicit instruction, as well as task analysis to isolate the steps involved in solving many mathematics problems. Three evidence-based instructional supports should be used with students with ASD: graphic organizers, manipulatives, and technology aided instruction. Graphic organizers can help students understand and make connections between related mathematics concepts, and guide them through problem-solving processes when working with word problems. Manipulatives can be used in conjunction with graphic organizers and explicit and systematic instruction to help students visualize and make sense of the mathematics concepts and tasks. Technology aided instruction (i.e., the use of calculators, video modeling, or computers) is also recommended to help students compensate for difficulties they may have with computation, and to help students connect mathematics topics to real-world applications.

Communication Interventions for Students with ASD

The National Autism Center's (NAC) National Standards Project (NSP; National Autism Center, 2015) has identified several language interventions that have an established level of evidence in treating students with ASD. Three intervention approaches have an established level of evidence for students with ASD in preschool and beyond: modeling, story-based interventions, and language training. In modeling, the communication partner, which could be an adult or a peer, demonstrates the desired behaviors. Video modeling has also been shown to have established efficacy, and story-based interventions been shown to be effective. In preschool populations, stories may be entirely visually based, and as a student begins to master literacy skills, words and sentences are added to the stories. For adolescents, this intervention may be a comic strip (Hutchins & Prelock, 2006) where they are also engaged in drawing the comic and adding the "thought" or "word" bubbles above the character's head. Story-based interventions help a student with ASD begin to take on the perspective taking as they engage with "others" in their stories. Language training may help improve communication, interpersonal skills, and interactive play skills. Strategies can include modeling, prompting (either verbally, visually, or gesturally, or a combination thereof) and the use of positive reinforcement to shape the language behavior.

Much of the research regarding communication in school-age children with ASD has focused on discrete rather than global or holistic social skills. Volkmar et al. (2014) also found that many of the social communication strategies were completed at the individual level, with few interventions completed at the small group or classroom levels. Some interventions were conducted on a playground as a way to encourage more natural communication. However, the authors of this review also found limited evidence for social-pragmatic interventions. The comprehensive review completed by The National Autism Center (2015) also designated social skills programs as having emerging evidence.

Providing direct instruction on written language skills has been shown to have some efficacy as an academic intervention for students with ASD. A literature review of 15 writing instruction studies indicated that direct instruction in the written use of story elements, narration, and spelling resulted in student improvements in these skills, which were maintained over time (Pennington & Delano, 2012).

Multicomponent Interventions to Address a Variety of Needs

Instructional strategies and interventions should match the individual student's needs and support access to the core curriculum (Spooner et al., 2019). As such, multicomponent interventions are often an appropriate way to meet students' needs, especially since there is a strong connection between social skills and academic performance (Fleury et al., 2014). Students with ASD may be receiving a variety of different support services, so it is essential that all relevant professionals be included when determining instructional or intervention plans for students with ASD (Leach & Duffy, 2009). Related professionals, including special education teachers, SLPs, occupational therapists, psychologists, behavior analysts, and parents (Leach & Duffy, 2009) should work together to identify the student's needs, strengths, and goals and to determine an appropriate multicomponent intervention. To help support students' long-term success, interventions should prioritize conversation ability and communication skills, which are associated with increased odds of pursuing college and declaring a science, technology, engineering, or mathematics major (Wei et al., 2017).

Factors Influencing Interdisciplinary Collaboration in Schools

Interdisciplinary collaboration relies on an understanding of the variety of school systems and structures that may influence the needs and services of students with ASD. Although the descriptions below are typical, school structures, personnel roles, and resources can vary. We recommend that practitioners consult with administrators and other key stakeholders in their settings to better understand the variables relevant to meeting the needs of students with ASD.

School Type

Public schools serve 90% of students in the US (National Center for Education Statistics [NCES], 2017). Public schools, including magnet and charter schools, are responsible per IDEA (2004) for identifying and serving students with disabilities under their jurisdiction. For public schools, this includes all students within their boundaries, and for charter schools, all enrolled students. Property taxes serve as the primary funding source for public schools (Hoffman, Anderson-Butcher, Fuller, & Bates, 2017), which may limit available resources to serve students with ASD in low-income urban and rural areas. Charter schools rely on state or federal government budgets to receive needed funds (Waitoller, Maggin, & Trzaska, 2017).

Private schools differ from public and charter schools. Since they charge tuition, private schools are more likely to have the necessary funds to serve students. Private schools are only required to provide accommodations to students with disabilities (Americans with Disabilities Act, 1990), not interventions since IDEA excludes private institutions. As a private institution, these schools have more flexibility to provide specialized curricula and services for students with ASD or other disorders. In the event a public school is unable to reasonably meet the needs of a student, they may refer parents to a private school with specialized services and pay the students' tuition (IDEA, 2004). A thorough understanding of students' educational needs and the resources of their public, charter, or private school is necessary for effective interdisciplinary care.

School Level

School level also influences the available resources of schools and the needs of students. At the primary level, students with ASD may still be unidentified or in the process of receiving individualized education plans (IEP) if needed (IDEA, 2004). With assessment and identification being the primary concern, school psychologists, SLPs, and other trained professionals are more heavily involved at this stage. School-based autism services most often focus on accessibility (e.g., transportation, adapting activities) and speech, physical, and behavioral interventions (Wei, Wagner, Christiano, Shattuck, & Yu, 2014).

At the secondary level, schools serve more students (NCES, 2017). Students are expected to be more independent, face more transitions within the school day and between days, and navigate a more complex social landscape (Rispoli, Lee, Nathanson, & Malcolm, 2019). ASD services include more social and emotional counseling than speech, physical, or behavioral interventions (Wei et al., 2014), as well as an increased focus on post-secondary transition (Rispoli et al., 2019). It also becomes increasingly difficult to coordinate services within the school compared to the elementary school where often only one general education teacher is serving a student at a time (Hedges et al., 2014). By middle and high school, a student may see upwards of four teachers a day, while only one is required to participate in the development of their IEP (IDEA, 2004), which may result in inconsistent implementation across teachers.

School Setting

The U.S. Census Bureau (2010) outlines two types of urban areas: urbanized areas, populated by over 50,000 people, and urban clusters, with between 2,500 and 50,000 inhabitants. These two definitions account for major cities, metropolitan areas, and suburbs. Together, in 2010, over 249 million people or 80.7% of the US population lived in these settings, including the majority of the nation's students. Urban schools are more likely to have greater ethnic and linguistic diversity and high dropout rates (Vaughn et al., 2019), and are more prone to racial segregation (Chapman, 2018). Urban schools also tend to be close to medical centers, universities, and clinics, which may help facilitate collaboration (Iadarola et al., 2015). Urban schools may face a variety of challenges: high rates of teacher burnout and relocation (Ouellette et al., 2018), lack of funding in poverty centers, and large student populations per school (Merillat, Corrigan, & Harper, 2018).

Though serving a very different demographic, rural schools face many of the same challenges. The U.S. Census Bureau (2010) defines a rural area as any region with a population of less than 2,500 people. An estimated 59.5 million people in the US, or 19.3% of the population, live in rural areas. Despite the smaller proportion of the population, rural land makes up the majority of the US, meaning greater distances between students and schools. Rural schools, like urban schools, may face financial constraints, high dropout rates, and poverty (Hoffman, Anderson-Butcher, Fuller, & Bates, 2017). Rural schools have less access to trained professionals due to distance, transportation constraints, and stigma toward help-seeking. Because of this, rural schools may be understaffed and struggle to implement multi-tiered systems or programs (Oyen & Wollersheim-Shervey, 2018), relying more heavily on parents and community members to meet student needs (Hoffman et al., 2017).

Though suburbs are not distinguished from urban areas by the U.S. Census Bureau (2010), research indicates they are distinct. Suburban schools have higher mathematics and reading performance scores, as well as greater rates of college attendance (Goforth, Yosai, Brown, & Shindorf, 2017). However, suburban schools carry a mix of the advantages and disadvantages of rural and urban areas. Namely, distances between trained professionals are greater compared to urban centers, but parental involvement and funding are more common than in other areas. Suburban schools traditionally share similar racial and ethnic compositions as rural schools but have larger student populations than they do.

How Interdisciplinary Collaboration Can Address Students' Needs

Because ASD is a complex and multi-faceted disorder, students with ASD may require intervention from those with expertise in a number of different areas. Effective collaboration among personnel and families working with students with ASD improves student outcomes, facilitates transitions and strengthens working relationships (Emmons & Zager, 2018). The following elements are essential for collaboration: commitment, communication, strong leadership from decision makers, understanding the culture of the collaborator, adequate resources, minimizing turf issues, and engaging in preplanning (Johnson, Zorn, Yung Tam, Lamontagne, & Johnson, 2003). Effective collaboration also relies on establishing shared priorities. Parents, educators, and specialists working with students with ASD identify students' academic learning and social–emotional needs as high priorities, and parents rank students' academic learning as a higher priority than educators. Each of these groups also note the need for transparency in translating research into practice, as well as the need for continuing education/training (Saggers et al., 2019).

Collaboration can be strengthened through the involvement of knowledgeable administrators, the use of family-centered care, and by increasing the self-efficacy of service providers. Administrators with an understanding of ASD and evidence-based treatments are more likely to foster collaboration, provide appropriate services, and ensure that all personnel have the necessary skills and training (Pazey, Gevarter, Hamrick & Rojeski, 2014). Family-centered care, specifically a medical home model, is associated with positive student outcomes, including reductions in negative behaviors, increased social responsiveness, and overall improvements in quality of life (Carbone, Behl, Azor, & Murphy, 2010; Dang et al., 2017). Increasing service providers' self-efficacy also results in more ease in collaborating with parents, as well as improved performance and reductions in problem behaviors (Emmons & Zager, 2018).

Applied Case Example—Interdisciplinary Supports Implemented Through MTSS

In the following section, we will illustrate how professionals and relevant stakeholders can work together to meet the academic needs of students with ASD, using a fictional applied case example. Throughout this example, we focus on how a structure of MTSS (see chapter 'Supporting Students with Autism Spectrum Disorder in Schools Through Multi-Tiered Systems of Support' for more information), which includes School-Wide Positive Behavior Interventions and Supports (SWPBIS) and Response to Intervention (RtI), can be utilized to facilitate interdisciplinary collaboration to meet the needs of students with ASD. Students with ASD, regardless of whether they are receiving special education services or not, may have needs that correspond with any tier within MTSS, and their needs may be fluid (i.e., in some areas they may require Tier 2 supports, while in others they may not require any; as students respond to interventions, they may not require additional supports beyond Tier 1).

Proactive and responsive approaches to promote academic success (Tier 1). Sierra Middle School (SMS) is an urban school that enrolls approximately 700 students. Sierra Middle School has been implementing MTSS for the last 7 years and places a high value on interdisciplinary collaboration to meet the needs of all students. At Sierra, Tier 1 implementation efforts are facilitated and monitored through a Leadership Team, which includes an administrator, department heads for each subject area and special education, a school counselor, a school psychologist, a social worker, and a representative from the parental advisory board. After reviewing school and student-level data, this team decided on several research-based Tier 1 approaches to implement school-wide (see list of Tier 1 approaches in Table 1).

During a data review at one of their regular meetings, the School Leadership Team noticed that several students with ASD had lower grades in several classes, and a higher rate of office discipline referrals due to inappropriate behavior. The Leadership Team invited an ASD expert to their meetings to assist in re-examining their Tier 1 supports. The ASD expert recommended that the school incorporate Universal Design for Learning (UDL) as a framework to organize proactive supports not only for students with ASD, but all students. Universal Design for Learning (UDL) involves intentionally incorporating a variety of instructional supports from the outset, as opposed to individualized supports for particular students (Ok, Rao, Bryant, & McDougall, 2017). The Center for Applied Special Technology (CAST), a leader in research, development, and implementation related to UDL, provides three guiding principles for UDL: (1) provide multiple means of engagement, (2) provide multiple means of representation, and (3) provide multiple means of action and expression (CAST, 2018).

Sierra Middle School utilized the resources on the CAST website (http://www.cast.org/) to enhance their existing Tier 1 supports. They provided professional development for their teachers to ensure that they had the knowledge and resources to effectively implement UDL in their classrooms, and established interdisciplinary professional learning communities that provided teachers, related school personnel, and administrators opportunities to share knowledge and resources to enhance the quality of UDL implementation. The School Leadership Team reviewed data after the school implemented UDL for several weeks, and found that the grades and behaviors of most students with and without ASD had improved since implementing UDL.

Targeted and individualized supports and interventions (Tier 2). Students with ASD may need additional targeted supports and interventions in addition to Tier 1. The specific form of these interventions can vary based on individual student factors, such as age, level of functional and academic performance, and the student's particular needs and preferences. For many students in preschool and early elementary grades, interventions are individualized and intensive, and are gradually faded or adjusted as students' skills develop. When faded or adjusted, such interventions

Table 1 Tier 1, 2, and 3 Academic Strategies and Interventions for Students with ASD

Tier 1	Tier 2	Tier 3
Estimated that 80% responsive to Tier 1 supports alone	*Estimated that 15–20% will need Tier 2 supports in addition to Tier 1*	*Estimated that 5% will need Tier 3 supports in addition to Tiers 1 and 2*
Engagement: • Group opportunities to respond • Physical opportunities to respond • Variety of response opportunities • Incorporate student interests in academic tasks • Incorporate a variety of instructional tasks and activities **Academic Instruction**: • Explicit and systematic instruction • Graphic organizers • Visual cues • Mnemonic devices **Self-management**: • Explicit strategy instruction • Goal setting • Self-monitoring	**Teach new (or adjust existing) social, communicative, or academic behaviors**: • Discrete trials • Massed trials • Naturalistic behavior • Peer mediation • Video modeling • Self-modeling (video recorded) • Differentiated assessments and class activities • Differential reinforcement of other behaviors • Extinction • Antecedent manipulation **Build communication skills**: • Assistive devices • Picture Exchange System • Use scripts to help students engage with peers and/or academic content • Role plays • Social stories	**Individualized interventions, determined based on students' needs and strengths. Approaches that may be incorporated include**: • Task analysis • System of least to most prompts, or most to least prompts • Use a model-teach-lead format of instruction and support • Time delay prompting • Adapt curricula or assessments • Conduct functional-behavioral analysis and develop individualized behavior support plan **Team responsible for developing and monitoring individualized intervention should meet regularly to review data related to fidelity of intervention implementation, social validity of the intervention, and the student's response to intervention**

Note: Content in this table relates primarily to academic supports and interventions. See chapter 'Supporting Students with Autism Spectrum Disorder in Schools Through Multi-Tiered Systems of Support' for behavior strategies. Citations for content in this table: Archer & Hughes (2011), Fleury et al., (2014), Hart and Whalon (2008), Lane, Menzies, Ennis, and Bezdek (2013); Leach and Duffy (2009), National Research Council (2001)

can be delivered in a group format or supported in inclusive instructional settings (National Research Council, 2001).

Sierra Middle School organizes Tier 2 and 3 implementation efforts using a Student Support Team. The Student Support Team includes an administrator, school psychologist, counselor, special educator, SLP, a teacher representing each grade level, and a member of the parental advisory board. The team meets bi-weekly to identify students who may need additional supports and determine which of their existing supports and interventions are appropriate for each student. Whenever possible, the team focuses on providing students with access to group-based interventions to facilitate transfer to inclusive settings. Based on recommendations from reviews of research on students with ASD, Sierra Middle School ensures that for Tier 2 and 3 interventions they have: (1) a continuum of supports that are readily implemented, and located within inclusive, as well as specialized instructional environments; (2) interventions focused on the needs of particular students, and reflective of the family's goals and wishes; (3) interventions with students with ASD that support the development of language, communication, social understanding, and peer interaction; (4) high-quality training for practitioners and caregivers to allow them to implement and/or support interventions implemented with students with ASD; (5) a formal protocol establishing and coordinating the responsibilities of the various professionals involved in providing interventions to students with ASD; and (6) a structured consultation process to recruit student input and involvement (Guldberg et al., 2011). Table 1 provides a list of common Tier 2 supports and interventions.

At the first student support team meeting following the implementation of UDL at Tier 1, the team identified five students who needed additional support. These students had failing grades in their content area classes (English Language Arts and Mathematics). Based on data collected by the students' teachers, all five students tended to be withdrawn and not participate during class activities, which was directly affecting their academic performance in class. The student support team identified a social skills group, facilitated by a school psychologist and SLP, that might help support these students in developing communication skills useful for engaging in classroom activities.

Intensive and individualized supports for students with ASD (Tier 3). A small percentage of students with ASD will need intensive, individualized supports to reach their academic goals. Most students will have their needs effectively met through Tier 1 and 2 supports. The Student Support Team at Sierra Middle School identifies students in need of Tier 3 supports by evaluating students' response to Tier 2 interventions and supports. If a student has not made enough improvement after receiving a Tier 2 intervention for a specified amount of time, the Student Support Team initiates a process for the student to access Tier 3 supports.

Because Tier 3 supports are individualized and intensive, they are typically determined by a team of professionals who focus on the particular student's strengths and needs. This team could be a student's Individualized Education Plan (IEP) team, which includes an administrator, the student's parents or guardians, the student, the student's special education case manager, each of the student's general and special education teachers, and any relevant service providers (e.g., SLP, school psychologist, social worker, occupational therapist, audiologist, behavior specialist, mathematics or reading specialist). This team meets to review the data, determine goals for the student, and to develop an individualized intervention plan. It is recommended that intensive interventions for students with ASD incorporate behavioral principles. At this level of support, interventions tend to include multiple components and may target several different areas of need (i.e., behavior as well as communication and academic skills; Fleury et al., 2014). Table 1 provides some common Tier 3 intervention approaches.

It is important to use research-validated interventions for students in need of individualized supports because of the time-intensive nature of interventions required at this level (Lane et al., 2013). Additionally, for some students with ASD, Tier 3 interventions may focus on priority areas of behavior and communication, but not specifically academic skills. In these cases, teachers can still include students with ASD who have more individualized needs in resource or core instruction by adapting curricula or materials. For example, teachers may adapt the reading material students are presented with to provide the student with more intensive needs with a shorter text at an easier reading level (Fleury et al., 2014). Another example is that teachers may adapt an academic task that involves students writing their responses to have the student provide responses orally (or through pictures or text to speech communication device), which may also help support the student's communication skills. The goal of adjusting academic tasks should primarily be to provide the student with the greatest access to grade level core content and their general education peers.

The Student Support Team at Sierra Middle School met to review the data two weeks following the start of the Tier 2 intervention for the five students who were identified as in need of additional support. While four of the students demonstrated excellent progress, one student, Steven, continued to have failing grades and be disengaged during class activities. The team decides that Steven needs Tier 3 supports and begins the process of scheduling a meeting with his parents, teachers, and related service personnel. This team, based on a review of Steven's data, develop an individualized intervention that involves the collaboration of Steven's special education case manager, teachers, a behavior specialist, an SLP, and a school psychologist. The team implements the intervention and meets regularly to review Steven's progress. Steven's grades improve, thanks to the interdisciplinary collaboration of his team.

Conclusion

Students with ASD can be effectively supported in reaching their academic goals when included in general education classrooms, especially when instructional planning occurs within a framework of UDL, and additional supports and interventions are delivered within a system of MTSS. To efficiently and effectively assist students with ASD in achieving academically, a team of educators and care providers must communicate effectively and collaborate closely.

References

American Psychiatric Association. (2013). *Diagnostic and statistical manual of mental disorders* (5th ed.). Arlington, VA: Author.

Americans With Disabilities Act of 1990, Pub. L. No. 101-336, 104 Stat. 328 (1990).

Archer, A. L., & Hughes, C. A. (2011). *Explicit instruction: Effective and efficient teaching*. New York, NY: The Guilford Press.
Baio, J., Wiggins, L., Christensen, D. L., Maenner, M. J., Daniels, J., Warren, Z., … Dowling, N. F. (2018). Prevalence of autism spectrum disorder among children aged 8 years —Autism and developmental disabilities monitoring network, 11 sites, United States, 2014. *MMWR. Surveillance Summaries, 67*(6), 1–23.
Bianco, M., Carothers, D. E., & Smiley, L. R. (2009). Gifted students with Asperger syndrome: Strategies for strength-based programming. *Intervention in School and Clinic, 44*(4), 206–215.
Broome, K., McCabe, P., Docking, K., & Doble, M. (2017). A systematic review of speech assessments for children with autism spectrum disorder: Recommendations for best practice. *American Journal of Speech-Language Pathology, 26,* 1011–1029.
Brown, H. M., Oram-Cardy, J., & Johnson, A. (2013). A meta-analysis of the reading comprehension skills of individuals on the Autism Spectrum. *Journal of Autism and Developmental Disorders, 43,* 932–955.
Carbone, P. S., Behl, D. D., Azor, V., & Murphy, N. A. (2010). The medical home for children with autism spectrum disorders: Parent and pediatrician perspectives. *Journal of Autism and Developmental Disorders, 40,* 317–324.
CAST (2018). Universal Design for Learning Guidelines version 2.2. Retrieved from http://udlguidelines.cast.org.
Chapman, T. K. (2018). Segregation, desegregation, segregation: Charter school options as a return to separate and unequal schools for urban families. *Peabody Journal of Education, 93*(1), 38–51.
Chiang, H. M., & Lin, Y. H. (2007). Mathematical ability of students with Asperger syndrome and high-functioning autism: A review of literature. *Autism, 11*(6), 547–556.
Chen, L., Abrams, D. A., Rosenberg-Lee, M., Iuculano, T., Wakeman, H. N., Prathap, S., Chen, T., & Menon, V. (2019). Quantitative analysis of heterogeneity in academic achievement of children with autism. *Clinical Psychological Science, 7*(2), 362–380.
Dang, K., Bent, S., Lawton, B., Warren, T., Widjaja, F., McDonald, M. G., … & Hendren, R. L. (2017). Integrating autism care through a school-based intervention model: A Pilot study. *Journal of Clinical Medicine, 6*(10), 97.
Davidson, M. M., Kaushanskaya, M., & Weismer, S. E. (2018). Reading comprehension in children with and without ASD: The role of word reading, oral language, and working memory. *Journal of Autism and Developmental Disorders, 48,* 3524–3541.
El Zein, F., Solis, M., Vaughn, S., & McCulley, L. (2014). Reading comprehension interventions for students with autism spectrum disorders: A synthesis of research. *Journal of Autism and Developmental Disorders, 44,* 1303–1322.
Emmons, C. L., & Zager, D. (2018). Increasing collaboration self-efficacy to improve educational programming for students with Autism. *Focus on Autism and Other Developmental Disabilities, 33*(2), 120–128.
Finnegan, E., & Mazin, A. L. (2016). Strategies for increasing reading comprehension skills in students with autism spectrum disorder: A review of the literature. *Education and Treatment of Children, 39,* 187–220.
Fleury, V. P., Hedges, S., Hume, K., Browder, D. M., Thompson, J. L., Fallin, K., …Vaughn, S. (2014). Addressing the academic needs of adolescents with autism spectrum disorder in secondary education. *Remedial and Special Education, 35,* 68–79.
Goforth, A. N., Yosai, E. R., Brown, J. A., & Shindorf, Z. R. (2017). A multi-method inquiry of the practice and context of rural school psychology. *Contemporary School Psychology, 21,* 58–70.
Guldberg, K., Parsons, S., MacLeod, A., Jones, G., Prunty, A., & Balfe, T. (2011). Implications for practice from 'international review of the evidence on best practice in educational provision for children on the autism spectrum'. *European Journal of Special Needs Education, 26*(1), 65–70.
Guthrie, R. M. (2017). *Effectiveness of Repeated Reading and Error Correction Strategies on the Reading Fluency Skills of Students with Autism Spectrum Disorder.* (Doctoral dissertation). Retrieved from digitalcommons.wku.edu. (Paper 136).

Hart, J. E., & Whalon, K. J. (2008). Promote academic engagement and communication of students with autism spectrum disorders in inclusive settings. *Intervention in School and Clinic, 44*(2), 116–120.

Hedges, S. H., Kirby, A. V., Sreckovic, M. A., Kucharczyk, S., Hume, K., & Pace, S. (2014). "Falling through the cracks": Challenges for high school students with autism spectrum disorder. *High School Journal.*

Hoffman, J. A., Anderson-Butcher, D., Fuller, M., & Bates, S. (2017). The school experiences of rural youths: A study in Appalachian Ohio. *Children and Schools, 39*(3), 147–155.

Holbrook, S. (in preparation). Validation of a brief prosody rating scale for school-age children with autism spectrum disorder.

Hua, Y., Hendrickson, J. M., Therrien, W. J., Woods-Groves, S., Ries, P. S., & Shaw, J. J. (2012). Effects of combined reading and question generation on reading fluency and comprehension of three young adults with autism and intellectual disability. *Focus on Autism and Developmental Disabilities, 27*(3), 135–146.

Hutchins, T. L., & Prelock, P. A. (2006). Using social stories and comic strip conversations to promote socially valid outcomes for children with autism. *Seminars in Speech and Language, 27*(1), 47–59.

Iadarola, S., Hetherington, S., Clinton, C., Dean, M., Reisinger, E., Huynh, L., … & Kasari, C. (2015). Services for children with autism spectrum disorder in three, large urban school districts: Perspectives of parents and educators. *Autism, 19*, 694–703.

IDEA. (2004). Individuals with Disabilities Education Improvement Act of 2004. Pub. L. no. 108–446. 108th Congress, 2nd Session.

Johnson, L. J., Zorn, D., Yung Tam, B. K., Lamontagne, M., & Johnson, S. A. (2003). Stakeholders views of factors that impact successful interagency collaboration. *Exceptional Children, 69*, 195–209.

Jones, C. R. G., Happé, F., Golden, H., Marsden, A. J. S., Tregay, J., … & Charman, T. (2009). Reading and arithmetic in adolescents with autism spectrum disorders: Peaks and dips in attainment. *Neuropsychology, 23*, 718–728.

Kamps, D., Heitzman-Powell, L., Rosenberg, N., Mason, R., Schwartz, I., & Romine, R. S. (2016). Effects of Reading Mastery as a small group intervention for young children with ASD. *Journal of Developmental and Physical Disabilities, 28*(5), 703–722.

Kasari, C., & Patterson, S. (2012). Interventions addressing social impairment in autism. *Current Psychiatry Reports, 14*(6), 713–725.

Kim, S. H., Bal, V. H., & Lord, C. (2018). Longitudinal follow-up of academic achievement in children with autism form age 2 to 18. *The Journal of child Psychology and Psychiatry, 59*(3), 258–267.

King, S. A., Lemons, C. J., & Davidson, K. A. (2016). Math interventions for students with autism spectrum disorder: A best-evidence synthesis. *Exceptional Children, 82*(4), 443–462.

Knight, V. F., & Sartini, E. (2015). A comprehensive literature review of comprehension strategies in core content areas for students with Autism Spectrum Disorder. *Journal of Autism and Developmental Disorders, 45*, 1213–1229.

Lane, K., Menzies, H. M., Ennis, R. P., & Bezdek. (2013). School-wide systems to promote positive behaviors and facilitate instruction. *Journal of Curriculum and Instruction, 7*(1), 6–31.

Leach, D., & Duffy, M. L. (2009). Supporting students with autism spectrum disorders in inclusive settings. *Intervention in School and Clinic, 45*(1), 31–37.

McDonald, C. A., Donnelly, J. P., Feldman-Alguire, A. L., Rodgers, J. D., Lopata, C., & Thomeer, M. L. (2019). Special education service use by children with Autism spectrum disorder. *Journal of Autism and Developmental Disorders, 49*, 2437–2446.

McIntyre, N. S., Solari, E. J., Gonzales, J. E., Solomon, M., Lerro, L. E., Novotny, S., et al. (2017). The scope and nature of reading comprehension impairments in school-aged children with higher-functional autism spectrum disorder. *Journal of Autism and Developmental Disorders, 47*(9), 2838–2860.

Merillat, B. D., Corrigan, D. G., & Harper, B. E. (2018). Reducing stereotype threat in urban schools. *Social Psychology of Education, 21,* 1–26.
Micai, M., Holly, J., Vulchanova, M., & Saldana, D. (2017). Strategies of readers with autism when responding to inferential questions: An eye-movement study. *Autism Research, 10,* 888–900.
Nation, K., Clarke, P., Wright, B., & Williams, C. (2016). Patterns of reading ability in children with autism spectrum disorder. *Journal of Autism and Developmental Disorders, 36,* 911–919.
National Autism Center. (2015). *Findings and conclusions: National standards project, Phase 2.* Randolph, MA: Author.
National Center for Education Statistics. (2017). Selected statistics from the public elementary and secondary education universe: School year 2015–2016.
National Research Council, (2001). *Educating Children with Autism (Committee on Educational Intervention for Children with Autism*, Catherine Lord and James P. McGee, eds. Division of Behavioral and Social Sciences and Education). Washington, DC: National Academy Press.
Nopprapun, M., & Holloway, J. (2014). A comparison of fluency training and discrete trial instruction to teach letter sounds to children with ASD: Acquisition and learning outcomes. *Research in Autism Spectrum Disorders, 8*(7), 788–802.
Norbury, C., & Nation, K. (2011). Understanding variability in reading comprehension in adolescents with autism spectrum disorders: Interactions with language status and decoding skill. *Scientific Studies of Reading, 15*(3), 191–210.
Ok, M. W., Rao, K. R., Bryant, B. R., & McDougall, D. (2017). Universal design for learning in pre-k to grade 12 classrooms: A systematic review of research. *Exceptionality, 25*(2), 116–138.
Oswald, T. M., Beck, J. S., Iosif, A. M., McCauley, J. B., Gilhooly, L. J., Matter, J. C., et al. (2016). Clinical and cognitive characteristics associated with mathematics problem solving in adolescents with autism spectrum disorder. *Autism Research, 9*(4), 480–490.
Ouellette, R. R., Frazier, S. L., Shernoff, E. S., Cappella, E., Mehta, T. G., Maríñez-Lora, A. … & Atkins, M. S. (2018). Teacher job stress and satisfaction in urban schools: Disentangling individual-, classroom-, and organizational-level influences. *Behavior Therapy, 49*, 494–508.
Oyen, K. A., & Wollersheim-Shervey, S. (2018). An examination of critical features of positive frameworks: Impact in rural environments for school-based practitioners. *Contemporary School Psychology*, 1–13.
Pazey, B. L., Gevarter, C., Hamrick, J., & Rojeski, L. (2014). Administrator views and knowledge of instructional practices for students with autism spectrum disorders. *Research in Autism Spectrum Disorders, 8,* 1253–1268.
Pennington, R. C., & Delano, M. E. (2012). Writing instruction for students with autism Spectrum disorders: A review of literature. *Focus on Autism and Other Developmental Disabilities, 27*(3), 158–167.
Prelock, P. A., & McCauley, R. J. (2012). *Treatment of autism spectrum disorders: evidence-based intervention strategies for communication and social interactions.* Baltimore: Paul H. Brookes Pub. Co.
Randi, J., Newman, T., & Grigorenko, E. L. (2010). Teaching children with autism to read for meaning: Challenges and possibilities. *Journal of Autism and Developmental Disorders, 40*(7), 890–902.
Reisener, C. D., Lancaster, A. L., McMullin, W. A., & Ho, T. (2014). A preliminary investigation of evidence-based interventions to increase oral reading fluency in children with autism. *Journal of Applied School Psychology, 30,* 50–67.
Rispoli, M., Lee, G. K., Nathanson, E. W., & Malcolm, A. L. (2019). The parent role in school-based teams for adolescents with autism spectrum disorder. *School Psychology, 34*(4), 458–467.
Saggers, B., Tones, M., Dunne, J., Trembath, D., Bruck, S., Webster, A., … & Wang, S. (2019). Promoting a collective voice from parents, educators and allied health professionals on the educational needs of students on the autism spectrum. *Journal of Autism and Developmental Disorders, 49*, 3845–3865.

Schatz, R. B. (2017). *Combining readers theater, story mapping and video self-modeling interventions to improve narrative reading comprehension in children with high-functioning autism.* (Doctoral dissertation). Retrieved from PsycINFO. (10599296).

Senokossoff, G. W. (2016). Developing reading comprehension skills in high-functioning children with autism spectrum disorder: A review of the research, 1990-2012. *Reading & Writing Quarterly: Overcoming Learning Difficulties, 32*(3), 223–246.

Spooner, F., Root, J. R., Saunders, A. F., & Browder, D. M. (2019). An updated evidence-based practice review on teaching mathematics to students with moderate and severe developmental disabilities. *Remedial and Special Education, 40*(3), 150–165.

Tirado, M. J., & Saldaña, D. (2016). Readers with autism can produce inferences, but they cannot answer inferential questions. *Journal of Autism and Developmental Disorders, 46*(3), 1025–1037.

U.S. Census Bureau. (2010). *2010 Census Urban and Rural Classification and Urban Area Criteria.* Retrieved from https://www.census.gov/programs-surveys/geography/guidance/geo-areas/urban-rural/2010-urban-rural.html.

Vaughn, S., Martinez, L. R., Williams, K. J., Miciak, J., Fall, A., & Roberts, G. (2019). Efficacy of a high school extensive reading intervention for English learners with reading difficulties. *Journal of Educational Psychology, 111*(3), 373–386.

Volkmar, F., Siegel, M., Woodbury-Smith, M., King, B., McCracken, J., & State, M. (2014). Practice Parameter for the assessment and treatment of children and adolescents with Autism Spectrum Disorder. *Journal of the American Academy of Child and Adolescent Psychiatry, 53*(2), 237–257.

Waitoller, F. R., Maggin, D. M., & Trzaska, A. (2017). A longitudinal comparison of enrollment patterns of students receiving special education in urban neighborhoods and charter schools. *Journal of Disability Policy Studies, 28*(1), 3–12.

Wass, S. V., & Porayska-Pomsta, K. (2014). The uses of cognitive training technologies in the treatment of autism spectrum disorders. *Autism, 18*(8), 851–871.

Wei, X., Christiano, E. R., Yu, J. W., Wagner, M., & Spiker, D. (2015). Reading and math achievement profiles and longitudinal growth trajectories of children with an autism spectrum disorder. *Autism, 19*(2), 200–210.

Wei, X., Wagner, M., Christiano, E. R., Shattuck, P., & Yu, J. W. (2014). Special education services received by students with autism spectrum disorders from preschool through high school. *The Journal of Special Education, 48*(3), 167–179.

Wei, X., Yu, J. W., Shattuck, P., & Blackorby, J. (2017). High school math and science preparation and postsecondary STEM participation for students with an autism spectrum disorder. *Focus on Autism and Other Developmental Disabilities, 32*(2), 83–92.

White, S. W., Elias, R., Salinas, C. E., Capriola, N., Conner, C. M., Asselin, S. B., … & Getzel, E. E. (2016). Students with autism spectrum disorder in college: Results from a preliminary mixed methods needs analysis. *Research in developmental disabilities, 56*, 29–40

Supporting Students with Autism Spectrum Disorder in Schools Through Multi-Tiered Systems of Support

Sarah E. Pinkelman, Kaitlin Bundock, and Kristen Rolf

Abstract This chapter describes multi-tiered systems of support (MTSS) as methods to implement school-wide evidence-based practice. This system includes examples like positive behavioral interventions and supports or response to intervention. These systems adapt the intensity of support for the population and need of students across behavioral and academic domains. The use of interdisciplinary teams through a multi-tiered framework allows schools to best serve student needs. Characteristics of MTSS schools and each of the three tiers are discussed.

Multi-tiered Systems of Support (MTSS) are frameworks for evidence-based practice (EBP) in schools. In MTSS, evidence-based prevention and intervention efforts are organized by population groups (Tier 1/primary, Tier 2/secondary, and Tier 3/tertiary) related to student need (Merrell & Buchanan, 2006). Across these groups, or "tiers," an increasing intensity of support is provided to students based on their need. This multi-tiered logic originated in the area of public health and disease prevention (Walker et al., 1996) as a way to prevent health problems and minimize the number of people who require intensive medical care at the tertiary level. Common examples of MTSS in schools include school-wide positive behavioral interventions and supports (SWPBIS) and response to intervention (RtI). Both of these frameworks are consistent with the MTSS logic, with SWPBIS focusing on student prosocial and problem behavior and RtI focusing on student academic achievement.

SWPBIS aims to improve the social culture in schools and provide effective behavior support to all students, with intensified support provided to students as needed (Horner, Sugai, & Fixsen, 2017; Sugai & Horner, 2009). The three tiers in SWPBIS encompass a variety of evidence-based behavior support strategies that improve student prosocial behavior and minimize student problem behavior. Tier 1 SWPBIS involves best practice in classroom management and instruction for all students, Tier 2 is supplemental support that is provided to individual students or groups of students, and Tier 3 includes individualized comprehensive interventions that teach socially appropriate behavior and address the function of the student's

S. E. Pinkelman (✉) · K. Bundock · K. Rolf
Department of Special Education and Rehabilitation, Utah State University, Logan, UT, USA
e-mail: sarah.pinkelman@usu.edu

M. B. McClain et al. (eds.), *Interprofessional Care Coordination for Pediatric Autism Spectrum Disorder*, https://doi.org/10.1007/978-3-030-46295-6_10

problem behavior (i.e., "why" the student engages in the problem behavior). RtI is a MTSS applied to academics (Freeman, Miller, & Newcomer, 2015; Harlacher, Sanford, & Nelson Walker, n.d.; Harn, Basaraba, Chard, & Fritz, 2015). In RtI, core academic curricula in the areas of reading and math are provided at Tier 1, and Tiers 2 and 3 involve intensifying the core instruction or using a research-validated supplemental or replacement curriculum or intervention (Fuchs & Fuchs, 2006; Harlacher, Sanford, & Nelson Walker, nd.). Both SWPBIS and RtI share common elements related to the intricacies of implementing MTSS in schools. These elements are described below. For more information on RtI and promoting academic success, see the chapter "Promoting Academic Success".

Hallmarks of MTSS in Schools

Contextual Fit

Contextual fit refers to how well practices align with the values, skills, and resources in a given setting (Albin, Lucyshyn, Horner, & Flannery, 1996). Related to values, SWPBIS and RtI start with identifying a school's valued outcomes, such as improving reading achievement scores or reducing disruptive behavior in the classroom. After defining the valued outcomes, school teams then collaboratively select research-validated practices that will result in achieving these outcomes with the majority of the student population (Horner & Sugai, 2015). Schools implementing SWPBIS and RtI also assess social validity, or the extent to which relevant stakeholders agree that the goals, procedures, and results (i.e., student outcomes) are acceptable and socially meaningful (Wolf, 1978). In SWPBIS, community stakeholders provide input related to a variety of program components, such as the school climate and the selection of school-wide rules and expectations. In RtI, families work with school teams to select a core academic curriculum that they feel is best suited for their particular student population. The second element of contextual fit, skills, refers to the skill set required by those who will be implementing the practice (e.g., teachers, paraprofessionals) and those overseeing implementation (i.e., school administrators). By assessing the skills needed to carry out these implementation and supervisory functions, school teams can determine if additional training and coaching is needed, and if so, develop a plan for how they will provide such support. Lastly, resources in contextual fit refer to the allocation of funding, time, and materials that are needed for successful implementation, and the school's capacity to provide ongoing support for implementation.

Evidence-Based Practice

Another hallmark of SWPBIS and RtI is evidence-based practice (EBP). EBP remains a hot topic in the fields of education and services for students with Autism Spectrum Disorder (ASD), and there are many descriptions of EBP available in the literature. Arguably, the definition of EBP most relevant to MTSS and serving children with ASD is the definition provided by Slocum et al. (2014), who describe EBP as a decision-making process that integrates the best available evidence, clinical expertise, values, and context. In SWPBIS and RtI, the best available evidence refers to research-validated practices that are likely to produce intended student outcomes under particular conditions when implemented with fidelity. Clinical expertise is the skill set of teachers and staff who are tasked with implementing the intervention, as well as those who will support the implementers (e.g., instructional coaches, special education director, principal). Values and context as described by Slocum et al. (2014) are similar to contextual fit and social validity that was briefly outlined above. Variables related to stakeholder values and particulars of the implementation setting (i.e., the classroom, school, district) have a significant impact on the extent to which practices are implemented with fidelity and the likelihood that the practice will produce intended student outcomes.

Data-Based Decision-Making

Data-based decision-making is a critical component of both SWPBIS and RtI. Data are collected on both student outcomes and fidelity of implementation at different levels of the system (e.g., individual, group, school-wide) across all three tiers. These data not only inform the extent to which interventions are being implemented with fidelity and impacting student behavior, but these data also allow school teams to determine the level of student need (i.e., Tier 1, Tier 2, or Tier 3) across domains (e.g., social behavior and academics). For example, in SWPBIS, system-level data are collected using assessment tools such as the Tiered Fidelity Inventory (TFI; Algozzine et al., 2019) to determine the extent to which the school-wide MTSS framework is in place. System-wide data are also collected on student behavior via proxy measures, such as office discipline referrals (ODRs). In Tier 3 SWPBIS and RtI, data are collected on individual student behavior and individual implementer (e.g., teacher, paraprofessional) behavior to assess if the student's plan is being implemented with fidelity and if the plan is having an impact on student behavior and academic achievement.

Continuum of Support

In SWPBIS and RtI, different levels of intervention intensity, or “tiers” are provided for students based on their academic and behavioral needs (Fuchs & Fuchs, 2006; National Center on Intensive Intervention, n.d.; Stecker, 2007). While MTSS can have any number of tiers of support, it is most common to have three (Freeman et al., 2015). Tier 1, also known as the primary tier, aims to prevent students from developing challenges in academics and social behavior by providing a level of support that allows for a minimum of 80% of the student population to be successful (Hawken, Vincent, & Schumann, 2008). For students who are not successful at Tier 1, Tier 2 is initiated. Ideally, no more than 15% of students will require Tier 2 supports. Tier 2 is designed to supplement what students already receive as part of Tier 1 (Hawken et al., 2008). For students who are not successful at Tiers 1 or 2, Tier 3 support is provided. It is estimated that approximately 5% of students in a school will require Tier 3 supports. In Tier 3, also known as the tertiary tier, students receive intensive, individualized support (Hawken et al., 2008). This may involve further intensifying interventions that are already in place as part of Tiers 1 and 2, layering on additional individualized interventions, or using interventions that replace what the student previously received at Tiers 1 and 2.

Teaming

Another hallmark of SWPBIS and RtI is the use of building-level teams, which are responsible for reviewing school-wide student data, making data-based decisions, reviewing data on the effectiveness of strategies, and planning future actions (Nellis, 2012). Schools often have leadership teams, behavior support teams, academic support teams, and grade-level teams. School leadership teams typically include administrators and at least one representative from each relevant school role (teachers, counselors, school psychologists). The school leadership team is responsible for guiding and overseeing MTSS implementation efforts. They are tasked with ensuring that strategies and interventions are being used with fidelity and that student outcomes are being achieved. This team collaboratively problem solves to determine what adjustments are necessary based on data, and also ensures that sufficient resources are available to support implementation (e.g., materials, funding, staff time allocation).

Student support teams (behavior and/or academic) make data-based decisions for groups of students (Tier 1 and Tier 2) and individual students (Tier 3). The structure and purpose of behavior support teams and academic support teams are similar. It is recommended that these teams be combined when possible (based on school size and structure) to help facilitate collaboration and consistency between behavior and academic intervention efforts (Harn et al., 2015). Support teams typically meet twice per month to review data and (a) determine the extent to which Tier 1 supports are effective for the majority of the student population, (b) examine whether specific students need Tier 2 or 3 intervention, and (c) discuss the progress of students who are receiving Tier 2 or 3 interventions to determine whether any adjustments should be made. It is recommended that student support teams are interdisciplinary and include an administrator, representatives from each grade level and content area (if middle or high school), school psychologists, social workers, and specialized personnel such as a Board Certified Behavior Analyst (BCBA) for behavior support teams, and reading or mathematics specialists for academic support teams.

Another team in SWPBIS and RtI are grade-level teams. Grade-level teams involve teachers from each grade level who meet to discuss curriculum and teaching practices and to review data to determine if there are students who are facing similar behavioral and/or academic difficulties in multiple contexts. If there is evidence that students are facing significant difficulties in multiple areas and they have not responded to Tier 1 support, grade-level teams may refer students to the student support team for additional support.

Systems Approach

SWPBIS and RtI focus on establishing systems to support the implementation of research-validated practices. Without effective systems in place, it is unlikely that schools will be able to implement practices with sufficient fidelity to improve student outcomes and sustain implementation over time (Fixsen, Naoom, Blase, Friedman, & Wallace, 2005). Systems are not simply the school policies, but include the coordination of relevant school personnel for processes such as general operating procedures, budget and staff time allocation, data systems, teaming, hiring, onboarding, evaluation, and ongoing coaching for staff. By working to maximize the system infrastructure, this improves the school's capacity to efficiently implement practices and sustain implementation over time (Horner, Sugai, & Fixsen, 2017).

Integrated MTSS Support Students with ASD

While SWPBIS and RtI were originally developed and implemented in isolation from one another, researchers and practitioners now recognize the importance of integrating behavioral and academic supports to efficiently and effectively meet student needs (Freeman et al., 2015; Harn et al., 2015; Hawken et al., 2008; McIntosh, Horner, Chard, Boland, & Good, 2006). It is important to prioritize the integration of academic and behavioral support efforts, primarily because academic and behavioral success are tied to one another, and because coordination of system-level efforts ensures more efficient and organized use of resources and personnel (Hawken et al., 2008). Research has found that students' academic performance influences the likelihood that they will receive ODRs, as well as the degree to which they will respond to behavioral interventions (McIntosh et al., 2006). Additionally, student behavior can also influence academic success. Students who face difficulty accessing academic material may engage in off-task behavior, which may escalate as academic demands increase. Similarly, students who are exposed to academic material that is too easy for them may also engage in problem behavior. Due to how closely behavior and academics are linked, it is important for professionals to consider both academic and behavioral factors when evaluating student performance and making data-based decisions about interventions.

Using an integrated and collaborative approach to academic and behavioral support also helps ensure that school resources are used efficiently, and that interventions do not conflict with one another. If it is determined that a student needs both behavioral and academic interventions, it is important to involve the school personnel related to the implementation of each intervention to ensure that they are compatible, and to streamline different intervention components when possible. For example, a student who needs an intensive reading intervention who also engages in frequent off-task behavior may benefit from an intervention that includes targeted skill building in reading and a dense schedule of reinforcement for on-task behavior and work completion. The student's needs will be most efficiently and effectively met if the reading specialist and behavior specialist collaborate when designing, implementing, and evaluating the intervention.

It is important to note that students could require different levels of support for academics and social behavior, and this is also true for students with ASD. For example, a student with ASD might require an additional 30 min/day of reading instruction above what they receive in the general education classroom (Tier 2), and also have an individualized behavior support plan (Tier 3) that allows them to be successful in the general education setting. Another student with ASD might be successful with core academic instruction (Tier 1), but require small group social skills instruction for skill building in social behavior (Tier 2). The supports provided across the multi-tiered framework for both academics and social behavior are outlined below.

Tier 1

Goals and aims of Tier 1. The primary goal of Tier 1 supports is to prevent academic and behavioral problems before they occur by implementing effective practices to promote positive academic, behavioral, and social outcomes aligned with school success (Lane, Menzies, Ennis, & Bezdek, 2013). As mentioned earlier in this chapter, it is estimated that approximately 80% of the student population will be responsive to Tier 1 efforts alone, as long as they are implemented with fidelity (Hawken et al., 2008; Lane et al., 2013). The key implementation features of Tier 1 supports include the identification of meaningful outcomes, establishing and investing in schoolwide systems, selecting and implementing contextually appropriate and research-validated practices, and collecting and using data for decision-making (Simonsen, Sugai, & Negron, 2008).

To identify meaningful outcomes, the school leadership team works with relevant stakeholders (e.g., teachers, staff, families, community members) to identify socially significant outcomes related to academic and behavioral success. At this stage, schools examine data related to their school and any existing school-improvement plans to select areas that are priorities for improvement. The team then sets observable, measurable, and feasible goals to focus their Tier 1 implementation efforts.

A number of schoolwide systems will facilitate effective Tier 1 implementation, such as school teams, clear policies for how students are identified and provided intervention, universal screening, data collection and evaluation systems, fidelity checks, and an ongoing commitment to SWPBIS from staff and administration at both the school and district levels will enhance implementation (Horner, Sugai, & Anderson, 2010). A leadership team should be built with relevant representatives from administration, teachers, special services, support staff, and community members (Simonsen et al., 2008). The leadership team is responsible for guiding the implementation of other system-level components of Tier 1, which includes gaining at least 80% buy-in from the school faculty and staff, establishing an efficient data collection and evaluation system, and pursuing training in effective implementation of academic and behavioral efforts (Simonsen et al., 2008). After initial implementation, the leadership team is responsible for evaluating the effectiveness and fidelity of Tier 1 practices, providing ongoing coaching and training to maintain practices, and evaluating progress on the school's established goals.

At the core of Tier 1 is the selection and implementation of contextually appropriate, research-validated practices that will be provided to all students in the school. Within the context of SWPBIS, this involves establishing clearly defined schoolwide rules and expectations along with a continuum of consequences for appropriate and inappropriate behavior (Hawken et al., 2008). For RtI, this entails selecting a research-validated curriculum in each core content area that will be implemented by all teachers (Hawken et al., 2008; Lane et al., 2013).

The final critical element related to the implementation of Tier 1 practices is the collection and use of data for decision-making. Data are collected to determine which students need additional supports (using universal screening), evaluate the fidelity with which Tier 1 practices are implemented, and assess the degree to which student needs are being met through Tier 1 efforts (Horner et al., 2010). If there is low fidelity, or if fewer than 80% of students are responsive to Tier 1 efforts, the leadership team should invest in coaching teachers on Tier 1 practices and/or adjusting Tier 1 practices to ensure that contextually appropriate and research-validated practices are being used effectively and meeting the needs of the majority of the student population (Hawken et al., 2008; Lane et al., 2013).

Tier 1 RtI. Tier 1 RtI includes the core instruction that is provided to all students. Tier 1 RtI often refers to English/language arts and math curricula that are provided to all students in general education classrooms (Lane et al., 2013). Additionally, Tier 1 involves the implementation of effective teaching practices that can be used with any curricula in any class (i.e., frequent opportunities to respond, the use of assessment data to guide instructional decision-making, etc.; Lane et al., 2013). Tier 1 instruction should be backed by research. Schools that implement Tier 1 instruction that is not research-validated risk creating a situation in which a disproportionate number of students require more intensive intervention. Tier 1 instruction is the first level of preventative support. Schools that successfully implement research-validated instructional programs at Tier 1 create an environment in which most students will meet grade-level standards (Fuchs & Fuchs, 2006; Stecker, 2007).

Data collection to monitor students' responsiveness to intervention at Tier 1 involves universal screening of all students three times per academic year at their grade level (Lane et al., 2013). Often, this involves giving students a quick, reliable, and valid assessment known as a curriculum-based measure (CBM). A variety of CBMs are available for reading, writing, and math (Deno, 1985; Fuchs & Fuchs, 2006; Shinn, 2007). Conducting universal screening at each student's grade level allows school leadership to make instructional decisions that will support the students to meet short and long-term goals (National Center on Response to Intervention, n.d.b). The interdisciplinary school leadership team should include teachers who provide general education and special education services, related service personnel (e.g., occupational therapists, speech/language pathologists, physical therapists, etc.), a school psychologist, a school counselor, a behavior specialist, and at least one administrator with authority to commit resources. Including all of these individuals will enable the school leadership team to quickly and effectively design supports that will benefit all students.

Tier 1 SWPBIS. Consistent with MTSS logic, Tier 1 SWPBIS aims to prevent problem behavior from developing through the implementation of research-validated classroom management for all students. Common Tier 1 practices in SWPBIS include (a) working with stakeholders to establish school-wide rules that can be applied to any school context (e.g., be safe, be respectful, be responsible), (b) operationally defining rule-following for all school environments (e.g., being safe, respectful, and responsible on the playground, in the classroom, etc.), (c) explicitly teaching students the rules and expectations across environments, (d) reinforcing student appropriate behavior, (e) providing a continuum of consequences for problem behavior, and (f) data-based decision-making (Horner et al., 2010).

Data are collected at Tier 1 to evaluate the fidelity with which Tier 1 practices are being implemented and also to assess the degree to which Tier 1 is impacting student behavior (Horner et al., 2010). Analyzing these data also allow school teams to determine if any student might benefit from additional support at Tier 2. Fidelity data at Tier 1 are collected using tools such as the TFI, as outlined earlier in this chapter. For student behavior, proxy measures such as ODRs are used to monitor student rule violations. School teams review ODR data regularly and analyze data to identify any patterns (e.g., by location, time of day, student) and assess the impact of Tier 1 on the student population. These interdisciplinary school teams include a representative sample of the teachers, related service personnel, staff, and administration who work in the school, as well as family and student representatives. Including all of these individuals on the team allows for relevant stakeholders to have an opportunity to provide feedback on Tier 1 practices, solve problem, and shape Tier 1 implementation in a manner that is in the best interest of all students in the school.

Tier 2

Goals and aims of Tier 2. The goal of Tier 2 is to provide students who are non-responsive at the Tier 1 level with additional supports (Hawken et al., 2008). It is anticipated that even with well-implemented Tier 1 efforts, approximately 15% of students will require additional support at the Tier 2 level (Hawken et al., 2008; Lane et al., 2013). Tier 2 efforts are designed to heighten the intensity of support by increasing the time allocated to instruction, increasing the frequency of opportunities to practice and opportunities for feedback, and providing targeted instruction in specific areas of need (Fairbanks, Simonsen, & Sugai, 2008; Hawken et al., 2008; Horner et al., 2010). It is important to note that Tier 2 supports should be implemented in addition to those at Tier 1, and not as a substitution for Tier 1 (Lane et al., 2013). Additionally, Tier 2 supports should be considered fluid and temporary, meaning that a student should only receive Tier 2 supports until they are responding to intervention and can be successful at Tier 1 without additional supports (Lane et al., 2013).

Tier 2 interventions should require minimal time to implement, have similar features across students, and be aligned with Tier 1 efforts to facilitate implementation and sustainability (Fairbanks et al., 2008; Hawken et al., 2008; Yong & Cheney, 2013). As such, Tier 2 interventions are often multicomponent in nature (address more than one skill or area of need), frequently involve the use of standardized protocols, and often are delivered to groups of students (Hawken et al., 2008; Yong & Cheney, 2013). Tier 2 interventions may include direct instruction on specific skills, the allocation of more minutes to instruction in a particular subject, increased structure, more precise feedback, and increased school to home communication (Fairbanks et al., 2008; Hawken et al., 2008; Horner et al., 2010; Rodriguez, Loman, & Borgmeier, 2016; Yong & Cheney, 2013).

There are several system components essential for the efficient implementation of Tier 2. These include the establishment of criteria for early identification based on universal screening, a progress monitoring system, team meetings with a goal of identifying and monitoring the progress of students in need of Tier 2 supports, allocating financial time and effort to coordinate intervention implementation, an administrative and team process for selecting interventions, and the use of fidelity data to guide and adjust implementation (Horner et al., 2010). Additionally, a plan for gradually fading Tier 2 interventions should be incorporated to help facilitate maintenance and generalization of skills targeted during the Tier 2 intervention (Rodriquez et al., 2016; Yong & Cheney, 2013).

Tier 2 RtI. Tier 2 support is provided to students who perform below the defined benchmark in an academic area (Hawken et al., 2008). Supports in this tier may involve intensifying the instruction provided as part of Tier 1 or providing a research-validated intervention that supplements core instruction. Tier 2 supports are often provided to small groups of students with similar academic needs, with the goal that they will respond well to the intervention and not require more intensive interventions (Fuchs & Fuchs, 2006; Harlacher, Sanford, & Nelson Walker, n.d.; Stecker, 2007).

Students who receive Tier 2 supports participate in the universal screening described as part of Tier 1 (Lane et al., 2013). This allows school personnel to monitor how students are performing relative to other students at their grade level (National Center on Response to Intervention, n.d.b). Students receiving Tier 2 supports also benefit from progress monitoring (Hawken et al., 2008). Progress monitoring involves frequently giving students reliable, valid, and relatively quick assessments in the relevant academic area at their instructional level (Fuchs & Fuchs, 2006; National Center on Response to Intervention, n.d.a). In Tier 2, administering a progress monitoring assessment every two to four weeks is usually sufficient, depending on how sensitively the particular assessment measures growth, the subject area, and the student's goals (Harlacher, Sanford, & Nelson Walker, n.d.). Progress monitoring data assist school personnel in setting appropriate goals for students, monitoring their progress toward short and long-term goals, and adjusting instruction.

As described previously regarding Tier 1 RtI, the school leadership team that is responsible for monitoring the progress of students receiving Tier 2 supports should be interdisciplinary. For example, a student with ASD receiving Tier 2 supports in reading may also require additional support in the area of mathematics, particularly, when engaging in mathematics with more intense reading demands (e.g., solving story problems). In a situation like this, the reading and mathematics teachers both need to participate in the school leadership team so that reading performance and its impact on mathematics may be monitored. If the school leadership team decides that the student would benefit from supplemental reading instruction, then the individual responsible for delivering the supplemental instruction should also be a member of the school leadership team. It is important to carefully consider the needs of the students who receive Tier 2 supports to ensure that all of the necessary individuals are involved in the school leadership team.

Tier 2 SWPBIS. Tier 2 behavioral interventions are appropriate for students who engage in frequent mild to moderate intensity behavior problems throughout the day, and who have not been responsive to Tier 1 supports alone. These students are considered at risk, and should be provided with efficient and effective interventions to prevent the development of more intensive behavior problems (Mitchell, Stormont, & Gage, 2011). Students are typically identified for Tier 2 support by the behavior support team based on data such as ODRs, high rates of absenteeism, or teacher/parent referral. With Tier 2 interventions, there is a high priority placed on quick intervention implementation following identification; it is recommended that students be able to access an appropriate Tier 2 intervention within five days of being identified as in need of support (Crone, Hawken, & Horner, 2010). The intervention should align with the area of need demonstrated by the student. For example, a student exhibiting frequent off-task or disruptive behavior could be a good candidate for Check-in Check-out (CICO), the most widely implemented Tier 2 intervention in schools (Mitchell et al., 2011; Rodriguez et al., 2016). On the other hand, a student who is not engaging in disruptive and off-task behavior, but is struggling with poor social skills and peer interactions would likely be a good candidate for a social skills intervention. Regardless of the specific Tier 2 intervention selected, interdisciplinary collaboration plays an important role in the selection and provision of services. The interdisciplinary student support team works collaboratively to collect and review data when determining which students require Tier 2 support and to identify appropriate Tier 2 interventions for each student. To ensure that Tier 2 interventions are implemented with fidelity, relevant school professionals communicate to identify who is responsible for both implementing the intervention and collecting data to monitor student progress. For example, when implementing CICO, the CICO coordinator plays an important role in facilitating interdisciplinary collaboration. The CICO coordinator is responsible for communicating with each student's teachers to help address any concerns they have and deliver feedback to teachers on how they are implementing the intervention. The CICO coordinator is also responsible for communicating with the student's family on a regular basis, as well as providing data to the student support team so they can evaluate student progress. In addition to communicating with teachers, the student support team, and students' families, the CICO coordinator also updates administrators on a regular basis and asks for their support in resolving issues or challenges as they arise.

Tier 2 behavioral interventions are typically directly linked to Tier 1 practices, provide students with more structure, include specific prompts, incorporate self-monitoring, and include reinforcement of appropriate behavior (Fairbanks et al., 2008; Hawken et al., 2008; Horner et al., 2010; Rodriguez et al., 2016). For example, CICO is structured to align with the school-wide expectations in place at Tier 1. A student is provided with (a) positive adult contact at the start of the day when they check-in with the CICO coordinator, (b) targeted and specific feedback from their teacher(s) throughout the day, (c) reinforcement through teacher attention and feedback for appropriate behavior, and (d) additional reinforcement at the end of the day from the CICO coordinator if they meet their daily point goal (Crone et al., 2010). Additionally, students can self-monitor the degree to which they meet expectations throughout the day, and have teachers validate or correct their ratings. This process can also be used to help fade the intervention once the student has made adequate progress, which is a goal of Tier 2 interventions to help ensure that students can be successful with Tier 1 supports only (Rodriguez et al., 2016).

Tier 3

Goals and aims of Tier 3. Tier 3 interventions target the estimated 5% of students who have the most intensive needs in schools and are non-responsive to Tier 1 and Tier 2 supports (Hawken et al., 2008; Lane et al., 2013). These students may have needs in multiple areas (academic and social behavior), and/or may have multiple risk factors. Tier 3 interventions typically incorporate individualized lesson plans and strategies to address an individual student's specific learning needs (Hawken et al., 2008). Because Tier 3 supports are individualized and intensive, they require a significant time investment and should be used only for students who have not been successful with Tier 1 and 2 supports. Tier 3 supports are implemented in addition to, not as a replacement for, Tier 1 and 2 supports.

Tier 3 interventions involve the use of systems features, including the behavior support team, a progress monitoring system, a process for evaluating intervention fidelity, a specified process for reporting intervention outcomes, access to specialized expertise, and use of data to guide implementation (Horner et al., 2010). The process for implementing Tier 3 support begins by organizing an interdisciplinary team of relevant school personnel, family member(s), and perhaps the student themselves. The team works together to examine what assessments might be needed to inform particulars of Tier 3 intervention, data to be collected, and the process and people involved in collecting those data. The data most typically collected in the process of creating individualized interventions is a strength-based assessment and a functional behavior assessment (FBA; Fairbanks et al., 2008; Horner et al., 2010). After data are collected, the team meets again to evaluate the data and develop a comprehensive plan of support (Fairbanks et al., 2008). Tier 3 typically involves intensive instruction, applied behavior analytic techniques, self-management strategies, person-centered planning, and often components of Tier 2 interventions discussed earlier in this chapter (i.e., increased instructional time, opportunities for practice and feedback, etc.; Hawken et al., 2008; Horner et al., 2010). The interdisciplinary Tier 3 team also determines (a) the specific frequency of intervention implementation, (b) team member roles related to intervention delivery, (c) a measurement process to evaluate student progress, (d) criteria for response to intervention, and (e) how fidelity of implementation will be monitored.

Tier 3 RtI. Tier 3 RtI may involve further intensifying the academic supports provided in Tiers 1 and 2 (Fuchs & Fuchs, 2006; Harlacher, Sanford, & Nelson Walker, n.d.; Stecker, 2007), or it may also involve replacing the core and supplemental interventions provided in Tiers 1 and 2 with a research-validated core replacement program. Tier 3 support is provided to individual students or small groups of students. It is important to note that there is no consensus within the field regarding how Tier 3 academic supports interact with special education services; in some cases, Tier 3 RtI is considered synonymous with special education services, while in others Tier 3 supports are separate from special education services, or considered a step prior to referral for special education services (Hawken et al., 2008).

Students receiving Tier 3 support typically participate in the same universal screening process as students who receive Tier 1 and Tier 2 supports. Again, this allows school personnel to assess performance relative to the grade-level standards (National Center on Response to Intervention, n.d.b). Occasionally, however, a team may decide that participating in universal screening at the student's grade level is not beneficial for the student, such as when a student's skill level is well below grade level. Regardless if a student participates in universal screening, progress monitoring is still used to measure academic achievement at the student's instructional level. Progress monitoring at Tier 3 uses the same types of assessments as progress monitoring in Tier 2. The main difference between Tier 2 and Tier 3 progress monitoring is the frequency with which the assessments are delivered. Depending on the assessments being used, the academic area, the skill(s) being monitored, and the amount of time required to administer the assessments versus the amount of instructional time available, progress monitoring assessments in Tier 3 are usually administered at least every one to two weeks (Busch & Reschly, 2007; Harlacher, Sanford, & Nelson Walker, n.d.; National Center on Response to Intervention, 2012).

An interdisciplinary team is critical to the successful implementation of Tier 3 RtI. As stated earlier in this chapter, many students who receive Tier 3 supports in one area also receive them in other areas. As such, a student with ASD who receives Tier 3 supports in reading may also require Tier 3 supports in writing, mathematics, and related services. The amount of individualized instruction necessary to support a student who needs Tier 3 supports in multiple areas requires that all of the student's teachers and related service personnel meet frequently and regularly to review progress monitoring data and plan instruction. These meetings provide opportunities for alignment of instruction across service providers. For example, the reading, writing, and mathematics teachers may collaborate with the speech/language pathologist to design instruction that is aligned across subject areas and uses the student's time efficiently by not being overly repetitive or unintentionally introducing skills and concepts in ways that contradict one another.

Tier 3 SWPBIS. Tier 3 SWPBIS involves individualized, function-based support for students whose problem behavior is not sufficiently responsive to Tier 1 or Tier 2 support. Tier 3 includes working on an interdisciplinary team to conduct a functional behavior assessment (FBA) to hypothesize the variables maintaining problem behavior (i.e., the function of problem behavior), and the conditions under which problem behavior is most and least likely to occur. The FBA process should include input from relevant professionals who can provide input with respect to the student's social behavior, academic performance, mental health, and any other areas relevant to the student's success (e.g., speech and language, occupational therapy, etc.). From these FBA data, the interdisciplinary team develops a comprehensive behavior support plan (BSP; also known as behavior intervention plan). The BSP outlines strategies to (a) influence the larger social context around the student (b) prevent problem behavior (antecedent manipulations), (c) teach function-matched replacement behavior and other skills, (d) reinforce appropriate behavior, and (d) respond to problem behavior (consequence manipulations; Horner, Sugai, & Anderson, 2010). A common misconception is that Tier 3 is reserved for students receiving special education services. While students with special needs, including students with ASD, often engage in problem behavior (Ala'i-Rosales, et al., 2019), it is erroneous to equate special education services with Tier 3 behavior support, as not all students who require Tier 3 behavior support receive special education services.

A challenge for effective Tier 3 behavior support is not only developing the BSP, but ensuring that the plan is implemented consistently and with sufficient fidelity that it will produce desired student outcomes (Pinkelman & Horner, 2017). As such, in addition to specific instructional and function-matched strategies, the BSP should also include an implementation and evaluation plan that details (a) team members responsible for implementing each component of the plan, (b) how team members will receive training to implement the plan, (c) a timeline for implementation, (d) data to be collected on both fidelity and student outcomes, and (e) when data will be reviewed to assess both the extent to which the BSP is being implemented with fidelity and the extent to which it is impacting student behavior.

Conclusion

MTSS provides a framework for schools to efficiently deliver evidence-based practice to all students, including students with ASD. The continuum of supports in MTSS (i.e., Tiers 1, 2, and 3) allow interdisciplinary school teams to match intervention intensity to student need. Integrated and interdisciplinary MTSS that include both academic and behavior support are maximally effective and allow school teams to collaboratively address the unique and varied needs of all students.

References

Ala'i-Rosales, S., Cihon, J. H., Currier, T. D. R., Ferguson, J. L., Leaf, J. B., Leaf, R., McEachin, J., & Weinkauf, S. (2019). The big four: Functional assessment research informs preventative behavior analysis. *Behavior Analysis in Practice, 12,* 222–234.

Albin, R. W., Lucyshyn, J. M., Horner, R. H., & Flannery, K. B. (1996). Contextual fit for behavior support plans. In L. K. Koegel, R. L. Koegel, & G. Dunlap (Eds.), *Positive behavioral support: Including people with difficult behavior in the community* (pp. 81–98). Baltimore: Brookes.

Algozzine, B., Barrett, S., Eber, L., George, H., Horner, R., Lewis, T., Putnam, B., Swain-Bradway, J., McIntosh, K., & Sugai, G (2019). School-wide PBIS Tiered Fidelity Inventory. OSEP Technical Assistance Center on Positive Behavioral Interventions and Supports. www.pbis.org.

Busch, T. W. & Reschly, A. L. (2007). Progress monitoring in reading: Using curriculum-based measurement in a response-to-intervention model. *Assessment for Effective Instruction, 32*(4), 223–230.

Crone, D. A., Hawken, L. S., & Horner, R. H. (2010). *Responding to problem behavior in schools: The behavior education program* (2nd ed.). New York, NY: Guilford.

Deno, S. (1985). Curriculum-based measurement: The emerging alternative. *Exceptional Children, 52*(3), 219–232.

Fairbanks, S., Simonsen, B., & Sugai, G. (2008). Classwide secondary and tertiary tier practices and systems. *Teaching Exceptional Children, 40*(6), 44–52.

Freeman, R., Miller, D., & Newcomer, L. (2015). Integration of academic and behavioral MTSS at the district level using implementation science. *Learning Disabilities: A Contemporary Journal, 13,* 59–72.

Fixsen, D. L., Naoom, S. F., Blase, K. A., Friedman, R. M., & Wallace, F. (2005). Implementation Research: A Synthesis of the Literature. Tampa, FL: University of South Florida, Louis de la Parte Florida Mental Health Institute, The National Implementation Research Network (FMHI Publication #231).

Fuchs, D., & Fuchs, L. S. (2006). Introduction to response to intervention: What, why, and how valid is it? *Reading Research Quarterly, 41,* 93–99.

Harlacher, J. E., Sanford, A., & Nelson Walker, N. (n.d.). Distinguishing between tier 2 and tier 3 instruction in order to support implementation of RTI. Retrieved

from http://www.rtinetwork.org/essential/tieredinstruction/tier3/distinguishing-between-tier-2-and-tier-3-instruction-in-order-to-support-implementation-of-rti.
Harn, B., Basaraba, D., Chard, D., & Fritz, R. (2015). The impact of schoolwide prevention efforts: Lessons learned from implementing independent academic and behavior support systems. *Learning Disabilities: A Contemporary Journal, 13*(1), 3–20.
Hawken, L. S., Vincent, C. G., & Schumann, J. (2008). Response to intervention for social behavior: Challenges and opportunities. *Journal of Emotional and Behavioral Disorders, 16,* 213–225.
Horner, R. H., & Sugai, G. (2015). School-wide PBIS: An example of applied behavior analysis implemented at a scale of social importance. *Behavior Analysis in Practice, 8,* 80–85.
Horner, R. H., Sugai, G., & Anderson, C. M. (2010). Examining the evidence base for school-wide positive behavior support. *Focus on Exceptional Children, 42*(8), 1–14.
Horner, R. H., Sugai, G., & Fixsen, D. L. (2017). Implementing effective educational practices at scales of social importance. *Clinical Child and Family Psychology Review, 20,* 25–35.
Lane, K. L., Menzies, H. M., Ennis, R. P., & Bezdek, J. (2013). School-wide systems to promote positive behaviors and facilitate instruction. *Journal of Curriculum and Instruction, 7,* 6–31.
McIntosh, K., Horner, R. H., Chard, D. J., Boland, J. B., & Good, R. H. (2006). The use of reading and behavior screening measures to predict nonresponse to school-wide positive behavior support: A longitudinal analysis. *School Psychology Review, 35,* 275–291.
Merrell, K. W., & Buchanan, R. (2006). Intervention selection in school-based practice: Using public health models to enhance systems capacity of schools. *School Psychology Review, 35,* 167–180.
Mitchell, B. S., Stormont, M., & Gage, N. A. (2011). Tier two interventions implemented within the context of a tiered prevention framework. *Behavioral Disorders, 36*(4), 241–261.
National Center on Intensive Intervention. (n.d.). Intensive intervention & multi-tiered system of supports (MTSS). Retrieved from https://intensiveintervention.org/intensive-intervention/multi-tiered-systems-support.
National Center on Response to Intervention. (n.d.a). Implementer series: What is progress monitoring? Retrieved from https://rti4success.org/video/implementer-series-what-progress-monitoring.
National Center on Response to Intervention. (n.d.b). Implementer series: What is screening? Retrieved from https://rti4success.org/video/implementer-series-what-screening.
National Center on Response to Intervention. (2012). RTI implementer series: Module 2: Progress monitoring. Retrieved from https://rti4success.org/sites/default/files/RTI%20PM%20Manual_web_w_handouts.pdf.
Nellis, L. M. (2012). Maximizing the effectiveness of building teams in response to intervention implementation. *Psychology in the Schools, 49,* 245–256.
Pinkelman, S. E., & Horner, R. H. (2017). Improving implementation of function-based interventions: Self-monitoring, data collection, and data review. *Journal of Positive Behavior Interventions, 19,* 228–238.
Rodriguez, B. J., Loman, S. L., & Borgmeier, C. (2016). Tier 2 interventions in positive behavior support: A survey of school implementation. *Preventing School Failure, 60,* 94–105.
Shinn, M. R. (2007). Identifying students at risk, monitoring performance, and determining eligibility within response to intervention: Research on education need and benefit from academic intervention. *School Psychology Review, 36*(4), 601–617.
Simonsen, B., Sugai, G., & Negron, M. (2008). Schoolwide positive behavior supports: Primary systems and practices. *Teaching Exceptional Children, 40*(6), 32–40.
Slocum, T. A., Detrich, R., Wilczynski, S. M., Spencer, T. D., Lewis, T., & Wolfe, K. (2014). The evidence-based practice of applied behavior analysis. *The Behavior Analyst, 37,* 41–56.
Stecker, P. M. (2007). Tertiary intervention: Using progress monitoring with intensive services. *Teaching Exceptional Children, 39*(5), 50–57.
Sugai, G., & Horner, R. H. (2009). Defining and describing schoolwide positive behavior support. In W. Sailor, G. Dunlap, G. Sugai, & R. Horner (Eds.), *Handbook of positive behavior support* (pp. 307–326). Issues in Clinical Child Psychology Series. New York, NY: Springer.

Walker, H. M., Horner, R. H., Sugai, G., Bullis, M., Sprague, J., Bricker, D., Kaufman, M. J. (1996). Integrated approaches to preventing antisocial behavior patterns among school-age children and youth. *Journal of Emotional and Behavioral Disorders, 4,* 194–209.

Wolf, M. M. (1978). Social validity: The case for subjective measurement or how applied behavior analysis is finding its heart. *Journal of Applied Behavior Analysis, 11,* 203–214.

Yong, M., & Cheney, D. A. (2013). Essential features of tier 2 social-behavioral interventions. *Psychology in the Schools, 50*(8), 844–861.

Partners in School: An Example of Care Coordination to Ensure Consistency of Evidence-Based Practices Across Home and School for Youth with Autism Spectrum Disorder (ASD)

Gazi F. Azad, Brianna J. Williams, Kyla E. Minton, Susan M. Sheridan, and David S. Mandell

Abstract The Individuals with Disabilities Education Act (IDEA, 2004) and the Every Student Succeeds Act (ESSA, 2015) mandate that families participate in shared decision-making with schools. For youth who receive special education services, such as those who have ASD, having parents and teachers aligned in their practices is even more crucial. Unfortunately, consistency of evidence-based practices (EBP) across home and school is rarely experienced. This chapter describes the development of *Partners in School*, an example of coordinating care between home and school settings for youth with ASD. The goal of *Partners in School* is to ensure that parents and teachers are implementing the same EBPs in the same way (i.e., consistently). It draws from the literature on school consultation, business negotiations, and health communication/shared decision-making. The scientific literature is merged with the perspectives of parents and teachers of elementary students with ASD from a large urban school district. The chapter begins by anchoring this approach on the empirical evidence for family–school partnerships, and then concludes by describing the implications of *Partners in School* for care coordination.

G. F. Azad (✉)
Division of Child and Adolescent Psychiatry, New York State Psychiatric Institute and Columbia University, New York, NY, USA
e-mail: gazi.azad@nyspi.columbia.edu

K. E. Minton
Center for Autism and Related Disorders, Kennedy Krieger Institute, Baltimore, MD, USA

B. J. Williams
Department of Counseling, Educational Psychology, and Special Education, Michigan State University, East Lansing, MI, USA

S. M. Sheridan
College of Education and Human Sciences, University of Nebraska Lincoln, Lincoln, NE, USA

D. S. Mandell
Center for Mental Health, Perelman School of Medicine, University of Pennsylvania, Philadelphia, PA, USA

M. B. McClain et al. (eds.), *Interprofessional Care Coordination for Pediatric Autism Spectrum Disorder*, https://doi.org/10.1007/978-3-030-46295-6_11

A family–school partnership can be defined as a student-centered relationship involving close communication and collaboration between parents and teachers, given their shared responsibilities in ensuring the academic, social, emotional, and behaviorial well-being of children (Christenson & Sheridan, 2001). The concept of family–school partnerships is grounded in ecological systems theory, which identifies five distinct areas that contribute to development. In this theoretical approach, families or schools are situated in the area characterized by direct contact, called the microsystem. The mesosystem focuses on the relationship between these different systems (Bronfenbrenner, 1992). Difficulties occur for youth when there is incongruity, such as a mismatch between the home and school systems. As a result, various professional organizations (e.g., National Parent-Teacher Association, 2009; State Support Network, 2018) have created guidelines to improve family–school partnerships, focusing on welcoming families, communicating effectively, establishing trust, sharing power, and providing professional development training.

Parents' involvement in their children's education is often based on the opportunities for participation presented by the school staff. The most effective programs targeting family-school partnerships work with parents directly to target specific skills or behaviors (Magnuson & Schindler, 2016). For example, the *Getting Ready for School* intervention targets families from traditionally underserved backgrounds and provides them with weekly workshops to prepare their preschoolers for the transition to school (Marti et al., 2018). Educating parents of developmental milestones may empower them to work with teachers to integrate developmentally appropriate opportunities into their daily routines at home (Magnuson & Schindler, 2016). When a strong family-school partnership is lacking, children may experience inconsistencies between expectations and responses to behaviors at home and at school, leading to higher levels of externalizing behaviors (Daley, Munk, & Carlson, 2011).

A strong family-school partnership is important for all children, and there are many reasons why it is particularly critical for youth with ASD who receive special education services. First, a diagnostic characteristic of youth with ASD is difficulty with change. In the area of restricted, repetitive patterns of behavior, the Diagnostic and Statistical Manual-Fifth Edition (DSM-5), makes references to an "insistence on sameness" and "inflexible adherence to routines" (American Psychiatric Association, 2013). Therefore, discontinuity of experiences across home and school may be particularly distressing for youth with ASD. Second, the challenges associated with ASD are often pervasive across home and school contexts (Azad & Mandell, 2016). For example, youth who struggle to transition from preferred to non-preferred activities often display this rigidity both at home and at school. Third, a comprehensive approach to addressing the needs of youth with ASD requires both parents and teachers to engage in EBPs at home and school, respectively. Accordingly, there has been a trend in the field of autism services toward parent-mediated interventions (Green et al., 2015; McConachie & Diggle, 2006; Oono, Honey, & McConachie, 2013; Rogers et al., 2014) or teacher coaching models (Kretlow & Bartholomew, 2010; Mandell et al., 2013; Wilson, Dykstra, Watson, Boyd & Crais, 2012) to ensure that the primary stakeholders in children's lives are engaging in scientifically supported practices. Unfortunately, there are limited models that effectively harness the power of both parents and teachers to improve outcomes for children with ASD.

Partners in School Development: Drawing from Multidisciplinary Research

The goal of *Partners in School* is to maximize continuity for children with ASD by ensuring that the same EBPs are used across home and school. This approach establishes bidirectional parent-teacher communication and takes them through a systematic problem-solving process with the goal of duplicating intervention components from the school to the home. To develop this comprehensive model, we drew from several scientific literatures including school consultation, business negotiations, and health communication/shared decision-making.

School Consultation

At the epicenter of school-based consultation models is the concept of problem-solving. There are four essential steps to problem-solving: (1) identifying the problem, (2) determining why it may be happening, (3) developing and then subsequently implementing an intervention, and (4) evaluating the effectiveness of that intervention. In Bergan & Kratochwill's, (1990) model of behavioral consultation (BC), a consultant (e.g., school psychologist) and consultee (i.e., teacher) collaboratively work through this problem-solving sequence to address a student's needs in the classroom.

Sheridan and colleagues expanded BC to include parents in Conjoint Behavioral Consultation (CBC). In CBC, consultants work with both parents and teachers (i.e., as consultees) to problem solve concerns about students. In both BC and CBC, the problem-solving process is implemented through a series of three or more interviews (Sheridan & Kratochwill, 2008). Several randomized controlled trials (RCTs) have confirmed that CBC is effective in improving behavior outcomes for typically developing children (Sheridan et al., 2012; Sheridan, Witte, Holmes, Coutts, et al., 2017; Sheridan, Witte, Holmes, Wu, et al., 2017). More specifically, parents who participated in CBC reported significantly fewer challenging behaviors in children when compared to a control group of parents (Sheridan et al., 2013). Further, students whose parents participated in CBC demonstrated increased "learning related" behaviors, such as following directions and decreased disruptive behaviors, such as excessive motor movement (Sheridan et al., 2017).

School-based consultation for youth with ASD has been led by Ruble and Colleagues (2010). Their approach, titled, "Collaborative Model for Promoting Competence and Success (COMPASS)," includes one preliminary parent-teacher consultation meeting, followed by four teacher coaching sessions. In randomized control trials, COMPASS has shown to be successful in helping children obtain their Individual Education Program (IEP) goals (Ruble, Dalrymple, & McGrew, 2010; Ruble, Dalrymple, & McGrew, 2012). Both CBC and COMPASS are impactful models that have greatly influenced the development of *Partners in School*.

Business Negotiations

The idea of problem-solving in school consultation has many similarities to the concept of negotiation in business. For example, Adair & Brett's (2005) four-stage model of transactional negotiation includes relational positioning, identifying the problem, generating solutions, and reaching an agreement. During these four stages, negotiators alternate between cooperative and competitive orientations. Business experts suggest that there is a relationship between a negotiator's emotional state and the outcome of the negotiation. More specifically, positive moods can increase a negotiator's tendencies to select a cooperative strategy (Forgas, 1998), whereas negative moods can make negotiators more competitive in their preferences (Loewenstein, Thompson, & Bazerman, 1989).

Experiencing positive emotions is related to the idea of a mental model. Based on language expectancy theory (Burgoon, Denning, & Roberts, 2002), a mental model is defined as a cognitive representation of the expected negotiation, which includes the self, the dyadic relationship, attributions about the other person, and knowledge of the bargaining process. Of particular importance is the notion that individuals who modified their initial perceptions (or mental models) did so at the onset of the interaction; otherwise, the fixed assumptions tended to persist throughout the interaction (Bazerman, Curhan, Moore, & Valley, 2000; Thompson & Hastie, 1990). A mechanism to modify these initial perceptions is to engage in positive violations of expectations. Positive violations occur when someone behaves better than expected or when someone initially evaluated negatively behaves according to social norms, cultural values, or situational demands (Burgoon et al., 2002). The negotiation literature suggests that people are more satisfied with a deal, and more likely to follow through with a deal, when they experience positive emotions, particularly at the beginning of the negotiation as a positive violation of their expectations. Therefore, in the *Partners in School* model, positive emotions in parents and teachers are elicited at the onset of their interaction.

Health Communication and Shared Decision-Making

Historically, there is much similarity between the patient-physician relationship and the parent-teacher relationship. Although both of these relationships have been predominately one-sided (Henderson, Hunt, & Day, 1993; Siminoff & Step, 2005; Work & Stafford, 1987), there are recent shifts that encourage a partnership approach. For example, medical-shared decision-making advocates for a *partnership* approach featuring the two-way exchange of information and preferences between patients and their physicians (Charles, Gafni, & Whelan, 1999). As mentioned previously, home-school *partnerships* advocate for a mutually beneficial relationship between parents and teachers around issues of communication, problem-solving, support, and overlapping goals (Christenson & Sheridan, 2001; Sheridan & Kratochwill, 2008).

Similar to business negotiation, experts in health communication have shown that initial experiences influence subsequent outcomes. In health communication, the nature of initial communication exchanges between a physician and his/her patient has a direct influence on patients' choices between treatment options and their subsequent adherence to treatment plans (Siminoff & Step, 2005). Unfortunately, when patients and physicians come together within the health context, their differences are immediately highlighted. When differences are highlighted, this sets the course of the interaction for both parties to solely focus on their own needs. One way to address this problem is to have communicators "discover" their similarities. Creating shared understandings and common interests are key to co-constructing the interaction. In general, people are more inclined to cooperate with other people who they perceive as similar to themselves (Siminoff & Step, 2005). These findings suggest that in the *Partners in School* model, it is necessary to direct parents' and teachers' attention to their similarities given the inclination to focus on their differences.

Partners in School Development: Perspectives of Parents and Teachers of Youth with ASD

Agreement on Concerns

In a previous study, researchers merged the scientific literature described above with the perspectives of parents and teachers of children with ASD from schools in a large urban public school district (Azad, Marcus, Sheridan, & Mandell, 2018). Their initial interest was to examine whether parents and teachers agreed about their concerns for the same child. They interviewed parents and teachers about their top three concerns for the child with ASD, and then subsequently gave them an opportunity to discuss their concerns during a dyad observation. Interview data showed that parent and teacher concerns clustered around eight general areas (e.g., following direction, difficulty transitioning, aggressive behaviors, etc.) Parents and teachers shared the same primary concern 28% of the time. More importantly, 69% of parents and teachers shared the same top two concerns, even if they were not in the same order. For example, a parent's first concern may have been the teacher's second concern, and vice versa. This finding is encouraging because it suggested that parents and teachers agreed with their concerns when multiple concerns are queried. Unfortunately, during the discussion of their concerns, 49% of the parent-teacher dyads discussed concerns that neither reported as their primary concern; 31% discussed concerns that neither reported as their primary or secondary concern. These findings indicated that although parents and teachers may agree about their concerns, they are unable to communicate about them effectively (Azad & Mandell, 2016). Therefore, in the *Partners in School* model, it became imperative to get parents and teachers talking about their most salient concerns.

Problem-Solving

Researchers were also interested in the extent to which parents and teachers could generate solutions about mutual concerns. Their data suggested that parents and teachers of children with ASD displayed limited use of the core elements of problem-solving (e.g., defining a mutual concern, setting goals, developing interventions to address their mutual concerns, discussing data collection methods), but moderate levels of behaviors that facilitated the problem-solving process (e.g., discussing students' strengths, providing background information about the home or school setting). Parents and teachers also were generally "nice" to each other, referred to as psychological involvement in problem-solving. For example, they communicated in a calm manner and used verbal and nonverbal cues to convey understanding (Azad, Kim, Marcus, Sheridan, & Mandell, 2016). These findings suggested that the *Partners in School* model would need to focus on the core elements of problem-solving with parents and teachers of children with ASD.

Given that this exploratory work was conducted in a diverse urban setting, researchers were interested in whether demographic characteristics of parents or teachers impacted their problem-solving skills. Data showed that lower income parents and parents interacting with white teachers displayed less problem-solving compared to higher income parents and parents interacting with non-white teachers (Azad et al., 2018). Based on these findings, it would be necessary to add explicit strategies that would "even the playing field," allowing parents and teachers equal opportunities to engage in the problem-solving process.

Central Themes

Given the limited work in this area, researchers aimed to gain a deeper understanding of what ideal collaborations would look like between parents and teachers. Content analyses suggested parents and teachers were concerned about different aspects of communication. Parents were more concerned about the content of their communication with teachers, such as what their child was learning at school (i.e., in order to create similar ex-periences at home). Teachers were more concerned about the mechanisms of communication and reported feeling frustrated with the communication methods (e.g., written and face-to-face) they attempted to use to stay connected with parents.

Further, parents and teachers did not want to ask the other person to be more involved because of the perceptions of their challenges (i.e., faced by the other person). Both attributed resistance from the other person as a lack of confidence in their own expertise. Although both parents and teachers valued parental presence, teachers wanted parents to be active partners in the education of their children (Azad, Wolk, & Mandell, 2018). These findings suggested that both the content and mechanisms of communication, as well as the expertise of parents and teachers would have to be considered in the *Partners in School* model.

Logistical Needs

Researchers asked parents and teachers how long meetings should be in the *Partners in School* model. For parents, 53.8% of the sample opted for 30–60 min. Approximately 46.2% of teachers wanted 15–30 min meetings. Accordingly, *Partners in School* has both 30- and 45-min meetings. Second, researchers queried about how the meetings should take place with face-to-face, phone, or a combination of these approaches provided as options. Parents wanted face-to-face (54%) or a combination of face-to-face and phone meetings (39%). Similarly, 48.7% of teachers wanted face-to-face meetings and 41% wanted a combination. Therefore, *Partners in School* includes both phone and face-to-face components.

There was also interest in how many meetings parents and teachers would actually participate in across a 10-week or approximately 2-month span, and what time of day those meetings should take place. Parents were variable in their opinions on the number of meetings, ranging from two (i.e., once a month; 23.1%), five (i.e., every 2 weeks, 30.7%), or 10 meetings (i.e., once a week; 17.9%). About half (51.3%) or slightly over a third (35.9%) of the parents wanted these meetings to take place either in the morning to early afternoon, or early to late afternoon, respectively. Many teachers wanted two meetings (23.1%) or five meetings (43.6%) over the course of the 10 weeks. Only a minority (10.3%) wanted these meetings to be after school or in the evenings and more than half (66.7%) wanted meetings to take place at variable times. To accommodate these preferences, *Partners in School* three face-to-face meetings scheduled during the day, and phone meetings scheduled at variable times.

The *Partners in School* Model

Partners in School is a four-step model that occurs over the course of 10 weeks. It is comprised of: (1) an individual pre-consultation phone interview; (2) an in-person consultant-facilitated parent-teacher consultation meeting; (3) implementation of the same student intervention plan at home and at school; and (4) an individual post-consultation phone interview. Pre- and post-consultation surveys are collected after the phone interviews. See Fig. 1 for a visual representation of the model.

Pre-consultation Phone Interview (30 Min)

Parents and teachers participate in a pre-consultation phone interview that is conducted separately with the consultant. The goals of pre-consultation are to: (a) build rapport with parents and teachers; (b) encourage parents and teachers to reflect on the other person's role; and (c) gain child-specific information that would facilitate the in-person consultation. To accomplish these goals, we begin by asking parents or teachers to identify a strength in the other person. In school-based meetings, parents and teachers are accustomed to reporting on the problems that they experience with students (Azad & Mandell, 2016), and therefore, this question is purposely intended to create a positive violation of expectations and trigger a more positive mood.

Next, the challenges faced by the other person are discussed. As mentioned previously, parents and teachers often do not want to ask the other person to be more involved given their (i.e., the other person's) challenges. This approach was a way for parents and teachers to acknowledge the other person's challenges openly, but not let these factors impede their ability to collaboratively work together. After these initial questions designed to build rapport and empathy, parents or teachers discussed preferences displayed by the child at home or school, respectively. Partners in School utilizes strength-based student intervention plans given the longstanding evidence of positive reinforcement in shaping behavior (MacNaul & Neely, 2018).

The last two components of the pre-consultation phone interview were related to baseline data collection. Using the eight concerns identified in the exploratory work, parents and teachers selected the concerns that were most relevant for the child. For the concerns that they endorsed, parents and teachers ranked ordered their top three concerns (prior work indicating 69% agreement when multiple concerns, regardless of the order, are queried). For each of the three concerns, parents and teachers rated the frequency and severity of that concern at home or school, respectively. Pre-consultation surveys targeting parent or teacher (e.g., self-efficacy), dyadic (e.g., communication), or child (e.g., behavior problems) outcomes were distributed after the interviews either by mail or in-person at the child's school.

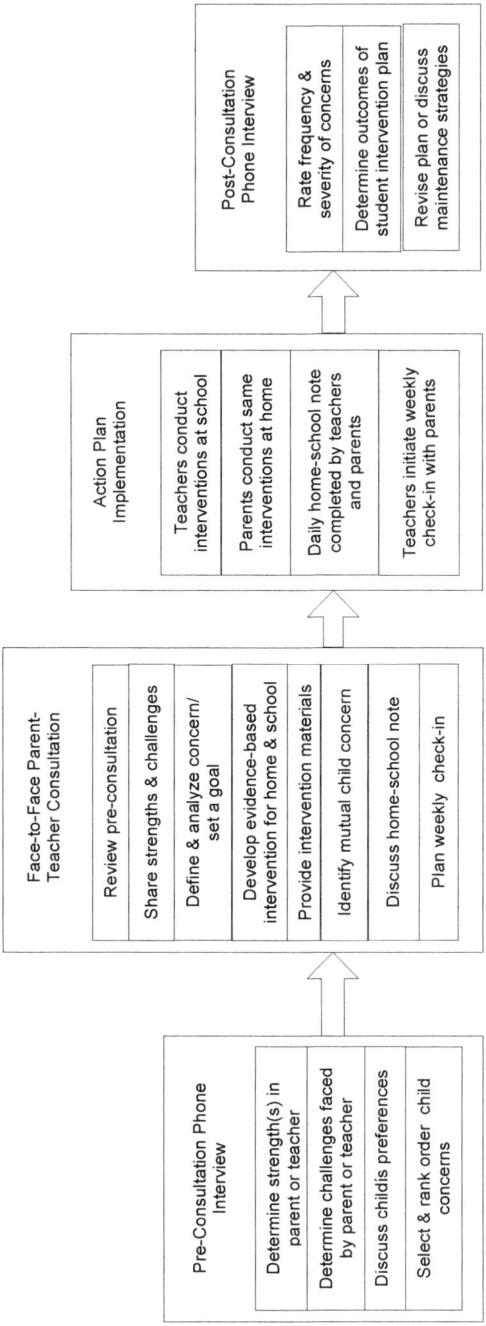

Fig. 1 Visual representation of the *partners in school* model

Face-to-Face Parent-Teacher Consultation (45 Min)

Parents and teachers were asked to bring their pre-consultation surveys to the face-to-face consultation meeting. The goals of the consultation meeting were to: (a) share information gathered during the pre-consultations; (b) collaboratively design an individualized student intervention plan to be implemented in the same way across home and school; and (c) develop a communication plan for parents and teachers to discuss intervention progress. The consultant began this meeting by providing parents and teachers with notes about the information that they shared during their separate pre-consultation phone interview. The initial part of the consultation was prescriptive to allow parents and teachers equal opportunities to speak (given the research showing that low-income parents and parents interacting with white teachers may engage in less problem-solving).

Parents and teachers shared the top three concerns that they identified in the child during the pre-consultation. They reported on these concerns rather than having the consultant report on the overlapping concern because of the emphasis on similarities at the onset of the interaction (i.e., target concern), rather than differences. Next, parents and teachers shared the strengths they identified in the other person with the intention of eliciting positive emotions. They shared their perspectives on the other person's challenges, so neither party would feel guilty about the other's involvement. Both of these brief shares were intended to be positive violations of expectations to alter the course of the discussion into a more cooperative (rather than competitive) interaction.

The next phase of the consultation meeting focused on the core components of problem-solving given that it was the areas where parents and teachers struggled the most. Parents and teachers provided more information on the target concern and set a goal to be achieved at home or school, respectively.

When developing the individualized student intervention plan to address the mutual concern, the consultant merged knowledge on the core principals of EBPs for ASD with the expertise of parents and teachers. Intervention research has established 27 EBPs that lead to positive educational outcomes in children with ASD (Wong et al., 2014). The goal of *Partners in School* is to help parents and teachers implement EBPs, and to do so consistently across settings. This approach is not wedded to a particular evidence-based program (e.g., JASPER [Kasari, Paparella, Freeman, & Jahromi, 2008]; Early Achievements [Landa, Holman, O'Neill, & Stuart, 2011]), rather it capitalizes on the large array of evidence-based approaches available (e.g., prompting, reinforcement, etc.). There were shared and nonshared EBPs in the student intervention plans developed during *Partners in School*. More specifically, all student intervention plans (i.e., the shared aspect) utilized visual supports (Knight, Sartini, & Spriggs, 2014) and positive reinforcement (MacNaul & Neely, 2018) given the evidence-base for these approaches. Other nonshared EBPs were used based on the needs of the student (Azad et al., 2018).

It was essential that parents and teachers felt like equal active partners in the process of developing the student intervention plan. The expertise of parents and teachers were valued, whether it was about the child's preferences or the different strategies that they previously used to address the mutual concern. All materials needed for the student intervention plan were provided to parents and teachers on the same day to facilitate immediate implementation.

In addition to the student intervention plan, there was a communication plan that parents and teachers co-constructed together. The first component of the communication plan was the daily home-school notes. Teachers were provided with 15 copies of the daily home-school note and a folder to keep the home-school notes in their classroom. Parents were provided with a folder to place in their child's backpack for the home-school notes to travel from school to home, and back to school. Parents and teachers also planned for a weekly check-in using any mode of communication (e.g., call or text) that they preferred.

For each day that the student intervention plan was implemented across home and school, parents and teachers completed a pre-populated home-school note that listed each of the steps in the student intervention plan generated during the consultation meeting. Teachers indicated whether the steps were completed at school and how much progress was made toward the goal. They also signed the form and sent it home to parents. Parents also indicated whether the same steps were completed at home and how much progress the child made toward their goal. Parents signed the form and returned it in their child's backpack to the teacher. A bidirectional form of communication was created to allow both parents and teachers to feel like equal active partners. At the end of the first and second week, the consultant emailed the teacher to remind him/her that it was their day to check-in with the parent. Teachers initiated a weekly check-in with parents using the mode of communication that they agreed upon during the consultation meeting. Teachers were provided with three semi-structured questions for the weekly check-in. At the end of the third week, the consultant collected the home-school notes to graph the student-level data and schedule the post-consultation phone interview. Parents and teachers implemented the student intervention plan in their respective settings for three weeks.

Post-consultation Phone Interview (30 Min)

The goals of the post-consultation phone interview were to discuss (a) the outcomes of the intervention plan; (b) the outcomes of the communication plan; and (c) changes to the student intervention plan or generalization strategies. This interview was conducted with parents or teachers, separately. The consultant began the phone interview by asking parents or teachers to rate the frequency and severity of the top three concerns that they identified during the pre-consultation phone interview. Next, they discussed the student-level data showing how much progress the student made toward their predetermined goal. Parents and teachers provided their perspectives on the communication plan, including the daily home-school notes and the weekly check-ins. Depending on how much progress the student made, the consultant discussed either alterations to the student intervention plan or strategies to generalize the plan (e.g., to a different time of the day).

Implications for Interdisciplinary Care Coordination

Children and adolescents with ASD require care in multiple settings, with home and school being the settings where these youth spend a majority of their time. Although the accumulated evidence on family-school partnerships suggests that coordinating care between home and school contexts is critical, there are limited empirically grounded approaches that attempt to do this effectively in educational practice. *Partners in School* is an example of how to effectively coordinate care between home and school settings. This approach is grounded in the literature from school consultation, business negotiation, and health communication/shared decision-making. This evidence was merged with mixed-method data from parents and teachers about their agreement on child concerns, the ability to problem solve, and perspectives on their ideal collaborations. Logistical information from parents and teachers also was gathered, and taken into consideration. The goal of *Partners in School* is to synchronize home and school settings, such that parents and teachers are implementing the same EBPs in the same way. Aligning parent and teacher practices increases children's access to EBPs by strengthening intervention dosage, intensity, and impact.

The *Partners in School* model has implications for interdisciplinary care coordination. Research has consistently shown that parents (Vohra, Madhavan, Sambamoorthi, & St. Peter, 2014) and professionals (Golnick, Ireland, & Borowsky, 2009) often report a lack of interdisciplinary care coordination as a major barrier in the provision of high-quality services for children with ASD. For example, Farmer et al., (2014) reported that less than one-third (29.9%) of families of children with ASD received coordinated care. Given that coordinated care across disciplines is difficult to achieve, parents often become the "messenger" by relaying information between professionals (e.g., providing school-based information from teachers to primary care providers). If parents and teachers are not synchronized, it is unlikely that care from other providers (e.g., pediatricians, psychologists, etc.) will be coordinated, and subsequently integrated into a comprehensive treatment plan. Coordinating care between parents and teachers may be particularly important for lower SES parents given that this vulnerable population has a higher risk of lacking interdisciplinary care coordination (Brown, Green, Desai, & Weitzman, 2014). Care coordination between home and school may be the first step in more interdisciplinary care coordination, and ultimately, better outcomes for youth with ASD.

References

Adair, W. L., & Brett, J. M. (2005). The negotiation dance: Time, culture, and behavioral sequences in negotiation. *Organization Science, 16,* 33–51.
American Psychiatric Association. (2013). *Diagnostic and statistical manual of mental disorders* (5th ed.). Washington, DC: Author.
Azad, G., & Mandell, D. S. (2016). Concerns of parents and teachers of children with autism in elementary school. *Autism, 40,* 435–441.
Azad, G., Kim, M., Marcus, S. C., Sheridan, S. M., & Mandell, D. S. (2016). Parent-teacher communication about children with autism spectrum disorder: An examination of collaborative problem-solving. *Psychology in the Schools, 53*(10), 1071–1084.
Azad, G., Gormley, S., Marcus, S., & Mandell, D. S. (2018a). Parent-teacher problem solving about concerns in children with autism spectrum disorder: The role of income and race. *Psychology in the Schools, 56*(2), 276–290.
Azad, G., Marcus, S., Sheridan, S., & Mandell, D. S. (2018b). Partners in school: An innovative parent-teacher consultation model for children with autism spectrum disorder. *Journal of Educational and Psychological Consultation, 28*(4), 460–486.
Azad, G., Wolk, C. B., & Mandell, D. S. (2018c). Ideal interactions: Perspectives of parents and teachers of children with autism spectrum disorder. *School Community Journal, 28,* 63–84.
Bazerman, M. H., Curhan, J. R., Moore, D. A., & Valley, K. L. (2000). Negotiation. *Annual Review of Psychology, 51,* 279–314.
Bergan, J. R., & Kratochwill, T. R. (1990). *Applied clinical psychology: Behavioral consultation and therapy*. New York, NY: Plenum Press.
Bronfenbrenner, U. (1992). Ecological systems theory. In R. Vasta (Ed.), *Six theories of child development: Revised formulations and current issues* (pp. 187–249). London, UK: Jessica Kinglsey Publishers.
Brown, N. M., Green, J. C., Desai, M. M., Weitzman, C. C., & Rosenthal, M. S. (2014). Need and unmet need for care coordination among children with mental health conditions. *Pediatrics, 133,* 530–537.
Burgoon, M., Denning, V. P., & Roberts, L. (2002). Language Expectancy Theory. In J. P. Dillard & M. Pfau (Eds.), *The SAGE handbook of persuasion: Developments in theory and practice* (pp. 117–136). Thousand Oaks, CA: Sage Publications.
Charles, C., Gafni, A., & Whelan, T. (1999). Decision-making in the physician-patient encounter: Revisiting the shared treatment decision-making model. *Social Science and Medicine, 49,* 651–661.
Christenson, S. L., & Sheridan, S. M. (2001). *Schools and families: Creating essential connections for learning*. New York, NY: Guilford Press.
Daley, T. C., Munk, T., & Carlson, E. (2011). A national study of kindergarten transition practices for children with disabilities. *Early Childhood Research Quarterly, 26*(4), 409–419.
Farmer, J. E., Clark, M. J., Mayfield, W. A., Cheak-Zamora, N., Marvin, A. R., Law, J. K., et al. (2014). The relationship between the medical home and the unmet needs for children with autism spectrum disorders. *Maternal and Child Health Journal, 18,* 672–680.
Forgas, J. P. (1998). On feeling good and getting your way: Mood effects on negotiator cognition and bargaining strategies. *Journal of Personality and Social Psychology, 74,* 565–577.
Golnick, A., Ireland, M., & Borowsky, I. (2009). Medical homes for children with autism: A physician survey. *Pediatrics, 123,* 966–971.
Green, J., Charman, T., Pickles, A., Wan, M. W., Elsabbagh, M., Slonims, V., et al. (2015). Parent-mediated intervention versus no intervention for infants at high risk of autism: A parallel, single-blind, randomized trial. *Lancet Psychiatry, 2,* 133–140.
Henderson, M. V., Hunt, S. N., & Day, D. (1993). Parent-teacher conferencing skills and pre-service programs. *Education, 114,* 71–73.

Kasari, C., Paparella, T., Freeman, S. N., & Jahromi, L. (2008). Language outcomes in autism: Randomized comparison of joint attention and play interventions. *Journal of Consulting and Clinical Psychology, 76,* 125–137.

Knight, V. F., Sartini, E., & Spriggs, A. (2014). Evaluating visual activity schedules as evidence-based practice for individuals with autism spectrum disorders. *Journal of Autism and Developmental Disorders, 45,* 157–178.

Kretlow, A. G., & Bartholomew, C. C. (2010). Using coaching to improve the fidelity of evidence-based practices: A review of studies. *Teacher Education and Special Education, 33*(4), 279–299.

Landa, R. J., Holman, K. C., O'Neill, A. H., & Stuart, E. A. (2011). Intervention targeting development of socially synchronous engagement in toddlers with autism spectrum disorder: A randomized controlled trial. *Journal of Child Psychology and Psychiatry, and Allied Disciplines, 52,* 13–21.

Loewenstein, G., Thompson, L., & Bazerman, M. (1989). Social utility and decision making in interpersonal context. *Journal of Personality and Social Psychology, 57,* 426–431.

MacNaul, H. L., & Neely, L. C. (2018). Systematic review of differential reinforcement of alternative behavior without extinction for individuals with autism. *Behavior Modification, 42,* 398–421.

Magnuson, K., & Schindler, H. (2016). Parent programs in pre-k through third grade. *The Future of Children, 26*(2), 207–221.

Mandell, D. S., Stahmer, A. C., Shin, S., Xie, M., Reisinger, E., & Marcus, S. C. (2013). The role of treatment fidelity on outcomes during a randomized field trial of an autism intervention. *Autism: The International Journal of Research and Practice, 17*(3), 281–295.

Marti, M., Merz, E. C., Repka, K. R., Landers, C., Noble, K. G., & Duch, H. (2018). Parent involvement in the getting ready for school intervention is associated with changes in school readiness skills. *Frontiers in Psychology, 9,* 759.

McConachie, H., & Diggle, T. (2006). Parent implemented early intervention for young children with autism spectrum disorder: A systematic review. *Journal of Evaluation in Clinical Practice, 13,* 120–129.

National Parent-Teacher Association. (2009). National standards for family-school partnerships. Retrieved from: https://www.pta.org/home/run-your-pta/National-Standards-for-Family-School-Partnerships.

Oono, I. P., Honey, E. J., & McConachie, H. (2013). Parent-mediated early intervention for young children with autism spectrum disorders (ASD). *Evidence-Based Child Health: A Cochrane Review Journal, 8*(6), 2380–2479.

Rogers, S. J., Vismara, L., Watner, A. L., McCormick, C., Young, G., & Ozonoff, S. (2014). Autism treatment in the first year of life: A pilot study of infant start, a parent-implemented intervention for symptomatic infants. *Journal of Autism and Developmental Disorders, 44*(12), 2981–2995.

Ruble, L. A., Dalrymple, N. J., & McGrew, J. H. (2010). The effects of consultation on individualized education program outcomes for young children with autism: The collaborative model for promoting competence and success. *Journal of Early Intervention, 32,* 286–301.

Ruble, L. A., Dalrymple, N. J., & McGrew, J. H. (2012). *Collaborative model for promoting competence and success for students with ASD.* New York, NY: Springer Science and Business Media.

Sheridan, S. M., & Kratochwill, T. R. (2008). *Conjoint behavioral consultation: Promoting family-school connections and interventions.* New York, NY: Springer.

Sheridan, S. M., Bovaird, J. A., Glover, T. A., Garbacz, S. A., Witte, A., & Kwon, K. (2012). A randomized trial examining the effects of conjoint behavioral consultation and the mediating role of the parent-teacher relationship. *School Psychology Review, 41,* 23–46.

Sheridan, S. M., Ryoo, J. H., Garbacz, S. A., Kunz, G. M., & Chumney, F. L. (2013). The efficacy of conjoint behavioral consultation on parents and children in the home setting: Results of a randomized controlled trial. *Journal of School Psychology, 51,* 717–733.

Sheridan, S. M., Witte, A. L., Holmes, S. R., Coutts, M. J., Dent, A. L., Kunz, G. M., et al. (2017a). A randomized trial examining the effects of conjoint behavioral consultation in rural schools:

Student outcomes and the mediating role of the teacher-parent relationship. *Journal of School Psychology, 61,* 33–53.
Sheridan, S. M., Witte, A. L., Holmes, S. R., Wu, C., Bhatia, S. A., & Angell, S. R. (2017b). The efficacy of conjoint behavioral consultation in the home setting: Outcomes and mechanisms in rural communities. *Journal of School Psychology, 62,* 81–101.
Siminoff, L. A., & Step, M. M. (2005). A communicative model of shared decision making: Accounting for cancer treatment decisions. *Health Psychology, 2,* 99–105.
State Support Network. (2018). Strategies for equitable family engagement. Retrieved from: https://statesupportnetwork.ed.gov/resources/strategies-equitable-family-engagement.
Thompson, L., & Hastie, R. (1990). Social perception in negotiation. *Organizational Behavior and Human Decision Processes, 47,* 98–123.
Vohra, R., Madhavan, S., Sambamoorthi, U., & St. Peter, C. (2014). Access to services, quality of care, and family impact for children with autism, other developmental disabilities, and other mental health conditions. *Autism, 18,* 815–826.
Wilson, K. P., Dykstra, J. R., Watson, L. R., Boyd, B. A., & Crais, E. R. (2012). Coaching in early education classrooms serving children with autism: A pilot study. *Early Childhood Education Journal, 40,* 97–105.
Wong, C., Odom, S. L., Hume, K., Cox, A., Fetting, W., Kucharczyk, S., … & Schultz, T. R. (2014). *Evidence-based practices for children, youth, and young adults with autism spectrum disorder.* Chapel Hill: The University of North Carolina, Frank Porter Graham Child Development Institute, Autism Evidence-Based Practice Review Group.
Work, W., & Stafford, L. (1987). Parent-teacher communication. *Communication Education, 36*(2), 182–187.

Transition from Adolescence to Adulthood in Those Without a Comorbid Intellectual Disability

Jessie Richard and Amie Duncan

Abstract Transitioning from adolescence to adulthood is a difficult journey for all adolescents, and it can be especially challenging for adolescents with autism spectrum disorder without a comorbid intellectual disability. Navigating the features associated with mastering daily living skills, understanding puberty and sexuality, transitioning from pediatric health care to adult health care, seeking out postsecondary education and vocational opportunities, and dealing with mental health issues can be challenging. It is important for parents, professionals, and school personnel to have an extensive understanding of the issues that may affect these adolescents in order to help them access resources and facilitate a successful adult outcome. This chapter highlights the challenges faced by adolescents in these areas, presents a case study, and provides resources and strategies that may aid adolescents in achieving independence and autonomy.

Clinical Phenotype of Adolescents with ASD Without an Intellectual Disability

Autism spectrum disorder (ASD) is a neurodevelopmental disorder characterized by deficits in the areas of social communication, including social interaction, speech, and nonverbal communication, as well as restricted and/or repetitive behaviors (APA, 2018). While current prevalence rates estimate that 1 in 59 children have ASD, approximately 44% of individuals with ASD do not have a comorbid intellectual disability (i.e., average to above-average cognitive abilities) (Baio et al., 2018). Despite their cognitive abilities, the outcomes of attending college, living independently, and being employed for individuals with ASD without a comorbid intellectual disability are extremely bleak (Henninger & Taylor, 2013), as they are less likely to be engaged

J. Richard (✉)
Nationwide Children's Hospital, Center for Autism Spectrum Disorders, Columbus, OH, USA
e-mail: Jessie.richard@nationwidechildrens.org

A. Duncan
Department of Pediatrics, Cincinnati Children's Hospital Medical Center, Cincinnati, OH, USA

M. B. McClain et al. (eds.), *Interprofessional Care Coordination for Pediatric Autism Spectrum Disorder*, https://doi.org/10.1007/978-3-030-46295-6_12

in any vocational or educational activities after high school even as compared to individuals with ASD and a comorbid ID (Taylor & Seltzer, 2011). Thus, despite having intact cognitive abilities, these adolescents with ASD may struggle to successfully transition to the adult world.

ASD is considered a lifelong disability; however, the manifestation of ASD symptoms change as an individual develops from childhood to adulthood. Among specific symptoms associated with ASD, verbal communication and social skills are two areas that typically improve in adolescence for individuals with average intelligence (Ratto & Mesibov, 2015). However, the social-communication skills of adolescents with ASD without a comorbid intellectual disability look qualitatively different from their same-aged peers. For example, an adolescent with ASD may not wait for a lull in conversation to join a group of people talking, but instead may jump into a conversation without reading the cues provided that indicate an appropriate time to enter, which may then lead to decreased friendships and a negative reputation. While there are improvements in these many symptom areas from childhood into adolescence, these improvements still remain impaired relative to typical peers. Due to social-communication deficits and other challenges associated with having a diagnosis of ASD (e.g., executive functioning deficits), opportunities to learn the skills needed to have a successful adult outcome in terms of independent living, postsecondary education, employment, community participation, relationships, and quality of life can be limited (Volkmar, Reichow, & McPartland, 2014).

Achieving Independence and Autonomy

Daily Living Skills

Daily living skills encompass foundational adaptive behaviors necessary for achieving independence and autonomy in adulthood. These skills, defined as behaviors necessary for age-appropriate, independent functioning in social, communication, daily living, or motor areas, are often significantly impaired in individuals with ASD compared to same-aged peers (Duncan & Bishop, 2015; Kanne et al., 2011). These daily living skills impairments become more distinct as individuals with ASD age (Smith, Maenner, & Malick Seltzer, 2012). Having appropriate adaptive behaviors increases the overall likelihood of achieving independence and autonomy in adulthood, thereby increasing the opportunity for young adults with ASD to live independently, obtain employment, and decrease some of the costs for parents that are associated with having a child with ASD (Bal, Kim, Cheong, & Lord, 2015).

Life skills include anything a person needs to be able to do, throughout their lifespan, to attend to his/her physical needs including hygiene (e.g., bathing, brushing teeth, eating, dressing), managing health care (e.g., making doctor appointments, taking medications), cooking (e.g., using stove, oven, microwave), housekeeping (e.g., laundry, cleaning the house), money management (e.g., checking accounts, saving accounts, debit/credit cards), and navigating the community (e.g., going grocery shopping, transportation). In individuals with ASD without a comorbid intellectual disability, there are several factors that may affect the development, mastery, and generalization of critical daily living skills. For example, executive functioning plays a role in life skill development (Pugliese et al., 2016) with regards to planning, organizing, initiation, regulating, and self-monitoring skills that are needed to achieve these tasks (e.g., remembering to start and complete all of the steps of one's morning routine before going to school or work).

A 2016 Government Accountability Office report on Youth with Autism identified life skills interventions as 1 of 14 services that need to be targeted during the transition to adulthood. The transition from adolescence to adulthood is complex, especially for adolescents with ASD and their families, and it is critical to provide adequate preparation to ensure that daily living skills are learned, practiced, and implemented (Stewart, Stavness, King, Antle, & Law, 2006). Directly teaching individuals with ASD is a key component for learning daily living skills and effective evidence-based strategies include direct instruction, task analysis, visual supports, technology, video modeling, and behavioral-based strategies such as reinforcement and prompting (Matson, Hattier, & Belva, 2012; Palmen, Didden, & Lang, 2012). Incorporating individual skills training, goal-setting, self-management, and family support are also important components to utilize when helping individuals with ASD learn daily living skills. Research shows that providing systematic individualized instruction to help achieve individual goals creates the opportunity for an individual with ASD to develop independence and autonomy with daily living skills (Foxx, 2008). While there are few manualized interventions that target daily living skills (Duncan, Ruble, Meinzen-Derr, Thomas, & Stark, 2017), it is clear that it is important to directly teach adolescents with ASD these daily living skills in various environments (e.g., home, school, community) and provide multiple opportunities to practice to improve the attainment and generalization of these new skills.

Puberty and Sexuality

Puberty is a typical experience all children go through including those with ASD. However, children with ASD do not always follow the traditional stages of development, especially in regards to how puberty interacts with the areas of social communication. This can have an adverse impact on their development of close relationships with peers and family members, romantic relationships, and sexuality later in adulthood due to the subtle rules associated with interactions pertaining to peer pressure, sexual feelings, relationships, and romantic desires (Cabral Fernandes et al., 2016). Adolescents with ASD receive less sexuality education than typically developing peers (Ballan & Burke Freyer, 2017), and caregivers are more likely to report problematic sexual behaviors such as inadequate self-care, difficulties in understanding privacy and boundaries, and repetitive patterns and sensory fascinations linked to sexuality (Corona, Fox, Christodulu, & Worlock, 2016). Recent research also suggests that individuals with ASD are just as likely or more likely to identify as lesbian, gay, bisexual, transgender, or queer/questioning (LGBTQ), which will be important for parents and professionals to address so that appropriate education and support can be provided to the adolescent with ASD (George & Stokes, 2018).

Individuals with ASD are often portrayed as uninterested in sexuality and relationships, but this is hardly true. Because of this misconception, adolescents with ASD are often not taught appropriate information about puberty and sexuality, thus they acquire their information from their own observations, social media, television and movies, and their parents (Ballan & Burke Freyer, 2017). It is important to directly teach and talk about issues pertaining to sexuality including sexual development, safe sex, contraception, sexually transmitted diseases, and social skills development (Corona et al., 2016). Providing direct, clear, specific descriptions and instruction combined with visual representations and visual supports is considered best-practice to address issues surrounding empathy and perspective-taking, privacy, self-care, abuse awareness and prevention, and social conventions (e.g., rules for flirting and dating) (Corona et al., 2016). Some useful strategies for having these conversations with adolescents with ASD include using behavioral principles to break abstract and complex ideas down into simpler concepts, social stories, and narratives to educate and address questions pertaining to relationships, and social behavior mapping to address internal self-regulation and internal motivations (Ballan & Burke Freyer, 2017).

Adolescents with ASD are more susceptible to increased physiological symptoms of anxiety, distress, and loneliness than typically developing peers when puberty and sexuality are not appropriately addressed (Pecora, Mesibov, & Stokes, 2016). Females with ASD experience more negative feelings associated with the desire for social relations and recognition that they are not fitting into social situations the same way as their typically developing peers. Females also carry an additional vulnerability when they are not taught appropriate sexual behaviors because the core symptoms of ASD can impact judgment of the character of potential sexual predators (Pecora et al., 2016). This misconception is impacted by limited social relationships and misinterpretation of nonsocial sources of sexual information. It is essential to provide accurate information regarding sexual knowledge and behaviors to adolescents with ASD to alleviate future concerns in adulthood regarding sexuality.

Health Care Transition

Transitioning from pediatric care to adult-centered care is a difficult process for all adolescents to go through, but there are added challenges faced by adolescents with ASD. The conversation surrounding health care transition should ideally begin with a child's pediatrician between the ages of 12–14; however, these are often overlooked and the conversations begin too late or do not happen at all. The process of health care transition focuses on the medical, psychological, social, educational, and vocational needs of adolescents as they transition from child-focused care to adult-focused care within the health care field (Kiely Law & Law, 2014). Only 40% of youth with special health care needs (YSHCN) receive transition services from their health care providers (Cheak-Zamora, Yang, Farmer, & Clark, 2013) despite the development of specific milestones for this health care transition (White et al., 2018).

When discussing the transition from pediatric to adult-focused care, it is important to discuss some key topics including shifting to an adult provider, health care needs of adults, health insurance retention, independence, and the adolescent's responsibility for their own health care needs (Kiely Law & Law, 2014). Many adolescents with ASD who transition to adulthood are at an increased risk of developing multiple health problems, mental illness, and behavioral problems (Cheak-Zamora & Teti, 2015), and they also have common comorbidities such as mental and behavioral health disorders, epilepsy, gastrointestinal problems, anxiety and depression, and respiratory, food, and skin allergies (Kuhlthau, Warfield, Hurson, Delahaye, & Crossman, 2015). More information regarding these comorbidities are discussed in the previous chapter titled "Medical Comorbidities in Pediatric Autism Spectrum Disorder" of this handbook. Without a transition plan in place, many of these adolescents may live without services that could impact their autonomy and independence.

Barriers are often experienced by families and adolescents that impact their ability to access health care transition services including age, gender, ethnicity, complexity of condition, family structure, parental education, household income, health insurance status, shared decision making, satisfaction with health care services, and the presence of a medical home (Cheak-Zamora et al., 2013). Families can aid the transition process by scheduling appointments with adult care providers during less busy times to allow time to acclimate to the new physician, organize pre-appointment visits to provide familiarity and practice, give choices (e.g., listen to lungs first or look in ears first, you pick), engage in role modeling scenarios for what will happen with the physician, and create a reward system for appropriate behavior (Kuhlthau et al., 2015). Parents of adolescents with ASD should also encourage their child to provide the doctor with information about why they are visiting. This could happen before transitioning to their adult health care provider, so they have more practice with the pediatrician they are already familiar with. If a parent or caregiver needs to add additional information that their adolescent may have missed, it is important to explain to them later why the gaps were filled to ensure understanding.

Another important piece to discuss with regards to health care transition is the issue of guardianship. When adolescents turn 18, parents lose the ability to make medical decisions on behalf of their child (Cheak-Zamora & Teti, 2015). Some adolescents would be better suited to having a guardian help with their medical decisions, and this is a topic that should be discussed thoroughly with an individual's health care team before they are 18 years old.

Individuals with ASD have unique needs in the health care field, and the need to individualize transition plans to address the specific needs of each adolescent is necessary because a one-size-fits-all model does not apply to ASD (Rogers & Zeni, 2015). It is crucial for families to begin this process early and address all the quintessential questions and needs of their child before the age of 18.

Vocational Skills and Employment

Recent studies have shown that around 50% of adults with ASD who do not have a comorbid intellectual disability are employed (Farley et al., 2009) and that we know little about the factors that prevent them from obtaining and maintaining employment or being underemployed (Walsh, Lydon, & Healy, 2014). Employment positively impacts an individual's health, well-being, and cognitive abilities. Being employed requires demonstrating independence, self-esteem, community engagement, and social understanding, which are areas individuals with ASD often show difficulties navigating. Particularly, social interactions, behavior management, stress, and anxiety can hinder an individual's ability to fully participate and succeed in the workplace (Wei et al., 2018). Understanding job interviews, workplace social dynamics, mixed communication styles as well as new situations and occasional changes in tasks and routines make maintaining employment for adults with ASD more difficult (Headly et al., 2018; Seaman & Cannella-Malone, 2016). These characteristics of work and the workplace environment are likely why more adults with ASD are unemployed or underemployed than individuals in similar disability groups (Wei et al., 2018).

There are multiple strategies to help adolescents with ASD transition successfully into the workforce as adults. It is important to assess an adolescent's skills, and match them with jobs that are compatible with the skills and expectations they have for themselves. It is also essential to teach soft skills, such as organization (e.g., knowing what tasks need to be done), customer and coworker interactions (e.g., handling feedback, maintaining relationships), and time management and prioritization of work tasks (Seaman & Cannella-Malone, 2016). These are skills associated with executive functioning, and individuals with ASD often show a greater need for direct teaching of these skills (e.g., how to determine which tasks are most critical and which tasks can wait to be completed) to be successful in various workplace tasks. In addition to direct teaching and supports, various modifications to the environment, such as wearing headphones, dimming lights, and pairing new employees with more experienced employees are useful strategies to use when transitioning into the workforce (Hedley et al., 2018). Using video modeling, prompting, and training on the job allows for more opportunities to practice the skills associated with a job, and can also be used to help teach pre-employment skills like resume writing (Seaman & Cannella-Malone, 2016).

Any opportunity to practice these skills during high school improves employment outcomes and there are interventions that are focused on building these skills in adolescence and early adulthood (e.g., Wehman et al., 2013). Understanding the importance of planning, paying attention to vulnerabilities that might impact youth with ASD, and getting institutional supports to support the integration of individuals with ASD into the workforce increases the likelihood of maintaining employment (Roux et al., 2013).

Postsecondary Education

Many adolescents with ASD have a desire to attend postsecondary education, but the US Department of Education has found that students with ASD in the U.S. have some of the lowest rates of enrollment (44%) at any postsecondary institution when compared to the general population (67%) and all disability groups (60%) (Anderson et al., 2017). There are many benefits to attending postsecondary education including better vocational outcomes, improved socialization, independence, self-awareness, and life skills (Accardo, 2017; Anderson et al., 2017). However, there are also many barriers that impact the success of an individual with ASD in college including mental health issues, stress, poor study skills, poor social skills, sensory sensitivities, and organization and time management skills (Anderson, Stephenson, & Carter, 2017).

Students with ASD have reported challenges with academics as well as nonacademic challenges. Some academic challenges include difficulty understanding abstract or ambiguous concepts, poor planning skills and concentration, difficulty with group work, and the social demands of class (Anderson et al., 2017). Some of these difficulties arise from individuals with ASD's executive functioning deficits and other difficulties arise from their difficulties comprehending social cues. Supports are available to help address these academic challenges including peer mentoring, subject-specific support (e.g., writing center), exam accommodations (e.g., extended time, quiet environment), help with note-taking, social clubs, and assistance with time management (Sarrett, 2018). Some nonacademic challenges identified by students with ASD include difficulties with social interactions outside of class, feelings of isolation and depression, sensory sensitivities, and daily living skills (Anderson et al., 2017). These areas can also be addressed by using peer or faculty mentors, social support groups, parents, friends, and individual or group counseling. It is important to provide adolescents a better understanding of all the factors that go into attending college before they arrive to ensure they have the tools and skills needed to succeed. There has been a significant increase in programs on college campuses that provide a range of supports to address challenges in the areas of academic, social, executive functioning, daily living skills, and mental health for undergraduates with ASD (Gelbar, Smith, & Reichow, 2014).

Preparing for college in a comprehensive manner is critical to ensuring success in college. It may be helpful to have adolescents with ASD engage in activities such as taking college courses in high school to better understand the expectations of college courses, deciding on the size of a university, which may help with class size and community engagement, and determining whether a 2- or 4- year college is more appropriate based on goals after college (Zeedyk, Tipton, & Blacher, 2016). Adolescents also need to be aware that it will be their responsibility to disclose their disability to the campus disability services office and to discuss any needed accommodations with their professors. Unlike high school, students will not receive any accommodations unless there is documentation through the school's disabilities services center (Roberts, 2010). In order to prepare for disclosing their diagnosis, the caregivers of adolescents with ASD could role-play how to do this (e.g., develop a social script on what to say regarding their diagnosis and strengths/challenges) and help them understand the importance of disclosing their disability. Many students do not disclose their ASD diagnosis to disability services for fear of being stigmatized, wanting to try college on their own without any supports, and a belief that accommodations would not help (Anderson et al., 2017). Without the necessary supports in place, students with ASD face the risk of being unsuccessful in college and possibly developing mental health issues such as depression and anxiety.

Mental Health

Mental health is an increasingly important area to be better aware of, especially with regards to adolescents and young adults with ASD. Research has found co-occurring mental health difficulties, including anxiety, depression, and loneliness, to be some of the most commonly reported experiences of students with ASD (Jackson, Hart, Theirfeld, & Volkmar, 2018). Identifying these co-occurring mental health issues is difficult as individuals with ASD may be less likely to directly express feelings of sadness, hopelessness, worry, low self-esteem, or suicidal ideation (Chandrasekhar & Sikich, 2015). Symptoms of mental health difficulties in individuals with ASD include a decreased interest in a preferred item or activity, refusal to attend structured activities, regression in self-care abilities, worsening hygiene or general appearance, increased social withdrawal, increased insistence on sameness, decreased concentration, increased agitation, aggression, and self-injury (Chandrasekhar & Sikich, 2015). Additionally, the physical symptoms associated with mental health issues often appear similar to the core symptoms of ASD, including flat or constricted affect, social withdrawal, or insistence on sameness.

As adolescents transition into adulthood, many of the skills and next steps discussed in this chapter are associated with an increased likelihood of mental health issues. As adolescents go through the changes associated with puberty, graduate high school and go to college or get a job, learn new daily living skills, and take on health care management, each of these new experiences brings stress and new challenges. Without the appropriate preventative strategies and training, individuals may begin to feel hopeless, worthless, and anxious about all the changes and tasks that are necessary for functioning as an adult. It is important for parents and professionals to be aware of and take notice when an individual is beginning to display some of these symptoms and determine how to provide appropriate support if mental health becomes an issue (e.g., working with an individual therapist, attending a support group, normalizing mental health difficulties). Utilizing strategies that help individuals with ASD navigate new situations, and providing support and treatment such as cognitive behavioral therapy to address depression or anxiety symptoms is an appropriate place to start (White et al., 2018). Accessing tutoring and mentoring services to help with school work, using a social script, planning social activities to increase community interaction, and providing written instructions with visuals to help complete a complex task that caused anxiety previously are all strategies that can be used.

Greater mental health difficulties are associated with poorer overall social skills and greater difficulties with social responsiveness (Radcliffe, Wong, Dossetor, & Hayes, 2015). Individuals with ASD often already have difficulty with social skills and social responsiveness; therefore, it is important to target these areas and keep the symptoms of mental health in mind as adolescents' transition into adulthood.

Summary

The transition to adulthood for adolescents with ASD without a comorbid intellectual disability can be difficult as they strive to develop and master critical daily living skills, go through puberty, understand their sexuality, move from the pediatric to adult health care system, seek to obtain and maintain employment, attend college, and deal with mental health challenges. In order to facilitate a successful adult outcome, it is critical for parents, professionals, and school personnel to have an in-depth understanding of the issues that may affect these adolescents and then access resources to address any difficulties or challenges. We have included a case study that represents how multiple disciplines can work together in order to assist the adolescent with ASD with transitioning to adulthood. There is an abbreviated list of resources at the end of this chapter.

Case Conceptualization

William is a 17-year-old male who has been previously diagnosed with autism spectrum disorder (ASD) and Attention Deficit Hyperactivity Disorder (ADHD)—Inattentive Type. He attends his local high school and is mainstreamed with an Individualized Education Plan (IEP). Through his IEP he receives biweekly speech therapy to address social-communication goals (i.e., engage in back and forth conversation with peers) and participates in a study skills class to assist with executive functioning deficits (e.g., organization, prioritization, time management).

William and his mother participated in an updated evaluation through the ASD Adolescent Assessment Clinic, which is an interdisciplinary clinic at his local hospital that includes a psychologist, psychiatrist, and speech-language pathologist who conduct thorough assessments of adolescents with ASD in order to facilitate a successful transition to adulthood. The role of the psychologist is to reevaluate symptoms of ASD and conduct updated assessments of cognitive abilities, adaptive behavior, executive functioning, internalizing and externalizing disorders, and social skills. The psychologist also conducts a clinical interview with the parent and the teen to discuss overall concerns and issues related to the upcoming transition from high school to the adult world (e.g., interest in postsecondary education and employment, applying for various adult services in the future, short-term and long-term goals). The role of the speech-language pathologist is to conduct updated language testing (i.e., receptive and expressive language) and assess pragmatic language skills. The role of the psychiatrist is to conduct a clinical interview with the parent and adolescent to obtain a comprehensive history and understanding of mental health concerns or diagnoses and discuss medication management issues. After the assessment, the interdisciplinary team meets to conceptualize how the patient's symptoms, strengths, and challenges fit with current diagnoses and determine if new diagnoses are warranted. Further, the team creates a holistic set of recommendations to address not only the needs of the adolescent with ASD, but also supports and services in areas such as postsecondary education, employment, independent living, social-communication skills, recreation and leisure, puberty and sexuality, driving, financial planning, guardianship, and adult services. The psychologist then conducts a feedback session with the adolescent with ASD and their family that includes a detailed discussion of their profile of strengths and difficulties, current diagnoses, and a prioritized list of recommended supports and services.

After participating in the ASD Adolescent Assessment Clinic, William continued to meet criteria for ASD and ADHD-Inattentive Type, but was also diagnosed with a generalized anxiety disorder (e.g., worried about his performance at school, worried about how classmates viewed him, became anxious when thinking about past failures). He had clear strengths such that he was actively participating in 2 extracurricular activities, had a good relationship with 1 classmate that he occasionally saw outside of school, had started to take driver's education classes, and was starting to actively participate in IEP meetings by asking questions and stating his preferences and goals for the future. However, William demonstrated clear challenges such that he struggled to perform basic daily living skills (e.g., completing morning hygiene routine, making snacks or meals for himself, doing laundry), continued to have difficulties organizing his belongings and keeping track of school assignments, frequently missed social cues (e.g., being too detailed in his conversations with others), and was not able to identify or cope with emotions such as frustration or anxiety. Thus, the treatment team prioritized the following supports: (1) begin individual cognitive behavioral therapy with a psychologist or social worker to help with emotion management and also build his social skills with a focus on his relationships with peers; (2) begin individual occupational therapy to address some of his daily living skills deficits and learn evidence-based strategies that could be applied to a range of skills (e.g., task analysis, video modeling); (3) learn about opportunities in the community to foster social skills (e.g., social skills groups, teen night offered through the local Autism Society); (4) continue medication management with his psychiatrist; and (5) provide resources about how to address executive functioning deficits in teens (e.g., books, apps, etc.). William was also referred to work with a developmental pediatrician in the Transition Clinic at the local hospital, which would assist him with the transition to the adult health care system (e.g., identifying an adult primary care provider) and with identifying what adult supports or agencies may be beneficial (e.g., Social Security Income, guardianship). He was also referred to a vocational education counselor through the local hospital to assist him with applying for Vocational Rehabilitation services and identifying supports to help him find and keep a part-time job. The treatment team also provided recommendations that were related to the long-term goals that William and his family had for him including: (1) a list of community colleges and 4-year colleges in the surrounding area that had support programs for students with ASD and/or executive functioning challenges; (2) social skills groups and support groups for adults with ASD; (3) resources on self-advocacy due to an interest in learning how to disclose his diagnosis of ASD to others while also communicating his unique set of strengths; (4) resources on building the critical skills that are needed to live on his own (e.g., budgeting, maintaining a household, navigating the community); and (5) resources to build social skills specific to the workplace. After the feedback session, William's family commented that they felt equipped with the tools and resources to help William meet his short-term and long-term goals as he transitioned from high school to the adult world.

Selected Resources

- Social-Communication Skills
  - *Social Skills for Teenagers with Developmental and Autism Spectrum Disorder: PEERS Treatment Manual* by Elizabeth Laugeson
  - *The Science of Making Friends: Helping Socially Challenged Teens and Young Adults* by Elizabeth Laugeson & John Elder Robison
  - *The Asperkids (Secret) Book of Social Rules: The Handbook of Not-So-Obvious Social Guidelines for Tweens and Teens with Asperger Syndrome* by Jennifer Cook O'Toole.
- Achieving Independence and Autonomy
  - *Taking Care of Myself -2: For Teenagers and Young Adults with ASD* by Mary Wrobel
  - *Smart but Scattered Teens: The Executive Skills Program for Helping Teens Reach Their Potential* by Guare, Dawson, & Guare
  - *The Complete Guide to Personal Finance: For Teenagers* by Tamsen Butler.
- Puberty and Sexuality
  - Organization for Autism Research's Sex Ed for Self-Advocates: https://researchautism.org/sex-ed-guide-sexual-orientation-gender-identity/
  - Healthy Bodies for Boys and Girls from the Kennedy Vanderbilt Center: http://kc.vanderbilt.edu/healthybodies/
  - Sexuality across the Lifespan for Children and Adolescents with Developmental Disabilities: An instructional guide for Parents/Caregivers of individuals with developmental disabilities. http://www.fddc.org/sites/default/files/file/publications/Sexuality%20Guide-Parents-English.pdf.
- Health Care Transition

  - Got Transition: https://www.gottransition.org/.

- Employment

  - *Teaching Pre-Employment Skills to 14-17-Year-Olds* by Joanne Lara
  - *Social Thinking at Work: Why Should I Care?* by Michelle Garcia Winner & Pamela Crooke
  - *Asperger's on the Job: Must Have Advice for People with Asperger's or HFA and their Employers, Educators, and Advocates* by Rudy Simone
  - Autism Speaks Employment Toolkit: www.autismspeaks.org.

- Post-secondary Education

  - College Autism Network: https://collegeautismnetwork.org/
  - Think College: (www.thinkcollege.org)
  - Indiana Resource Center for Autism - Academic Supports for College Students with Autism: http://www.iidc.indiana.edu/?pageId=3417
  - *Parties, Dorms, and Social Norms: A Crash Course on Safe Living in Young Adults on the Autism Spectrum* by Lisa Meeks & Tracy Loye Masterson
  - *The Parent's Guide to College for Students on the Autism Spectrum* by Brown, Wolf, King, & Bork
  - *Developing College Skills in Students With Autism and Asperger's Syndrome* by Sarita Freedman.

- Mental Health

  - *Living Well on the Spectrum* by Valerie Gaus
  - *Cognitive-Behavioral Therapy for Adult Asperger Syndrome (Guides to Individualized Evidence Based Treatment Series)* by Valerie Gaus
  - *CBT for Children and Adolescents with High-Functioning Autism Spectrum Disorders* by Scarpa, White, & Attwood
  - Cognitive Behavioral Therapy interactive website for teens: www.anxietybc.com.

References

Accardo, A. L. (2017). College-bound young adults with ASD: Self-reported factors prompting and inhibiting success. *College of Education Faculty Scholarship, 9,* 1–12.

American Psychiatric Association. (2018). What is autism? Retrieved from https://www.psychiatry.org/patients-families/autism/what-is-autism-spectrum-disorder.

Anderson, A. H., Stephenson, J., & Carter, M. (2017). A systematic literature review of the experiences and supports of students with autism spectrum disorder in post-secondary education. *Research in Autism Spectrum Disorders, 39,* 33–53.

Baio, J., Wiggins, L., Christensen, D. L., Maenner, M. J., Daniels, J., Warren, Z., et al. (2018). Prevalence of autism spectrum disorder among children aged 8 years—autism and developmental disabilities monitoring network, 11 sites, United States, 2014. *MMWR Surveillance Summaries, 67*(6), 1–23.

Bal, V. H., Kim, S.-H., Cheong, D., & Lord, C. (2015). Daily living skills in individuals with autism spectrum disorder from 2 to 21 years or age. *Autism, 19,* 774–784.

Ballan, M. S., & Burke Freyer, M. (2017). Autism spectrum disorder, adolescence, and sexuality education: Suggested interventions for mental health professionals. *Sexuality and Disability, 35,* 261–273.

Cabral Fernandes, L., Gillberg, C. I., Cedarlund, M., Hagberg, B., Gillberg, C., & Billstedt, E. (2016). Aspects of sexuality in adolescents and adults diagnosed with autism spectrum disorders in childhood. *Journal of Autism and Developmental Disorders, 46,* 3155–3165.

Chandrasekhar, T., & Sikich, L. (2015). Challenges in the diagnosis and treatment of depression in autism spectrum disorders across the lifespan. *Dialogues in Clinical Neuroscience, 17,* 219–227.

Cheak-Zamora, N. C., & Teti, M. (2015). "You think it's hard now ... It gets much harder for our children": Youth with autism and their caregiver's perspectives of health care transition services. *Autism, 19,* 992–1001.

Cheak-Zamora, N. C., Yang, X., Farmer, J. E., & Clark, M. (2013). Disparities in transition planning for youth with autism spectrum disorder. *Pediatrics, 131,* 447–454.

Corona, L. L., Fox, S. A., Christodulu, K. V., & Worlock, J. A. (2016). Providing education on sexuality and relationships to adolescents with autism spectrum disorder and their parents. *Sexuality and Disability, 34,* 199–214.

Duncan, A. W., & Bishop, S. L. (2015). Understanding the gap between cognitive abilities and daily living skills in adolescents with autism spectrum disorders with average intelligence. *Autism, 19,* 64–72.

Duncan, A. W., Ruble, L. A., Meinzen-Derr, J., Thomas, C. L., & Stark, L. J. (2017). Preliminary efficacy of a daily living skills intervention for adolescents with high-functioning autism spectrum disorder. *Autism, 22,* 983–994.

Farley, M. A., McMahon, W. M., Fombonne, E., Jenson, W. R., Miller, J., Gardner, M., et al. (2009). Twenty-year outcome for individuals with autism and average or near-average cognitive abilities. *Autism Research, 2,* 109–118.

Foxx, R. M. (2008). Applied behavior analysis treatment of autism: The state of the art. *Child and Adolescent Psychiatric Clinics of North America, 17,* 821–834.

Gelbar, N. W., Smith, I., & Reichow, B. (2014). Systematic review of articles describing experience and supports of individuals with autism enrolled in college and university programs. *Journal of Autism and Developmental Disorders, 44,* 2593–2601.

George, R., & Stokes, M. A. (2018). Sexual orientation in autism spectrum disorder. *Autism Research, 11,* 133–141.

Hedley, D., Cai, R., Uljarevic, M., Wilmot, M., Spoor, J. R., Richdale, A., et al. (2018). Transition to work: Perspectives from the autism spectrum. *Autism, 22,* 528–541.

Henninger, N. A., & Taylor, J. L. (2013). Outcomes in adults with autism spectrum disorders: A historical perspective. *Autism, 17,* 103–116.

Jackson, S. L. J., Hart, L., Theirfeld Brown, J., & Volkmar, F. R. (2018). Brief report: Self-reported academic, social, and mental health experiences of post-secondary students with autism spectrum disorder. *Journal of Autism and Developmental Disorders, 48,* 643–650.

Kanne, S. M., Gerber, A. J., Quirmbach, L. M., Sparrow, S. S., Cicchetti, D. V., & Saulnier, C. A. (2011). The role of adaptive behavior in autism spectrum disorders: Implications for functional outcome. *Journal of Autism and Developmental Disorders, 41,* 1007–1018.

Kiely Law, J., & Law, P. A. (2014). Health care transition services for youth with autism spectrum disorders. *Rehabilitation Psychology, 59,* 340–348.

Kuhlthau, K. A., Warfield, M. E., Hurson, J., Delahaye, J., & Crossman, M. K. (2015). Pediatric provider's perspectives on the transition to adult health care for youth with autism spectrum disorder: Current strategies and promising new directions. *Autism, 19,* 262–271.

Matson, J. L., Hattier, M. A., & Belva, B. (2012). Treating adaptive living skills of persons with autism using applied behavior analysis: A review. *Research in Autism Spectrum Disorders, 6,* 271–276.

Palmen, A., Didden, R., Lang, R. A. (2012). Systematic review of behavioral intervention research on adaptive skill building in high-functioning young adults with autism spectrum disorder. *Research in Autism Spectrum Disorders,* 6602–6617.

Pecora, L. A., Mesibov, G. B., & Stokes, M. A. (2016). Sexuality in high-functioning autism: A systematic review and meta-analysis. *Journal of Autism and Developmental Disorders, 46,* 3519–3556.

Pugliese, C. E., Anthony, L. G., Strang, J. F., Dudley, K., Wallace, G. L., Naiman, D. Q., et al. (2016). Longitudinal examination of adaptive behavior in autism spectrum disorders: Influence of executive function. *Journal of Autism and Developmental Disorders, 46,* 467–477.

Ratcliffe, B., Wong, M., Dossetor, D., & Hayes, S. (2015). The association between social skills and mental health in school-aged children with autism spectrum disorder, with and without intellectual disability. *Journal of Autism and Developmental Disabilities, 45,* 2487–2496.

Ratto, A. B., & Mesibov, G. B. (2015). Autism spectrum disorders in adolescence and adulthood: Long-term outcomes and relevant issues for treatment and research. *Science China Life Sciences, 58,* 1010–1015.

Roberts, K. D. (2010). Topic areas to consider when planning transition from high school to post-secondary education for students with autism spectrum disorders. *Focus on Autism and Other Developmental Disabilities, 25,* 158–162.

Rogers, K., & Zeni, M. (2015). Systematic review of medical home models to promote transitions to primary adult health care for adolescents living with autism spectrum disorder. *Worldview on Evidence-Based Nursing, 12,* 98–107.

Roux, A. M., Shattuck, P. T., Cooper, B. P., Anderson, K. A., Wagner, M., & Narendorf, S. C. (2013). Postsecondary employment experiences among young adults with an autism spectrum disorder. *Journal of the American Academy of Child and Adolescent Psychiatry, 52,* 931–939.

Sarrett, J. C. (2018). Autism and accommodations in higher education: Insights from the autism Community. *Journal of Autism and Developmental Disorders, 48,* 679–692.

Seaman, R. L., & Cannella-Malone, H. I. (2016). Vocational skills interventions for adults with autism spectrum disorder: A review of the literature. *Journal of Developmental and Physical Disabilities, 28,* 479–494.

Smith, L. E., Maenner, M. J., & Malick Seltzer, M. (2012). Developmental trajectories in adolescents and adults with autism: The case of daily living skills. *Journal of the American Academy of Child and Adolescent Psychiatry, 51,* 622–631.

Stewart, D., Stavness, C., King, G., Antle, B., & Law, M. (2006). A critical appraisal of literature reviews about the transition to adulthood for youth with disabilities. *Physical & Occupational Therapy in Pediatrics, 26,* 5–24.

Taylor, J. L., & Seltzer, M. M. (2011). Employment and post-secondary educational activities for young adults with autism spectrum disorders during the transition to adulthood. *Journal of Autism and Developmental Disorders, 41,* 566–574.

Volkmar, F. R., Reichow, B., & McPartland, J. C. (2014). *Adolescents and adults with autism spectrum disorder*. New York: Springer.

Walsh, L., Lydon, S., & Healy, O. (2014). Employment and vocational skills among individuals with autism spectrum disorder: Predictors, impact, and interventions. *Review Journal of Autism and Developmental Disorders, 1,* 266–275.

Wehman, P., Schall, C., McDonough, J., Molinelli, A., Riehle, E., Ham, W., et al. (2013). Project SEARCH for youth with autism spectrum disorders: Increasing competitive employment on transition from high school. *Journal of Positive Behavior Interventions, 15,* 144–155.

Wei, X., Yu, J. W., Wagner, M., Hudson, L., Roux, A. M., Shattuck, P., et al. (2018). Job searching, job duration, and job loss among young adults with autism spectrum disorder. *Journal of Vocational Rehabilitation, 48,* 1–10.

White, P. H., Cooley, W. C., American Academy of Pediatrics, & American Academy of Family Physicians. (2018). Supporting the health care transition from adolescence to adulthood in the medical home. *Pediatrics*, *142*, e20182587.

White, S. W., Simmons, G. L., Gotham, K. O., Conner, C. M., Smith, I. C., Beck, K. B., et al. (2018). Psychosocial treatments targeting anxiety and depression in adolescents and adults on the autism spectrum: Review of the latest research and recommended future directions. *Current Psychiatry Reports, 20,* 82.

Zeedyk, S. M., Tipton, L., & Blacher, J. (2016). Educational supports for high functioning youth with ASD: The postsecondary pathway to college. *Focus on Autism and Other Developmental Disabilities, 31,* 37–48.

Clinical and School Identification and Intervention for Youth with ASD: Culturally and Linguistically Responsive Interdisciplinary Considerations

Bryn Harris, Nuri Reyes, and Trenesha Hill

Abstract Despite dramatic demographic changes over the past five decades specifically, culturally and lingustically diverse (CLD) children are more likely to receive delayed diagnosis and misidentification of ASD as well as experience significant barriers to obtaining ASD services in general. Delays in ASD identification or intervention provision can negatively impact future outcomes and may indicate that professionals are missing important cultural or linguistic considerations when providing services to CLD children and families. Strong interdisciplinary care practices can improve the outcomes of CLD children and their families with ASD. This chapter presents the challenges and successes to the facilitation of interdisciplinary care among CLD children. As services for ASD most often occur in clinical and school-based settings, the chapter will focus on both settings. Recommendations for culturally and linguistically responsive interdisciplinary care for children with ASD are provided.

Racial/ethnic diversity in the United States (U.S.) has changed rapidly, particularly in the past five decades. In 1965, the non-Hispanic White population was 84% of the U.S. population (Pew Research Center, 2015). By 2015, this percentage fell to 62% (Pew Research Center, 2015) and by mid-century, the non-Hispanic White population is expected to be less than 50% of the U.S. population (U.S. Census Bureau, 2017). Alternatively, the size of non-White populations across the U.S. has been increasing nationwide, with some states experiencing more growth than others. For example, California, Hawaii, New Mexico, and Texas identify themselves as states where the non-Hispanic White population is considered the minority population.

B. Harris (✉)
School of Education and Human Development, Department of Pediatrics, University of Colorado Denver, Denver, CO, USA
e-mail: Bryn.Harris@ucdenver.edu

N. Reyes
Departments of Pediatrics and Psychiatry, University of Colorado School of Medicine, Anschutz Medical Campus, Aurora, CO, USA

T. Hill
Pediatric Mental Health Institute, Children's Hospital Colorado, Aurora, CO, USA

M. B. McClain et al. (eds.), *Interprofessional Care Coordination for Pediatric Autism Spectrum Disorder*, https://doi.org/10.1007/978-3-030-46295-6_13

Alternatively, the states of Maine, Vermont, New Hampshire, West Virginia, New Hampshire each have less than 10% of the population that identifies as non-White, the lowest percentages in the U.S. (Maciag, 2015). Children under the age of 18 in the U.S. are more likely to identify as non-White than the adult population and projections indicate that the child population is expected to be increasingly racially diverse in future decades. In 2018, 50% of U.S. children were non-Hispanic White, 25% were Hispanic, 14% were Black, 5% were Asian, and 5% were "all other races" (Federal Interagency Forum on Child and Family Statistics, 2019).

The U.S. has long been a country of linguistic diversity although compiling records pertaining to languages spoken did not begin until the 1980 U.S. Census. Since this date, the American Community Survey of the U.S. Census has gathered this data every decade (e.g., 1980, 1990, 2000, 2010). The findings of the 2010 report detailed a dramatic decrease over time of English-only households in the United States (89.1% of the population in 1980–79.7% in 2010). Persons age 5 and older that speak a language other than English rose from 11 to 20.3% during that same time period. Over two-thirds of the people that report speaking another language identify as Spanish speakers (Rambaut & Massey, 2013). Children are more likely to live in a linguistically diverse household than adults, and 22% of children in the U.S. (ages 5–17) report speaking Spanish in the home. Furthermore, there are almost 500 languages spoken in the U.S. (U.S. Census Bureau, 2010). Similar to racial/ethnic diversity, states within the U.S. vary extensively pertaining to the language use of their population. For example, California reported 43.3% of their population speaks a language other than English. Alternatively, West Virginia, Mississippi, Kentucky, Montana, North Dakota, and Alabama, identified between 2 and 5% of their population as those that speak another language besides English (Rambaut & Massey, 2013).

Notably, the authors would like to acknowledge that there are many terms utilized in this chapter pertaining to race/ethnicity, culture and language. Often, we use the terms utilized in the cited literature. When possible, we attempt to use strengths-based and culturally responsive terms. For example, we prefer the term "bilingual" or "multilingual" children when possible as these terms speak to the additive benefit of being bilingual and more accurately describe the child than other common terms (such as English language learner). The authors would also like to state that this chapter will focus on race/ethnicity and language diversity; however, we acknowledge that there are many other culturally diverse populations that are not represented in this chapter. More research is needed in all areas of diversity within the field of ASD, and we encourage all future research to consider its potential impact on diverse contexts and populations.

The following chapter will describe considerations when providing interdisciplinary school and clinical services to children from culturally and linguistically diverse (CLD) families including diagnostic assessments and intervention services. The recommendations provided within may assist with reducing ASD service disparities in both clinical and school settings and ultimately improve the outcomes of children with ASD from CLD populations.

Disparities in ASD Identification and Service Utilization

ASD Identification and Diagnosis

It is imperative that children with ASD receive an early diagnosis so that they can receive early intervention services and potentially improve later outcomes (Bryson, Rogers, & Fombonne, 2003; Rogers & Vismara, 2008; Stahmer & Mandell, 2007). Often, parents of children with ASD identify first concerns in their children when they are around 12–24 months (Guinchat et al., 2012; Herlihy, Knoch, Vibert, & Fein, 2015; Kozlowski, Matson, Horovitz, Worley, & Neal, 2011). However, on average, children with ASD tend to receive an ASD diagnosis at age 4 (Baio et al., 2018).

The age of diagnosis tends to increase when children are from racially/ethnically diverse backgrounds, living in rural areas, foreign-born, or lower SES (Daniels & Mandell, 2014; Fountain, King, & Bearman, 2011; Kogan et al., 2009; Mandell, Novak, & Zubritsky, 2005; Sansosti, Lavik, & Sansosti, 2012; Valicenti-McDermott, Hottinger, Seijo, & Shulman, 2012). In fact, two recent studies reported that White children are approximately 30 and 50% more likely to have an ASD diagnosis at age 8 years than African American or Hispanic children, respectively (Baio, 2014); and Latino children are less likely to have a school identification of ASD or a comprehensive evaluation by age 3 than their White and African American peers (Baio et al., 2018). Finally, parents from non-English primary language households with children with ASD tend to describe their child's ASD symptoms as more severe than parents from homes where English is the primary language (Lin & Stella, 2015; Reyes et al., 2018). These results may indicate that parents of children from culturally diverse backgrounds are less likely to seek diagnostic services if their children display mild symptoms of ASD.

Researchers have also identified several cultural factors that may influence parent first concerns pertaining to ASD symptomatology. For example, in studies of parents of children with ASD, American and Japanese parents reported that they were first concerned about delayed speech (De Giacomo & Fombonne, 1998; Ohta et al., 1987), whereas urban Indian parents reported that they were primarily concerned about their child's impaired social functioning (Daley, 2004). In addition, cultural variations in communication exist. Zhang, Oetzel, Gao, Wilcox, and Takai (2007) conducted research to investigate nonverbal communication methods and their different cultural meanings in China. The researchers found that pointing with the index finger and eye contact with adults are considered inappropriate behaviors within the Chinese culture (Zhang et al., 2007). These behaviors are commonly assessed within ASD assessments to confirm the presence of ASD. Furthermore, Norbury and Sparks (2013) provided a review of potential cultural differences within ASD assessment including pretend play, public displays of emotion, and the extent to which children (especially boys) play with toy dolls. The researchers found cultural differences to the extent that adults engage in pretend play with children and adult discusson of emotional states (Norbury & Sparks, 2013). Furthermore, Pachter and Dworkin (1997) found that Puerto Rican mothers anticipated certain social milestones, such as recognizing the mother and smiling at others, later in age than Caucasian mothers indicating that there are cultural differences in developmental milestone expectations. These differences in cultural values and expectations likely have an impact on family access to clinical early intervention and school-based services, ASD identification, and professional interpretation of ASD assessment data.

Access to Clinical and School Services

As soon as children receive an ASD diagnosis, families are encouraged to seek intervention services. It is often recommended that children diagnosed with ASD receive at least 25 h per week of academic and intervention services (National Research Council, NRC, 2001; Odom, Boyd, & Hall, 2010a, Odom, Collet-Klingenberg, Rogers, & Hatton et al., 2010b). However, it is well documented that children with ASD do not receive the recommended amount of services that they need (Magaña, Lopez, Aguinaga, & Morton, 2013; Siller, Reyes, Hotez, Hutman, & Sigman, 2014; Thomas, Ellis, McLaurin, Daniels, & Morrissey, 2007). Moreover, families of children with ASD often report having more difficulties accessing clinical services than families with children with other developmental disabilities (Chiri & Warfield, 2012; Montes, Halterman, & Magyar, 2009; Vohra, Madhavan, Sambamoorthi, & Peter, 2014).

Disparities in accessing clinical intervention services have also been reported in ASD. For instance, families from minority backgrounds, with low parental education, and living in rural areas tend to receive fewer intervention services than their peers (Leigh, Grosse, Cassady, Melnikow, & Hertz-Picciotto, 2016; Magaña et al., 2013; Murphy & Ruble, 2012; Thomas et al., 2007). For example, Latino children from families with low SES tend to receive fewer clinical intervention services than their White and more affluent counterparts (Liptak et al., 2008). Overall, access to intervention services for children with ASD has been reported to be particularly limited for racial and ethnic minorities and those with low parental education.

Although the reasons for these disparities are likely to be complex, barriers to accessing an ASD diagnosis and intervention services in families from diverse backgrounds have been identified, including psychosocial, economic, political, and healthcare factors (Iland, Weiner, & Murawski, 2012). Specifically, regarding ASD diagnosis, Latino families have reported several barriers to obtaining clinical diagnostic assessments for ASD, including having limited knowledge about ASD, understanding of the medical system, and knowing where to go for help (Zuckerman et al., 2017). With respect to clinical services, Latino parents have also reported barriers, such as increased community stigma, limited care services due to poverty, limited English proficiency, and an inability to take advantage of services (Zuckerman et al., 2014).

Despite the aforementioned challenges with disparities in accessing ASD services among CLD populations, school settings may be one potential institution that can reduce these disparities (Harris et al., 2019). A large percentage of children (38%)

with ASD are identified through educational evaluations and do not receive a clinical diagnosis of ASD (Pettygrove et al., 2013). For CLD children, schools may be the only place where ASD services are accessible to families. In school settings, evaluations and services are federally mandated (when eligible) and are provided at no cost. Thus, for CLD children, schools may potentially contribute to earlier identification and accessible service allocation. However, despite an increase in access to ASD assessment and intervention within school settings over time, some researchers have found that disparities in ASD school identification persist (Pettygrove et al., 2013).

Assessment of ASD in Clinical Settings

Since no biological markers exist for diagnosing ASD, the diagnosis is made based on caregiver information and behavioral observations (Centers for Disease Control and Prevention, 2020). Clinicians use ASD-specific screeners and diagnostic tools to identify social impairments by comparing an individual's social behavior to operational definitions of "normative" social behavior. However, because culture defines what is typical and atypical, there is cross-cultural variation in normative social behavior (i.e., what is considered typical in one culture may be atypical in another culture). The operational definitions of normative social behavior that are included in ASD-specific screeners and diagnostic tools are often based on the majority culture of the U.S. and fail to account for the variability in social norms across cultures, resulting in measures that may lack sensitivity to cross-cultural variation in social behavior.

First, given the central role that culture plays in the establishment of normative social behaviors, we must carefully consider if and when variation in social behaviors is truly deviant and warrants a diagnosis of a disorder (Norbury & Sparks, 2013). For example, abnormalities in social communication, including eye contact, are a core feature of ASD, with the absence of (or poor) eye contact suggestive of ASD. However, cross-cultural differences in the use of eye contact in social interactions are well documented (Fugita, Wexley, & Hillery, 1974; Uono & Hietanen, 2015), and may significantly impact an individual's performance on ASD-specific measures. In fact, a recent study found that Black and Hispanic children were more likely to have atypical (i.e., higher) scores on the Unusual Eye Contact item on the ADOS-2 than White children, which may lead to inaccurate estimations of social impairments among Black and Hispanic children (Harrison, Long, Tommet, & Jones, 2017). Without careful assessment practices, the use of culturally loaded measures may place culturally and linguistically diverse (CLD) children at-risk for being over- or under-identified with ASD.

Moreover, another factor to disparities in ASD identification is the assessment practices and interpretation utilized by professionals conducting ASD evaluations. All ASD evaluation tools are culturally loaded, which impacts the performance and applicability of children from diverse cultural groups (Harris, Barton, & Albert, 2014). Cultural variations in behavior may contribute to inappropriate assessment practices and data interpretation. For example, Zhang et al. (2007) found that eye contact with adults and pointing with the index finger are considered inappropriate behaviors within the Chinese culture (Zhang et al., 2007). These behaviors are commonly assessed within ASD evaluation and are directly assessed on the Autism Diagnostic Observation Schedule (ADOS) as the absence of these behaviors may indicate the presence of ASD. Norbury and Sparks (2013) conducted a review of potential cultural differences within ASD assessment. The authors found that pretend play, public displays of emotion, and the extent to which children (especially boys) play with toy dolls varies based on cultural factors. These differences may impact the interpretation of ASD assessments and potentially contribute to misidentification or delayed identification (Norbury and Sparks, 2013).

Also, while some of the ASD-specific screening and diagnostic tools that were developed in Western, English-speaking countries have undergone cultural adaptations for use across cultural groups, such adaptations have mainly involved surface-level adaptations, such as translation to facilitate use in non-English-speaking populations (Al-Maskari, Melville, & Willis, 2018). It is important to note that measures that have been translated but not normed or standardized with a given population may not be valid for the population as the translation does not ensure that the English and non-English versions of the measures are functionally equivalent (Soto et al., 2015). For example, although most of the activities in the Autism Diagnostic Observation Schedule, Second Edition 2 (ADOS-2), a commonly used ASD diagnostic tool that has been translated into several languages, was found to be culturally appropriate for a sample of Afrikaans-speaking individuals residing in the Western Cape of Africa, some elements of the ADOS-2 were unfamiliar to this population, and would benefit from adaptation to make the elements culturally appropriate (Smith, Malcom-Smith, & de Vries, 2017). These findings highlight the need to examine the validity and cultural appropriateness of measures that have only undergone surface-level adaptations (e.g., translation) and lack diverse norms for use in CLD populations.

Finally, the administration, scoring, and interpretation of commonly utilized and researched ASD diagnostic tools (i.e., ADOS-2 and the Autism Diagnostic Interview [ADI-R]) require substantial training. In addition to concerns related to the cultural appropriateness and validity of ASD-specific screeners and diagnostic tools for use in CLD populations, the assessment of ASD in CLD populations is also negatively impacted by a shortage of professionals who have sufficient training to conduct ASD assessments (Marrus et al., 2014). Moreover, the number of professionals who have training and experience in conducting ASD assessments with CLD populations is even smaller. Thus, although several tools are available for the screening and diagnosis of ASD, several factors can hinder the accurate and timely diagnosis of ASD among CLD populations.

ASD Assessment in School Settings

Children may qualify for special education services under the Autism[1] eligibility category per the Individuals with Disabilities Education Act (IDEA) within the educational setting. Receiving a medical diagnosis of ASD does not guarantee a child will receive an education identification of Autism as the child must demonstrate an educational impact of the disability to qualify for school-based services (IDEA law, Section 300.8 (c)). There are several challenges associated with the educational identification of Autism. First, while school personnel likely have access to ASD-specific screeners, access to psychometrically stronger diagnostic tools (e.g., ADOS and ADI-R) may not be readily available or feasible for school personnel as these measures are costly and time-intensive. Second, schools may lack or have few qualified professionals who are trained to conduct ASD assessments, particularly among culturally and linguistically diverse populations (Harris et al., 2019). That is, school districts may lack the resources needed to provide school personnel with the comprehensive training necessary to reliably administer ASD assessments (Campbell, Ruble, & Hammond, 2014). Third, there is no clearly defined process that exists for the educational identification of Autism. As such, it is the responsibility of individual school districts and state boards to establish procedures and processes for the educational identification of Autism that align with federal law and state guidelines for students with disabilities.

Using IDEA special education eligibility data, Sullivan (2013) found the prevalence rate for educational identification of Autism in school settings to be 1 in 228. While this prevalence rate is lower than the CDC's ADDM prevalence rate, clinical diagnosis and educational identification of ASD are two different processes and cannot be equated. However, this rate is problematic as it is much lower than the general prevalence rate, varies extensively by state (see Barton et al., 2016), and consists of significant disparities among CLD populations. For example, Hispanic and American Indian/Alaskan Native students were less likely to be identified with ASD compared to White students while Asian/Pacific Islander students were more likely to be identified with ASD than their White counterparts (Sullivan, 2013). In summary, White and Asian children are more likely to receive an educational identification of ASD than other racial groups, mirroring disparities in the clinical diagnosis of ASD.

Culturally and linguistically responsive identification and evaluation of students with ASD is a critical first step for professionals in providing effective school-based services (Harris et al., 2019). Evaluations in the school context can be completed as early as age 3, when children are first eligible to receive school-based services under IDEA Part C (Dilly & Hall, 2019). Professional organizations (i.e., the American Psychological Association [APA]) have not specifically outlined recommendations for ASD assessment of CLD children; however, they do provide some guidance. Both the American Psychological Association (2014) and National Association of School Psychologists (2010) recommend that psychologists utilize evidence-based

[1] For the purpose of increased clarity, the term "Autism" will be used to describe an educational identification and "ASD" will be used to describe a medical/clinical diagnosis.

assessment practices. Specific to ASD, evidence-based assessment practices should include the use of reliable and valid measures in a comprehensive, multisource developmental assessment (Campbell, Ruble, & Hammond, 2014; Huerta & Lord, 2012; Wilkinson, 2014).

Limited research has been conducted regarding school-based ASD assessment practices, particularly with CLD populations. A recent mixed-methods study investigated the self-reported experiences of school psychologists when conducting ASD evaluations with CLD students (Harris et al., 2019). There were many perceived barriers that school psychologists endorsed regarding implementing culturally and linguistically responsive ASD assessment. One of the most striking results was the limited endorsement of engaging families in the ASD assessment process. Because of this potential low level of involvement, it is also possible that families lack sufficient knowledge pertaining to school systems to best advocate for their children's needs. Regarding ASD methods specifically, the use of observations was minimally endorsed by school psychologists. The utilization of native language and English within an ASD assessment was also minimally endorsed. In addition, few respondents endorsed utilizing interdisciplinary practices when engaging in ASD evaluation among CLD children. Multiple school psychologists also stated that they have limited or poor assessment tools for CLD populations and that they are not confident regarding interpreting data from children that are CLD. School psychologists also commonly reported that language barriers were a challenge when conducting ASD evaluations (Harris et al., 2019). This study highlights that school psychologists face multiple barriers when conducting ASD assessment with CLD families, and these barriers may indeed contribute to access to timely and accurate identification of ASD.

Although there are challenges associated with conducting ASD assessments in schools (e.g., fewer qualified school personnel to conduct ASD assessments), schools play a critical role in identifying children with ASD, particularly those who may have been "missed" by the healthcare system (Pettygrove et al., 2013). Moreover, there are several benefits of conducting ASD assessments in schools. First, schools provide greater and more equitable access to services for CLD students and their families than specialty clinical settings (Broder-Fingert, Shui, Pulcini, Kurowski, & Perrin, 2013). Second, unlike clinical settings, there are no waitlists for ASD assessments in schools as IDEA mandates that school-aged assessments are conducted within 60 days of signed parent consent to evaluate. Third, school personnel have the ability to conduct more naturalistic observations of students, especially peer-to-peer interactions. Fourth, IDEA mandates the use of interpretation services when necessary; therefore, linguistically diverse students and families may have easier access to a linguistically appropriate assessment in school settings than clinical settings.

When conducting evaluations for the educational identification of Autism, utilizing a multidisciplinary approach is not only best practice, but also required by IDEA. Each of the team members, who may include school psychologists, teachers, English language acquisition support staff, and speech therapists (among many others), provide unique perspectives and guidance to the evaluation process and eligibility determination. Teams are also required to include parents, as engaging families in this process is critical. Families may have diverse experiences and understanding of disabilities such as ASD or have varied cultural values and beliefs pertaining to behavior and communication. As such, the collaboration between multidisciplinary team members is critical during the evaluation process, as it allows team members to compare and share assessment findings (Kroncke, Willard, & Huckabee, 2016).

ASD Assessment in Clinical/Community Settings

Due to a shortage of adequately trained professionals, families often wait months to receive a comprehensive diagnostic assessment in clinical and community settings (Bisgaier, Levinson, Cutts, & Rhodes, 2011). Moreover, diagnostic assessments conducted in clinical settings often are time-consuming, and require multiple visits to complete (Kalb et al., 2012). Given the challenges associated with receiving timely diagnostic assessments in clinical settings, efforts have been made to develop accurate and efficient strategies for the screening and assessment (please refer to chapters 'Screening and Surveillance' and 'Interdisciplinary Evaluation of Autism Spectrum Disorder' for more information about screening and interdisciplinary evaluation) of ASD in clinical settings.

Training established for community providers in the screening and evaluation of ASD has demonstrated effectiveness in increasing access to diagnostic assessments in community settings. For example, ECHO (Extension for Community Health Outcomes) Autism STAT is a hybrid model for training primary care providers (PCP), who work in underserved areas in the screening and diagnosis of children at-risk for ASD using the STAT assessment (Stone et al., 2004). ECHO Autism STAT combines ECHO Autism (Mazurek, Brown, Curran, & Sohl, 2017), a videoconference-based collaboration that connects PCPs to an interdisciplinary team of autism experts (see chapter 'ECHO Autism' for additional information on ECHO Autism), and the Screening Tool for Autism in Toddlers and Young Children (STAT; Stone et al., 2004), an autism diagnostic training for pediatric medical providers. The implementation of ECHO Autism STAT was shown to increase PCP's administration of autism screeners and their self-efficacy in autism screening and identification, autism referral and resources, assessment and treatment of psychiatric comorbidities, and additional aspects of care for autism (Mazurek, Curran, Burnette, & Sohl, 2019).

Partnering with community agencies has also been proven effective in promoting local, timely access to comprehensive ASD evaluations. One such program, the Autism Diagnosis Education Project (ADEP; OCALI, n.d.), facilitates unique partnerships between community-based primary care practices and professionals providing early intervention and early childhood services in Ohio to conduct local comprehensive multidisciplinary ASD evaluations. Through ADEP, children suspected of having ASD receive a psychoeducational evaluation from a local early intervention team. Then, children receive a medical evaluation from a community medical provider, who either diagnoses or rules out ASD. That is, instead of experiencing long wait times and driving long distances for a comprehensive diagnostic evaluation, families of children suspected of having ASD are able to receive more timely diagnostic services through local community providers. The implementation of ADEP has resulted in the reduction in the average age of ASD diagnosis of children in Ohio from 62 months to 30 months for the evaluation of 1,078 children between 2013 and 2018.

Another evidence-based strategy for increasing access to diagnostic assessments in clinical settings, particularly among minority and low-income populations, involves the use of patient navigators. Patient navigation, which has a strong evidence-base in adult oncology, involves providing individualized assistance to patients, caregivers, and families to help overcome healthcare system barriers and facilitate timely access to quality care (Freeman & Rodriguez, 2011). Recent studies have found that the use of patient navigators is a feasible and effective practice to address barriers that impede timely ASD diagnosis among low-income families. For example, Feinberg et al. (2016) found that children who received patient navigation were significantly more likely to complete an ASD diagnostic evaluation than children who received routine clinic care. Additionally, children who received patient navigation underwent diagnostic evaluations earlier than those who received routine clinic care. The Screening and Linkage Services for Autism (SaLSA) is another promising practice that aims to improve access to autism screening follow-up, diagnostic evaluation, and early intervention services for ASD among predominantly Spanish-speaking, low-income families through autism patient navigators (Project SaLSA, HRSA Grant R40MC27702, 2014).

Community providers may find resources to gain competency in conducting ASD assessments in CLD populations through professional organizations. For example, the American Psychological Association (APA) and the American Education Research Association provide ethical requirements for the assessments of individuals from diverse populations. Additionally, the CDC's "Learn the Signs. Act Early" campaign has resources and materials for community providers, educators, and families. Additionally, the Ohio Center for Autism and Low Incidence (OCALI), which is primarily funded by the Ohio Department of Education, has online and in-person training that are designed to assist school evaluation teams and other school personnel with identifying and serving students with ASD.

In addition to finding resources through professional organizations and community agencies, community providers are also encouraged to collaborate with other clinical providers when conducting ASD evaluations in CLD populations. Given the complexities and variability in symptoms of ASD, collaboration with other clinical providers is beneficial as it allows clinicians to gather information to make differential and/or comorbid diagnoses. Community providers may decide to collaborate with a number of providers from various disciplines, including speech and language pathologists, developmental pediatricians, audiologists, occupational therapists, and geneticists. For example, collaborating with a speech and language pathologist or can be used to determine if a child's communication deficits are due to ASD, a language disorder, or being a bilingual learner; the latter is important for children with limited English language exposure.

Questions to Consider When Conducting ASD Diagnostic Assessments with Diverse Populations

The following questions are presented to aid professionals in utilizing culturally and linguistically sensitive ASD assessment practices.

1. Are the social-communicative impairments the result of typical variations of cultural norms? That is, are the social-communicative impairments observed due to differences in cultural expectations and/or values?
2. Are language impairments accounting for observed social-communicative impairments?
3. Is the assessment culturally and linguistically responsive?
   a. Do the caregivers and children understand the concepts and questions that are being asked?
   b. Are cultural and/or linguistic factors impacting the child's performance and/or the validity of information gathered during the assessment?
4. Have personal biases that may influence the assessment process been identified and addressed?
5. Are evidence-based assessment practices being employed?
6. Is data being collected from multiple sources including standardized and qualitative information?
7. Are multiple professionals involved in a collaborative assessment process?
8. When interpreting the assessment data, are considerations pertaining to culture and language discussed as potential influences?

ASD Intervention: Considerations for Culturally and Linguistically Diverse Children and Families

Substantial research has identified the benefit of early intervention on future outcomes for children with ASD (e.g., Fernell, Eriksson, & Gillberg, 2013; Kuppens & Onghena, 2012; Magiati, Tay, & Howlin, 2014). Although there are numerous evidence-based interventions for ASD, the selection of such will be warranted by symptom severity and family needs. Across all interventions, evidence supports combining parent-mediated interventions with professional-implemented interventions to maximize outcomes (Landa, 2018). Typically, evidence-based intervention falls into two categories: Naturalistic Developmental Behavioral Interventions (e.g., Schreibman et al., 2015) and those that are more commonly referred to as Applied Behavior Analysis (ABA; see chapter 'Coordinating ABA Services') utilizing a foundation of discrete trial training formats. However, limited research has been conducted pertaining to CLD children and ASD intervention. Furthermore, researchers acknowledge the limited inclusion of CLD children in ASD research which greatly impacts knowledge pertaining to evidence-based practices (see Wong et al., 2015). Furthermore, behavioral interventions for children with ASD that are effective for one population, may not be effective for other populations (Buzhardt et al., 2015). Thus, the influence of cultural factors on the utility, implementation, and design of these interventions is generally unknown. More research on evidence-based interventions for CLD children with ASD is critical.

There are numerous challenges reported pertaining to providing optimal ASD intervention to CLD children and families. One of the challenges pertaining to current ASD intervention practice is the reliance on translating materials into another language. While this practice has good intentions, translation alone does not improve cultural factors that may not be considered. For example, Buzhardt et al. (2015) found that translating an evidence-based intervention into Spanish may not improve "cultural congruence" for Latinos. Instead, interventions need to be analyzed for potential alignment with cultural values, expectations, and perceptions (DuBay et al., 2018). Historically, families from CLD families have reported higher levels of discontent with early intervention services. This may be due to this aforementioned cultural incongruence as well as other factors such as language barriers that may impact the ability to create strong relationships with professionals (Iland et al, 2012).

Given that ASD is a complex disorder, in recent years, a wide range of professionals often work with this population and collaboration among interventionists is critical to effectively serve families (American Academy of Pediatrics, 2014; Strunk, Leisen, and Schubert, 2017; World Health Organization, 2010). In fact, children with ASD are often served by psychologists, social workers, speech and language pathologists, occupational therapists, physical therapists, teachers, nurses, dietitians, psychiatrists, and developmental pediatricians (Myers & Johnson, 2007). Thus, working in collaboration is described as a best practice model and one that can increase culturally and linguistically responsive services (D'Amour, Ferrada-Videla, San Martin Rodriguez, & Beaulieu, 2005).

An example of that approach is the Treatment and Education of Autistic and Related Communication Handicapped CHildren (TEACCH), which was one of the first programs that included an interdisciplinary approach, including clinical services, family involvement, and counseling. TEACCH shows some promising results in being effective as an interdisciplinary intervention, although early intensive behavioral intervention shows the strongest evidence-base for children with ASD (Virués-Ortega, Arnold-Saritepe, Hird, & Phillios, 2017). Although this research is in its infancy (Carbone, Behl, Azor, & Murphy 2010; Soares, Baum, & Frick, 2015), it is likely that using an interdisciplinary approach will improve treatment planning and service coordination when providing services to children with ASD from traditionally underserved groups.

Despite limited research on this topic, a recent review of 18 studies investigated the effects of utilizing the heritage language (i.e., native language) in ASD intervention. The majority of the studies found demonstrated small effects for utilizing the heritage language in ASD intervention. The authors also found problematic research designs in many studies; thus, the implications of these studies should be interpreted with caution. However, these findings indicate that utilizing the heritage language of the child can demonstrate favorable outcomes and should be considered during intervention design (Lim et al., 2019).

While there are benefits to obtaining ASD intervention in clinical and home settings, ASD intervention within the school setting offers the family the ability to receive services with reduced barriers (e.g., transportation, cost). Intervention for ASD in a school setting may look different from clinical settings for a variety of reasons as school professionals tailor special education intervention to goals in the Individualized Education Plan. There are many advantages to providing school-based interventions to children with ASD as the child is in a natural environment, with peers, and intervention can occur within multiple school settings and in real time during structured (such as the classroom setting) and unstructured settings (such as recess or lunch).

Strengthening Partnerships with Culturally and Linguistically Diverse Families

Evidence-based practices for ASD often require heavy family involvement and resources to implement them consistently. Although evidence-based practices (EBPs) have been shown to be promising in addressing and alleviating some ASD symptoms and related difficulties, some families with a child with ASD might struggle to include these interventions in their daily lives (Hume, Bellini, & Pratt, 2005; Wainer, Hepburn, & Griffith, 2017; Williams & Wishart, 2003). Specifically, it is well documented that families of children with ASD often experience increased levels of stress; navigating and accessing services might also be a source of stress for them (Sanders & Morgan, 1997). For some families, they may have to modify their work schedules or stop working altogether because several evidenced-based interventions require family involvement (Karst & Van Hecke, 2012). For other families, they may feel that they have minimal involvement in the planning or implementation of these interventions (Kohler, 1999; Wainer et al., 2017). Also, after receiving an ASD diagnosis, families may face other challenges, including their own mental and physical health issues, marital problems, parent-child relationships, sibling relationships, family resources, parent copying styles, parental self-efficacy, and social support (Karst & Van Hecke, 2012). Families from CLD backgrounds may experience similar difficulties when caring for a child with ASD (Kheir et al., 2012; Moh & Magiati, 2012; Pakenham et al., 2005; Sivberg, 2002; Wang, Michaels, & Day, 2011).

Families may also face an increased number of barriers that may widen disparities in accessing ASD services (Zuckerman et al., 2018). Thus, several factors might need to be considered when working with diverse or traditionally underserved families. For example, when delivering evidence-based interventions to families from different linguistic and ethnic background it may be important to include bilingual and bicultural staff to communicate effectively with families (Barnett, Gonzalez, Miranda, Chavira, & Lau, 2018), or at least provide adequate interpreter services.

Also, it may be useful to understand the family's beliefs and views about their child as well as family values (Al Anbar, Dardennes, Prado-Netto, Kaye, & Contejean, 2010; Reyes et al., 2018; Zuckerman, Lindly, Sinche, & Nicolaidis, 2015). Families may also benefit from information on how to navigate their health care system, early intervention, and school services (Moody et al., 2019). To increase family satisfaction, it may also be beneficial to include and involve families in the treatment planning (Wainer et al., 2017) and to include culturally informed interventions (Lopez, Magaña, Morales, & Iland, 2019). Moreover, families may find it helpful to participate in interventions designed to address their own difficulties when raising a child with ASD (Mirza, Krischer, Stolley, Magaña, & Martin, 2018). Finally, with families from rural areas, it might be valuable to include telehealth services to provide services that they otherwise would not have access to (Hepburn, Blakeley-Smith, Wolff, & Reaven, 2016; Ingersoll, & Berger, 2015; Lindgren et al., 2016; Vismara, McCormick, Young, Nadhan, & Monlux, 2013; Wacker et al., 2013).

In both the clinical and school settings, family support resources will be accessible to all families. In the school setting specifically, schools will have resources such as family liaisons and parent organizations, however, the focus on supporting CLD families will vary by school and district. School districts are legally mandated to provide a family advocacy office where families can receive educational advocacy support. If a child has an educational identification of Autism, the family can also access state legal advocacy resources through federally mandated offices. Although these resources exist, research surrounding the effectiveness of these resources with CLD families is not currently available.

In the clinical/community setting, families have additional opportunities for resources by accessing parent training programs. Parent training programs are effective for families of children with ASD to reduce caregiver mental health concerns, improve family knowledge of ASD, and increase caregiver self-advocacy (Matson, Mahan & Matson, 2009; McConachie & Diggle, 2007; Matson et al., 2009). For example, Magaña et al. (2017) found that Spanish-speaking Latinx mothers of children with ASD that participated in a parent training program reported improvements in understanding of ASD, awareness of their child's strengths and needs, knowledge of their child's rights, support systems, access within the community, and efficacy of evidence-based strategy implementation. In addition, children with ASD had reduced impaired language between pre- and post-test (Magaña, Lopez, & Machalicek, 2017).

One specific example of an evidence-based parent training program is the Parents Taking Action (PTA) program by Magaña et al. (2017). This parent training program was created for Spanish-speaking families to address disparities for Latinx children with ASD. The researchers utilized the ecological validity model to adapt and develop their materials in the PTA program (Bernal, Bonilla & Bellido, 1995). In this model, there are eight cultural domains that are considered when creating interventions, not only for interventions for ASD. These include language, persons, metaphors, content, concepts, goals, methods, and context. This model can be of assistance when professionals would like to evaluate, modify, or align existing evidence-based interventions within culturally or linguistically diverse populations. Magaña et al.

(2017) found various positive effects of the PTA program not only within the families, but also the ASD symptoms of the children.

Magaña et al. (2017) found that the use of promotoras was essential to the change reported by Spanish-speaking parents enrolled in the parent training program. Promotoras, also known as promotores de salud, is the Spanish term for "community health worker." Promotoras are typically employed in clinical settings such as hospitals and agencies, and are sometimes referred to as family navigators. The focus of the promotoras is to work within a Spanish-speaking community as a lay health worker, disseminating resources to families. This resource can be provided at a low cost and, by definition, will provide culturally and linguistically responsive support (Rotheram-Borus, Swendeman, & Chorpita, 2012).

Questions to Consider When Conducting ASD Intervention with CLD Populations

The following questions are presented to aid professionals in utilizing culturally and linguistically responsive ASD intervention practices.

(1) Serve as an advocate. Does the family have knowledge of ASD, ASD service providers, and agencies/institutions for ASD services? Are there parent training programs? Promotoras? If not, can you utilize telehealth services to access these resources?
(2) What does the family desire for their child's current interventions and future outcomes?
(3) What are language considerations of the family? Is an interpreter or translator required? Are materials needed in the native language?
(4) In what ways are school and clinical intervention service providers collaborating? What are the barriers to effective collaboration? How can this collaboration be improved?

Interpretation and Translation Services

Interpretation and translation services are required in both medical and school settings, although to varying degrees. Interpretation refers to oral communication, and translation refers to written communication. While there are multiple laws that ensure proper interpretation and translation services in the medical setting, few laws pertaining to these services exist in the school setting. If a family requires interpretation or translation services under IDEA services (also known as special education services) in the school setting, these services are provided by the school district. However, schools generally use their discretion regarding the use of interpretation/translation services at other times outside of IDEA services (e.g., parent–teacher conferences, parent association meetings). In the medical setting, interpretation requires more specific coursework and certification; interpretation in the school setting requires the certification of the school district, and district practices vary extensively.

Professionals will likely utilize interpreters for family interviews and multidisciplinary meetings. It is recommended that professionals hold a pre-meeting with the interpreter to plan for the session and discuss technical words that may be challenging to interpret. In addition, discussions around the manner of interpretation are important. For example, some interpreters use simultaneous interpretation while other models will require the speaker to pause and allow for time for interpretation. Professionals should note that the direct interpretation of standardized assessments into other languages voids standardization and is not recommended by professional associations (American Educational Research Association, 2014).

Discussion

Disparities in ASD services by CLD children and families exist, and ultimately contribute to poorer outcomes. Interdisciplinary collaboration can increase cultural and linguistic responsiveness of ASD services. When practitioners are trying to rule out the difference from disability, it is important that substantial data is collected in a culturally and linguistically responsive manner, multiple perspectives are considered and various professionals and family members are involved.

Currently, evidence-based ASD identification practices exist, although have not been comprehensively researched within culturally and linguistically diverse populations. Thus, professionals have the responsibility of considering the impact of culture and language throughout their evaluation and to interpret their data with caution due to potential biases. Partnering with families in the assessment process cannot be understated, as cultural and linguistic factors must be considered throughout the evaluation. Professionals must also consider when it is appropriate to report standardized scores and how the lack of standardized measures for CLD children and families may influence assessment data. Assessment data should be compiled comprehensively with a team, and with the intention of supporting family, child and school intervention goals.

While there is more emerging research pertaining to ASD intervention practices within CLD families, there continues to be a disproportionate amount of ASD research on non-White children and families. This limits the ability of professionals to identify evidence-based practices with the families and children they serve, likely impacting appropriate service allocation. Some promising practices exist, such as the use of promotoras and parent training programs, although this research is emerging and includes small segments of CLD families. Ultimately, professionals have limited research regarding potential cultural or linguistic influences on the performance of all interventions deemed evidence-based for treating ASD.

As disparities occur in both school and clinical settings among CLD children, the collaboration between settings can potentially improve disparities and the outcomes of children with ASD. Future research should focus on innovative ways to collaborate between settings to aid in timelier ASD identification and service allocation. Furthermore, training programs and professional development that is designed to be collaborative and completed in multidisciplinary teams can also be beneficial. Ultimately, it is critical that all professionals serve first and foremost as advocates so that all children can access appropriate and individually tailored services. Both clinical and school settings serve important roles in this process, and should be viewed as complementary.

References

AERA, APA, & NCME. (2014). Standards for educational and psychological testing. Washington, DC: AERA.

Al Anbar, N. N., Dardennes, R. M., Prado-Netto, A., Kaye, K., & Contejean, Y. (2010). Treatment choices in autism spectrum disorder: The role of parental illness perceptions. *Research in Developmental Disabilities, 31*(3), 817–828.

Al Maskari, T. S., Melville, C. A., & Willis, D. S. (2018). Systematic review: Cultural adaptation and feasibility of screening for autism in non-English speaking countries. *International Journal of Mental Health Systems, 12*(1), 22.

American Academy of Pediatrics. (2014). Policy statement: AAP Publications reaffirmed or retired. *Pediatrics, 134,* e1520.

American Community Survey: Race/Ethnicity and American Indian & Alaska Native documentation. (2010). Retrieved from https://www.census.gov/programs-surveys/acs/technical-documentation/race-ethnicity-aian.2010.html.

American Educational Research Association, American Psychological Association, & National Council on Measurement in Education, & Joint Committee on Standards for Educational and Psychological Testing. (2014). *Standards for Educational and Psychological Testing*. Washington, DC: AERA.

Baio, J. (2014). Prevalence of autism spectrum disorder among children aged 8 years-autism and developmental disabilities monitoring network, 11 sites, United States, 2010.

Baio J., Wiggins, L., Christensen, D. L., Maenner, M., Daniels, J., Warren, Z., …, Dowling, N. (2018). Prevalence of autism spectrum disorder among children aged 8 years—Autism and developmental disabilities monitoring network, 11 sites, United States, 2014. *MMWR Surviellence, 67*(No. SS-6), 1–23.

Barnett, M. L., Gonzalez, A., Miranda, J., Chavira, D. A., & Lau, A. S. (2018). Mobilizing community health workers to address mental health disparities for underserved populations: A systematic review. *Administration and Policy in Mental Health and Mental Health Services Research, 45*(2), 195–211.

Barton, E., Harris, B., Leech, N., Stiff, L., Choi, G., & Joel, T. (2016). An Analysis of State Autism Educational Assessment Practices and Requirements. *Journal of Autism and Developmental Disorders*.

Bernal, G., Bonilla, J., & Bellido, C. (1995). Ecological validity and cultural sensitivity for outcome research: Issues for the cultural adaptation and development of psychosocial treatments with Hispanics. *Journal of abnormal child psychology, 23*(1), 67–82.

Bisgaier, J., Levinson, D., Cutts, D. B., & Rhodes, K. V. (2011). Access to autism evaluation appointments with developmental-behavioral and neurodevelopmental subspecialists. *Arch Pediatric Adolescent Medicine, 165*(7), 673–674.

Broder-Fingert, S., Shui, A., Pulcini, C. D., Kurowski, D., & Perrin, J. M. (2013). Racial and ethnic differences in subspecialty service use by children with autism. *Pediatrics, 132*(1), 94–100.

Bryson, S. E., Rogers, S. J., & Fombonne, E. (2003). Autism spectrum disorders: Early detection, intervention, education, and psychopharmacological management. *The Canadian Journal of Psychiatry, 48*(8), 506–516.

Buzhardt, J., Rusinko, L., Heitzman-Powell, L., Trevino-Maack, S., & McGrath, A. (2016). Exploratory evaluation and initial adaptation of a parent training program for Hispanic families of children with autism. *Family process, 55*(1), 107–122.

Campbell, J. M., Ruble, L. A., & Hammond, R. K. (2014). Comprehensive developmental assessment model. In L. A. Wilkinson (Ed.), *School psychology book series. Autism spectrum disorder in children and adolescents: Evidence-based assessment and intervention in schools* (pp. 51–73). Washington, DC: American Psychological Association.

Carbone P., Behl D., Azor V., & Murphy N. (2010). The medical home for children with autism spectrum disorders: parent and pediatrician perspectives. *Journal of Autism and Developmental Disorders, 40*, 317e324.

Centers for Disease Control and Prevention. (2020). *What is autism spectrum disorder?* Retrieved from https://www.cdc.gov/ncbddd/autism/facts.html.

Chiri, G., & Warfield, M. E. (2012). Unmet need and problems accessing core health care services for children with autism spectrum disorder. *Maternal and Child Health Journal, 16*(5), 1081–1091.

D'Amour D., Ferrada-Videla M., San Martin Rodriguez L., & Beaulieu M. (2005). The conceptual basis for interprofessional collaboration: Core concepts and theoretical frameworks. *Journal of Interprofessional Care, 1*, 116e131.

Daniels, A. M., & Mandell, D. S. (2014). Explaining differences in age at autism spectrum disorder diagnosis: A critical review. *Autism, 18*(5), 583–597.

Daley, T. (2004) From symptom recognition to diagnosis: Children with autism in urban India. *Social Science & Medicine, 58*(7), 1323–1335.

De Giacomo, A., & Fombonne, E. (1998). Parental recognition of developmental abnormalities in autism. *European Child and Adolescent Psychiatry, 7*(3), 131–136. https://doi.org/10.1007/s007870050058.

Dilly, L. J., & Hall, C. M. (2019). Autism spectrum disorder assessment in schools. New York, NY: Routledge.

DuBay, M., Watson, L. R., & Zhang, W. (2018). In search of culturally appropriate autism interventions: Perspectives of Latino caregivers. *Journal of autism and developmental disorders, 48*(5), 1623–1639.

Feinberg, E., Abufhele, M., Sandler, J., Augustyn, M., Cabral, H. D., Chen, N., … & Silverstein, M. (2016). Reducing disparities in timely autism diagnosis through family navigation: Results from a randomized pilot trial. *Psychiatric Services, 67*(8), 912–5.

Federal Interagency Forum on Child and Family Statistics (2019). America's children: Key national indicators of well-being. Retrieved from https://www.childstats.gov/americaschildren/demo.asp.

Fernell, E., Eriksson, M. A., & Gillberg, C. (2013). Early diagnosis of autism and impact on prognosis: a narrative review. *Clinical Epidemiology, 5*, 33.

Fountain, C., King, M. D., & Bearman, P. S. (2011). Age of diagnosis for autism: Individual and community factors across 10 birth cohorts. *Journal of Epidemiology and Community Health, 65*(6), 503–510.

Freeman, H. P., & Rodriguez, R. L. (2011). History and principles of patient navigation. *Cancer, 117*(S15), 3537–3540.

Fugita, S. S., Wexley, K. N., & Hillery, J. M. (1974). Black-white differences in nonverbal behavior in an interview setting. *Journal of Applied Social Psychology, 4*(4), 343–350.

Guinchat, V., Chamak, B., Bonniau, B., Bodeau, N., Perisse, D., Cohen, D., et al. (2012). Very early signs of autism reported by parents include many concerns not specific to autism criteria. *Research in Autism Spectrum Disorders, 6*(2), 589–601.

Harris, B., Barton, E. E. & Albert, C. (2014). Evaluating autism diagnostic and screening tools for cultural and linguistic responsiveness. *Journal of Autism and Developmental Disorders, 44*(6), 1275–1287.

Harris, B., McClain, M., Haverkamp, C., Benallie, K., Benny, K. & Cruz, R. (2019). School-based autism assessment of culturally and linguistically diverse children. *Professional Psychology: Research and Practice*.
Harrison, A. J., Long, K. A., Tommet, D. C., & Jones, R. N. (2017). Examining the role of race, ethnicity, and gender on social and behavioral ratings within the autism diagnostic observation schedule. *Journal of Autism and Developmental Disorders, 47*(9), 2770–2782.
Hepburn, S. L., Blakeley-Smith, A., Wolff, B., & Reaven, J. A. (2016). Telehealth delivery of cognitive-behavioral intervention to youth with autism spectrum disorder and anxiety: A pilot study. *Autism, 20*(2), 207–218.
Herlihy, L., Knoch, K., Vibert, B., & Fein, D. (2015). Parents' first concerns about toddlers with autism spectrum disorder: Effect of sibling status. *Autism, 19*(1), 20–28.
Huerta, M., & Lord, C. (2012). Diagnostic evaluation of autism spectrum disorders. *Pediatric Clinics of North America, 59*(1), 103–111. https://doi.org/10.1016/j.pcl.2011.10.018.
Hume, K., Bellini, S., & Pratt, C. (2005). The usage and perceived outcomes of early intervention and early childhood programs for young children with autism spectrum disorder. *Topics in Early Childhood Special Education, 25*(4), 195–207.
Iland, E. D., Weiner, I., & Murawski, W. W. (2012). Obstacles faced by Latina mothers of children with autism. *Californian Journal of Health Promotion, 10*(SI-Latino), 25–36.
Ingersoll, B., & Berger, N. I. (2015). Parent engagement with a telehealth-based parent-mediated intervention program for children with autism spectrum disorders: predictors of program use and parent outcomes. *Journal of Medical Internet Research, 17*(10), e227.
Kalb, L. G., Freedman, B., Foster, C., Menon, D., Landa, R., Kishfy, L., et al. (2012). Determinants of appointment absenteeism at an outpatient pediatric autism clinic. *Journal of Developmental and Behavioral Pediatrics, 33*(9), 685–697.
Karst, J. S., & Van Hecke, A. V. (2012). Parent and family impact of autism spectrum disorders: A review and proposed model for intervention evaluation. *Clinical Child and Family Psychology Review, 15*(3), 247–277.
Kheir, N., Ghoneim, O., Sandridge, A. L., Al-Ismail, M., Hayder, S., & Al-Rawi, F. (2012). Quality of life of caregivers of children with autism in Qatar. *Autism, 16*(3), 293–298.
Kogan, M. D., Blumberg, S. J., Schieve, L. A., Boyle, C. A., Perrin, J. M., Ghandour, R. M., … & van Dyck, P. C. (2009). Prevalence of parent-reported diagnosis of autism spectrum disorder among children in the US, 2007. *Pediatrics, 124*(5), 1395–1403.
Kohler, F. W. (1999). Examining the services received by young children with autism and their families: A survey of parent responses. *Focus on Autism and Other Developmental Disabilities, 14*(3), 150–158.
Kozlowski, A. M., Matson, J. L., Horovitz, M., Worley, J. A., & Neal, D. (2011). Parents' first concerns of their child's development in toddlers with autism spectrum disorders. *Developmental Neurorehabilitation, 14*(2), 72–78.
Kroncke, A. P., Willard, M., & Huckabee, H. (2016) School-based assessment. In Kroncke et al. (Eds.), *Assessment of Autism spectrum disorder. Contemporary issues in psychological assessment*. Switzerland: Springer, Cham.
Kuppens, S., & Onghena, P. (2012). Sequential meta-analysis to determine the sufficiency of cumulative knowledge: The case of early intensive behavioral intervention for children with autism spectrum disorders. *Research in Autism Spectrum Disorders, 6*(1), 168–176.
Landa, R. J. (2018). Efficacy of early interventions for infants and young children with, and at risk for, autism spectrum disorders. *International Review of Psychiatry, 30*(1), 25–39.
Leigh, J. P., Grosse, S. D., Cassady, D. L., Melnikow, J., & Hertz-Picciotto, I. (2016). Spending by California's department of developmental services for persons with autism across demographic and expenditure categories. *PLoS One, 11*(3), e0151970. https://doi.org/10.1371/journal.pone.0151970.
Lim, N., O'Reilly, M. F., Sigafoos, J., Ledbetter-Cho, K., & Lancioni, G. E. (2019). Should heritage languages be incorporated into interventions for bilingual individuals with neurodevelopmental disorders? A systematic review. *Journal of Autism and Developmental Disorders, 49*(3), 887–912.

Lin, S. C., & Yu, S. M. (2015). Disparities in healthcare access and utilization among children with autism spec.

Lindgren, S., Wacker, D., Suess, A., Schieltz, K., Pelzel, K., Kopelman, T., … , & Waldron, D. (2016). Telehealth and autism: Treating challenging behavior at lower cost. *Pediatrics, 137*(Suppl. 2), S167–S175.

Liptak, G. S., Benzoni, L. B., Mruzek, D. W., Nolan, K. W., Thingvoll, M. A., Wade, C. M., et al. (2008). Disparities in diagnosis and access to health services for children with autism: Data from the National Survey of Children's Health. *Journal of Developmental and Behavioral Pediatrics, 29*(3), 152–160.

Lopez, K., Magaña, S., Morales, M., & Iland, E. (2019). Parents Taking Action: Reducing disparities through a culturally informed intervention for Latinx parents of children with autism. *Journal of Ethnic & Cultural Diversity in Social Work, 28*(1), 31–49.

Maciag, M. (2015). Gentrification in America report. Retrieved from https://www.governing.com/gov-data/census/gentrification-in-cities-governing-report.html.

Magiati, I., Tay, X. W., & Howlin, P. (2014). Cognitive, language, social and behavioural outcomes in adults with autism spectrum disorders: a systematic review of longitudinal follow-up studies in adulthood. *Clinical psychology review, 34*(1), 73–86.

Magaña, S., Lopez, K., Aguinaga, A., & Morton, H. (2013). Access to diagnosis and treatment services among latino children with autism spectrum disorders. *Intellectual and Developmental Disabilities, 51*(3), 141–153. https://doi.org/10.1352/1934-9556-51.3.141.

Magaña, S., Lopez, K., & Machalicek, W. (2017). Parents taking action: A psycho-educational intervention for Latino parents of children with autism spectrum disorder. *Family process, 56*(1), 59–74.

Mandell, D. S., Novak, M. M., & Zubritsky, C. D. (2005). Factors associated with age of diagnosis among children with autism spectrum disorders. *Pediatrics, 116*(6), 1480–1486.

Matson, M. L., Mahan, S., & Matson, J. L. (2009). Parent training: A review of methods for children with autism spectrum disorders. *Research in Autism Spectrum Disorders, 3*(4), 868–875.

Marrus, N., Veenstra-VanderWeele, J., Hellings, J. A., Stigler, K. A., Szymanski, L., King, B. H., …, Cook, E. (2014). The American Academy of Child Adolescent Psychiatry (AACAP) Autism and Intellectual Disability Committee. Training of child and adolescent psychiatry fellows in autism and intellectual disability. *Autism, 18*(4), 471–475.

Mazurek, M. O., Brown, R., Curran, A., & Sohl, K. (2017). ECHO autism: A new model for training primary care providers in best-practice care for children with autism. *Clinical Pediatrics, 56*(3), 247–256.

Mazurek, M. O., Curran, A., Burnette, C., & Sohl, K. (2019). ECHO autism STAT: Accelerating early access to autism diagnosis. *Journal of Autism and Developmental Disorders, 49*(1), 127–137.

McConachie, H., & Diggle, T. (2007). Parent implemented early intervention for young children with autism spectrum disorder: A systematic review. *Journal of evaluation in clinical practice, 13*(1), 120–129.

Mirza, M., Krischer, A., Stolley, M., Magaña, S., & Martin, M. (2018). Review of parental activation interventions for parents of children with special health care needs. *Child: Care, Health and Development, 44*(3), 401–42

Moh, T. A., & Magiati, I. (2012). Factors associated with parental stress and satisfaction during the process of diagnosis of children with autism spectrum disorders. *Research in Autism Spectrum Disorders, 6*(1), 293–303.

Montes, G., Halterman, J. S., & Magyar, C. I. (2009). Access to and satisfaction with school and community health services for US children with ASD. *Pediatrics, 124*(Supplement 4), S407–S413.

Moody, E. J., Kaiser, K., Sharp, D., Kubicek, L. F., Rigles, B., Davis, J., … & Rosenberg, C. R. (2019). Improving Family Functioning Following Diagnosis of ASD: A Randomized Trial of a Parent Mentorship Program. *Journal of Child and Family Studies, 28*(2), 424–435.

Murphy, M. A., & Ruble, L. A. (2012). A comparative study of rurality and urbanicity on access to and satisfaction with services for children with autism spectrum disorders. *Rural Special Education Quarterly, 31*(3), 3–11.
Myers S., & Johnson C. (2007). Management of children with autism spectrum disorder. *Pediatrics, 120*(5), 1162e1182.
National Association of School Psychologists Principles for Professional Ethics. (2010). *School Psychology Review, 39*(2), 302–319.
National Research Council (NRC). (2001). *Educating children with Autism.* Washington, DC: National Academic Press.
Norbury, C. F., & Sparks, A. (2013). Difference or disorder? Cultural issues in understanding neurodevelopmental disorders. *Developmental Psychology, 49*(1), 45–58.
OCALI. (n.d). Autism diagnosis education project. Retrieved from https://www.ocali.org/project/adep.
Odom S., Boyd B., & Hall, L. (2010a) Evaluation of comprehensive treatment models for individuals with autism spectrum disorders. *Journal of Autism and Developmental Disorders, 40*(4): 425–436.
Odom, S. L., Collet-Klingenberg, L., Rogers, S. J., & Hatton, D. D. (2010b). Evidence-based practices in interventions for children and youth with autism spectrum disorders. Preventing school failure: *Alternative Education for Children and Youth, 54*(4), 275–282.
Ohta, M., Nagai, Y., & Hara, H. et al. (1987). Parental perception of behavioral symptoms in Japanese autistic children. *Journal of Autism and Developmental Disorders, 17*, 549–563. https://doi.org/10.1007/BF01486970.
Pakenham, K. I., Samios, C., & Sofronoff, K. (2005). Adjustment in mothers of children with Asperger syndrome: An application of the double ABCX model of family adjustment. *Autism, 9*(2), 191–212.
Pachter, L., & Dworkin, P. (1997). Maternal expectations about normal child development in 4 cultural groups. *Archives of Pediatrics and Adolescent Medicine, 151*, 1144–1150.
Pettygrove, S., Pinborough-Zimmerman, J., Meaney, F. J., Van Naarden Braun, K., Nicholas, J., Miller, L., …, Rice, C. (2013). Predictors of ascertainment of autism spectrum disorders across nine US communities. *Journal of Autism and Developmental Disorders, 43*(8), 1867.
Pew Research Center. (2015). *Modern immigration wave brings 59 million to U.S., driving population growth and change through 2065: Views of immigration's impact on U.S. society mixed.* Washington, DC: Pew Research Center. Accessed January 29, 2018. http://www.pewhispanic.org/2015/09/28/modern-immigration-wave-brings-59-million-to-u-s-driving-population-growth-and-change-through-2065.
Project SaLSA, HRSA Grant R40MC27702. (2014). Retrieved from http://www.ucdenver.edu/academics/colleges/medicalschool/programs/JFKPartners/projects/Pages/Project-SaLSA.aspx.
Rambaut, R., & Massey, D. (2013). Immigration and Language Diversity in the United States. *Daedalus, 142*(3), 141–154.
Reyes, N. M., Lindly, O. J., Chavez, A. E., Folan, A., Macias, K., Smith, K. A., Reynolds, A., & Zuckerman, K. (2018). Maternal beliefs about autism: A link between intervention services and autism seve.
Rogers, S. J., & Vismara, L. A. (2008). Evidence-based comprehensive treatments for early autism. *Journal of Clinical Child & Adolescent Psychology, 37*(1), 8–38.
Sanders, J. L., & Morgan, S. B. (1997). Family stress and adjustment as perceived by parents of children with autism or Down syndrome: Implications for intervention. *Child & Family Behavior Therapy, 19*(4), 15–32.
Sansosti, F. J., Lavik, K. B., & Sansosti, J. M. (2012). Family experiences through the autism diagnostic process. *Focus on Autism and Other Developmental Disabilities, 27*(2), 81–92.
Sivberg, B. (2002). Family system and coping behaviors: A comparison between parents of children with autistic spectrum disorders and parents with non-autistic children. *Autism, 6*(4), 397–409.
Schreibman, L., Dawson, G., Stahmer, A. C., Landa, R., Rogers, S. J., McGee, G. G., ... & McNerney, E. (2015). Naturalistic developmental behavioral interventions: Empirically validated treatments for autism spectrum disorder. *Journal of autism and developmental disorders, 45*(8), 2411–2428.

Siller, M., Reyes, N., Hotez, E., Hutman, T., Sigman, M. (2014). Longitudinal change in the use of services in autism spectrum disorder: Understanding the role of child characteristics, family demographics, and parent cognitions. *Autism, 18*(4):433–446. https://doi.org/10.1177/1362361313476766.

Smith, L., Malcolm-Smith, S., & de Vries, P. J. (2017). Translation and cultural appropriateness of the autism diagnostic observation schedule-2 in Afrikaans. *Autism, 21*(5), 552–563.

Soares N., Baum R., & Frick K. (2015). Improving developmental-behavioral pediatric care workflow. *Journal of Developmental & Behavioral Pediatrics, 36(*1), 45e52.

Soto, S., Linas, K., Jacobstein, D., Biel, M., Migdal, T., & Anthony, B. J. (2015). A review of cultural adaptations of screening tools for autism spectrum disorders. *Autism, 19*(6), 646–661.

Stone, W., Coonrod, E., & Turner, L. (2004). Psychometric properties of the STAT for early autism screening. *Journal of Autism and Developmental Disorders, 34,* 691–701.

Strunk, J., Leisen, M., & Schubert, C. (2017). Using a multidisciplinary approach with children diagnosed with autism spectrum disorder. *Journal of Interprofessional Education & Practice, 8,* 60–68.

Sullivan, A. L. (2013). School-based autism identification: Prevalence, racial disparities, and systemic correlates. *School Psychology Review, 42*(3), 298–316.

Thomas, K. C., Ellis, A. R., McLaurin, C., Daniels, J., & Morrissey, J. P. (2007). Access to care for autism-related services. *Journal of Autism and Developmental Disorders, 37*(10), 1902–1912.

Uono, S., & Hietanen, J. K. (2015). Eye contact perception in the west and east: A cross-cultural study. *PLoS ONE, 10*(2), e0118094–e0118094.

U.S. Census Bureau. (2017). New Census Bureau Report Analyzes U.S. Population Projections. Retrieved from https://www.census.gov/newsroom/press-releases/2015/cb15-tps16.html.

Valicenti-McDermott, M., Hottinger, K., Seijo, R., & Shulman, L. (2012). Age at diagnosis of autism spectrum disorders. *The Journal of Pediatrics, 161*(3), 554–556.

Virués-Ortega, J., Arnold-Saritepe, A., Hird, C., Phillips, K. (2017). The TEACCH program for people with Autism: Elements, outcomes, and comparison with competing models. In J. Matson (Ed.), *Handbook of treatments for Autism spectrum disorder. Autism and child psychopathology series*. Switzerland: Springer, Cham.

Vismara, L. A., McCormick, C., Young, G. S., Nadhan, A., & Monlux, K. (2013). Preliminary findings of a telehealth approach to parent training in autism. *Journal of Autism and Developmental Disorders, 43*(12), 2953–2969.

Vohra, R., Madhavan, S., Sambamoorthi, U., & St Peter, C. (2014). Access to services, quality of care, and family impact for children with autism, other developmental disabilities, and other mental health conditions. *Autism, 18*(7), 815–826.

Wilkinson, L. A. (2016). A best practice guide to assessment and intervention for autism spectrum disorder in schools. Jessica Kingsley Publishers.

Williams, K. R., & Wishart, J. G. (2003). The Son-Rise Program 1 intervention for autism: An investigation into family experiences. *Journal of Intellectual Disability Research, 47*(4–5), 291–299.

Wacker, D. P., Lee, J. F., Dalmau, Y. C. P., Kopelman, T. G., Lindgren, S. D., Kuhle, J., … , & Waldron, D. B. (2013). Conducting functional communication training via telehealth to reduce the problem behavior of young children with autism. *Journal of Developmental and Physical Disabilities, 25*(1), 35–48.

Wainer, A. L., Hepburn, S., & McMahon Griffith, E. (2017). Remembering parents in parent-mediated early intervention: An approach to examining impact on parents and families. *Autism, 21*(1), 5–17.

Wang, P., Michaels, C. A., & Day, M. S. (2011). Stresses and coping strategies of Chinese families with children with autism and other developmental disabilities. *Journal of Autism and Developmental Disorders, 41*(6), 783–795.

Wong, C., Odom, S. L., Hume, K. A., Cox, A. W., Fettig, A., Kucharczyk, S., … & Schultz, T. R. (2015). Evidence-based practices for children, youth, and young adults with autism spectrum

disorder: A comprehensive review. *Journal of Autism and Developmental Disorders, 45*(7), 1951–1966.
World Health Organization. (2010). *Framework for action on interprofessional education & collaborative practice*. Retrieved from https://www.who.int/hrh/resources/framework_action/en/.
Zhang, J., Wheeler, J. J., & Richey, D. (2006). Cultural validity is assessment instruments for children with autism from a Chinese cultural perspective. *International Journal of Special Education, 21*, 109–113.
Zuckerman, K. E., Lindly, O. J., Reyes, N. M., Chavez, A. E., Macias, K., Smith, K. N., et al. (2017). Disparities in diagnosis and treatment of autism in Latino and non-Latino white families. *Pediatrics, 139*(5), e20163010.
Zuckerman, K. E., Lindly, O. J., Sinche, B. K., & Nicolaidis, C. (2015). Parent health beliefs, social determinants of health, and child health services utilization among US school-age children with autism. *Journal of Developmental and Behavioral Pediatrics, 36*(3), 146.
Zuckerman, K. E., Sinche, B., Mejia, A., Cobian, M., Becker, T., & Nicolaidis, C. (2014). Latino parents' perspectives on barriers to autism diagnosis. *Academic Pediatrics, 14*(3), 301–308.
Zuckerman, K. E., Lindly, O. J., Reyes, N. M., Chavez, A. E., Cobian, M., Macias, K., ... & Smith, K. A. (2018). Parent perceptions of community autism spectrum disorder stigma: measure validation and associations in a multi-site sample. *Journal of Autism and Developmental Disorders, 48*(9), 3199–3209.

International Perspectives in Coordinated Care for Individuals with ASD

Ashley J. Harrison, Luodi Yu, and John-Joe Dawson-Squibb

Abstract In spite of recent attention and initiatives, international dissemination of ASD services still requires substantial effort to meet the needs of families. Although the importance of interdisciplinary care coordination remains important in moving progress forward, in the global context this may manifest in different ways. Parents currently play more prominent roles to promote improvements in international ASD service provision but coordination with a range of stakeholders at all levels is required for meaningful progress. Currently, providers must engage in creative approaches to ensure that best practices reach families. This occurs through thoughtful adaptation and translation, careful consideration of cross-cultural differences in social behaviors, and attention to the role of culture in the assessment and therapeutic context. To make more impactful strides research is needed in a wide range of areas such as incorporating cross-cultural variability into the assessment process and in the domain of implementation science.

Service provision for individuals with autism spectrum disorder (ASD) faces unique challenges in many international contexts. ASD-specific initiatives have called for the need to (a) understand the etiology of ASD from a global perspective, (b) increase the availability of evidence-based intervention across the lifespan, and (c) increase ASD knowledge and decrease stigma particularly in low- and middle-income countries (LMIC; Khan et al., 2012). To meet these important goals, essential global policy

A. J. Harrison (✉)
Educational Psychology Department, University of Georgia, Athens, GA, USA
e-mail: ashley.harrison@uga.edu

L. Yu
Autism Research Center, School of Psychology, South China Normal University, Guangzhou, China

Department of Speech-Language-Hearing Sciences, University of Minnesota Twin Cities, Minneapolis, MN, USA

J.-J. Dawson-Squibb
Center for Autism Research in Africa, Division of Child and Adolescent Psychiatry, University of Cape Town, Cape Town, South Africa

M. B. McClain et al. (eds.), *Interprofessional Care Coordination for Pediatric Autism Spectrum Disorder*, https://doi.org/10.1007/978-3-030-46295-6_14

changes, increased numbers of trained support personnel across a range of professional disciplines, and greater coordination of care must all occur (Hahler & Elsabbagh, 2015; Khan et al., 2012). Additionally, though only a modest amount of research has examined how culture impacts global ASD service provision (Daley, 2002), this type of science is an essential first step to successfully improving interdisciplinary quality of care for individuals with ASD.

Increasing research shows that a failure to account for known cultural differences in behavior can result in diagnostic and treatment seeking inequities (Harrison, Long, Tommet, & Jones, 2017; Ravindran & Myers, 2012). Thus, considering the role of culture should be at the forefront of efforts to globally disseminate best practices for individuals with ASD and should shape how clinicians adapt interventions and interact with families. Research and clinical efforts have resulted in some international dissemination in domains of ASD screening and surveillance, diagnostic evaluation, and intervention, thus these will be the focus of the current chapter.

The successful efforts to improve ASD quality of care across the international landscape arise from a necessary partnership between stakeholders and providers of all backgrounds. Although coordination of care remains at the forefront of best practices for individuals with ASD, this concept has a different meaning in LMIC, where shortages in medical, psychological, behavioral, and educational providers have been documented in countries around the world such as Tanzania (Manji & Hogan, 2014), Kenya (Ndetei et al., 2007), Nepal (Shrestha & Santangelo, 2014), Ethiopia (Tilahun et al., 2017), and China (Wu Cai Lu Autism Research Institute, 2019). Parents in these resource-low countries play a particularly important role, not only with regard to service coordination for their own child, but also in making gains to increase (a) local ASD research, (b) empirically supported treatments, and (c) positive beliefs and knowledge about ASD (Silverman & Brosco, 2007). One strategy emphasizes that meaningful progress toward improving ASD global care comes from a combination of bottom-up and top-down participation from families, professionals, local leadership, non-government organizations (NGOs), and government agencies (Wallace et al., 2012).

Global Considerations in Screening and Surveillance

Early intervention for individuals with ASD increases opportunities for optimal developmental outcomes (Estes et al., 2015), and is more cost-effective compared to late-start intervention (Koegel, Koegel, Ashbaugh, & Bradshaw, 2014). A prerequisite for early intervention is early identification. Although early identification has been vigorously promoted in high-income Western countries by means involving screening and surveillance systems (Zwaigenbaum et al., 2015), there are still many challenges to overcome globally.

Best Practices in Screening

Timing of early identification: Interracial and international disparities. In the United States (US), it is recommended by the American Academy of Pediatrics (AAP) that young children should be screened for ASD at 18 and 24 months of age (Zwaigenbaum et al., 2015). However, there is not always a seamless transition between initial identification and diagnostic confirmation. Research consistently reports large gaps between initial identification and actual diagnosis (2.7–3.7 years; Shattuck et al., 2009). Significantly, many non-pathological factors were shown to impact the timeliness of early identification, including race/ethnicity, cultural background, and social-economic status. In the US, disparities were found such that Black children with autistic disorder received a diagnosis and entered the mental health system at a later age compared to White peers (Mandell, Listerud, Levy, & Pinto-Martin, 2002). Moreover, having ≥ 4 primary care physicians preceding diagnosis delayed diagnosis by 6 months, which indicates the importance of pediatric care continuity (Mandell, Novak, & Zubritsky, 2005). Overall, reliable and timely early detection rely on the coherence and coordination within and across standardized screening system and specialized care provision (see also, chapter "Screening and Surveillance").

The same concern may apply to countries/regions, where ASD prevalence estimates have been historically lower compared to Western developed countries (Elsabbagh et al., 2012). Unfortunately, it is virtually impossible to report the timing of early identification of ASD in most non-Western developing countries/regions due to the scarcity of reliable population-based surveillance. Nonetheless, lower prevalence estimates and tendency of late diagnosis in these countries have been documented (Onaolapo & Onaolapo, 2017), which are often associated with limited service availability (Pang et al., 2018). Also, standardized primary care developmental screening for ASD is limited to nonexistent in many lower income countries/regions, for instance, Pakistan (Imran & Azeem, 2014), Nepal (Shrestha & Santangelo, 2014), China (Huang, Jia, & Wheeler, 2013), and sub-Saharan Africa (Chambers et al., 2017).

Different roles of distinct providers in conducting screenings. There are often shortages of health facilities and personnel in lower income and/or remote areas (Huang et al., 2013; Janvier et al., 2016; Oro, Esmer, & Navarro-Calvillo, 2014). Ideally, each toddler should be screened for ASD and developmental delays at routine pediatric checkup following AAP recommendations; however, this model is infeasible in many countries (Huang et al., 2013; van de Vijver & Tanzer, 2004). Integrating screening into routine primary health care is an important target for expanding care access (Collins et al., 2011). One potential solution is to have other service providers participate in various forms of developmental surveillance in community settings. In Australia, health nurses were trained to identify behavioral red flags of ASD in infants as part of a developmental surveillance system. This approach capacitated the community to accurately identify ASD as early as 12 months (Barbaro & Dissanayake, 2010). Janvier et al. (2016) explored the feasibility of early screening administered by childcare providers in underserved communities and demonstrated promising results. Finally, community health care workers providing decentralized mental health care in Ethiopia have begun receiving ASD screening training to help with broader identification (Tilahun et al., 2017). These models and those in chapter "Developmental Screening in Community-Based Settings" provide examples for innovative approaches for increasing early detection.

Cross-culturally adapted measures. Second only to the timing of screening, the method of screening is of great importance, and a range of empirically supported early screening instruments exist (Dumont-Mathieu & Fein, 2005). Given that most early identification instruments were developed under Western cultures in English speaking countries, it is important to keep in mind potential biases in behavior sampling and cross-cultural validity of these instruments (Norbury & Sparks, 2013). One widely used ASD-specific screening tool is the Modified Checklist for Autism in Toddlers (M-CHAT; Robins, Fein, Barton, & Green, 2001). This measure has demonstrated high sensitivity and specificity for the early identification of young children with ASD (Robins et al., 2014; Robins et al., 2001).

The M-CHAT has been translated to multiple languages. However, lower positive predictive value (PPV) has been observed in Spain, Japan, and Sri Lanka (Canal-Bedia et al., 2011; Inada, Koyama, Inokuchi, Kuroda, & Kamio, 2011; Perera, Wijewardena, & Aluthwelage, 2009). These differences might reflect comparably lower prevalence in the distinct or be indicative that the M-CHAT was simply not adequate in describing ASD-specific behaviors of unique cultural contexts. A Chinese study demonstrated adding a short observation checklist significantly improved sensitivity, specificity, and PPV (Wong et al., 2004). The above studies suggest that when applying a measure internationally, caution should be taken regarding the cross-cultural validity in its description of ASD-specific behaviors.

Best Practices for Cultural Adaptation and Validation

Developing a novel, high-quality assessment requires abundant expertise and labor. Using culturally adapted measures is often much easier for many researchers and practitioners but is also time intensive. Readying an instrument for use in a new cultural contexts often begins with translation, for which specific considerations should be taken: (1) using simple sentences; (2) avoiding pronouns; (3) avoiding metaphors; (4) avoiding passive tense; (5) avoiding hypothetical phrasing (Werner & Campbell, 1970). Bracken and Barona (1991) recommended a combination of adaptation and translation in alignment with the following steps: (1) Translation from original to target language by a bilingual who is sufficiently knowledgeable; (2) blind back-translation and a repetition of this step if necessary; (3) Bilingual review committee to minimize cultural and linguistic inappropriateness; (4) pilot testing; (5) field testing; (6) norm development; (7) cross-cultural validation examining psychometric properties. It is important to note that the function of back-translation is to check semantic equivalence between the original and translated measures, thus it should only be done after a thorough scrutiny of the translation by experts and target population (Borsa, Damásio, & Bandeira, 2012).

Other Cultural Variables: Knowledge and Stigma

Culture influences how people accept and view disabilities such as ASD (Ravindran & Myers, 2012). For instance, a survey discovered that in China 53–69% of people conceptualized autistic children as intellectually disabled and extremely impaired, whereas in the US only 13–21% of people did so (Yu, Stronach, & Harrison, Submitted). Negative perceptions of ASD or ASD stigma can greatly impact early identification efforts. High proportions of Ethiopia parents of autistic children experienced stigma (45.1%) and tried to hide the condition of their child (Tilahun et al., 2016). In South Korea, a study showed that parents were afraid of disclosing the needs of their autistic child due to fear of losing educational opportunities (Grinker et al., 2012).

In many instances stigma derives from low levels of ASD knowledge. For example, stigma often accompanies beliefs of the spiritual causation of ASD in many African countries that exemplify low ASD resource regions. Historically there has been a lack of access to knowledge and training for professionals and caregivers (Ruparelia et al., 2016). In settings where screening and surveillance systems are yet to be established, detection of ASD usually depends on the sensitivity of caregivers and other stakeholders at the community level who may delay diagnosis due to reasonable concerns about stigmatization. Thus, it is important for researchers and care providers to be aware of the cultural variables that can hinder early ASD screening efforts, as well as later diagnosis and treatment seeking. At the community level, public education campaigns in LMIC are needed to reduce misunderstanding and stigma. At the institutional level, coordinated effort should be made to establish the infrastructure for early screening and referral systems and to promote their importance (Ruparelia et al., 2016).

Diagnostic Evaluation in the International Context

Similar to ASD early screening, several meaningful issues arise when applying diagnostic classification approaches developed in high-income, Western countries to other global contexts. Individuals across a range of disciplines must consider how to adapt ASD evaluations, while maintaining important psychometric rigor. Additionally, given the social nature of ASD symptoms, careful attention must be paid to how symptom presentation may vary across cultural and linguistic contexts (see chapter "Clinical and School Identification and Intervention for Youth with ASD: Culturally and Linguistically Responsive Interdisciplinary Considerations"). Importantly, the evolution of the ASD diagnostic criteria over time and the variability between diagnostic classification systems impacts the process of conducting ASD diagnostic evaluations across the international canvas.

Global Perspectives in ASD Diagnostic Criteria

Global Diagnostic Classification Systems. ASD criteria vary depending on adherence to the US classification system, the Diagnostic and Statistical Manual (DSM-5; American Psychiatric Association, 2013), or the more internationally used criteria published by the World Health Organization, the International Classification of Diseases: tenth revision, 2nd edition (ICD-10; World Health Organization, 2004). The more recent publication of the DSM-5 resulted in noteworthy changes to the ASD diagnostic criteria, which results in a lack of synchronization with ICD-10 (Doernberg & Hollander, 2016). These differences impact how countries report health statistics, healthcare processes (i.e., insurance billing codes), and clinical diagnostic procedures, thus resulting in different diagnostic profiles (Clark, Cuthbert, Lewis-Fernández, Narrow, & Reed, 2017). Although the DSM-5 changes represent important evidence-based forward progress in many domains, cultural considerations were not necessarily at the forefront of the ASD criteria revision (Clark et al., 2017), which can introduce bias in the diagnostic process from the outset.

ASD Diagnostic Evaluation Best Practices. ASD diagnostic evaluation is a complex process comprised of multiple components, and often most effective from the perspective of an interdisciplinary team involving both parents and professionals (Prelock, Beatson, Bitner, Broder, & Ducker, 2003). A core ASD diagnostic assessment battery includes both an observation-based ASD diagnostic instrument and ASD-specific parent interviews and questionnaires to evaluate for the presence of the ASD symptoms (Ozonoff, Goodlin-Jones, & Solomon, 2005). Measures of cognition, language, and adaptive functioning provide additional essential information for evaluating the dimensional level of clinical impairment. Additional domains of frequent impairment in ASD that may also require evaluation include neuropsychology, attention, executive functioning, academic achievement, and psychiatric comorbidities (Ozonoff et al., 2005). Implementation of the core battery might necessitate multiple providers with distinct training, but an evaluation of additional domains would inevitably require the expertise of an interdisciplinary team.

Unfortunately, in many parts of the world, great challenges exist trying to identify one professional with ASD expertise let alone multiple providers to serve on an interdisciplinary evaluation team. Parents from LMIC report challenges with identifying multidisciplinary ASD specialist teams and finding sufficient ASD services (e.g., Divan, Vajaratkar, Desai, Strik-Lievers, & Patel, 2012; Shrestha & Santangelo, 2014). A general shortage of ASD specialists in LMIC has a clear foundation in the literature (Manji & Hogan, 2014; Ndetei et al., 2007).

Cross-Cultural Variability in ASD Diagnosis

Sociocultural variability in behavior. Different cultures promote different norms in social behavior. Thus, considering the sociocultural context is particularly important in identifying a disorder, such as ASD, with social impairment at the core. Differences arise in a myriad of behaviors included as core aspects of the ASD differential diagnostic picture, such as eye contact, pragmatic language, emotion expression and recognition, and nonverbal communication. These differences result in part, because young children from different culture groups use distinct cultural and linguistic norms to guide their social communicative actions and perceptions (Tomasello, Kruger, & Ratner, 1993).

More specifically, different cultures have specific norms for when and how to engage in eye contact and other nonverbal communication (Collett, 1971; Knapp, Hall, & Horgan, 2013). Known cultural differences in emotion recognition also exist (Elfenbein, 2013; Elfenbein, Beaupré, Lévesque, & Hess, 2007). This may be attributable to attentional face processing differences or differences in aligning facial cues with basic emotions (Jack, Garrod, Yu, Caldara, & Schyns, 2012). Finally, many aspects of language, particularly pragmatic language, have known cultural variations (Carter et al., 2005).

Cultural Biases in ASD Diagnostic Instruments. Despite the documentation of these differences, little research has quantified sociocultural differences in young children in a way that can be meaningfully applied to assessment development. This poses a particular problem for ASD diagnostic tools often reliant on directly observing behavior to diagnose ASD and comparing it to operational definitions of typical and atypical behavior. Unfortunately, as is common in the field, much of the research to develop ASD diagnostic instruments and collect normative data has relied primarily on samples comprised of White, Western males that represent one, narrow sociocultural group (Hilton et al., 2010). This narrow definition of typical behavior can result in important measurement biases in widely used ASD diagnostic instruments (Harrison et al., 2017) and thus, a tendency to over pathologize behaviors that may simply reflect different cultural norms (Norbury & Sparks, 2013). As such, the field should prioritize research from a range of disciplines that helps to better understand the nature of sociocultural differences and how to account for this variability in instrument development and adaptation.

Cultural Biases in the Diagnostic Context. Meaningful bias can also occur in the interactive evaluation context. In the US, contributing to diagnostic timing disparities, Black children have a higher likelihood of receiving an incorrect initial diagnosis of Attention Deficit/Hyperactivity Disorder (ADHD) or conduct disorder rather than ASD (Mandell, Ittenbach, Levy, & Pinto-Martin, 2007). This pattern of misdiagnosis may reflect implicit clinician biases resulting in a tendency to assume behavior is the result of externalizing behavior disorders rather than ASD. In addition to ethnic minority disparities, females with autistic symptoms often do not receive a diagnosis due to a clinician's tendency to narrowly view the presentation of ASD

(Kirkovski, Enticott, & Fitzgerald, 2013). Caregiver perception of behavior and personal values have cultural underpinnings that can also impact the diagnostic process in how readily parents endorse problems (e.g., Matson et al., 2017). Mandell et al. (2009) reported that lower maternal education decreased the odds of documented ASD. Promoting increased awareness of how cultural differences impact the diagnostic process among clinicians can help buffer biased interactions (Ennis-Cole, Durodoye, & Harris, 2013).

Global Dissemination of ASD Interventions

The term intervention in relation to ASD includes a broad range of approaches including child-based approaches, parent-focused interventions or sometimes a combination. There is growing evidence supporting a range of ASD-specific interventions, which highlights the importance of coordinated care (Bearss, Burrell, Stewart, & Scahill, 2015). We will examine global issues related to: (a) Cultural Considerations in Implementation, (b) Cross-Cultural Adaptation of interventions, and (c) Parent-Based Interventions.

Cultural Considerations in Intervention Implementation

Implementation science is increasingly gaining attention as researchers seek to better understand the barriers and facilitators that enable evidence-based interventions to be effectively provided in multiple and diverse settings (Schlebusch et al., in press; Stahmer, Dababnah, & Rieth, 2019). Implementation science is a method of enquiry designed to support investigators in determining whether interventions or approaches have utility in real-world settings (Damschroder et al., 2009). The evidence for the majority of ASD interventions results from research conducted in high-income countries despite the majority of those with ASD living in LMIC (Franz, Chambers, von Isenburg, & de Vries, 2017). The significant treatment gap that exists in most LMIC countries necessitates an increased focus on how best to implement, adapt, and disseminate evidence-based treatments in settings that are different to those for which they were originally intended (Damschroder et al., 2009).

The impact of culture on ASD treatment-seeking. An array of research has highlighted that diverse cultural groups have differing perspectives on the etiology of ASD (Ennis-Cole et al., 2013; Hebert & Koulouglioti, 2010). The etiological understanding of ASD will inevitably inform beliefs about treatment. For example, some minority parents may regard problems with social skills or language delays as a temporary phenomenon that will be outgrown (Danseco, 1997) and some Latino mothers have reportedly viewed ASD as a gift from God that enables them to serve others (Wilder, Dyches, Obiakor, & Algozzine, 2004). With such beliefs, parents may not seek treatment. Differences also exist in thresholds for treatment seeking.

For example, Asian Americans are reportedly less likely to seek professional help until they are unable to manage (Dyches, Wilder, Sudweeks, Obiakor, & Algozzine, 2004).

In addition to the difference in initial treatment seeking behaviors, individuals from different cultural groups may seek treatment from different types and combinations of sources (Sue & Sue, 2008). For example, African Americans tend to first seek aid from personal connections and Latino Americans may work with folk healers instead of medical professionals. Given the number of cultural groupings worldwide, significantly more research is required in this area to understand variability in culturally linked treatment seeking behaviors (Ennis-Cole et al., 2013).

Cultural Considerations for ASD Providers. If therapists and educators are to work effectively with caregivers and parents from culturally diverse and nondominant cultures an understanding of the impact of culture on their communication and learning is needed (Trembath, Balandin, & Rossi, 2005). Both patient and provider cultural impact the course of treatment. Thus, professionals working with individuals with ASD should employ approaches that creatively meet the needs of the culturally diverse groupings they serve through increased personal awareness, cultural knowledge, and flexible use of skills (Ennis-Cole et al., 2013).

Culturally Appropriate ASD Intervention Implementation Approaches

Cross-cultural adaptation of clinician-based interventions. Given the significant treatment gaps described previously in the majority of LMIC, the consideration of cross-cultural adaptation of clinician-based interventions is increasingly regarded as a priority (Chambers & Norton, 2016; Schlebusch, in press). More than 200 members of the International Society for Autism Research (INSAR) helped to identify ASD research priorities and knowledge gaps (Vivanti et al., 2018). Of the six key issues raised, five are pertinent to cross-cultural adaptation and highlight the need for increased awareness of implementation and cultural diversity in this area of research. The relevant key issues summarized include: (a) a focus on the feasibility of treatment procedures and alignment with stakeholder values, (b) research designs that compare different interventions and formats, (c) use of community-partnered participatory research to guide adaptation, (d) inclusion of implementation constructs in treatment trials, and (e) an iterative approach to the progression of knowledge from intervention development to implementation.

Cultural adaptations can be required when the target audience is different from that of the original intervention or program (Schlebusch et al., in press). The aim of any adaptation, including clinician-based, is to improve the effectiveness of the intervention by ensuring accessibility, feasibility, and acceptability for the cultural group though still maintaining fidelity (Chambers & Norton, 2016; Schlebusch et al., in press).

A good example of identifying stakeholder perspectives, feasibility, adaptation, and implementation in adaptation is the research on the parent perceptions of a parent-implemented Naturalistic Developmental Behavioral Intervention (NBDI; Stahmer et al., 2019). While NDBI have been shown to have positive effects, effectiveness in community settings has had little examination (Kasari et al., 2014). After following 13 families as they received training in a specific NDBI, one study concluded that such a training by community providers is feasible and well received, and explored adaptation of specific elements of the program based on participant feedback (Stahmer et al., 2017). Although this study is limited by a small sample, it provides an important example of how research investigating stakeholders' perspectives leads to program adaptation and can facilitate successful implementation in different communities or cultures.

Emphasizing the Use of Parent/Caregiver-based Interventions. Developing effective treatments that can be used by nonspecialists is regarded among the top research priorities for improving the lives of those with intellectual disabilities and lower functioning ASD (Reichow, Servili, Yasamy, Barbui, & Saxena, 2013). Research supports the efficacy of delivery by nonspecialist providers and the importance of such approaches given the previously mentioned scarcity of specialists in LMIC. There is an increasing focus on empowering parents to provide and engage in a range of intervention approaches (Irwin, Siddiqi, & Hertzman, 2007; Kasari et al., 2014; Nevill, Lecavalier, & Stratis, 2016).

Bearss et al. (2015) provide a useful taxonomy to distinguish between the myriad of ASD interventions and training involving parents/caregivers. The framework outlines a distinction between "Parent Support" programs, "Parent/Caregiver-Mediated Interventions", as well as interventions with a component of both known as Parent Education & Training (PET; Dawson-Squibb & de Vries, 2019). A recent scoping review of PET interventions outside of the US identified a highly diverse range of programs from 20 countries and all continents except South America (Dawson-Squibb et al., 2019). This review highlighted the diversity and range of programs that are delivered around the globe, but also revealed the need for methodological quality improvements due to a failure to consider implementation factors and a lack of research focus on cultural factors. This gap is an important barrier to these needed interventions being successfully disseminated in culturally diverse settings.

Cultural Adaptation and Translation of Outreach Materials on Autism Spectrum Disorder. Adaptation of interventions to ensure their acceptability and accessibility is required in different cultural settings (Bernal & Rodriguez, 2012) and should align with previously discussed published translation and adaptation standards (e.g., Bracken & Barona, 1991). This process for interventions may require even greater time and input from a diverse group of stakeholders. Grinker et al. (2015) provide a useful illustration of the cultural adaptation through qualitative methods and translation of a US parent intervention (Autism Speaks First 100 days kit) into another language (Korean). The importance of cultural consensus modeling was determined as necessary and provided information about barriers to care. This emphasizes the importance of including relevant stakeholders when considering cultural adaptations, ensures the prioritization of intervention acceptability, and provides a clear conceptual model and methodology for adapting programs to make them culturally acceptable.

Final Overview

In line with the World Health Organization (2013) report, international ASD service provision progress requires substantial attention, particularly in LMIC. Improving global ASD assessment and intervention remains a key focus for researchers, policy-makers, clinicians, educators, and families and must occur through coordinated efforts. To inform progress, research needs to focus on diverse, international samples to more clearly delineate cultural differences in ASD beliefs and stigmas, sociocultural variability in symptom domains, and treatment attitudes. A failure to understand these culture differences and how they impact the diagnostic assessment process and treatment-seeking can result in diagnostic inaccuracies and delays in essential early treatment. Efforts to ensure an awareness of how culture impacts on the uptake of assessments and interventions, and how best they should be adapted for diverse cultures and communities should be considered a priority. This complex area requires the attention of relevant stakeholders from a range of disciplines to come up with creative ways to meet the significant needs of many underserved and marginalized communities and is critical to the successful implementation of empirically supported services. Cultural factors should be considered from the early development of assessments and interventions, and cross-cultural transadaptation should be done in conjunction with stakeholders who can ensure it is accessible and acceptable. This process of engagement and finding ways to creatively meet the needs of communities should be considered an ongoing process that engages individuals involved in all levels of ASD care. Wider implementation of models like the Global Autism Public Health initiative that focuses on the engagement of a wide range of stakeholders to most effectively promote change aligns with this goal (Wallace et al., 2012). Similarly, work to establish universally cross-culturally applicable assessment and intervention approaches like World Health Organization recent progress developing a parent training approach is an important step forward (Hamdani et al., 2017).

References

American Psychiatric Association. (2013). *Diagnostic and statistical manual of mental health disorders* (5th ed.). Washington, DC: American Psychiatric Association Publishing.

Barbaro, J., & Dissanayake, C. (2010). Prospective Identification of Autism spectrum disorders in infancy and toddlerhood using developmental surveillance: The social attention and communication study. *Journal of Developmental and Behavioral Pediatrics, 31,* 376–385.

Bearss, K., Burrell, T. L., Stewart, L., & Scahill, L. (2015). Parent training in autism spectrum disorder: What's in a name? *Clinical Child and Family Psychology Review, 18,* 170–182.

Bernal, G. E., & Rodriguez, M. M. D. (2012). *Cultural adaptations: Tools for Evidence-Based Practice with Diverse Populations*. Washington, DC.

Borsa, J. C., Damásio, B. F., & Bandeira, D. R. (2012). Adaptação e validação de instrumentos psicológicos entre culturas: algumas considerações. *Paidéia (Ribeirão Preto), 22,* 423–432.

Bracken, B. A., & Barona, A. (1991). State of the art procedures for translating, validating and using psychoeducational tests in cross-cultural assessment. *School Psychology International, 12,* 119–132.

Canal-Bedia, R., García-Primo, P., Martín-Cilleros, M. V., Santos-Borbujo, J., Guisuraga-Fernández, Z., Herráez-García, L., et al. (2011). Modified checklist for Autism in toddlers: Cross-cultural adaptation and validation in Spain. *Journal of Autism and Developmental Disorders, 41,* 1342–1351.

Carter, J. A., Lees, J. A., Murira, G. M., Gona, J., Neville, B. G., & Newton, C. R. (2005). Issues in the development of cross-cultural assessments of speech and language for children. *International Journal of Language & Communication Disorders, 40,* 385–401.

Chambers, D. A., & Norton, W. E. (2016). The adaptome: Advancing the science of intervention adaptation. *American Journal of Preventive Medicine, 51,* S124–S131.

Chambers, N. J., Wetherby, A. M., Stronach, S. T., Njongwe, N., Kauchali, S., & Grinker, R. R. (2017). Early detection of autism spectrum disorder in young isiZulu-speaking children in South Africa. *Autism, 21,* 518–526.

Clark, L. A., Cuthbert, B., Lewis-Fernández, R., Narrow, W. E., & Reed, G. M. (2017). Three approaches to understanding and classifying mental disorder: ICD-11, DSM-5, and the national institute of mental health's research domain criteria (RDoC). *Psychological Science in the Public Interest, 18,* 72–145.

Collett, P. (1971). Training englishmen in the non-verbal behaviour of Arabs. *International Journal of Psychology, 6,* 209–215.

Collins, P. Y., Patel, V., Joestl, S. S., March, D., Insel, T. R., Daar, A. S., et al. (2011). Grand challenges in global mental health. *Nature, 475,* 27–30.

Daley, T. C. (2002). The need for cross-cultural_research on the pervasive developmental disorders. *Transcultural Psychiatry, 39,* 531–550.

Damschroder, L. J., Aron, D. C., Keith, R. E., Kirsh, S. R., Alexander, J. A., & Lowery, J. C. (2009). Fostering implementation of health services research findings into practice: A consolidated framework for advancing implementation science. *Implementation Science, 4,* 50.

Danseco, E. R. (1997). Parental beliefs on childhood disability: Insights on culture, child development and intervention. *International Journal of Disability, Development and Education, 44,* 41–52.

Dawson-Squibb, J.-J., & de Vries, P. J. (2019). Developing an evaluation framework for parent education and training in Autism Spectrum Disorder: Results of a multi-stakeholder process. *Journal of Autism and Developmental Disorders, 49,* 4468–4481.

Divan, G., Vajaratkar, V., Desai, M. U., Strik-Lievers, L., & Patel, V. (2012). Challenges, coping strategies, and unmet needs of families with a child with Autism spectrum disorder in Goa, India. *Autism Research, 5*(3), 190–200.

Doernberg, E., & Hollander, E. (2016). Neurodevelopmental disorders (ASD and ADHD): DSM-5, ICD-10, and ICD-11. *CNS Spectrums, 21*(4), 295–299.

Dumont-Mathieu, T., & Fein, D. (2005). Screening for autism in young children: The modified checklist for Autism in toddlers (M-CHAT) and other measures. *Mental Retardation and Developmental Disabililies Research Reviews, 11*(3), 253–262.

Dyches, T. T., Wilder, L. K., Sudweeks, R. R., Obiakor, F. E., & Algozzine, B. (2004). Multicultural issues in Autism. *Journal of Autism and Developmental Disorders, 34,* 211–222.

Elfenbein, H. A. (2013). Nonverbal dialects and accents in facial expressions of emotion. *Emotion Review, 5,* 90–96.

Elfenbein, H. A., Beaupré, M., Lévesque, M., & Hess, U. (2007). Toward a dialect theory: Cultural differences in the expression and recognition of posed facial expressions. *Emotion, 7,* 131.

Elsabbagh, M., Divan, G., Koh, Y. J., Kim, Y. S., Kauchali, S., Marcín, C., et al. (2012). Global prevalence of autism and other pervasive developmental disorders. *Autism Research, 5,* 160–179.
Ennis-Cole, D., Durodoye, B. A., & Harris, H. L. (2013). The impact of culture on Autism diagnosis and treatment: Considerations for counselors and other professionals. *The Family Journal, 21,* 279–287.
Estes, A., Munson, J., Rogers, S. J., Greenson, J., Winter, J., & Dawson, G. (2015). Long-term outcomes of early intervention in 6-year-old children with Autism spectrum disorder. *Journal of the American Academy of Child and Adolescent Psychiatry, 54,* 580–587.
Franz, L., Chambers, N., von Isenburg, M., & de Vries, P. J. (2017). Autism spectrum disorder in sub-saharan africa: A comprehensive scoping review. *Autism Research, 10,* 723–749.
Grinker, R. R., Chambers, N., Njongwe, N., Lagman, A. E., Guthrie, W., Stronach, S., et al. (2012). "Communities" in community engagement: Lessons learned from Autism research in South Korea and South Africa. *Autism Res, 5,* 201–210.
Grinker, R. R., Kang-Yi, C. D., Ahmann, C., Beidas, R. S., Lagman, A., & Mandell, D. S. (2015). Cultural adaptation and translation of outreach materials on Autism spectrum disorder. *Journal of Autism and Developmental Disorders, 45,* 2329–2336.
Hahler, E.-M., & Elsabbagh, M. (2015). Autism: A global perspective. *Current Developmental Disorders Reports, 2,* 58–64.
Hamdani, S. U., Akhtar, P., Zill-e-Huma, U., Nazir, H., Minhas, F. A., Sikander, S., ... Rahman, A. (2017). WHO Parents Skills Training (PST) programme for children with developmental disorders and delays delivered by Family Volunteers in rural Pakistan: study protocol for effectiveness implementation hybrid cluster randomized controlled trial. *Global Mental Health, 4,* e11.
Harrison, A. J., Long, K. A., Tommet, D. C., & Jones, R. N. (2017). Examining the role of race, ethnicity, and gender on social and behavioral ratings within the Autism diagnostic observation schedule. *Journal of Autism and Developmental Disorders, 47,* 2770–2782.
Hebert, E. B., & Koulouglioti, C. (2010). Parental beliefs about cause and course of their child's Autism and outcomes of their beliefs: A review of the literature. *Issues in Comprehensive Pediatric Nursing, 33,* 149–163.
Hilton, C. L., Fitzgerald, R. T., Jackson, K. M., Maxim, R. A., Bosworth, C. C., Shattuck, P. T., et al. (2010). Brief report: Under-representation of African Americans in autism genetic research: A rationale for inclusion of subjects representing diverse family structures. *Journal of Autism and Developmental Disorders, 40,* 633–639.
Huang, A. X., Jia, M., & Wheeler, J. J. (2013). Children with Autism in the people's Republic of China: Diagnosis, legal issues, and educational services. *Journal of Autism and Developmental Disorders, 43,* 1991–2001.
Imran, N., & Azeem, M. W. (2014). Autism spectrum disorders: Perspective from Pakistan. In V. Patel, V. Preedy, & C. Martin (Eds.), *Comprehensive guide to Autism* (pp. 2483–2496). New York, NY: Springer.
Inada, N., Koyama, T., Inokuchi, E., Kuroda, M., & Kamio, Y. (2011). Reliability and validity of the Japanese version of the modified checklist for autism in toddlers (M-CHAT). *Research in Autism Spectrum Disorders, 5,* 330–336.
Irwin, L. G., Siddiqi, A., & Hertzman, C. (2007). *Early child development: A powerful equalizer.* Switzerland: Retrieved from Geneva.
Jack, R. E., Garrod, O. G., Yu, H., Caldara, R., & Schyns, P. G. (2012). Facial expressions of emotion are not culturally universal. *Proceedings of the National Academy of Sciences, 109,* 7241–7244.
Janvier, Y. M., Harris, J. F., Coffield, C. N., Louis, B., Xie, M., Cidav, Z., & Mandell, D. S. (2016). Screening for autism spectrum disorder in underserved communities: Early childcare providers as reporters. Autism: Advance online publication.
Kasari, C., Lawton, K., Shih, W., Barker, T. V., Landa, R., Lord, C., et al. (2014). Caregiver-mediated intervention for low-resourced preschoolers with Autism: An RCT. *Pediatrics, 134,* e72.
Khan, N. Z., Gallo, L. A., Arghir, A., Budisteanu, B., Budisteanu, M., Dobrescu, I., et al. (2012). Autism and the grand challenges in global mental health. *Autism Res, 5,* 156–159.

Kirkovski, M., Enticott, P. G., & Fitzgerald, P. B. (2013). A review of the role of female gender in autism spectrum disorders. *Journal of Autism and Developmental Disorders, 43,* 2584–2603.

Knapp, M. L., Hall, J. A., & Horgan, T. G. (2013). *Nonverbal communication in human interaction.* Boston, MA: Wadsworth Cengage Learning.

Koegel, L. K., Koegel, R. L., Ashbaugh, K., & Bradshaw, J. (2014). The importance of early identification and intervention for children with or at risk for autism spectrum disorders. *International Journal of Speech-Language Pathology, 16,* 50–56.

Mandell, D. S., Listerud, J., Levy, S. E., & Pinto-Martin, J. A. (2002). Race differences in the age at diagnosis among Medicaid-eligible children with autism. *Journal of the American Academy of Child & Adolescent Psychiatry, 41*(12), 1447–1453. https://doi.org/10.1097/01.CHI.0000024863.60748.53.

Mandell, D. S., Ittenbach, R. F., Levy, S. E., & Pinto-Martin, J. A. (2007). Disparities in diagnoses received prior to a diagnosis of Autism spectrum disorder. *Journal of Autism and Developmental Disorders, 37,* 1795–1802.

Mandell, D. S., Novak, M. M., & Zubritsky, C. D. (2005). Factors associated with age of diagnosis among children with Autism spectrum disorders. *Pediatrics, 116,* 1480.

Mandell, D. S., Wiggins, L. D., Carpenter, L. A., Daniels, J., DiGuiseppi, C., Durkin, M. S., et al. (2009). Racial/ethnic disparities in the identification of children with autism spectrum disorders. *American Journal of Public Health, 99,* 493.

Manji, K. P., & Hogan, M. N. (2014). Identifying gaps in knowledge, prevalence and care of children with autism spectrum disoders in Tanzania—A qualitative review article. *Tanzania Medical Journal, 26,* 7–17.

Matson, J. L., Matheis, M., Burns, C., Esposito, G., Venuti, P., Pisula, E., et al. (2017). Examining cross-cultural differences in autism spectrum disorder: A multinational comparison from Greece, Italy, Japan, Poland, and the United States. *European Psychiatry, 42,* 70–76.

Ndetei, D., Ongetcha, F., Mutiso, V., Kuria, M., Khasakhala, L., & Kokonya, D. (2007). The challenges of human resources in mental health in Kenya. *African Journal of Psychiatry, 10,* 33–36.

Nevill, R. E., Lecavalier, L., & Stratis, E. A. (2016). Meta-analysis of parent-mediated interventions for young children with autism spectrum disorder. *Autism, 22,* 84–98.

Norbury, C. F., & Sparks, A. (2013). Difference or disorder? Cultural issues in understanding neurodevelopmental disorders. *Developmental Psychology, 49,* 45.

Onaolapo, A. Y., & Onaolapo, O. J. (2017). Global data on Autism spectrum disorders prevalence: a review of facts, fallacies and limitations. *Universal Journal of Clinical Medicine, 5,* 14–23.

Organization, W. H. (2013). *Autism spectrum disorders and other developmental disorders: From raising awareness to building capacity.* Retrieved from Geneva.

Oro, A. B., Esmer, C., & Navarro-Calvillo, M. E. (2014). Autism spectrum disorders in Mexico. In V. Patel, V. Preedy, & C. Martin (Eds.), *Comprehensive guide to Autism* (pp. 2469–2482). New York, NY: Springer.

Ozonoff, S., Goodlin-Jones, B. L., & Solomon, M. (2005). Evidence-based assessment of autism spectrum disorders in children and adolescents. *Journal of Clinical Child and Adolescent Psychology, 34,* 523–540.

Pang, Y., Lee, C. M., Wright, M., Shen, J., Shen, B., & Bo, J. (2018). Challenges of case identification and diagnosis of Autism spectrum disorders in China: A critical review of procedures, assessment, and diagnostic criteria. *Research in Autism Spectrum Disorders, 53,* 53–66.

Perera, H., Wijewardena, K., & Aluthwelage, R. (2009). Screening of 18–24-month-old children for Autism in a semi-urban community in Sri Lanka. *Journal of Tropical Pediatrics, 55,* 402–405.

Prelock, P. A., Beatson, J., Bitner, B., Broder, C., & Ducker, A. (2003). Interdisciplinary assessment of young children with Autism spectrum disorder. *Language, Speech, and Hearing Services in Schools, 34,* 194–202.

Ravindran, N., & Myers, B. J. (2012). Cultural influences on perceptions of health, illness, and disability: A review and focus on Autism. *Journal of Child and Family Studies, 21,* 311–319.

Reichow, B., Servili, C., Yasamy, M. T., Barbui, C., & Saxena, S. (2013). Non-specialist psychosocial interventions for children and adolescents with intellectual disability or lower-functioning Autism spectrum disorders: A systematic review. *PLOS Medicine, 10,* e1001572.
Robins, D. L., Casagrande, K., Barton, M., Chen, C.-M. A., Dumont-Mathieu, T., & Fein, D. (2014). Validation of the modified checklist for Autism in toddlers, revised with follow-up (M-CHAT-R/F). *Pediatrics, 133,* 37.
Robins, D. L., Fein, D., Barton, M. L., & Green, J. A. (2001). The modified checklist for Autism in toddlers: An initial study investigating the early detection of autism and pervasive developmental disorders. *Journal of Autism and Developmental Disorders, 31,* 131–144.
Ruparelia, K., Abubakar, A., Badoe, E., Bakare, M., Visser, K., Chugani, D. C., et al. (2016). Autism spectrum disorders in Africa: Current challenges in identification, assessment, and treatment: A report on the international child neurology association meeting on ASD in Africa, Ghana. *Journal of Child Neurology, 31,* 1018–1026.
Schlebusch, L., Chambers, N., Dawson-Squibb, J. J., Harty, M., Franz, L., & de Vries, P. J. (in press). Challenges and opportunities of implementing early interventions for autism spectrum disorders in resource-limited settings: A South African example. In M. Hodes, S. Shur-Fen Gau, & P. de Vries (Eds.), *In Starting at the beginning: Laying the Foundation for lifelong mental health.*
Shattuck, P. T., Durkin, M., Maenner, M., Newschaffer, C., Mandell, D. S., Wiggins, L., et al. (2009). The timing of identification among children with an Autism spectrum disorder: Findings from a population-based surveillance study. *Journal of the American Academy of Child and Adolescent Psychiatry, 48,* 474–483.
Shrestha, M., & Santangelo, S. L. (2014). Autism: Challenge in Nepal. In V. Patel, V. Preedy, & C. Martin (Eds.), *Comprehensive guide to Autism* (pp. 2497–2507). NY: Springer.
Silverman, C., & Brosco, J. P. (2007). Understanding autism: Parents and pediatricians in historical perspective. *Archives of Pediatrics and Adolescent Medicine, 161,* 392–398.
Stahmer, A. C., Brookman-Frazee, L., Rieth, S. R., Stoner, J. T., Feder, J. D., Searcy, K., & Wang, T. (2017). Parent perceptions of an adapted evidence-based practice for toddlers with autism in a community setting. *Autism, 21*(2), 217–230. https://doi.org/10.1177/1362361316637580.
Stahmer, A. C., Dababnah, S., & Rieth, S. R. (2019). Considerations in implementing evidence-based early autism spectrum disorder interventions in community settings. *Pediatric Medicine, 2,* 18.
Sue, D., & Sue, D. (2008). *Counselling the culturally diverse: Theory and practice (5th ed.)* NY.
Tilahun, D., Fekadu, A., Tekola, B., Araya, M., Roth, I., Davey, B., et al. (2017). Ethiopian community health workers' beliefs and attitudes towards children with autism: Impact of a brief training intervention. *Autism, 23,* 39–49.
Tilahun, D., Hanlon, C., Fekadu, A., Tekola, B., Baheretibeb, Y., & Hoekstra, R. A. (2016). Stigma, explanatory models and unmet needs of caregivers of children with developmental disorders in a low-income African country: A cross-sectional facility-based survey. *BMC Health Services Research, 16,* 152.
Tomasello, M., Kruger, A. C., & Ratner, H. H. (1993). Cultural learning. *Behavioral and Brain Sciences, 16,* 495–511.
Trembath, D., Balandin, S., & Rossi, C. (2005). Cross-cultural practice and autism. *Journal of Intellectual & Developmental Disability, 30,* 240–242.
van de Vijver, F., & Tanzer, N. K. (2004). Bias and equivalence in cross-cultural assessment: An overview. *Revue Européenne de Psychologie Appliquée/European Review of Applied Psychology, 54,* 119–135.
Vivanti, G., & Stahmer, A. (2018). Early intervention for autism: Are we prioritizing feasibility at the expenses of effectiveness? A cautionary note. *Autism, 22*(7), 770–773. https://doi.org/10.1177/1362361318803043.
Wallace, S., Fein, D., Rosanoff, M., Dawson, G., Hossain, S., Brennan, L., et al. (2012). A global public health strategy for autism spectrum disorders. *Autism Research, 5,* 211–217.

Werner, O., & Campbell, D. T. (1970). Translating, working through interpreters, and the problem of decentering. *A Handbook of Method in Cultural Anthropology, 398,* 420.

Wilder, L. K., Dyches, T. T., Obiakor, F. E., & Algozzine, B. (2004). Multicultural perspectives on teaching students with Autism. *Focus on Autism and Other Developmental Disabilities, 19*(2), 105–113.

Wong, V., Hui, L.-H. S., Lee, W.-C., Leung, L.-S. J., Ho, P.-K. P., Lau, W.-L. C., et al. (2004). A modified screening tool for Autism (Checklist for Autism in toddlers [CHAT-23]) for Chinese children. *Pediatrics, 114*(2), e166–e176.

World Health Organization. (2004). *ICD-10: International statistical classification of diseases and related health problems: Tenth revision* (2nd ed).

Wu Cai Lu Autism Research Institute. (2019). *Report on the development of China's Autism education rehabilitation industry*. Retrieved from Beijing, China.

Yu, L., Stronach, S., & Harrison, A. J. (Submitted). Public Knowledge and stigma of Autism spectrum disorder: Comparing China with the United States. *Autism: International Journal of Research and Practice*.

Zwaigenbaum, L., Bauman, M. L., Fein, D., Pierce, K., Buie, T., Davis, P. A., et al. (2015). Early screening of Autism spectrum disorder: Recommendations for practice and research. *Pediatrics, 136*(Supplement 1), S41.

Coordinating ABA Services

Kristen Padilla, Jessica S. Akers, and Marie Kirkpatrick

Abstract Interventions based on the principles of applied behavior analysis (ABA) have been found to be effective for targeting skills across multiple domains for children with autism spectrum disorder (ASD). Interventions address critical skills including increased communication, adaptive and social behavior, as well as reductions in challenging behavior. Targeting these skills leads to increased independence and improved quality of life for children with ASD. Behavior analytic services may be offered in multiple settings including various types of clinics, schools, and in the home. Given that children with ASD often receive services from different service providers, it is imperative for those providing behavior analytic services to collaborate with others to provide optimal care for the child and family. Behavior analysts have a specific skill set and expertise that allows them to provide valuable contributions while participating as a member of an interdisciplinary team. This chapter will outline the implementation of ABA services across settings and describe the way in which caregivers and other professionals can work together to provide better coordination of care for the child.

Applied Behavior Analysis

Applied behavior analysis (ABA) is a science that seeks to address socially significant issues including increasing appropriate behavior in individuals with autism spectrum disorder (ASD; Cooper, Heron, & Heward, 2019). One of the underlying principles of ABA is that behavior is a function of its consequences; thus, in order to alter behavior, one must first alter the environment to introduce new consequences. According to this approach, learning occurs because environmental consequences strengthen (reinforce) specific responses. Overall, this approach is positive in that it assumes that all individuals can learn (including those with disabilities) as long as the contingencies are arranged to support learning. Within ABA there is an emphasis on observable, measurable behavior. Target behaviors are operationally defined with

K. Padilla (✉) · J. S. Akers · M. Kirkpatrick
Department of Educational Psychology, Baylor University, Waco, TX, USA
e-mail: Kristen_Padilla-Mainor@baylor.edu

M. B. McClain et al. (eds.), *Interprofessional Care Coordination for Pediatric Autism Spectrum Disorder*, https://doi.org/10.1007/978-3-030-46295-6_15

clear definitions so that others should be able to identify occurrences of the behavior based on the definition alone. These definitions include descriptions of multiple dimensions of the behavior (e.g., duration and intensity) as well as examples and nonexamples. Another key feature of ABA is the strong reliance on data to make informed decisions regarding the implementation of interventions. These data are graphed and visually analyzed to determine the effectiveness or ineffectiveness of procedures.

Individuals who practice within the field of ABA are referred to as behavior analysts. Behavior analysts are certified by the Behavior Analyst Certification Board (BACB) and there are four levels of certification that correspond to the level of education (BACB, n.d.). Board Certified Behavior Analysts (BCBAs) hold a master's degree and generally provide oversight of the implementation of behavioral strategies with individuals with ASD. BCBA-Ds hold a doctoral degree and serve in a similar role as master's level BCBAs. The Board Certified Assistant Behavior Analyst (BCaBA) certification requires an undergraduate degree and the Registered Behavior Technician (RBT) certification requires a high school diploma. BCaBAs and RBTs are usually the individuals providing direct services to children with ASD under the supervision of a BCBA or BCBA-D.

It is important to recognize the differences in certifications as their roles within the interdisciplinary team vary. BCaBAs and RBTs will often be more familiar with the client as they interact with them more frequently; however, given a BCBA's advanced training and expertise, their input regarding treatment planning within the interdisciplinary team should be given due consideration. In the event that other professionals are interacting with BCaBAs or RBTs, keep in mind that they generally do not have the advanced expertise to make changes to their client's treatment plan; discussions related to such changes should include the BCBA. In addition to certification, behavior analysts may be licensed by the state in which they reside. Licensure is important for seeking compensation from insurance companies and it adds another level of legitimacy for behavior analysts which better protects individuals receiving ABA services (Dorsey, Weinburg, Zane, & Guigi, 2009). Regulatory bodies (e.g., licensing boards) are distinct for each state, thus licensure requirements and procedures vary across states ("Licensure and Other Regulations of ABA Practitioners", n.d.).

Although all professionals participating in the interdisciplinary team ultimately want what is best for the client, they may disagree on the way in which treatment should progress. These disagreements may relate to the selection of goals, development of interventions as well as evaluation of the effectiveness of the interventions. These distinctions often arise based on differences in philosophical orientations for each of the team members. It could be argued that behavior analysts' philosophy is the most disparate from the philosophies of the other team members; behavior analysts must learn how to behave flexibly as a team member without violating their own ethical guidelines (discussed below). There is empirical support and guidance for behavior analysts on how to navigate these situations (Kelly & Tincani, 2013). Brodhead (2015) provides a decision-making model that can be used as a tool for behavior analysts when encountering suggestions to introduce nonbehavioral treatments. Within this paper, Brodhead stressed the importance of behavior analysts becoming familiar with the proposed treatment as well as other treatments commonly implemented by professionals from other disciplines. In addition, the model emphasizes the continuous assessment of the possible risk to the client with every treatment decision. Similarly, one way to improve collaboration between different professionals is to increase understanding of the philosophical underpinnings, the scope of practice, and training of the other professions. LaFrance, Weiss, Kazemi, Gerenser, and Dobres (2019) provide an in-depth description of each of these components for behavior analysis, psychology, speech-language pathology, and occupational therapy. There are areas of overlap between the professions, but also areas of distinction which highlight the need for collaboration. Mutual understanding of philosophy and practice can promote respect and enhance communication across professionals.

The professionals with whom behavior analysts interact as well as the practical considerations for collaboration vary slightly across settings. We will now outline considerations and suggestions for integrating behavior analysts as members of an interdisciplinary team in clinic, school, and home settings.

Clinic-Based Services

Many children with ASD receive ABA services in clinical settings. These clinics may be affiliated with universities and hospitals or be privately owned and operated. Universities and hospitals house professionals from several different fields of study, therefore collaborations across professions can be facilitated with fewer practical difficulties based on the close physical proximity and the similarity of administrative procedures. These units often contain research and clinical training programs for university students as well. In clinical settings, behavior analysts often collaborate with psychiatrists, physicians, speech-language pathologists, physical therapists, and occupational therapists. These professionals may be employed within the same agency or collaborate as external providers. It is important for behavior analysts to clearly communicate their agency's purpose, service provisions, operations, and procedures as well as their diagnostic and treatment model. Additionally, behavior analysts should be forthcoming with information regarding compensation for services, as payment options and procedures for billing insurance may vary across settings.

There are two primary categories of services that may be provided by behavior analysts within clinical settings. These include behavior acquisition programs (e.g., early intensive behavioral intervention, social skills groups) and behavior reduction programs (e.g., severe challenging behavior services, food selectivity/refusal). We will highlight one example from each of the categories.

Early Intensive Behavioral Intervention (EIBI)

Assessment. Prior to developing goals, the behavior analyst will conduct a skills-based assessment and gather input from the caregivers and other team members (e.g., speech-language pathologist). This information can be obtained using questionnaires (presented orally or written), educational reports (e.g., Individualized Education Program [IEP]), or observations in specific environments (e.g., classroom).

Goal development. Goals for children receiving EIBI services are focused on teaching new communication, social, academic, and adaptive skills. Goals include specific mastery criteria, different objectives to support mastery of the goal, and stipulations for correct responses. Developing EIBI goals should constitute a group effort as input from multiple team members will result in the most comprehensive goals. For example, the behavior analyst may write a goal related to walking up and downstairs based on the recommendation of the physical therapist. The behavior analyst can ensure the goal is regularly practiced and the physical therapist can periodically check into evaluate progress and provide recommendations. It is important for behavior analysts to collaborate with caregivers during the goal development phase. Caregivers should regularly provide input on treatment priorities. This helps caregivers feel involved and empowered in their child's treatment plan and promotes the client's generalization of skills across settings.

Caregiver involvement. Throughout the child's participation in the EIBI program, caregivers should be kept abreast of progress and the introduction of new goals. Regular caregiver meetings are imperative for providing the most effective services. There are teaching strategies that the behavior analyst should ensure the caregiver can implement prior to the child's discharge. These strategies include chaining, setting up naturalistic learning opportunities, prompting correct responses, and providing reinforcement contingent on appropriate behavior. These procedures are important in teaching communication, promoting adaptive behavior, and avoiding future child engagement in challenging behavior.

Generalization across settings. One of the benefits of conducting EIBI in a clinical setting is access to other peers with and without ASD. The presence of multiple children allows for group activities (e.g., circle time), teaching peer play, and increasing the child-to-therapist ratio to better approximate other learning environments (e.g., classroom). It is essential for the behavior analyst to obtain input from the other team members and peers when arranging these situations to ensure they accurately mirror the natural environment. For instance, if the child will be expected to participate in cooperative groups with four peers in the classroom, the behavior analyst should try to organize a similar arrangement in the clinical setting. Prior to transitioning from EIBI to a different therapeutic or classroom setting, it is important to develop a formalized transition process. The transition process should document goals, mastery criteria, and phases of transition (e.g., progressive duration in a new setting, pairing, short-term objectives, and reinforcement schedule) prior to transitioning to the next setting.

Severe Challenging Behavior Services

Goal development. At the onset of services, target challenging behavior should be identified and goals for reduction should be determined. The referral concerns (i.e., target challenging behavior) should be clearly delineated by the caregiver or by the referring party in the event that is not the caregiver (e.g., the teacher refers to challenging behavior in the classroom). Once the referral concerns are clearly defined in measurable terms, the team must set a terminal goal for reduction in challenging behavior. A common goal for reduction is a 90% decrease in challenging behavior; however, the goal should be determined based on input from caregivers, teachers, and other individuals who interact with the child on a daily basis. The input from these related parties is essential because they have a clear understanding of the expectations of the situations to which the child will be exposed.

Prior to conducting assessments, the behavior analyst should discuss any ongoing procedures being implemented by other professionals and request that these procedures remain consistent throughout the child's admission in the clinical setting. If strict consistency is not possible, the behavior analyst will request that the professional alert them to any changes. This is necessary to verify that any change in the child's behavior is due to the behavioral intervention as opposed to a side effect from a procedure being implemented by the caregiver or another professional. This is especially important when the child is receiving services from a psychiatrist as medication changes can result in substantial changes in behavior.

Assessment. Assessment procedures for children with ASD who engage in severe challenging behavior begin with an interview with caregivers (or other referring party) describing the topography of the challenging behavior (i.e., what it looks like) and the conditions under which challenging behavior often occurs. After gathering this information, behavior analysts will conduct a function-based assessment to determine the consequences which are maintaining the challenging behavior (i.e., the purpose of the behavior). During this assessment, the behavior analyst provides different consequences (e.g., access to attention) contingent on challenging behavior to see which consequences lead to elevated levels of challenging behavior. Behavior analysts often conduct these assessments; however, in some cases, challenging behavior may not occur when the behavior analyst provides consequences and it may be necessary to have caregivers conduct the assessment. In the event that the caregiver is conducting the assessment, the behavior analyst will provide feedback to the caregiver and ensure the safety of the caregiver by absorbing instances of aggression if necessary.

Following the completion of these assessments an intervention must be developed. The most commonly implemented function-based intervention is functional communication training (FCT; Fisher, Greer, Fuhrman, & Querim, 2015). When implementing FCT, the behavior analyst ensures that the consequence, which previously followed the challenging behavior, is provided when the individual engages in the appropriate communication response. For example, if the behavior analyst determines that the child is engaging in challenging behavior in order to gain access to a tablet, the behavior analyst will ensure the tablet is withheld following challenging behavior and is provided following an appropriate request such as "tablet please". Collaboration with caregivers and other professionals, particularly the speech language pathologist, should begin with the selection of the communication response. These responses may be vocal, signs, produced via an augmentative communication device, or a card exchange (Tiger, Hanley, & Bruzek, 2008). There is research to suggest that initially teaching a response that can be physically guided (e.g., card exchange) reduces the amount of time the child is exposed to the aversive condition (e.g., denied access to the tablet) and thus may result in lower levels of challenging behavior (Fisher et al., 2018). However, the caregiver's opinion should be thoughtfully considered prior to the selection of the response.

Generalization across settings. Initially, the functional communication response is reinforced every time the child emits the response. This schedule is impossible to maintain in the natural environment; thus, the behavior analyst must ensure the child can appropriately endure periods of time in which the reinforcer is unavailable. One way to achieve this is to introduce stimuli to signal when the reinforcer is or is not available. These established stimuli have been shown to facilitate rapid transfer of treatment effects to novel implementers (Fisher et al., 2015). Specifically, researchers found that once the child responded appropriately in the presence of the stimuli (e.g., requests the tablet when the green bracelet is visible and refrains from requesting when the red bracelet is visible) the stimuli remained effective when used by different therapists in different settings. In addition to this procedure, the behavior analyst should introduce a variety of novel situations to evaluate the effectiveness of the intervention. These situations can include having unfamiliar individuals implement the intervention, having unfamiliar individuals (e.g., peers) in close proximity while the intervention is implemented, and implementing the interventions in new settings (e.g., an outside play area).

Caregiver involvement. Prior to discharge, the behavior analyst should conduct intensive training in the clinic for caregivers and other professionals (e.g., teachers). Once the caregiver implements the final treatment plan with 90% accuracy, treatment should transfer to the natural environment. The behavior analyst should visit the home, school, and any other locations in which the child regularly spends time to ensure the treatment remains effective.

School-Based Services

Within schools, behavior analysts provide a variety of direct and indirect services that address difficulties experienced by students with ASD. The selection of services is centered on the student's needs as well as school resources and personnel availability. Chapter "Promoting Academic Success" covers specific components to promote school and academic success for children with ASD but here we focus on behavior analytic services in school settings. The reader is encouraged to align recommendations from various chapters to meet the needs of their child and family. In educational settings, behavior analysts typically collaborate with teachers, paraprofessionals, speech-language pathologists, occupational therapists, and adaptive physical education instructors. Team members and service providers need to clearly communicate service duration and frequency, goals, and intervention components in order to monitor progress efficiently. There are three primary types of services which are likely to be provided by the behavior analyst in school settings. These include: school-wide behavioral support services, specialized services through special education or Section 504, and teacher and caregiver consultation and coaching.

School-Wide Positive Behavioral Support (SWBPS)

School-Wide Positive Behavior Supports (SWPBS) is a research-based, highly effective, approach to teaching and reinforcing students' social, emotional, and academic learning skills. The goal of SWPBS is to establish a predictable, consistent, and positive school culture for all students and school personnel. SWBPS incorporates a framework based on a multitiered system providing a continuum of support for academic and behavioral needs for students. When implementing SWBPS, schools establish clearly defined behavioral expectations, deliver direct instruction to teach the desired behaviors, and reinforce appropriate behaviors in the school setting (Sugai & Horner, 2006).

Tier 1 of SWPBS entails curriculum and positive preventative supports for systematic training of expected social behaviors. Behavior analysts can facilitate or support the implementation of a Tier 1 program by providing training and coaching to teachers, school personnel, and students on system implementation, procedures, and principles of positive behavior support to help students with ASD be more successful in inclusive settings. Tier 2 of SWPBS is for students who require additional support beyond Tier 1, which may include group-based interventions, additional instruction, and caregiver collaboration (Sugai & Horner, 2006). Within Tier 2, behavior analysts can consult with teachers on classroom management strategies, provide small-group social skills lessons, and provide recommendations regarding positive behavior strategies to support students with ASD in the classroom. Tier 3 is for students that require more intensive, individualized services in order to be successful in the school setting (Sugai & Horner, 2006). Behavior analysts may be more involved in the direct implementation of procedures at this level because they conduct function-based assessments, develop intervention plans, and provide more individualized supports for students with ASD.

Specialized Student Support Services

Behavior analysts may work for school districts directly or be contracted as consultants or direct service providers. Their involvement in school districts may include participating in goal development and progress monitoring with team planning for special education services or services provided under Section 504. Consultation from a behavior analyst is often specifically requested when a student engages challenging behavior that interferes with academic, social, or behavioral progress. Per request of the IEP team, the behavior analyst conducts a function-based assessment and develops a behavior intervention plan (BIP) based on the results of the assessment (Lloyd, Weaver, & Staubitz, 2016). The behavior analyst presents the results of the assessment and the BIP to the IEP team. The responsibility of the behavior analyst then shifts to providing training to the personnel responsible for upholding the BIP on the student's campus (e.g., teachers, paraprofessionals, administrators). Following training, the behavior analyst collects treatment fidelity data on the implementation of the intervention to ensure that the BIP is being followed correctly and provides follow-up consultation and support as needed (Traub, Joslyn, Kronfli, Peters, & Vollmer, 2017).

Collaborating with Professionals Across Disciplines

Behavior analysts have extensive training and a specific set of skills that are applicable to many behavioral concerns occurring in both general and special education classrooms. These concerns can include class-wide disruptive behavior, individual student challenging behavior, academic concerns, and treatment adherence. The strengths of the behavior analyst can complement the strengths of other school professionals allowing them to serve as a valuable member of the team (Gadke, Stratton, Kazmerski, & Rossen, 2016). Although, professionals may not initially agree on the specific treatment recommendations, the team must find common language and collaborate to develop the best treatment plan for the student. Regardless of the placement setting, behavior analysts can work with other professionals to select the appropriate accommodations, modifications, and services to help the student succeed in the school setting.

Caregiver Involvement

From the initiation of services, behavior analysts must intentionally plan for target skills to generalize to other settings and maintain once the behavior analyst is no longer providing services. This is particularly important for students who engage in challenging behavior. Behavior analysts may be responsible for broaching the topic of the need for caregiver training during IEP meetings to facilitate behavior reduction in the home setting. School administrators may request for the behavior analyst to provide training to the caregivers directly or to ensure that the teacher is sufficiently trained such that he or she may provide training to the caregiver (Traub et al., 2017). The Individuals with Disabilities Education Act (IDEA, 2004) specifies collaborative partnerships between caregivers and schools which can enhance communication and mutual trust. When working with families, it is crucial for all service providers to be cognizant of the family dynamics and any cultural factors which may influence relationships between caregivers and other professionals (Taber-Doughty & Bouck, 2012). Collaborative relationships among school personnel, external service providers, and caregivers are important for the child's school, home, and community success. Chapter "Partners in School: An Example of Care Coordination to Ensure Consistency of Evidence-Based Practices Across Home and School for Youth with Autism Spectrum Disorder (ASD)" provides illustrative approaches to promote family-school partnerships.

Home-Based Services

Children with ASD may receive services in their homes from one or more service providers given the individualized needs of the child and available resources within the community. Home-based services may be supplemental to school-based or clinic-based services or it may be a standalone service. When providing in-home services, behavior analysts often collaborate with teachers, speech language pathologists, and occupational therapists. A large portion of children receiving EIBI services under the supervision of a BCBA receives these services in the home setting (Love, Carr, Almason, & Petursdottir, 2009). According to IDEA Part C, young children with developmental delays should receive early intervention services to the greatest extent possible in the natural environment (i.e., home setting; IDEA, 2004). Although behavior analysts are not generally funded through IDEA, providing services to young children in the home is a practice observed by many behavior analysts. In-home services generally can be categorized as short-term consultation services or long-term EIBI services.

Consultation Services

Behavior analysts often receive requests to provide in-home consultation services related to specific challenges encountered by the child with ASD. Examples of these specific challenges include toilet training, addressing difficulties with sleep, developing interventions to target challenging behavior, and increasing independence with daily routines. During the initial visit, the behavior analyst will conduct an in-depth interview with the caregiver to determine the target behavior, the current procedures being implemented (e.g., scheduled sit times for toileting), and the desired outcome of the consultation services. The behavior analyst will recruit information from other related service providers to aide in their development of intervention goals. For example, the behavior analyst may contact the classroom teacher to obtain information related to toileting behavior in the school setting or contact the occupational therapist to obtain information regarding fine motor skills for self-feeding. Typically, when providing short-term consultation services, the behavior analyst uses behavioral skills training to teach the caregiver to directly implement the intervention with their child. Behavioral skills training consists of providing clear instructions regarding implementation of the intervention, modeling implementation of the intervention and then requiring the caregiver to role-play implementation of the intervention. Once the caregiver initiates the intervention with their child, the behavior analyst will provide consistent feedback regarding accurate and inaccurate implementation. Therapy sessions continue until the caregiver demonstrates mastery in implementing the intervention with fidelity and the child reaches the predetermined mastery criteria for their engagement in the newly acquired behavior.

EIBI

EIBI services provided in the home follow similar assessment and goal development practices as to when these services are provided in clinic settings. Thus, collaboration with other professionals and caregivers should occur when conducting skills-based assessments as well as when selecting goals. The primary difference between EIBI services provided in clinic settings and in-home settings is the level of caregiver involvement during therapy. Although behavior analysts strive to promote caregiver involvement in clinic settings, it is generally easier to do so in the home setting as the caregiver must remain at home during therapy sessions.

Caregiver Involvement

According to several research studies, caregivers of children with ASD experience significantly more stress than caregivers of children without ASD (Dunn, Burbine, Bowers, & Tantleff-Dunn, 2001). Child engagement in challenging behavior further increases stress which can impact community inclusion and increase the probability of the caregiver experiencing anxiety or depression (Lai, Goh, Oei, & Sung, 2015). Caregivers' self-efficacy regarding their ability to change their child's behavior also affects stress levels and successful generalization of skills across settings. An encouraging finding is that caregivers have reported improved quality of life for their entire family after their child begins receiving ABA services (McPhilemy & Dillenburger, 2013).

Behavior analysts who provide in-home services ensure caregivers are involved in therapy sessions in the form of (a) observing the behavior analyst implement procedures or (b) aiding in the implementation of procedures. Behavior analysts often provide direct training to caregivers to ensure the caregiver can accurately implement the target teaching procedures. Once the primary caregiver receives sufficient coaching from the behavior analyst, the primary caregiver may serve as the trainer for other family members (Kuhn, Lerman, & Vorndran, 2003), thus, promoting generalization. In addition to including caregivers within therapy sessions, behavior analysts often incorporate siblings into session activities (Leaf, Leaf, McEachin, Cihon, & Ferguson, 2018). This can be especially valuable when teaching play and social skills.

Although providing therapy to children in the home setting has several benefits, there are some special considerations to which the behavior analyst must attend. As discussed earlier, behavior analysts must demonstrate cultural awareness when collaborating with caregivers. This is particularly important when providing services in the home setting as the behavior analyst is entering into the family's personal space. Some caregivers express concerns related to the lack of privacy that comes with in-home services (Leaf et al., 2018). Other caregivers may feel unsure as to what their role should be within therapy sessions. Thus, direct communication related to roles and designated therapy areas should be discussed at the onset of services.

Telehealth Services

Delivering health services via telehealth has become more prominent in the past decade as the use of technology has increased in the daily lives of consumers (Tomlinson, Gore, & McGill, 2018). The field of ABA has followed the trend set forth by other behavioral fields (e.g., psychiatry and psychology) by using videoconferencing to provide services to families for whom services may be difficult to access due to physical location or as a means to reduce the cost of services (Lindgren et al., 2016; Vandenbos & Williams, 2000). It is important that behavior analysts use a videoconferencing platform that is compliant with the Health Insurance Portability and Accountability Act (HIPAA; Pollard, Karimi, & Ficcaglia, 2017). Researchers have evaluated telehealth as a service delivery model for families of individuals with ASD for both behavior reduction and behavior acquisition programs (Wacker et al., 2013; Wainer & Ingersoll, 2015). Telehealth services allow behavior analysts to provide synchronous feedback, coaching, and modeling correct implementation of skills via a two-way video and audio feed (Pollard et al., 2017). Families who have received services through telehealth have indicated high levels of satisfaction regarding the use of telehealth for delivery of services and training (Machalicek, et al., 2016). With the continuous demand for ABA services to be provided by or overseen by BCBAs, telehealth is an appealing option for situations in which in-person therapy may not be feasible.

Coordinating care within telehealth services is particularly important given there may be minimal interactions across service providers. Pollard and colleagues (2017) recommend having a quality assurance program that involves ongoing communication and review of programs with all professionals involved in a child's care. It is also recommended that behavior analysts participate in frequent virtual meetings involving all members of the interdisciplinary team, lead regularly scheduled caregiver meetings, and continuously monitor caregiver satisfaction (Pollard et al., 2017). There is detailed information regarding telehealth services in the chapter "Telehealth Approaches to Care Coordination in Autism Spectrum Disorder".

Additional Considerations

Caregiver Consent and Buy-In

As mentioned throughout the chapter, it is imperative that all those providing services to individuals with ASD have an equal understanding of the goals for treatment and the interventions being implemented. Within the team, client and caregiver input should be prioritized as they are the individuals most impacted by treatment decisions. Therefore, it should be an emphasis on the behavior analyst to pursue caregiver "buy-in" and obtain consent for all assessment and services provided. In the past, caregivers have noted that at the initiation of ABA services they were not convinced that the treatment was appropriate for their family. Specifically, they stated that the use of difficult terminology and procedures were obstacles for them in integrating ABA into their daily lives (Maurice, Mannion, Letso, & Perry, 2001). Due to these concerns, the BACB requires behavior analysts to use client-friendly language when explaining assessments and behavior-change programs (BACB, 2014). By explaining goals and procedures in a way that is easy for them to understand, it is likely that the caregivers will consent to treatment and be more willing to incorporate the procedures across multiple environments.

Communication Across Providers

In order to encourage communication across professionals without violating HIPAA requirements, behavior analysts must obtain caregiver consent to share information with other interdisciplinary team members. For example, a behavior analyst who is conducting a function-based assessment in the home setting may seek information regarding challenging behavior from the speech language pathologist, which would require the behavior analyst to first request consent from the caregiver (United States, 2004). Having the opportunity to exchange information among interdisciplinary team members will not only relieve the caregiver of the burden of relaying information across professionals, it also allows the professionals to work together to provide the best interdisciplinary care for the child. Consent to share information allows professionals to be able to establish common language, promote generalization of goals, share effective teaching and intervention strategies, and learn from one another about how others provide specific treatment plans from various perspectives.

Ethical Guidelines for Behavior Analysts

Behavior analysts are bound by the ethical guidelines set forth by the BACB (BACB, 2014). The ethical code includes several guidelines that address a number of areas of practice and there are a few which directly relate to participating as a member of an interdisciplinary team. Behavior analysts have a responsibility to always behave in the best interest of their client, which may include collaborating with other professionals (BACB Code 2.03). Support for collaboration can also be found in the guideline addressing behavior analysts practicing within their scope of competence (BACB Code 1.02). This code specifically delineates that behavior analysts must only provide services for which they have received training. Therefore, it is often necessary for behavior analysts to participate within an interdisciplinary team in order to provide the best services for their client without practicing beyond their scope of competence. Once a collaboration has been established, the ethical guidelines call for behavior analysts to collaborate with other professionals in a manner that promotes clinically relevant improvement for their client (BACB Code 2.09). Within this collaboration, behavior analysts should ensure treatments are based on sufficient scientific evidence as well as effective for the specific client. When working with professionals from other disciplines it is important for behavior analysts to model ethical and appropriate behavior in order to foster a productive collaboration (BACB Code 2.09).

Team Coordination and Resource Management

Children with ASD often receive services from multiple providers employed at various agencies (e.g., schools, university-based clinics). Given these multifaceted dynamics, we recommend identifying a case manager or liaison to maintain ongoing communication among service providers and caregivers. Moreover, including a social worker as a member of the team will likely aid in team collaboration as well as help identify valuable resources for the family.

Community Inclusion for Children with ASD

To best support the child and family, behavior analysts along with other team members must find ways to promote community involvement and inclusion. This can be accomplished by providing training to adults involved with community agencies to promote awareness and inclusion for children with ASD. In service of this goal, professionals and community organizations have helped to create awareness and acceptance of children with ASD by providing workshops and specialized training. For example, several studies have reported training of airport staff (Skillicorn, 2013), law enforcement (Laan, Ingram, & Glidden, 2013), and youth club leaders

(McConkey, Mullan, & Addis, 2012). These are prime examples of how behavior analysts can use their skill set to train and consult with community stakeholders to promote inclusive practices for children with ASD.

In order for children with ASD to successfully participate in extracurricular activities with their peers, behavior analysts need to educate and train coaches and group leaders on the characteristics of ASD and strategies that will help the child perform in the target environment. Additionally, behavior analysts can create specific goals and intervention strategies to help the child learn the necessary behaviors to actively and appropriately participate.

Research has shown that successful inclusive recreational programs incorporate recruiting appropriate support personnel, training relevant adults and peers, and ensuring consistent communication with families. Additionally, behavior analysts must provide ongoing feedback and training for support personnel, identify individualized behavioral and social goals, and develop interventions that are appropriate for the setting (Brookman et al., 2003). Andrews, Falkmer, and Girdler (2014) recommend that programs include components that (a) facilitate friendships and recreational participation, (b) include peers, (c) incorporate activity preferences of all children, and (d) accommodate individual needs through adaptive leisure activities.

Conclusion

In conclusion, we believe behavior analysts have the skills to contribute as a valuable member of an interdisciplinary team given their emphasis on identifying socially significant goals that are client and family-driven. These goals are well defined to meet the specific needs of the client and family, which allows all team members to accurately monitor the progress that ensures the teaching techniques and interventions are effective. Throughout this chapter, we described common practices across settings and provide suggestions for collaboration between the behavior analyst and other interdisciplinary team members.

References

Andrews, J., Falkmer, M., & Girdler, S. (2014). Community participation interventions for children and adolescents with a neurodevelopmental intellectual disability: A systematic review. *Journal of Disability and Rehabilitation, 37,* 825–833.

Behavior Analyst Certification Board Certification. (n.d.). Retrieved from https://www.bacb.com/.

Behavior Analyst Certification Board. (2014). Professional and ethical compliance code for behavior analysts. Littleton, CO: Author. Retrieved from https://www.bacb.com/wpcontent/uploads/BACB-Compliance-Code-english_190318.pdf.

Brodhead, M. T. (2015). Maintaining professional relationships in an interdisciplinary setting: Strategies for navigating nonbehavioral treatment recommendations for individuals with autism. *Behavior Analysis in Practice, 8,* 70–78.

Brookman, L., Boettcher, M., Klein, E., Openden, D., Koegel, R. L., & Koegel, L. K. (2003). Facilitating social interactions in a community summer setting for children with autism. *Journal of Positive Behavior Interventions, 5,* 249–252.

Cooper, J. O., Heron, T. E., & Heward, W. L. (2019). *Applied behavior analysis* (3rd ed.). ISBN-10: 0134752554.

Dorsey, M. F., Weinberg, M., Zane, T., & Guidi, M. M. (2009). The case for licensure of applied behavior analysts. *Behavior Analysis in Practice, 2,* 53–58.

Dunn, M. E., Burbine, T., Bowers, C. A., & Tantleff-Dunn, S. (2001). Moderators of stress in parents of children with autism. *Community Mental Health Journal, 37,* 39–52.

Fisher, W. W., Greer, B. D., Mitter, D. R., Fuhrman, A. M., Romani, P. W., & Zangrillo, A. N. (2018). Further evaluation of differential exposure to establishing operations during functional communication training. *Journal of Applied Behavioral Analysis, 51,* 360–373.

Fisher, W. W., Greer, B. D., Fuhrman, A. M., & Querim, A. C. (2015). Using multiple schedules during functional communication training to promote rapid transfer of treatment effects. *Journal of Applied Behavior Analysis, 48,* 713–733.

Gadke, D. L., Stratton, K. K., Kazmerski, J. S., & Rossen, E. (2016). Understanding the board certified behavior analyst credential. *Communique, 45,* 18–19.

Individuals with Disabilities Education Improvement Act of 2004., 20 U.S.C. §1400 *et seq.* (2004).

Kelly, A., & Tincani, M. (2013). Collaborative training and practice among applied behavior analysts who support individuals with autism spectrum disorder. *Education and Training in Autism and Developmental Disabilities, 48,* 120–131.

Kuhn, S. A. C., Lerman, D. C., & Vorndran, C. M. (2003). Pyramidal training for families of children with problem behavior. *Journal of Applied Behavior Analysis, 36,* 77–88.

Laan, J. M., Ingram, R. V., & Glidden, M. D. (2013). Law enforcement training on mental health disorders and autism spectrum disorders in the southeastern United States. *Journal of Global Intelligence & Policy, 6,* 51–67.

Lai, W. W., Goh, T. J., Oei, T. P. S., & Sung, M. (2015). Coping and well-being in parents of children with autism spectrum disorder (ASD). *Journal of Autism and Developmental Disorders, 45,* 2582–2593.

LaFrance, D. L., Weiss, M. J., Kazemi, E., Gerenser, J., & Dobres, J. (2019). Multidisciplinary teaming: Enhancing collaboration through increased understanding. *Behavior Analysis in Practice.*

Leaf, J. B., Leaf, R., McEachin, J., Cihon, J. H., & Ferguson, J. L. (2018). Advantages and challenges of a home- and clinic-based model of behavioral intervention for individuals diagnosed with autism spectrum disorder. *Journal of Autism and Developmental Disorders, 48,* 2258–2266.

Licensure and Other Regulations of ABA Practitioners. (n.d.). Retrieved from https://www.apbahome.net/general/recommended_links.asp.

Lindgren, S., Wacker, D., Suess, A., Schieltz, K., Pelzel, K., Kopelman, T., … Waldron, D. (2016). Telehealth and autism: Treating challenging behavior at lower cost. *Pediatrics, 137,* S167–S175.

Lloyd, B., Weaver, E., & Staubitz, J. (2016). A review of functional analysis methods conducted in public school classroom settings. *Journal of Behavioral Education, 25,* 324–356.

Love, J. R., Carr, J. E., Almason, S. M., & Petursdottir, A. I. (2009). Early and intensive behavioral intervention for autism: A survey of clinical practices. *Research in Autism Spectrum Disorders, 3*(421–428), 3.

Machalicek, W., Lequia, J., Pinkelman, S., Knowles, C., Raulston, T., Davis, T., Alresheed, F. (2016). Behavioral telehealth consultation with families of children with autism spectrum disorder. *Behavioral Interventions, 31,* 223–250.

Maurice, C., Mannion, K., Letso, S., & Perry, L. (2001). Parent voices: Difficulty in accessing behavioral intervention for autism; working toward solutions. *Behavioral Interventions, 16,* 147–165.

McConkey, R., Mullan, A., & Addis, J. (2012). Promoting the social inclusion of children with autism spectrum disorders in community groups. *Early Child Development and Care, 182,* 827–835.

McPhilemy, C., & Dillenburger, K. (2013). Parents' experiences of applied behavior analysis (ABA)-based interventions for children diagnosed with autistic spectrum disorder. *British Journal of Special Education, 40,* 154–161.

Pollard, J. S., Karimi, K. A., & Ficcaglia, M. B. (2017). Ethical considerations in the design and implementation of a telehealth service delivery model. *Behavior Analysis: Research and Practice, 17,* 298–311.

Skillicorn, K. (2013). A review of airport accessibility programs for individuals diagnosed with autism spectrum disorders: Recommendations for the development of a program at Portland international airport (Master's thesis, Pacific University). Retrieved from http://commons.pacificu.edu/spp/468.

Sugai, G., & Horner, R. (2006). *Adoption, implementation, durability, & expansion of SW-PBS.* Paper presented at the Third Annual International Association for Positive Behavior Supports Convention. Reno, NV. Retrieved from http://www.SWPBS.org/pastconferencepresentations.htm.

Taber-Doughty, T., & Bouck, E. (2012). Family support and involvement throughout the school years. In D. Zager, M. L. Wehmeyer, & R. L. Simpson (Eds.), *Education students with autism spectrum disorders: Research-based principles and practices* (pp. 262–277). New York, NY: Routledge.

Tiger, J. H., Hanley, G. P., & Bruzek, J. (2008). Functional communication training: A review and practical guide. *Behavior Analysis in Practice, 1,* 16–23.

Tomlinson, S. R. L., Gore, N., & McGill, P. (2018). Training individuals to implement applied behavior analytic procedures via telehealth: A systematic review of the literature. *Journal of Behavioral Education, 27,* 172–222.

Traub, M. R., Joslyn, P. R., Kronfli, F. R., Peters, K. P., & Vollmer, T. R. (2017). A model for behavioral consultation in rural school districts. *Rural Special Education Quarterly, 36,* 5–16.

United States. (2004). *The health insurance portability and accountability act (HIPAA).* Washington, DC: U.S. Dept. of Labor, Employee Benefits Security Administration.

Vandenbos, G. R., & Williams, S. (2000). The internet versus the telephone: What is telehealth, anyway? *Professional Psychology: Research and Practice, 31,* 490–492.

Wacker, D. P., Lee, J. F., Dalmau, Y. C. P., Kopelman, T. G., Lindgren, S. D., Kuhle, J., … Waldron, D. B. (2013). Conducting functional communication training via telehealth to reduce the problem behavior of young children with autism. *Journal of Developmental and Physical Disabilities, 25,* 35–48.

Wainer, A. L., & Ingersoll, B. R. (2015). Increasing access to an ASD imitation intervention via a telehealth parent training program. *Journal of Autism and Developmental Disorders, 45,* 3877–3890.

Coordinating Speech-Language Pathology Services for Youth with Autism Spectrum Disorder

Lisa Wisman Weil

Abstract This chapter discusses the importance of coordinating speech-language services in the community, school, and home settings for youth with autism spectrum disorder (ASD). The role of the speech-language pathologist (SLP) is discussed relative to assessment and treatment of youth with ASD, over the course of development. Practical recommendations are provided for ways that the SLP can work with other community members to build inclusive communities. Interprofessional practice and other models of collaboration are considered, including case scenarios and resources to support successful evidence-based practice collaborations between SLPs and other professionals when supporting individuals with ASD.

Autism spectrum disorder (ASD) is a complex neurodevelopmental disorder (Betancur, 2011; Pelphrey, Shultx, Hudac, & Vander Wyk, 2011). Individuals with ASD meet a defined set of clinically diagnostic criteria (e.g., DSM-5; American Psychiatric Association, 2013), and yet they comprise a heterogeneous and neurodiverse group of individuals. The continuum of language and communication profiles of individuals with ASD is particularly diverse, and can range from nonverbal to minimally verbal to verbally fluent with language impairment to verbally fluent without language impairment (Kasari, Brady, Lord, & Tager-Flusberg, 2013; Kjelgaard & Tager-Flusberg, 2001; McGregor et al., 2012; Tager-Flusberg & Joseph, 2003). Deficits in social communication skills (including pragmatic language) are one of the core features of ASD. Children with ASD may also experience co-occurring deficits in the other domains of language: phonology, semantics, morphology, and syntax. Speech-language pathologists (SLPs) are important members of the service delivery team for youth with ASD and contribute unique knowledge and skills, especially in the areas of language and social communication.

According to the American Speech-Language-Hearing Association (ASHA, 2016), SLPs are professionals who support people with communication disorders and differences across the lifespan. Collaboration is one of eight key service delivery

L. Wisman Weil (✉)
Department of Communication Sciences and Disorders, Emerson College, Boston, MA, USA
e-mail: lisa_wismanweil@emerson.edu

M. B. McClain et al. (eds.), *Interprofessional Care Coordination for Pediatric Autism Spectrum Disorder*, https://doi.org/10.1007/978-3-030-46295-6_16

domains for SLPs, along with counseling, prevention and wellness, screening, assessment, treatment, modalities and technology, and populations and systems. "SLPs share a responsibility with other professionals for creating a collaborative culture" (ASHA, 2016, p. 8). A collaborative culture is especially important when coordinating speech-language pathology services for individuals with ASD (see additional resources in Appendix A).

SLPs are not typically the professionals who diagnose ASD (ASHA, n.d.), but may be the professionals who first notice signs and symptoms of ASD in young children, especially those enrolled in early intervention for late language emergence. In a prospective study of young children at risk for ASD, the earliest signs and symptoms of ASD emerge between 6 and 12 months of age (Ozonoff et al., 2010). The earliest signs and symptoms appear in the social communication domain, and include reduced gaze to faces, social smiles, directed vocalizations, and social engagement in children with ASD compared to those without ASD. One of the earliest red flags for ASD that caregivers notice, as a disruption in social communication, is reduced response to name at around 9–12 months of age (e.g., when the child is looking down at a toy and does not turn to look at his mother when she calls his name from behind). Delayed emergence of first words, less frequent canonical babbling (reduplication of consonant and vowel sounds; e.g., baba), and reduced gesture use are additional early signs of concern that many times warrant referral to a team of early intervention professionals, including an SLP. In the early developmental period, it is critical that the SLP know how to differentially diagnose language disorders and know when to collaborate, consult, and/or refer to other developmental specialists if an ASD diagnosis is suspected.

SLPs are the experts who assess language and communication for children who have ASD or who are at risk for ASD. SLPs may work as part of an interdisciplinary or interprofessional autism diagnostic team in healthcare and educational settings. In these models, the SLP is a member of the team along with other service providers (e.g., developmental pediatrician, occupational therapist, physical therapist, and psychologist) and the individual with ASD. Interdisciplinary teams involve professionals assessing the child in their area of expertise and then coming together to discuss the results of each of their individual assessments (Johnson, 2016). In comparison, interprofessional teams are more collaborative, including assessments where members of the team work together to plan and administer the assessment (Johnson, 2016). Communication is regular and ongoing. Families benefit from high-quality communication among team members because the results of the assessment are more likely to be explained the same way by all members of the team.

Interprofessional SLP Collaborations Across the Lifespan

Early Intervention

It is important for SLPs and the general population to know the signs of ASD. For children seeking an early intervention evaluation and for those already enrolled in early intervention for speech and language services, the SLP is often the first person to notice the signs and symptoms of ASD. An early diagnosis of ASD comes with the added benefit of early intervention services.

In early intervention, the SLP collaborates with families and caregivers to support wellness and development for the child with ASD. Support includes prevention and wellness activities, such as making appropriate and informed referrals to other healthcare providers and educators. Early intervention is critical to successful long-term language and communication outcomes for children with ASD. As reported by Koegel, Koegel, Ashbaugh, and Bradshaw (2014), fewer than 10% of children with ASD remained nonverbal after early intervention, whereas 50% of children who did not enroll in early intervention remained nonverbal.

Wagner, Wallace, and Rogers (2014) recommend several developmental treatment approaches for young children with ASD (e.g., Early Start Denver Model, Milieu Teaching, and Hanen More than Words). Developmental approaches to treatment meet five criteria: (1) follow the sequence of typical development, (2) reference research on typical development to guide clinical decision-making, (3) focus on child–adult interpersonal relationships, (4) use child-centered approaches, and (5) use play as the context for intervention (Wagner et al., 2014). In developmental approaches to intervention, a speech-language pathologist is often part of an interdisciplinary team of occupational therapists, physical therapists, behavior analysts, child psychologists, special educators, and physicians. The team of professionals works together to conduct assessments and develop treatment plans. Goals may target prelinguistic skills (e.g., gesture or directed eye gaze) or language and social communication skills, depending on the individualized needs of the child.

The Preschool Years

During the preschool years (ages 3–5 years), children with ASD who continue to need intervention transition from home-based early intervention to school and/or center-based services. A child who had an individualized family service plan (IFSP) and continues to qualify for intervention services in the public schools, will likely receive an individualized education plan (IEP). The IFSP and IEP documents are created via collaboration with other rehabilitation and education professionals, since young children with ASD often require intervention services from several different professionals.

During the preschool years, children with ASD often work with an SLP on their language and social-pragmatic communication development. Given the range of language abilities in children with ASD, from nonverbal to verbally fluent, treatment goals will be individualized to address the language and communication needs of the child. For a child who is nonverbal or minimally verbal, augmentative and alternative communication systems may be utilized to support communication. The SLP may consult with other educators regarding ways to facilitate social communication and interaction while using the child's AAC system. For children with ASD who are verbal communicators, intervention targets may focus on building pragmatic language skills, receptive and expressive vocabulary, increasing comprehension and use of a variety of developmentally appropriate grammatical morphemes and syntactic forms, phonology, preliteracy skills, and/or speech sound intelligibility.

One example of assessment and treatment collaboration among preschool professionals may include the SLP, classroom teacher, and reading intervention specialist. Some children with ASD develop average reading skills, while others demonstrate difficulty learning to read. Preschoolers with ASD who demonstrate poor phonological awareness and emergent literacy skills tend to be at risk for reading impairments, and those with co-occurring spoken language impairments are at even higher risk (Davidson & Ellis Weismer, 2014; Dynia, Bean, Justice, & Kaderavek, 2019). SLPs can work together with classroom teachers, special education teachers, and reading intervention specialists to assess all areas of phonological awareness, plan for treatment and write appropriate literacy goals, and implement the intervention plan for preschoolers with ASD who are at risk for reading impairments (Langer & Watson, 2008). SLPs can provide explicit classroom instruction on phonological awareness.

School-Age and Beyond

Many evidence-based intervention practices are available to target social and communication skills in children with ASD ages 6–14 years; however, fewer evidence-based intervention options are available for individuals with ASD who are high school age or older (Prelock & McCauley, 2012; Wong et al., 2015). Life-long support may be required for many individuals with ASD. Adolescents and adults with ASD struggle with social isolation: fewer than 10% have reciprocal friendships with peers, and nearly half have no peer relationships (Orsmond et al., 2004). It is critical that SLPs work together with other professionals, care providers and the individual with ASD to promote social-pragmatic and communication development during the school-age years. A team approach to transition planning for life beyond high school may also promote optimal social-communication outcomes and reduced social isolation during adolescence and adulthood.

Intervention for language, literacy, and communication during the school-age years may take place in an educational or outpatient setting. SLPs in the public schools are part of individualized education plan (IEP) teams, help with planning multitiered systems of support (MTSS) and response to intervention (RTI), consistent with the individuals with disabilities education improvement act (IDEA, 2004; Hollenbeck 2007; Leach, 2018). SLPs who work in outpatient hospital or community clinics may run social skills groups or work with individuals one-on-one to target social communication, language, and/or literacy.

During the school years, SLPs must work together with other school personnel to ensure that assessments and treatments are curriculum-based and educationally relevant. In a systematic review, compelling evidence was found to support SLPs and classroom educators in collaboration around curriculum-based target vocabulary and phonological awareness preliteracy activities in early elementary school (Archibald, 2017). The development of literacy skills is as important for children with ASD as they are for any other school-age child. Literacy skill development includes a progression from learning to decode and read to the establishment of good reading fluency and reading comprehension skills (Lanter & Watson, 2008). Fluent readers with ASD may experience less difficulty with fact-finding literacy tasks, but more difficulty with reading questions that require taking the perspective of characters in the story, making inferences from the story, and considering the beliefs and perspectives of characters in a story (Lanter & Watson, 2008).

SLPs collaborate and consult with families to support the child's communication development at school and home. Alli, Abdoola, and Mupawsoe (2015) surveyed nine parents of children with ASD (average age 11.8 years), who described that the communication challenges that existed within their families impacted their ability to participate in activities outside of the home. Alli and colleagues encouraged SLPs to work together with families to support improved understanding when new modes of communication are introduced in therapy (e.g., picture exchange communication system [PECS]), and to educate families on effective communication strategies. In-service events for caregivers of children with ASD provide an excellent opportunity for SLPs to partner with teachers and other school professionals around teaching effective communication strategies to use at home and school (e.g., teaching caregivers to repeat and explain new vocabulary, or to increase wait time before expecting a response to aid comprehension).

When working with youth with ASD who have severe disabilities, Bruce and Bashinski (2017) encourage an interprofessional practice approach that includes the learner, the communication partner, and the environment. A collaborative team approach is especially important with children with severe disabilities because each child is likely to have a unique set of co-occurring medical, educational, and communicative needs. No one professional is likely to be expert in all of the child's areas of need; yet when working collaboratively, each professional, the learner and the communication partners can all contribute their expert knowledge in order to optimize outcomes. The SLP, for example, can recommend ways to augment and enhance communication but the communication partners (e.g., parents, teachers, and paraprofessionals) are likely to be the experts on the everyday communication routines within the child's environment and can suggest communication situations that require augmentation. Additional examples of interprofessional practice collaborations when working with children with ASD are provided in Appendix B.

Building Inclusive Communities

Community Connections

When communities actively work to include children with ASD, stronger communities are created. SLPs can work to build inclusive communities for children with ASD via advocacy and outreach activities. These activities can include work to build relationships between children with ASD, neurotypical peers, and their families. Inclusion of children with ASD in community activities provides all community members with more experiences with neurodiversity. A focus on relationship building can create communities with greater acceptance and understanding of similarities and differences, and stronger community support systems as a result of intentional peer and family relationship building. For example, communities may come together around autism awareness day (see Fig. 1) to support increased public awareness of ASD and community inclusion.

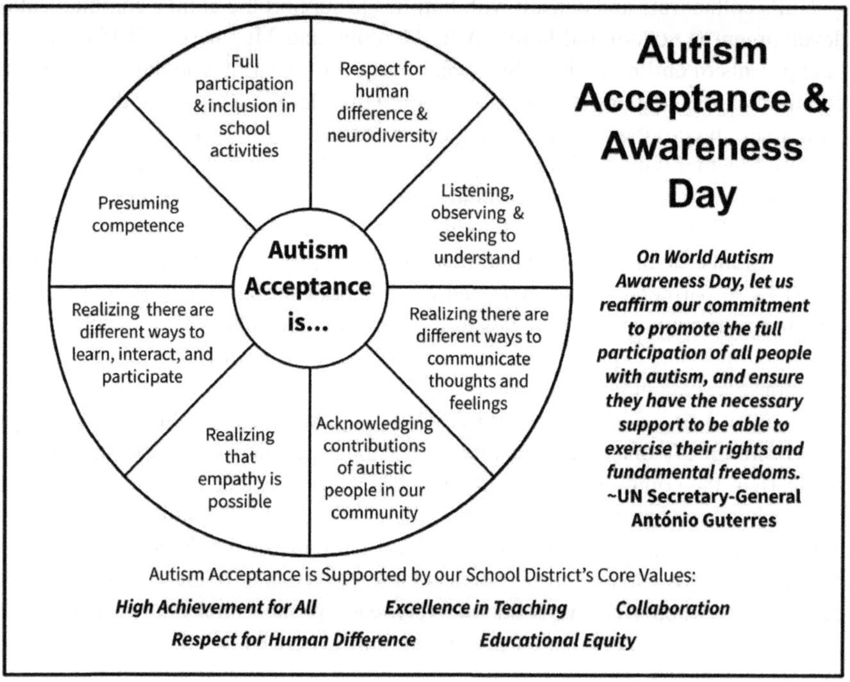

Fig. 1 Example of collaboration with parents of children with autism spectrum disorder in a school district to celebrate World Autism Awareness Day. Parents were asked, "what important messages do you want to be heard in a handout to celebrate world autism awareness day?" spokes of the wheel were filled with messages contributed by parents of children with autism

Play Dates

Positive relationships between peers with and without ASD enhance social and academic outcomes for all children. For children with ASD, play dates with peers, including neurotypical peers, can enhance positive peer relationships, friendship building, and social outcomes (Koegel, Werner, Vismara, & Koegel, 2005). SLPs can work together with classroom teachers and paraprofessionals, to facilitate positive peer relationships and friendship building at school, and can provide caregivers with training and suggestions for play dates and socializing outside of school time. In a multiple-baseline case study, Koegel et al. (2005) found improved reciprocal social interactions (verbal initiations, verbal responses, nonverbal eye contact, and joint engagement) during play dates that included contextual support: mutually reinforcing activities and adult-facilitated cooperative arrangements. Activities and locations that are likely to be mutually reinforcing for school-age children might include making crafts, baking and decorating cookies, playing a game, or structured play outside. In order to facilitate a cooperative arrangement between the children, ensure that both children have important roles to play in the activity and scaffold and support their back-and-forth interactions, as needed (e.g., when making cookies together, the adult can give each child a role, like having one child use the cookie cutters and the other child use the spatula to put the cookies on a pan).

Recreational Activities

Community-based unified sports teams provide opportunities for SLPs to collaborate with physical therapists, physical education teachers, applied behavioral analysis professionals, coaches, and families to support successful participation by youth with ASD. In an adapted soccer program for youth ages 5–19 years, children with ASD were partnered with neurotypical high school "buddies", who volunteered to support full participation of the children with ASD in the soccer practices and games (Hayward et al., 2016). Youth with ASD utilized individualized picture schedules and/or picture exchange communication systems (PECS) and token reinforcements to support communication and participation. After participating in the adapted soccer program, participants improved their physical fitness and soccer skills, and they built positive relationships with their "buddy" (Hayward et al., 2016).

In a survey of parents of children with ASD, 91% of the parents surveyed reported that "development of social skills" (p. 22) was their top goal for a sports program for their child (Alexander & Leather, 2013). The parents also tended to prefer a unified sports setting (59%; one with children with and without disabilities paired together for participation), rather than segregated settings (22%; one where all of the children have a disability) or inclusive settings (20%; one where most children do not have a disability but those with disabilities may participate).

In a study examining the impact of unified sports programs for individuals with intellectual disability, across five different countries (Germany, Hungary, Poland, Serbia, and Ukraine), the athletes with ongoing participation reported improved social inclusion (McConkey, Dowling, Hassan, & Menke, 2013). In particular, the athletes with intellectual disabilities and the partners without intellectual disabilities reported benefits to interpersonal communication skills, especially confidence in talking with one another and building friendships (McConkey et al., 2013). For individuals with ASD and co-occurring intellectual disability, these results may be suggestive of similar gains in social inclusion during participation in unified sports programs. While this study has not been replicated with individuals with ASD, the benefits to improved social communication skills of the athletes with intellectual disability are noteworthy.

SLPs can encourage participation in community recreational athletic events for children with ASD. SLPs may also play a critical role in supporting communication to allow for participation in recreational activities, including adapting AAC equipment to include relevant functional communication messages for athletes with ASD. Key benefits of athletic programs that include youth with and without disabilities playing together, include improved social communication skills, social inclusion, and relationship building among community members.

Interprofessional Education and Interprofessional Practice (IPE/IPP)

Intersectionality: Interprofessional Practice and "Best-Practice"

In the school setting, students benefit when SLPs work collaboratively with other educators, using co-teaching models (Heisler & Thousand, 2019; Justice, McGinty, Guy, & Moore, 2009). Heisler and Thousand (2019) describe four approaches to co-teaching: supportive, parallel, complementary, and team. Co-teaching methods are appropriate for children in preschool through high school.

In a supportive co-teaching model, one professional teaches a lesson while the other circulates to support student learning (Heisler & Thousand, 2019). For example, the SLP may provide a whole-class lesson on social communication skills in an inclusion classroom with children who have ASD and those without ASD. During the lesson, the general education teacher may circulate to support all of the students' learning during the lesson.

In a parallel co-teaching model, one professional works with a group of children while the other professional works with the remaining children simultaneously (Heisler & Thousand, 2019). If the lesson is about social communication skills, children may circulate around stations in the room that each focus on different components of social communication. The stations could focus on areas of social communication difficulty for both children with ASD and for children with language impairments (see Gerber, Brice, Capone, Fujiki, & Timler, 2012), who are likely to be in inclusion classrooms together. The SLP and classroom teacher should work together to identify areas of social communication to target based on the cohort of children in the classroom. Areas of focus may include verbal and nonverbal pragmatic skills (e.g., reading body language and facial expressions, making polite requests, taking turns when making comments, and providing polite feedback) and social communication situations (e.g., joining a conversation, working cooperatively, and resolving conflicts).

Complementary co-teaching involves one professional supporting differentiated instruction while the other provides the general classroom lesson (Heisler & Thousand, 2019). For example, the classroom teacher may be teaching the students a science lesson and the SLP may serve as the complementary co-teacher to explain figurative language, identify new or difficult vocabulary words, help the students to stop and think about what they are learning, and model ways for students to self-advocate when repeated instruction or further explanation is required (Heisler & Thousand, 2019).

Team co-teaching involves co-responsibility for teaching a class of students together (Heisler & Thousand, 2019). In the team co-teaching model, both professionals take responsibility for teaching all of the students in the classroom, not just the students on IEPs. SLPs involved in co-teaching would plan all lessons together with the co-teacher and may use supportive, parallel, or complementary co-teaching methods when teaching the students. In particular, the SLP can contribute to the lesson planning by recommending specific ways to target the goals of the children on IEPs while planning the lesson for the entire class together with the co-teacher (Heisler & Thousand, 2019).

Limitations and Conclusions

Interprofessional and interdisciplinary practice requires many resources (time and money related to service delivery and continuing education) in order to provide comprehensive and collaborative assessment and treatment (Archibald, 2017; Bauer et al., 2010; Gotham, Bishop, & Lord, 2011). Baker, Egan-Lee, Martimianakis, & Reeves (2011) interviewed nurses, OTs, pharmacists, PTs, SLPs, and social workers regarding the collaboration of health care. Results indicated that "inappropriate consultations" may result from professionals who do not understand each other's roles and scopes of practice.

Research investigating the clinical effectiveness of interprofessional practice compared to other models of collaboration (e.g., multidisciplinary and interdisciplinary) is limited (Archibald, 2017; Cirrin et al., 2010). Available studies tend to focus on the explanation of service delivery approaches rather than fidelity measures and effectiveness outcomes (Bruce & Bashinski, 2017; Ogletree, 2017; Pfeiffer et al., 2019). Professionals who practice collaboratively need to demonstrate clinical competence in their professional area of expertise, knowledge of the professional scope of practice of their team members, openness to inquiry and collaborative problem-solving, frequent communication among team members, and a focus on caring for optimal client/patient/student outcomes (Ogletree, 2017). Clinical SLPs are encouraged to use reason-based practice and local outcomes data to inform clinical decision-making, in the absence of available evidence to inform best practice regarding models of collaboration (Archibald, 2017; Cirrin et al., 2010).

Interprofessional practice and best practice are likely to become more synonymous in the coming decade. ASHA has created a 2018–2025 initiative to increase interprofessional education, practice, and research in the fields of speech-language pathology and audiology. ASHA has adopted the World Health Organization definition of interprofessional collaborative practice (IPP; WHO, 2010). ASHA's definition of IPP is "when multiple service providers from different professional backgrounds provide comprehensive healthcare or educational services by working with individuals and their families, caregivers, and communities- to deliver the highest quality of care across settings" (ASHA practice portal, n.d.). The focus of IPP is not on one professional field but on collaboration across disciplines, in all settings. Clinicians and researchers working in the field of ASD are well suited for excellence in interprofessional practice and with further research, current effective collaborative clinical practice models for youth with ASD are likely to inform future best practice in the fields of speech-language pathology, occupational therapy, physical therapy, education, psychology, and more.

Acknowledgement Thank you to Kristine Philbin, OT, OTR, MS for contributing examples of clinical collaborations including occupational therapy and speech-language pathology services.

Appendix A

Resources to further your study of speech-language pathology interprofessional practice service coordination for individuals with autism spectrum disorder:

ASHA Interprofessional Practice Resources

- Video about interprofessional practice service coordination for students with autism spectrum disorders: https://www.scsha.net/asha-ipp-autism-spectrum-disorders
- Interprofessional practice case vignette of a kindergartener with autism spectrum disorder: https://www.asha.org/uploadedFiles/Kindergarten-ASD-Vignette.pdf
- Interprofessional practice case rubric for a kindergartener with autism spectrum disorder: https://www.asha.org/uploadedFiles/Kindergarten-ASD-Rubric.pdf

- American Journal of Speech-Language Pathology (Wilkinson, 2017) clinical forum on interprofessional collaborative practice for individuals with severe disabilities, including those with ASD and co-occurring conditions (e.g., intellectual disability): https://pubs.asha.org/toc/ajslp/26/2.

Appendix B

Case Examples

Case Collaboration Example 1: Cooking Group

Once a week, three middle-school-age boys with autism participated in a cooking group. The boys attended their local public middle school with IEPs and were learning in a sub-separate classroom with minimal to no inclusion time with peers learning in general education classrooms. The speech-language pathologist, occupational therapist, and special education teacher joined the three boys weekly for a cooking group, to work collaboratively on communication, activities of daily living, and academic goals. The cooking supplies and materials were set up in order to facilitate communication, fine motor development, sensory regulation, and learning of mathematical concepts. One set of measuring cups was shared so that the students had opportunities to practice making verbal requests to peers and teachers. A variety of ingredients were measured, poured, and stirred to encourage bilateral hand skills, tolerance to sensory experiences, and self-regulation during the group. Ingredients were measured and counted to encourage mathematical practices. The SLP, OT, and special education teacher were all responsible for supporting the students and collaborated to ensure that each goal area was addressed during each cooking group session.

Case Collaboration Example 2: Executive Summary Cards

In a public school with a specialized unit for children on the autism spectrum, maladaptive behaviors increased when regular staff members were absent and substitutes were in the classroom. The substitute teachers often felt overwhelmed, and complained that they could not easily find the information needed to follow the behavior plans on the students' IEPs because it was buried in password-protected online systems and/or lengthy printed IEP documents. The special education teachers, occupational therapist, speech language pathologist, and behavioral specialist collaborated to create an "Executive Summary" for each student, formatted in an easy to follow bulleted list, including pictures of the students, successful behavior strategies with specific phrasing, triggers, and behaviors to watch for (e.g., running away or hair-pulling). Each student's individual schedule was also included in the one-page executive summary. The executive summary was then kept in a special folder for substitutes, which they could access and take with them for the day.

The executive summary also facilitated increased communication and collaboration among team members after the team came together to create cards for each child.

Appendix C

Once a week, three middle-school-age boys with autism participated in a cooking group. The boys attended their local public middle school with IEPs and were learning in a sub-separate classroom with minimal to no inclusion time with peers learning in general education classrooms. The speech-language pathologist, occupational therapist, and special education teacher joined the three boys weekly for a cooking group, to work collaboratively on communication, activities of daily living, and academic goals. The cooking supplies and materials were set up in order to facilitate communication, fine motor development, sensory regulation, and learning of mathematical concepts. One set of measuring cups was shared so that the students had opportunities to practice making verbal requests to peers and teachers. A variety of ingredients were measured, poured, and stirred to encourage bilateral hand skills, tolerance to sensory experiences, and self-regulation during the group. Ingredients were measured and counted to encourage mathematical practices. The SLP, OT, and special education teacher were all responsible for supporting the students and collaborated to ensure that each goal area was addressed during each cooking group session.

In a public school with a specialized unit for children on the autism spectrum, maladaptive behaviors increased when regular staff members were absent and substitutes were in the classroom. The substitute teachers often felt overwhelmed, and complained that they could not easily find the information needed to follow the behavior plans on the students' IEPs because it was buried in password-protected online systems and/or lengthy printed IEP documents. The special education teachers, occupational therapist, speech language pathologist, and behavioral specialist collaborated to create an "Executive Summary" for each student, formatted in an easy to follow bulleted list, including pictures of the students, successful behavior strategies with specific phrasing, triggers, and behaviors to watch for (e.g., running away or hair-pulling). Each student's individual schedule was also included in the one-page.

References

Alexander, M. G. F., & Leather, R. C. (2013). Parents' perspectives on appropriate sports programs for children with autism spectrum disorders. *Palestra, 27*(4), 20–24.

Alli, A., Abdoola, S., & Mupawose, A. (2015). Parents' journey into the world of autism. *South African Journal of Child Health, 9*(3), 81–84.

American Psychiatric Association. (2013). *Diagnostic and statistical manual of mental disorders* (5th ed.). Washington, DC: Author.
American Speech-Language-Hearing Association. (2016). Scope of practice in speech-language pathology [Scope of Practice]. www.asha.org/policy.
American Speech-Language-Hearing Association. (n.d.). Interprofessional education/interprofessional practice. https://www.asha.org/Practice/Interprofessional-Education-Practice/
Archibald, L. M. (2017). SLP-educator classroom collaboration: A review to inform reason-based practice. *Autism & Developmental Language Impairments, 2,* 1–17.
Baker, L., Egan-Lee, E., Martimianakis, M. A., & Reeves, S. (2011). Relationships of power: implications for interprofessional education. *Journal of Interprofessional Care, 25*(2), 98–104.
Bauer, K. L., Iyer, S. N., Boon, R. T., & Fore, C. (2010). 20 ways for classroom teachers to collaborate with Speech-Language Pathologists. *Intervention in School and Clinic, 45,* 333–337.
Betancur, C. (2011). Etiological heterogeneity in autism spectrum disorders: More than 100 genetic and genomic disorders and still counting. *Brain Research, 1380,* 42–77.
Binns, A. V., & Oram Cardy, J. (2019). Developmental social pragmatic interventions for preschoolers with autism spectrum disorder: A systematic review. *Autism & Developmental Language Impairments, 4*(1), 1–18.
Bruce, S. M., & Bashinski, S. M. (2017). The trifocus framework and interprofessional collaborative practice in severe disabilities. *American Journal of Speech-Language Pathology, 26*(2), 162–180.
Cirrin, F. M., Schooling, T. L., Nelson, N. W., Diehl, S. F., Flynn, P. F., Staskowski, M., et al. (2010). Evidence-based systematic review: Effects of different service delivery models on communication outcomes for elementary school-age children. *Language, Speech, and Hearing Services in Schools, 41,* 223–264.
Davidson, M. M., & Ellis Weismer, S. (2014). Characterization and prediction of early reading abilities in children on the autism spectrum. *Journal of Autism and Developmental Disorders, 44*(4), 828–845.
Dynia, J. M., Bean, A., Justice, L. M., & Kaderavek, J. N. (2019). Phonological awareness emergence in preschool children with autism spectrum disorder. *Autism & Developmental Language Impairments, 4,* 1–15.
Gerber, S., Brice, A., Capone, N., Fujiki, M., & Timler, G. (2012). Language use in social interactions of school-age children with language impairments: An evidence-based systematic review of treatment. *Language, Speech, and Hearing Services in Schools, 43,* 235–249.
Gotham, K., Bishop, S. L., & Lord, C. (2011). Diagnosis of autism spectrum disorders. In D. Amaral, D. Geshwind, & G. Dawson (Eds.), *autism spectrum disorders* (pp. 30–43). New York: Oxford University Press.
Hayward, L. M., Fragala-Pinkham, M., Johnson, K., & Torres, A. (2016). A community-based, adaptive soccer program for children with autism: Design, implementation, and evaluation. *Palaestra, 30*(4), 44–50.
Heisler, L. A., & Thousand, J. S. (2019). A guide to co-teaching for the SLP: A tutorial. *Communication Disorders Quarterly*, 1–6.
Hollenbeck, A. F. (2007). From IDEA to implementation: A discussion of foundational and future responsiveness-to-intervention research. *Learning Disabilities Research & Practice 22*(2), 137–146.
Individuals with Disabilities Education Improvement Act (IDEA) of 2004, PL 108–446, 20 USC §§ 1400 et seq.
Johnson, A. (2016). *Interprofessional education and interprofessional practice in communication sciences and disorders: An introduction and case-based examples of implementation in education and health care settings*. Rockville, MD: American Speech-Language-Hearing Association. Retrieved from https://www.asha.org/uploadedFiles/IPE-IPP-Reader-eBook.pdf.
Justice, L. M., McGinty, A., Guo, Y., & Moore, D. (2009). Implementation of responsiveness to intervention in early education settings. *Seminar in Speech Language Pathology, 30,* 59–74.

Kasari, C., Brady, N., Lord, C., & Tager-Flusberg, H. (2013). Assessing the minimally verbal school-aged child with autism spectrum disorder. *Autism Research, 6*(6), 479–493.
Kjelgaard, M. M., & Tager-Flusberg, H. (2001). An investigation of language impairment in autism: Implications for genetic subgroups. *Language and Cognitive Processes, 16*(2–3), 287–308.
Koegel, R. L., Werner, G. A., Vismara, L. A., & Koegel, L. K. (2005). The effectiveness of contextually supported play date interactions between children with autism and typically developing peers. *Research and Practice for Persons with Severe Disabilities, 30*(2), 93–102.
Koegel, L. K., Koegel, R. L., Ashbaugh, K., & Bradshaw, J. (2014). The importance of early identification and intervention for children with or at risk for autism spectrum disorders. *International Journal of Speech-Language Pathology, 16*(1), 50–56.
Lanter, E., & Watson, L. R. (2008). Promoting literacy in students with ASD: The basics for the SLP. *Language, Speech, and Hearing Services in Schools., 39*(1), 33–43.
Leach, D. (2018). Using multi-tiered systems of support for students with autism spectrum disorders in inclusive classrooms. *Journal of the Division on Autism and Developmental Disabilities, 5*(1), 6–17.
McConkey, R., Dowling, S., Hassan, D., & Menke, S. (2013). Promoting social inclusion through Unified Sports for youth with intellectual disabilities: A five-nation study. *Journal of Intellectual Disability Research, 57*(10), 923–935.
McGregor, K. K., Berns, A. J., Owen, A. J., Michels, S. A., Duff, D., Bahnsen, A. J., et al. (2012). Associations between syntax and the lexicon among children with or without ASD and language impairment. *Journal of Autism and Developmental Disorders, 42*(1), 35–47.
Ogletree, B. T. (2017). Addressing the communication and other needs of persons with severe disabilities through engaged interprofessional teams: Introduction to a clinical forum. *American Journal of Speech-Language Pathology, 26*(2), 157–161.
Orsmond, G. I., Krauss, M. W., & Seltzer, M. M. (2004). Peer relationships and social and recreational activities among adolescents and adults with autism. *Journal of Autism and Developmental Disorders, 34*(3), 245–256.
Ozonoff, S., Iosif, A. M., Baguio, F., Cook, I. C., Hill, M. M., Hutman, T., … & Steinfeld, M. B. (2010). A prospective study of the emergence of early behavioral signs of autism. *Journal of the American Academy of Child & Adolescent Psychiatry, 49*(3), 256–266.
Pelphrey, K. A., Shultz, S., Hudac, C. M., & Vander Wyk, B. C. (2011). Research review: Constraining heterogeneity: The social brain and its development in autism spectrum disorder. *Journal of Child Psychology and Psychiatry, 52*(6), 631–644.
Pfeiffer, D. L., Pavelko, S. L., Hahs-Vaughn, D. L., & Dudding, C. C. (2019). A national survey of speech-language pathologists' engagement in interprofessional collaborative practice in schools: Identifying predictive factors and barriers to implementation. *Language, Speech, and Hearing Services in Schools, 50*(4), 639–655.
Prelock, P. A., & McCauley, R. J. (2012). *Treatment of Autism Spectrum Disorders*. Baltimore: Brooks Publishing.
Tager-Flusberg, H., & Joseph, R. M. (2003). Identifying neurocognitive phenotypes in autism. *Philosophical Transactions of the Royal Society of London. Series B: Biological Sciences, 358*(1430), 303–314.
Tracy-Bronson, C. P., Causton, J. N., & MacLeod, K. M. (2019). Everybody has the right to be here: Perspectives of related service therapists. *International Journal of Whole Schooling, 15*(1), 132–174.
Wagner, A. L., Wallace, K. S., & Rogers, S. J. (2014). Developmental approaches to treatment of young children with autism spectrum disorder. *Handbook of Early Intervention for Autism Spectrum Disorders* (pp. 393–427). New York, NY: Springer.
Wilkinson, K. M. (Ed.). (2017) Clinical forum: Interprofessional collaborative practices in service delivery for individuals with severe disabilities [Special issue]. *American Journal of Speech Language Pathology, 26*(2).
Wong, C., Odom, S. L., Hume, K. A., Cox, A. W., Fettig, A., Kucharczyk, S., … & Schultz, T. R. (2015). Evidence-based practices for children, youth, and young adults with autism spectrum

disorder: A comprehensive review. *Journal of autism and developmental disorders, 45*(7), 1951–1966.

World Health Organization. (2010). Framework for action on interprofessional education and collaborative practice. World Health Organization.

World Health Organization. (2013). Interprofessional collaborative practice in primary health care: nursing and midwifery perspectives: six case studies. *Human Resources for Health Observer, 13*, 1–24.

Care Coordination in Primary Care

Tyanna C. Snider, Kristen E. Beck, and Rebecca A. Baum

Abstract Families embarking on the journey of ASD evaluation and treatment face a complex road ahead, and the Primary Care Clinician (PCC) can play a key role in navigating that journey successfully in the context of the medical home. Given the high frequency at which children visit their PCCs in early childhood, PCCs participate in early identification through developmental surveillance and screening and provide referrals for children who require further evaluation. Throughout childhood, PCCs facilitate crucial linkages to community resources and specialty providers while also providing routine preventive care to children with Autism Spectrum Disorder (ASD). To varying degrees, PCCs provide direct care for co-occurring medical or mental conditions and assist families in securing treatment services. To execute this role effectively, modifications to the medical home may be necessary. This chapter provides an overview of the knowledge, processes, and skills necessary to provide comprehensive care coordination for children with ASD in the medical home setting.

Care coordination is defined by the American Academy of Pediatrics (AAP) as a "process that facilitates linkage of children and their families with appropriate services and resources in a coordinated effort to achieve good health" (AAP Council on Children with Disabilities, 2005; p. 1238). Primary Care Clinicians (PCCs) recognize the need for care coordination, particularly for children with special healthcare needs; however, PCCs report a need for increased knowledge and training, time, and resources to provide high-quality and effective care coordination (AAP Council

T. C. Snider (✉)
Division of Pediatric Psychology and Neuropsychology, Nationwide Children's Hospital, Columbus, OH, USA
e-mail: tyanna.snider@nationwidechildrens.org

K. E. Beck
Clinical Assistant Professor of Pediatrics, Nationwide Children's Hospital, The Ohio State University College of Medicine, Columbus, OH, USA

R. A. Baum
Clinical Associate Professor of Pediatrics, Division of Developmental Behavioral Pediatrics, Nationwide Children's Hospital, The Ohio State University College of Medicine, Columbus, OH, USA

M. B. McClain et al. (eds.), *Interprofessional Care Coordination for Pediatric Autism Spectrum Disorder*, https://doi.org/10.1007/978-3-030-46295-6_17

on Children with Disabilities, 2005; Lobar, 2015). Care coordination is a dynamic process and may vary for each individual, child, or family. As such, the roles and responsibilities for a PCC in a care coordination team are also dynamic, making collaboration and coordination even more challenging. The AAP (2005; p. 1239) suggests that PCCs be aware of "the array of available subspecialty services, know when these services are needed, know how to gain access to and advocate for subspecialty care within health plans, and know how to use subspecialists' recommendations and communicate" this information to families and patients. Recent figures indicate that 11 out of every 1,000 children cared for in the medical home by the PCC have, or will eventually receive, a diagnosis of autism spectrum disorder (ASD; Will et al., 2013; Baio, 2008). Effective care coordination for this population of children includes the use of developmental screeners to aid in early identification of delays and symptoms of ASD, organizing care activities such as linking with treatment or referrals for evaluations or to specialty providers, and sharing and communicating concerns or information with the treatment team to ensure safe, appropriate, high-quality, and effective care. Well-executed care coordination can improve outcomes for the patient and family, treatment team members, and payers (Agency for Healthcare Research and Quality, 2018). This is particularly important for children with ASD as this population has increased mortality rates and greater healthcare utilization (Myers & Johnson, 2007). In order to provide effective care coordination, education and training related to identification, evaluation, and intervention for children with ASD is crucial. This chapter highlights the role of the PCC in care coordination between the patient's medical home, school, community, and other specialty providers.

Developmental Screening in the Pediatric Primary Care Center

The medical home is the cornerstone in identifying, evaluating, and providing services to children with ASD. The concept of the medical home has been in development for several decades and emphasizes the importance of developing a continuous partnership between the PCC, child, and family characterized by mutual responsibility and trust (AAP Medical Home Initiatives for Children with Special Needs Project Advisory Committee, 2002; Sia, Tonniges, Osterhus, & Taba, 2004). The AAP recommends that care in the medical home be accessible, continuous, comprehensive, family centered, coordinated, compassionate, and culturally effective (AAP, 2008; AAP Medical Home Initiatives for Children with Special Needs Project Advisory Committee, 2002). This includes developmental surveillance and screening to identify children with developmental delays, including ASD. When developmental surveillance and/or screening reveals a concern, the PCC assists with linkage to community-based services (e.g., early intervention, the educational system, or specialty providers). By collaborating with related service sectors (early intervention programs, early childhood education and childcare programs, public and private community agencies), PCCs can ensure that the needs of the child and family are addressed and that services are coordinated to realize maximum benefit for children with special healthcare needs (Rushton, 2005).

The AAP developed the Bright Futures guidelines as a set of principles and strategies to improve the health and well-being of all children. Bright Futures recommends developmental surveillance at each well-child check (newborn through 36 months). In addition, standardized developmental screening should be performed at ages 9, 18, and 30 months and ASD-specific screening should be performed at ages 18 and 24 months to assist with early identification and management of developmental concerns (Chlebowski, Robins, Barton, & Fein, 2013; AAP Committee on Children with Disabilities, 2001a, 2001b; Hagan, Shaw, & Duncan, 2017).

Developmental surveillance has been defined by Dworkin (1993; p. 533) as "a flexible, continuous process whereby knowledgeable professionals perform skilled observations of children during the provision of health care. Developmental surveillance includes eliciting and attending to parental concerns, obtaining a relevant developmental history, making accurate and informative observations of children, and sharing opinions and concerns with other relevant professionals." Developmental surveillance is a cumulative process, leveraging the trusted relationship that develops between the PCC, child, and family over time (Dworkin, 1993).

When performing developmental surveillance, PCCs should pay particular attention to communication and social development in children over the age of 1. Speech delays are the most common developmental concern for parents of children between 1 and 3 years old and warrant additional evaluation for hearing concerns, speech disorders, and ASD (AAP Committee on Children with Disabilities, 2001a, 2001b). Specific red flags include failure to respond to name, poor eye contact, lack of response to speech directed toward the child, delay in language development, or impairment in joint attention skills (i.e., child's lack of showing and pointing or failure to follow a caregiver's gaze or pointing; AAP Committee on Children with Disabilities, 2001a, 2001b; Dworkin, 1993; Hagan et al., 2017; Johnson & Myers, 2007; Richards, Mossey, & Robins, 2016).

Bright Futures also recommends all children be screened for developmental delays through the use of standardized developmental screening tools at 9 months, 18 months, and 30 months or if there is a concern (see chapter "Screening and Surveillance" for further information; AAP Committee on Children with Disabilities, 2001a, 2001b, 2006; Hagan et al., 2017). Screening refers to the use of a brief, standardized tool to identify children at risk for developmental delays and who require further evaluation (Marks & LaRosa, 2012). Standardized screening is more sensitive than relying on developmental surveillance alone, even for experienced practitioners (AAP Committee on Children with Disabilities, 2001a, 2001b). Periodic use of general developmental and social-emotional screening tools have been shown to identify two to six times more children with suspected delays than surveillance alone, leading to increased eligibility rates for early intervention and special education services (Marks & LaRosa, 2012). Screening may be the first indication a child warrants further evaluation for ASD (Rushton, 2005). PCCs have noted barriers to screening, including lack of familiarity with tools, difficulty with scoring, and lack of office-based systems for making referrals and monitoring outcomes (Zwaigenbaum et al., 2015a, 2015b).

Developmental Screening Instruments (See Table 1 for Summary of Developmental Screeners)

Ages and Stages Questionnaires. The Ages and Stages Questionnaire, Third Edition (**ASQ-3**) is an assessment tool that screens five developmental areas in children of 1–66 months of age: (1) communication, (2) gross motor, (3) fine motor, (4) problem-solving, and (5) personal-social skills. Caregivers indicate the child's developmental skills on 30 items plus overall concerns (Squires & Bricker, 2009).

The Ages and Stages Questionnaire: Social-Emotional, Second Edition (ASQ:SE-2) is an assessment tool for children between 1 and 72 months of age which evaluates self-regulation, compliance, social-communication, adaptive functioning, autonomy, affect, and interaction with people. Caregivers answer 31 developmental questions about their child and 3 questions about overall concerns. An ASD-specific screener should be used in addition to the ASQ screens at 18 and 24 months of age (Squires, Bricker, & Twombly, 2015).

Survey of Well-being of Young Children (SWYC). The SWYC measures three domains: (1) developmental milestones, (2) behavioral/emotional development, and (3) family risk factors. Ten questions ask about motor, language, social and cognitive development. A scoring chart based on the child's age in months determines whether the child's total score falls into the "Needs Review" or "Appears to Meet Age Expectations" category. If a child's score falls into the "Needs Review" category, the PCC must consider how far from the threshold the score is, interview the caregiver to confirm the answers, and then decide if active monitoring or referral is warranted. Of note, cutoff scores are not available for the 2- and 60-month forms (Perrin, Sheldrick, Visco, & Mattern, 2016).

To assess behavioral/emotional development, caregivers complete the Baby Pediatric Symptom Checklist (BPSC) or the Preschool Pediatric Symptom Checklist (PPSC) as part of the SWYC. The BPSC consists of 12 items divided into three subscales, each with 4 items. A 9-item questionnaire assesses family risk factors, including tobacco and substance use in the home, food insecurity, and caregiver depression. A positive answer in this section requires further discussion with the caregiver to determine the appropriate intervention. Finally, caregivers complete two questions asking for their concerns, which can be used to facilitate further discussion (Sheldrick et al., 2012a, 2012b).

Parents' Evaluations of Developmental Status (PEDS). The Parents' Evaluations of Developmental Status (PEDS) consists of 10 questions eliciting parents' verbatim concerns about learning, development, behavior, speech, gross motor, fine motor, and social relationships. The same 10 questions are used across the age range of PEDS from birth to 8 years, and the scoring form identifies which concerns predict problems. An interpretation form provides an algorithm of evidence-based next steps for deciding whether to refer, screen further, monitor, counsel parents, or provide reassurance. The interpretation form provides a place to record and track these decisions and action steps (Glascoe, 2018).

Parents' Evaluation of Developmental Status: Developmental Milestones (PEDS: DM) was designed to replace milestone checklists. It consists of 6–8 multiple choice items at each age level. Each item measures a different domain: fine/gross motor, self-help, academics, expressive and receptive language, and social-emotional skills. Parents are then encouraged to read their child a short story that is presented in the book on the opposite page. These stories focus on child development and positive parenting practices. Performing at or below the 16th percentile is the cutoff value for referral (Glascoe, 2018).

ASD Specific Screeners

In addition to general developmental screeners, specific screening for ASD should be performed at 18 and 24 months of age (AAP Council on Children with Disabilities, 2006). Early identification and referral of children with ASD result in improved prognosis (AAP Council on Children with Disabilities, 2006; Hagan et al., 2017). Two common screening tools discussed below are the Modified Checklist for Autism in Toddlers, Revised with Follow-Up (MCHAT-R/F) and POSI. Both the MCHAT-R/F and POSI have had numerous validation studies (Chlebowski et al., 2013; Robins et al., 2014; Sanchez-Garcia, Galindo-Villardon, Nieto-Librero, Martin-Rodero, & Robins, 2019; Salisbury et al., 2018; Smith, Sheldrick, & Perrin, 2013).

Modified Checklist for Autism in Toddlers, Revised with Follow-up (MCHAT-R/F). The MCHAT-R/F is a 2-stage caregiver-report screening tool to assess risk for ASD and should be administered to children between 16 and 30 months of age. The screening tool consists of 20 yes/no questions (Robins, 2019). A score of 0–2 is low risk for ASD. The child is screened negative and no additional action is needed at that visit. If the child is less than 24 months of age at the time of the initial screen, a second screen should be performed at 24 months of age. Even in light of a negative screen, referral for early intervention services and/or diagnostic evaluation is still indicated if developmental surveillance suggests risk for ASD. A score of 3–7 is moderate risk for ASD. The next step should be to administer the MCHAT-R/F follow-up screen and refer the child for early intervention services and a diagnostic evaluation as needed. A score of 8–20 is high risk. The child should be referred for diagnostic evaluation and early intervention services (Robins, 2019). Approximately 54% of children who screened positive on the M-CHAT and M-CHAT-R/F were diagnosed with ASD, and 98% presented with clinically significant developmental concerns warranting intervention (Chlebowski et al., 2013).

Parent's Observations of Social Interactions (POSI). A second specific screening tool for ASD is the Parent's Observations of Social Interactions (POSI). This

Table 1 Developmental screener comparison table

	ASQ-3; ASQ:SE-2	SWYC	PEDS; PEDS: DM
Age range	1–66 months	2–60 months	Birth–8 years
Questionnaire items	21 age-specific questionnaires	Subscales on developmental milestones, behavior, and family risk factors. For certain ages, a section for autism-specific screening (POSI) is included.	10 open-ended questions for all ages PEDS: DM 6–8 milestones type items
Developmental domains	ASQ3: communication, gross motor, fine motor, problem-solving, and personal-social skills; ASQ:SE-2: self-regulation, compliance, adaptive functioning, autonomy, affect, social communication, and interaction with others	Cognitive, language, motor, behavior, social-emotional interaction	Expressive language, receptive language, fine motor, gross motor, social-emotional, self-help, academics in both reading and math (older children)
Time to complete	10–15 min	10 min	2–5 min
Time to score	2–3 min	2–3 min to scores	1–2 min
Sensitivity	86%	76% (SWYC Milestones) Above 70% (PPSC) 93.6% (POSI 6–30 months) 75% (POSI 31–48 months)	74–80%
Specificity	85%	77% (SWYC Milestones) Above 70% (PPSC) 40.8% (POSI 6–30 months) 47.8% (POSI 31–48 months)	70–80%
Reading level	4th–6th grade	Unknown	PEDS: 4th–5th grade DM: 1st–2nd grade

(continued)

Table 1 (continued)

	ASQ-3; ASQ:SE-2	SWYC	PEDS; PEDS: DM
Cost	ASQ-3 Starter Kit: $295.00. Includes: ASQ-3 User's Guide, ASQ3 Quick-Start Guide, and a photocopiable print master set of 21 questionnaires and scoring sheets, as well as a CD-ROM with printable PDF questionnaires. No ongoing costs	Free	PEDS: DM plus PEDS: $346.00. Includes the PEDS: DM starter kit plus 100 PEDS Response Forms and the PEDS Brief Guide The PEDS: DM Recording Form (100 supplied with each order) includes the PEDS Scoring/Interpretation Form, PEDS Response Forms (pad of 50): $19.50. PEDS Score/Interpretation Forms (pad of 50): $19.50 PEDS: DM Recording Forms (100): $57.00
Languages	English, Spanish, Arabic, Chinese, French, and Vietnamese	English, Spanish, Khmer, Burmese, Nepali, Portuguese Haitian Creole, and Arabic	English and Spanish. Additional languages available to license
Training Options	DVD training: ASQ-3 Scoring and Referral, ASQ on a Home Visit; on-site customized seminars offered through Brookes On Location professional development program; annual "train-the-trainer" institutes	Instructions are included in the SWYC User's Manual, available online	Using PEDS: DM instructional video, PowerPoint slide shows, and additional downloadable training material available on website
Publisher	Brookes Publishing	Tufts Medical Center	PEDStest, LLC

Note Ages and Stages Questionnaire, Third edition (ASQ-3) is from Squires and Bricker (2009); the Ages and Stages Questionnaire: Social Emotional, Second edition (ASQ:SE-2) is from Squires et al. (2015); the Screening for Well-being of Young Children (SWYC) is from Perrin et al. (2016); the Parent's Observation of Social Interaction (POSI) is from Smith et al. (2013); the Parents' Evaluation of Developmental Status (PEDS) is from Glascoe et al. (2018); the Parents' Evaluation of Developmental Status: Developmental Milestones (PEDS: DM) is from Glascoe et al. (2018)

screen is part of the SWYC developmental milestones domain and consists of seven questions about social interactions. The POSI is administered between 16 and 35 months of age and is part of the 18-, 24-, and 30-month SWYC forms. Caregivers choose responses on a Likert scale for the first five questions and a range of developmental skills for the last two questions. A scoring guide is provided to identify positive responses. There is a maximum of seven potential points for this screening tool. A score of 3 or more indicates that a child is "at risk" and needs further evaluation or investigation (Smith et al., 2013).

Diagnostic Evaluation for Autism Spectrum Disorder

For some families, discussing concerns about the possibility of ASD can be difficult. This discussion may arise as part of the screening process during health supervision visits or because parents, family members or friends, or other professionals have voiced concerns. Families may approach the discussion with relief, as a possible explanation for their child's behavior, or with resistance or surprise (DePape & Lindsay, 2015).

Additional aspects unique to ASD can further complicate the evaluation process. The range of functioning and challenging behavior in children with ASD is vast, and a comprehensive evaluation can assist in clarifying the child's current strengths and challenges (Charman et al., 2011; McGuire et al., 2016). However, wait times for specialty evaluation are often long, leaving concerned parents with unanswered questions for months (Stein et al., 2018). Best practices suggest that an ASD evaluation be comprehensive, taking into account the child's level of cognition, communication, social-emotional skills, mental health, and behavior, as well as medical factors such as sleep and nutrition (Volkmar et al., 2014). This type of evaluation is best performed by an interprofessional team (e.g., speech and language pathology, developmental-behavioral pediatrics, neurology, and psychology). In addition to a comprehensive history based on Diagnostic and Statistical Manual of Mental Disorders, 5th Edition (DSM-5) criteria, the evaluation should ideally include measures of intelligence, adaptive functioning, and communication (American Psychiatric Association, 2013). The evaluation may also include the Autism Diagnostic Observation Schedule-2 (ADOS-2) which is a semi-structured, play-based assessment used to characterize a child's behavior to provide a more standardized determination of autistic features (Lord et al., 2012; see chapter "Interdisciplinary Evaluation of Autism Spectrum Disorder" for more information).

These best practices may be difficult to access in some communities due to workforce shortages, payment issues, or transportation difficulties (Baller et al., 2016; Ning et al., 2019; US Department of Health and Human Services, 2018). Evaluation teams may be comprised of different team members in different communities. Partnerships between specialists, PCCs, the educational system and/or early intervention have been developed in some communities in an effort to improve access to interprofessional evaluation. For inter-agency collaboration to be most effective, additional layers of planning are necessary, such as identifying processes to exchange protected health information, defining roles and responsibilities, determining procedures for billing and chart documentation.

Given the reality of long wait times for a possibly life-changing diagnosis, PCCs can assist families by providing recommendations for what families *can* do while a referral is pending. For children ages 0–3, families should contact their state's early intervention program for evaluation, intervention, and care coordination services that are available regardless of income. For children of age 3 and older, evaluation and intervention services are available through the child's local school district. High-quality resource materials on early identification, the evaluation process, and recommended interventions should be readily available in a variety of different formats. Some families prefer print materials, video clips, websites, or even talking with another family who has been through a similar experience. Identifying these resources ahead of time can make a difficult visit go more smoothly and provide the family with a sense of agency.

As families face a seemingly daunting journey, knowing that their PCC will be helping them navigate the process can be comforting. Identifying ways for the practice to "lighten the load" can make a complex process seem more manageable. Increasingly, practices are finding ways to define and implement care coordination services to provide families with assistance in managing payment denials, transportation issues, and referral linkage. These services may also be available through community agencies and sometimes through payers, so being aware of local resources is important. Identifying a "resource coordinator" at the practice to ensure that resources are kept current and are of high quality can be a useful way of managing this information. Other, more formal processes include parent navigators (Feinberg et al., 2016; Roth et al., 2016).

Support After Diagnosis

The PCC's roles extend beyond recognition and evaluation and encompass ongoing care and medical management, including yearly preventive care, management of acute illnesses, and other unique medical conditions that frequently co-occur with ASD (Myers & Johnson, 2007). Patients and families benefit greatly when the pediatric medical home can provide support after diagnosis, yet this may vary between individual practices and communities (Monz, Houghton, Law, & Loss, 2019; Todorow, Connell, & Turchi, 2018). Practices in rural or underserved areas may play a larger role in ongoing care than those close to specialty centers. Because access to specialty services is often limited, the medical home is frequently called upon to help coordinate or in some cases provide some direct care for co-occurring conditions.

In an effort to support coordinated, best practice for children with ASD, changes to the medical home may be necessary (Shahidullah, Azad, Mezher, McClain, & McIntyre, 2018). PCCs should strive to maintain the schedule and content of health supervision visits, including developmentally appropriate anticipatory guidance for topics such as sleep, feeding, and safety issues while also considering the unique needs of children with ASD. Visits with immunizations or long wait times may be difficult. Scheduling these visits toward the end of a session may allow for extra time or resources, and staff may benefit from additional training (Van Cleave et al., 2018). Practices should become familiar with ASD management and the role of the medical home; a variety of resources are available through the Center for Disease Control and Prevention (CDC) at https://www.cdc.gov/ncbddd/autism/index.html. Family advisory groups can also be an important tool for practices to ensure they are meeting the needs of children and families (National Institute for Children's Health Quality). PCCs may wish to connect with community-based organizations or local chapters of national organizations that support children and families affected by ASD.

Children with ASD will require ongoing developmental monitoring and support, and the longitudinal nature of services delivered in primary care clinic provides an ideal setting. Children with ASD may qualify for special education services through the educational system, which provides a comprehensive evaluation to determine if a child qualifies for services, goal creation and monitoring, and periodic re-evaluation. These records provide valuable information and can be obtained from the school system once parental consent is obtained, as per the Family Educational Rights and Privacy Act (FERPA; US Department of Education, 1974). Children with ASD may benefit from additional services outside of the school system (e.g., speech therapy, occupational therapy, physical therapy, or social skills training). PCCs can assist with referrals and help caregivers prioritize intervention based upon their goals for their child.

The transition from childhood to adulthood bears a particular mention. Youth and families have much to consider during this time, including the promotion of health literacy, assessment of living arrangements and guardianship, accessing medical and subspecialty care, and navigating social relationships. Children who receive special education services may be eligible to remain in the educational system until their 22nd birthday (US Department of Education, 2017). Adolescence can be a difficult time for some individuals with ASD as they begin to recognize their limitations compared to peers and siblings. Higher functioning individuals may be able to participate in post-secondary education, and many individuals with ASD may be able to participate in vocational training (see chapter "Transition from Adolescence to Adulthood in Those Without a Comorbid Intellectual Disability").

Treatment and Intervention

While there is no cure for ASD, the goal for intervention is to address the core symptoms of ASD and management of associated features or deficits to promote optimal development and functioning (see chapter "Management" for more information; Myers & Johnson, 2007; Zwaigenbaum et al., 2015a, 2015b). A growing body of the literature identifies evidence-based practice and empirically supported treatments for ASD (Myers & Johnson, 2007; Maglione, Gans, Das, Timbie, & Kasari, 2012; Zwaigenbaum et al., 2015a, 2015b). As the core deficits of ASD impact multiple settings and areas of functioning, the treatment team should be comprised of specialists across multiple disciplines. Ensuring that treatment team members communicate with each other and share information is vital to the child's progress and helps alleviate family distress (Zwaigenbaum et al., 2015a, 2015b).

One of the primary developmental delays observed in children with ASD is expressive or receptive language delays. Caregivers may present to the PCC with concerns that their child is not responding to their name or has limited to no use of meaningful verbal language. Referrals to audiology and speech-language pathology initiated by the PCC may be the first steps in the evaluation process. Evaluation by early intervention or the educational system does not require a diagnosis of ASD or other developmental delay, and referrals to these services is an appropriate early step. Some speech language pathologists have expertise in the evaluation and management of feeding difficulties, which are common in children with ASD (see chapter "Coordinating Speech-Language Pathology Services for Youth with Autism Spectrum Disorder"; Marí-Bauset, Zazpe, Mari-Sanchis, Llopis-González, & Morales-Suárez-Varela, 2014).

Similarly, referrals to Occupational Therapy (OT) may be necessary in order to target fine motor delays or sensitivities to loud noises, lights, or specific textures of clothes or food that can be associated with ASD. Sensory activities may also be utilized as rewards or motivators for desired behaviors or help calm a child (Myers & Johnson, 2007). Like speech language pathologists, occupational therapists may also have expertise in evaluating and treatment feeding difficulties related to sensory challenges.

Specific Treatments for ASD

Over the past 30 years, intensive interventions and programs for young children have been developed and evaluated for efficacy and effectiveness (Myers & Johnson, 2007). These programs can be divided into three categorizations: behavioral or behavior analytic, developmental, and structured teaching. Programs may include more "eclectic" interventions and may utilize strategies or techniques from each approach as well as include complementary or alternative therapies (Myers & Johnson, 2007; Warren et al., 2011).

Behavioral. Behavioral interventions are often the cornerstone of treatment for children with an ASD diagnosis. One notable approach for behavioral treatment is Applied Behavior Analysis (ABA; Autism Speaks Autism Treatment Network, 2018; Centers for Disease Control and Prevention, 2019; Warren et al., 2011). ABA is "based on the principles of learning and behavior derived from experimental psychology" in order to increase positive behaviors and decrease negative or even harmful behaviors (Myers & Johnson, 2007; CDC 2019). ABA-based interventions are considered an evidence-based "best" practice by the American Psychology Association (APA) and US Surgeon General and have become widely accepted and used in school and other treatment settings (Autism Speaks Autism Treatment Network, 2018). Children who receive early intensive ABA-based therapies demonstrate substantial gains in cognitive functioning, language and communication skills, and adaptive and social behavior, however, methodological concerns exists (Autism Speaks Autism Treatment Network, 2018; Myers & Johnson, 2007; Warren et al., 2011). The AAP recommends a minimum of 25 h per week of high-quality comprehensive treatment intervention (Myers & Johnson, 2007; see chapter "Coordinating ABA Services" for more information).

Developmental. Developmental models use developmental theory to identify and help address deficits of the child with ASD. One well-known developmental intervention for young children is the Early Start Denver Model (ESDM; see chapter "The Early Start Denver Model (ESDM)"), which also includes the use of ABA techniques in a developmental framework. Recently, the ESDM has shifted toward a home or school-based delivery model in which teachers or caregivers can be trained by a therapist to implement and utilize this intervention (Myers & Johnson, 2007; Warren et al., 2011).

Greenspan and Wieder's (1999) Developmental, Individual-difference, and Relationship-based model (DIR) is another example of a developmental intervention model. Sometimes referred to as "floor-time," this intervention uses floor-time play sessions to foster emotional and relational development through social interactions (Center for Disease Control and Prevention; Greenspan & Wieder, 1999). It is important to note that evidence supporting the efficacy of DIR is limited and has methodological flaws (Myers & Johnson, 2007).

Structured teaching. The Treatment and Education of Autistic and related Communication-handicapped Children (TEACCH) is an example of a structured teaching intervention. This intervention recognizes the unique learning needs of children with ASD and emphasizes the use of external changes and supports to the physical environment to manage deficits in attention and executive functioning, use of visual cues combined with verbal communication, and structured activities and support to promote social communication. TEACCH is typically delivered in an educational setting but more recently it has been adapted for home-based delivery with caregivers as co-therapists alongside autism professionals (Mesibov & Shopler, 2004).

Intervention in the School Setting

At the age of 3, the educational system may serve as a primary setting in which interventions are provided for children with ASD (see chapter "Transition to Early Schooling for Children with ASD"). Early intervention services provided through an Individual Family Service Plan (IFSP) are transitioned to the local school district.

At this juncture, families are faced with making several decisions regarding schooling, primarily, the decision to send their child to a private school, a specialized or specific-ASD school, or the public school district. The Individuals with Disabilities Education Act (IDEA) mandates that children with disabilities, including an ASD, are entitled to a Free and Appropriate Public Education (FAPE) that meets that child's unique needs (US Department of Education IDEA, 1990). The IDEA (1990) also states that children should receive education in the "Least Restrictive Environment" (LRE). Commonly, this is referred to as inclusion or mainstreaming, which allows children with disabilities opportunities to interact with typically developing peers and participate in the general educational curriculum as long as the child can be successful in this setting (US Department of Education IDEA, 1990). Although some children with ASD can be successful in this type of setting, others require more substantial supports and may benefit from special education programs or consideration of private school options. When making educational decisions, families will want to consider multiple factors and variables specific to their child (e.g., verbal abilities, cognitive functioning, and frequency or severity of challenging behaviors including aggressive or self-injurious behaviors) and specific to the local public school district and other private or specialized private schools in the area (see chapter "Promoting Academic Success" for more information).

Managing Co-occurring Conditions

Children with ASD frequently have unique healthcare needs due to co-occurring conditions. Emotional and behavioral difficulties including irritability, aggression and self-harm, anxiety, depression, and ADHD-like symptoms are more (Greenlee, Mosley, Shui, Veenstra-VanderWeele, & Gotham, 2016; Mansour, Dovi, Lane, Loveland, & Pearson, 2017; Vasa et al., 2016) common in children with ASD than their typical peers. Suicidal and homicidal ideations also occur in children with ASD and can be difficult to assess due to the communication difficulties and challenges in assessing the child's level of intent or insight. McGuire et al. (2016) present a framework for the evaluation and management of irritability and problem behaviors such as aggression in the primary care setting. Key points of the framework include assessment of safety, the child's developmental level, and contributing factors (e.g., psychosocial stressors and underlying medical problems). Possible interventions include improving communication, environmental modifications, counseling, and medication (McGuire et al., 2016).

Children with ASD experience certain co-occurring medical conditions more frequently than children without ASD, including difficulties with sleep, gastrointestinal functioning, and feeding (McElhanon, McCracken, Karpen, & Sharp, 2014; Marí-Bauset et al., 2014; Souders et al., 2017). Toolkits on co-morbid medical conditions developed by Autism Intervention Research Network on Physical Health/Autism Speaks provide practical strategies for use by families and primary care practitioners (see http://airpnetwork.org/what-we-do/toolkits; see chapter "Medical Comorbidities in Pediatric Autism Spectrum Disorder" for more information).

PCCs may have the ability to refer and transfer treatment to subspecialty providers to provide ongoing treatment for specific conditions or diagnoses. However, in more rural or underserved areas where specialty medical providers may not be available or may not be accessible or feasible for the family, the PCC may be more involved in the management of these concerns. Even in resource-rich areas, demand often outnumbers supply, resulting in long wait lists and poor access to care. This is particularly true for mental health specialists, and PCCs may be called upon to address psychiatric concerns. PCCs can become more familiar with pharmacotherapy through consultative efforts such as child psychiatry access lines (see http://web.jhu.edu/pedmentalhealth/index.html), and Project Extension for Community Healthcare Outcomes (ECHO; see chapter "ECHO Autism"), which link communities with specialty hubs through telehealth (see chapter "Telehealth Approaches to Care Coordination in Autism Spectrum Disorder"), providing education and case discussion (see https://echo.unm.edu/). In general, medications used to treat typically developing children with the above conditions are also used to treat children with ASD, although efficacy is usually somewhat decreased in the ASD population (Vasa et al., 2016).

Community or Neighborhood Resources and Interventions

Children with ASD may benefit from federally or state-funded programs including home health care, supplemental nutrition program for women, infants, and children (WIC), and other community-based programs such as camps, respite care, and childcare. Community team members may have varying levels of knowledge or experience caring for children with ASD. PCCs often serve as educators or navigators for families regarding the various community services that may be an integral part of the treatment team and provide support to the family, either financially or emotionally.

References

Agency for Healthcare Research and Quality. (2018, August). *Care coordination*. Retrieved from http://www.ahrq.gov/ncepcr/care/coordination.html.

American Academy of Pediatrics, Council on Children with Disabilities. (2005). Care coordination in the medical home: Integrating health and related systems of care for children with special health care needs. *Pediatrics, 116*, 1238–1244.

American Academy of Pediatrics Publications Reaffirmed and Retired. (February and May, 2008). *Pediatrics,* 122, 450.

Applied Behavior Analysis: A Parent's Guide (2018). Autism Speaks Autism Treatment Network, Autism Intervention Research Network on Physical Health. Retrieved from https://www.autismspeaks.org/sites/default/files/2018-08/Applied%20Behavior%20Analysis%20Guide.pdf.

Baio, J. (2008). Centers for Disease Control & Prevention. Prevalence of autism spectrum disorders-autism, & developmental disabilities monitoring network, 14 sites, United States. *Morbidity and Mortality Weekly Report*, Surveillance Summaries, 61.

Baller, J. B., Barry, C. L., Shea, K., Walker, M. M., Ouellette, R., & Mandell, D. S. (2016). Assessing early implementation of state autism insurance mandates. *Autism, 20,* 796–807.

Centers for Disease Control and Prevention. (2019, September 23). *Autism spectrum disorder (ASD), treatment for autism spectrum disorder.* Retrieved from https://www.cdc.gov/ncbddd/autism/treatment.html.

Charman, T., Pickles, A., Simonoff, E., Chandler, S., Loucas, T., & Baird, G. (2011). IQ in children with autism spectrum disorders: data from the Special Needs and Autism Project (SNAP). *Psychological Medicine, 4,* 619–627.

Chlebowski, C., Robins, D. L., Barton, M. L., & Fein, D. (2013). Large-scale use of the modified checklist for autism in low-risk toddlers. *Pediatrics, 131,* e1121–e1127.

Committee on Children with Disabilities. (2001a). American Academy of Pediatrics: The pediatrician's role in the diagnosis and management of autistic spectrum disorder in children. *Pediatrics, 107,* 1221–1226.

Committee on Children with Disabilities. (2001b). American Academy of Pediatrics: Developmental surveillance and screening of infants and young children. *Pediatrics, 108,* 192–196.

Council on Children with Disabilties. (2006). Identifying infants and young children with developmental disorders in the medical home: An algorithm for developmental surveillance and screening. *Pediatrics, 118,* 405–420.

DePape, A., & Lindsay, S. (2015). Parents' experiences of caring for a children with autism spectrum disorder. *Qualitative Health Research, 25,* 569–583.

Dworkin, P. H. (1993). Detection of behavioral, developmental, and psychosocial problems in pediatric primary care practice. *Current Opinion in Pediatrics, 5,* 531–536.

Feinberg, E., Abufhele, M., Sandler, J., Augustyn, M., Cabral, H., Chen, N., ... Silverstein, M. (2016). Reducing disparities in timely autism diagnosis through family navigation: results from a randomized pilot trial. *Psychiatric Services, 67,* 912–915.

Glascoe, F. P. (2018). *PEDStest.* Retrieved from https://pedstest.com.

Greenlee, J. L., Mosley, A. S., Shui, A. M., Veenstra-VanderWeele, J., & Gotham, K. O. (2016). Medical and behavioral correlates of depression history in children and adolescents with autism spectrum disorder. *Pediatrics, 137*(Supplement 2), S105–S114.

Greenspan, S. I., & Wieder, S. (1999) The developmental individual-difference, relationship-based (DIR/Floortime) model approach to autism spectrum disorders. In E. Hollander & E. Anagnostou (Eds.), *Clinical manual for the treatment of autism* (pp. 179–209). American Psychiatric Publishing, Inc.

Hagan, J., Shaw, J. S., & Duncan, P. M. (Eds.). (2017). *Bright futures: Guidelines for health supervision of infants, children, and adolescents* (4th ed.). American Academy of Pediatrics.

Johnson, C. P., & Myers, S. M. (2007). American Academy of Pediatrics Council on Children with, identification and evaluation of children with autism spectrum disorders. *Pediatrics, 120,* 1183–1215.

Lobar, S. L. (2015). DSM-V changes for autism spectrum disorders (ASD): Implications for diagnosis, management, and care coordination for children with ASDs. *Journal of Pediatric Health Care, 30,* 359–365.

Lord, C., Rutter, M., DiLavore, P. C., Risi, S., Gotham, K., & Bishop, S. L. (2012). Autism Diagnostic Schedule, Second Edition (ADOS-2), Western Psychological Services.

Maglione, M. A., Gans, D., Das, L., Timbie, J., & Kasari, C. (2012). Nonmedical interventions for children with ASD: Recommended guidelines and further research needs. *Pediatrics, 130,* S169–S178.

Mansour, R., Dovi, A. T., Lane, D. M., Loveland, K. A., & Pearson, D. A. (2017). ADHD severity as it relates to comorbid psychiatric symptomatology in children with autism spectrum disorders. *Research in Developmental Disabilities, 60,* 52–64.

Marí-Bauset, S., Zazpe, I., Mari-Sanchis, A., Llopis-González, A., & Morales-Suárez-Varela, M. (2014). Food selectivity in autism spectrum disorders: A systematic review. *Journal of Child Neurology, 29,* 1554–1561.

Marks, K. P., & LaRosa, A. C. (2012). Understanding developmental-behavioral screening measures. *Pediatrics in Review, 33,* 448–457; quiz 457–458.

McElhanon, B. O., McCracken, C., Karpen, S., & Sharp, W. G. (2014). Gastrointestinal symptoms in autism spectrum disorder: A meta-analysis. *Pediatrics, 133,* 872–883.

McGuire, K., Fung, L. K., Hagopian, L., Vasa, R. A., Mahajan, R., Bernal, P., … Whitaker, A. H. (2016). Irritability and problem behavior in autism spectrum disorder: A practice pathway for pediatric primary care. *Pediatrics, 137*(Supplement 2), S136–S148.

Medical Home Initiatives for Children with Special Needs Project Advisory Committee. (2002). American Academy of Pediatrics, the medical home. *Pediatrics, 110,* 184–186.

Mesibov, G. B. S. V., & Shopler, E. (2004). *The TEACCH approach to autism spectrum disorders (issues in clinical child psychology).* USA: Plenum Publish Corporation.

Monz, B. U., Houghton, R., Law, K., & Loss, G. (2019). Treatment patterns in children with autism in the United States. *Autism Research, 12,* 517–526.

Myers, S. M., & Johnson, C. P. (2007). American Academy of Pediatric Council on Children with Disabilities. Management of children with autism spectrum disorders. *Pediatrics, 120,* 1162–1182.

National Institute for Children's Health Quality. *Creating a patient and family advisory council: A toolkit for pediatric practices.* Retrieved from https://www.nichq.org/sites/default/files/resource-file/PFAC%20Toolkit.pdf.

Ning, M., Daniels, J., Schwartz, J., Dunlap, K., Washington, P., Kalantarian, H., … Wall, D. P. (2019). Identification and quantification of gaps in access to autism resources in the United States: An infodemiological study. *Journal of Medical Internet Research, 21,* e13094.

Perrin, E. C., Sheldrick, C., Visco, Z., & Mattern, K. (2016). *The survey of well-being of young children (SWYC) user's manual.* Floating Hospital for Children at Tufts Medical Center. Retrieved from www.floatinghospital.org/The-Survey-of-Wellbeing-of-Young-Children.

Richards, M., Mossey, J., & Robins, D. L. (2016). Parents' concerns as they relate to their child's development and later diagnosis of autism spectrum disorder. *Journal of Developmental & Behavioral Pediatrics, 37,* 532–540.

Robins, D. L. (2019). *M-CHAT.* Retrieved from mchatscreen.com.

Robins, D. L., et al. (2014). Validation of the modified checklist for autism in toddlers, revised with follow-up (M-CHAT-R/F). *Pediatrics, 133,* 37–45.

Roth, B. M., Kralovic, S., Roizen, N. J., Spannagel, S. C., Minich, N., & Knapp, J. (2016). Impact of autism navigator on access to services. *Journal of Developmental and Behavioral Pediatrics, 37,* 188–195.

Rushton, F. E., Jr. (2005). American Academy of Pediatrics Committee on Community Health, the pediatrician's role in community pediatrics. *Pediatrics, 115,* 1092–1094.

Salisbury, L. A., et al. (2018). Sensitivity and specificity of 2 autism screeners among referred children between 16 and 48 months of age. *Journal of Developmental and Behavioral Pediatrics, 39,* 254–258.

Sanchez-Garcia, A. B., Galindo-Villardon, P., Nieto-Librero, A. B., Martin-Rodero, H., & Robins, D. L. (2019). Toddler screening for autism spectrum disorder: A meta-analysis of diagnostic accuracy. *Journal of Autism Developmental Disorders, 49,* 1837–1852.

Shahidullah, J. D., Azad, G., Mezher, K. R., McClain, M. B., & McIntyre, L. L. (2018). Linking the medical and educational home to support children with autism spectrum disorder: Practice recommendations. *Clinical Pediatrics, 57,* 1496–1505.

Sheldrick, R. C., Henson, B. S., Merchant., S., Neger, E. N., Murphy, J. M., & Perrin, E. C. (2012a). The preschool pediatric symptom checklist (PPSC): Development and initial validated of a new social-emotional screening instrument. *Academic Pediatrics, 12,* 456–467.

Sheldrick, R. C., Henson, B. S., Neger, E. N., Merchant, S., Murphy, J. M., & Perrin, E. C. (2012b). The baby pediatric symptom checklist (BPSC): Development and initial validation of a new social-emotional screening instrument. *Academic Pediatrics, 13,* 72–80.

Sia, C., Tonniges, T. F., Osterhus, E., & Taba, S. (2004). History of the medical home concept. *Pediatrics, 113,* 1473–1478.

Smith, N., Sheldrick, R. C., & Perrin, E. C. (2013). An abbreviated screening instrument for autism spectrum disorders. *Infant Mental Health Journal, 34,* 149–155.

Souders, M. C., Zavodny, S., Eriksen, W., Sinko, R., Connell, J., Kerns., C., … Pinto-Martin, J. (2017). Sleep in children with autism spectrum disorder. *Current Psychiatry Reports, 19,* 34.

Squires, J., & Bricker, D. (2009). *Ages and stages questionnaire®, third edition (ASQ®-3).* Paul H. Brookes Publishing, LLC. Retrieved from https://agesandstages.com.

Squires, J., Bricker, D., & Twombly, E. (2015). *Ages and stages questionnaires, social-emotional, second edition (ASQ:SE-2).* Paul H. Brookes Publishing, LLC. Retrieved from https://agesandstages.com/products-pricing/asqse-2/.

Stein, R. E. K., Silver, E. J., Augustyn, M. C., Blum, N. J., High, P., & Roizen, N. J. (2018). Private versus medicaid patients referred to developmental behavioral pediatricians: Do they differ? A DBPNet study. *Journal of Developmental and Behavioral Pediatrics, 39,* 325–334.

Todorow, C., Connell, J., & Turchi, R. M. (2018). The medical home for children with autism spectrum disorder: An essential element whose time has come. *Current Opinion in Pediatrics, 30,* 311–317.

U.S. Department of Education. (1974). *Family Educational Rights and Privacy Act (FERPA)* 34 CFR § 99.31. Retrieved from https://www2.ed.gov/policy/gen/guid/fpco/ferpa/index.html.

U.S. Department of Education. (1990). *Individuals with Disabilities Education Act (IDEA).* Retrieved from https://sites.ed.gov/idea/.

U.S. Department of Education, Department Office of Special Education and Rehabilitative Services. (2017). *A transition guide to postsecondary education and employment for students and youth with disabilities.* Retrieved from http://www2.ed.gov/about/offices/list/osers/transition/products/postsecondary-transition-guide-2017.pdf.

U.S. Department of Health and Human Services Health Resources and Services Administration Bureau of Health Workforce and the National Center for Health Workforce Analysis. (2018). *The US health workforce chartbook: Part IV: Behavioral and allied health.*

Van Cleave, J., Holifield, C., Neumeyer, A. M., Perrin, J. M., Powers, R., Van, L., & Kuhlthau, K. A. (2018). Expanding the capacity of primary care to treat co-morbidities in children with autism spectrum disorder. *Journal of Autism and Developmental Disorders, 48,* 4222–4230.

Vasa, R. A., Mazurek, M. O., Mahajan, R., Bennett, A. E., Bernal, M. P., Nozzolillo, A. A., … Coury, D. L. (2016). Assessment and treatment of anxiety in youth with autism spectrum disorders. *Pediatrics, 137*(Supplement 2), S115–S123.

Volkmar, F., Siegel, M., Woodbury-Smith, M., King, B., McCracker, J., State., M., & American Academy of Child and Adolescent Psychiatry Committee on Quality Issues. (2014). Practice parameter for the assessment and treatment of children and adolescents with autism spectrum disorder. *Journal of the American Academy of Child Adolescent Psychiatry, 53,* 237–257.

Warren, Z., McPheeters, M. L., Sathe, N., Foss-Feig, J. H., Glasser, A., & Veenstra-Vanderweele, J. (2011). A systematic review of early intensive intervention for autism spectrum disorders. *Pediatrics, 127,* e1303–e1311.

Will, D., Barnfather, J., & Lesley, M. (2013). Self-perceived autism competency of primary care nurse practitioners. *Journal for Nurse Practitioners, 9,* 350–355.

Zwaigenbaum, L., Bauman, M. L., Choueiri, R., et al. (2015a). Early intervention for children with autism spectrum disorder under 3 years of age: Recommendations for practice and research. *Pediatrics, 136,* S60–S81.

Zwaigenbaum, L., et al. (2015b). Early screening of autism spectrum disorder: Recommendations for practice and research. *Pediatrics, 136*(Supplement 1), S41–S59.

American Psychiatric Association. (2013). Diagnostic and statistical manual of mental disorders (5th ed.). Washington, DC: Author.

Interprofessional Roles to Support Psychotropic Medication Prescribing for ASD

Cody A. Hostutler, Jeffrey D. Shahidullah, Rebecca A. Baum, and Brigid K. Groves

Abstract While developmental and behavioral interventions are the primary treatment methods for youth with ASD, psychotropic medications are often prescribed by psychiatrists, developmental-behavioral pediatricians, and sometimes primary care clinicians (PCCs) to manage co-occurring disorders and symptoms. To maximize the effectiveness of these medications, collaborations across family, medical, community, and school systems are needed. However, there are numerous barriers unique to interprofessional collaboration around psychotropic prescribing for children with ASD. As such, this chapter aims to discuss these unique barriers, outline models of interprofessional care, and describe specific interprofessional and collaborative roles between prescribers and non-prescribers to support effective psychotropic management for children with ASD.

As evidenced throughout this book, children diagnosed with ASD do best when professionals use a team-based approach to care. The treatment team for a child with ASD spans several systems including medical, school, family, community, and sometimes legal systems. Approximately half of the children with ASD are prescribed medications to manage comorbid or co-occurring emotional and behavioral symptoms (Madden et al., 2018). While psychiatrists, pediatricians, and developmental-behavioral pediatricians may be involved in prescribing psychotropic medications,

---

C. A. Hostutler (✉)
Pediatric Psychology and Neuropsychology, Nationwide Children's Hospital, Columbus, OH, USA
e-mail: cody.hostutler@nationwidechildrens.org

C. A. Hostutler · R. A. Baum
Department of Pediatrics, The Ohio State University College of Medicine, Columbus, OH, USA

J. D. Shahidullah
Department of Psychiatry, University of Texas at Austin Dell Medical School, Austin, TX, USA

R. A. Baum
Department of Developmental Behavioral Pediatrics, Nationwide Children's Hospital, Columbus, OH, USA

B. K. Groves
Department of Pharmacy, Columbus, OH, USA

M. B. McClain et al. (eds.), *Interprofessional Care Coordination for Pediatric Autism Spectrum Disorder*, https://doi.org/10.1007/978-3-030-46295-6_18

collaborative and interprofessional teams are often needed to maximize the benefits of psychotropic medication. Thus, the aim of this chapter is to describe the current state of prescribing, identify barriers to interprofessional collaboration around psychotropic medication management, and explore models that can be used to increase collaboration. The reader is referred to the chapter "Psychopharmacology of Autism Spectrum Disorder" for a detailed review of psychopharmacological therapies for use with ASD.

Current State of Prescribing

Developmental and behavioral therapies are the primary treatments for youth with autism spectrum disorder (ASD) to address the core impairments that characterize ASD: (1) deficits in social communication and social interaction and (2) restricted repetitive patterns of behavior, interests, and activities. However, psychotropic medications may be considered to manage co-occurring behavioral health conditions such as ADHD, anxiety and mood disorders, OCD, tics, sleep disorders, and associated problem behaviors or symptoms such as irritability associated with ASD. In fact, children and adolescents with ASD may be at increased risk for depression, anxiety, and bipolar disorders compared with peers without ASD (Kirsch et al., 2020). Accordingly, the use of psychotropic medications is more prevalent in children with ASD (48.5%) as compared to children without ASD (7.7%; Madden et al., 2018). The most common classes of medications prescribed for youth with ASD include stimulants, alpha-agonists, or atomoxetine (30.2%); antipsychotics (20.5%); and antidepressants (17.8%). Children with ASD are also substantially more likely to be prescribed more than one psychotropic medication at a time (i.e., polypharmacy) compared to non-ASD youth (Frazier et al., 2011; Logan et al., 2012), which can raise concern for medication side effects, treatment of side effects with additional medications, or drug–drug interactions. Due to the national shortage of child neurologists, child and adolescent psychiatrists, and developmental-behavioral pediatricians, particularly in rural areas (Health Resources and Services Administration [HRSA], 2015), the burden of first-line treatment often falls upon the patient's primary care clinician (PCC).

Barriers to Collaboration

While many agree that interprofessional collaboration is important in the treatment of children with complex health needs such as ASD (e.g., Myers & Johnson, 2007; Swiezy et al. 2008), this work often remains fragmented across siloed systems of care, and psychotropic medication management is no exception. The chapter "Interprofessional Education and Training" covers the barriers and facilitators to interprofessional care in significant depth and breadth, yet some barriers unique to psychotropic medication management in children with ASD bear separate mention.

Schools are required by federal law to administer, monitor, and support children who are prescribed psychotropic medication when indicated (IDEA, 2004; Section 504 of the Rehabilitation Act of 1973). However, a few states explicitly address the monitoring of treatment response or side-effects of psychotropic medications in their policies (Ryan et al., 2014). Teachers are often unaware that a child has been prescribed psychotropic medication or if the dose is being adjusted (Koegel, Krasno, Taras, Koegel, & Frea, 2014). Communication between the prescriber and teacher is uncommon, and often systems are not in place for this type of communication to occur. While school psychologists are often uniquely positioned to integrate and coordinate information across family, school, and medical systems (e.g., DuPaul & Franklin, 2019; Power et al., 2003), fewer than 20% of school psychologists report receiving formal coursework in child psychopharmacology (Gureasko-Moore, DuPaul, & Power, 2005).

Primary care is a fitting access point for management of developmental and behavioral health needs including ASD, as primary care is often the first and only contact for a majority of families who seek and receive mental health services (Polaha et al., 2011). Unfortunately, PCCs report a lack of confidence and knowledge in ASD treatment, and parents report that PCCs often appear unprepared to fully support the needs of children with ASD (Brachlow, Ness, McPheeters, & Gurney, 2007; Carbone et al., 2013; Kogan et al., 2008). Specialty training for pediatric residents in ASD typically consists of a required 4-week developmental-behavioral pediatrics rotation during the 3 years of residency training. Over one-third (36.6%) of pediatric residency training directors rate the quality of behavioral health training within the 4-week development and behavior rotation as suboptimal or below, and 62.8% rate the quality of behavioral health training within the pediatric residency program as a whole to be suboptimal or below (Shahidullah et al., 2018b). Other clinicians who often provide primary care to children and adolescents (family physicians, pediatric nurse practitioners, and physicians assistants) typically receive no to limited formal training in developmental-behavioral pediatrics.

Even for those pediatric clinicians who feel confident in the management of behavioral health concerns in ASD, additional system issues can serve as barriers to care delivery. These barriers include time, reimbursement, inefficient office workflows, challenging patient behavior, and limited infrastructure to support communication and trust between providers (Carbone, Behl, Azor, & Murphy, 2010; Carbone et al., 2013; Van Cleave et al., 2018). The primary care service sector is best positioned to address brief and straightforward complaints; addressing behavioral health concerns pose a challenge given that these visits typically take more time to complete with additional post-visit work, yet result in lower reimbursement rates (Meadows et al., 2011). Given the brevity of most primary care visits, it is challenging for clinicians to deliver the necessary standard of care for behavioral health conditions that encompasses a broad spectrum of empirically based biological, social, and psychological management considerations. It is thus not surprising that many PCCs feel the management of developmental and behavioral conditions, with the exception of ADHD, is outside of their primary responsibility (Heneghan et al., 2008).

Models of Collaborative Care Across Systems

Several models of care have been developed to improve the collaborative management of children with behavioral health needs such as ASD. Parents, specialists, and PCCs report a preference for effective communication between specialists and PCCs, as it allows specialists to efficiently share their expertise, particularly when children are not already connected to a comprehensive ASD treatment center (Van Cleave et al., 2018).

Coordinated telephonic consultation models such as the Massachusetts Child Psychiatry Access Project (MCPAP) provide direct consultation with specialists to support management within primary care (Straus & Sarvet, 2014). Taking this one-to-one telephonic consultation a step further, Project Extension for Community Healthcare Outcomes (Project ECHO®) includes an interdisciplinary group of specialists (termed a hub team) and provides didactics and case-based consultation to a group of community providers (e.g., Mazurek, Brown, Curran, & Sohl 2017; Sohl et al., 2017; see chapter "ECHO Autism" for more information). This extends the consultation model through transactional learning between specialists and groups of community providers rather than one community provider at a time. While traditionally used with community PCCs, the Project ECHO model is designed to be an open learning extension model that can be adapted to address any topic or profession.

While these telephonic consultation models have demonstrated positive outcomes (e.g., Sarvet et al., 2010; Wegner et al., 2008), PCCs report that their ability to implement this knowledge is often limited by behavioral aspects of care delivery (e.g., not tolerating medication, difficulty swallowing pills, behavioral difficulties during office visits; Van Cleave et al., 2018). Co-located, collaborative care and integrated care models involve the placement of behavioral health experts on-site to support the primary care team in addressing behavioral health needs within primary care (Njoroge et al., 2016). In co-located models, a specialist conducts a concurrent clinic in a shared space (e.g., primary care office, and school) which can increase access to care for patients. Collaborative care models typically screen for a specific, high need condition (e.g., ASD) and a care manager (e.g., nurse, social worker) who provides a protocol-driven process (i.e., stepped care) that may include consultation with specialty providers, direct intervention with families, and/or patient tracking through the use of a registry (e.g., Katon et al., 1995). Highly integrated care models typically involve the co-treatment of patients during a single visit with multiple providers (e.g., a psychologist and a PCC conducting a joint appointment for a child with ASD). Psychologists within these roles are able to support diagnostic clarity, provide information to families, clarify and improve treatment plans, coordinate care across systems, address barriers to adherence (e.g., pill swallowing, stigma, motivation, and organization), as well as evaluate and monitor medication effects. The involvement of behavioral health clinicians in primary care visits significantly reduces the time burden experienced by providers (Riley et al., 2019).

In addition to the integration of specialists within primary care centers, there is an emerging trend to integrate behavioral health specialists within schools. Integration of these specialists, including psychiatrists, within the school has been shown to increase access to care, be effective at improving symptoms, and was found to be acceptable by parents, teachers, and students (Herman, Cho, Marriott, & Walker, 2018). Having psychiatrists located within schools also affords easier coordination between school staff, parents, and psychiatrists. Integrating medical providers, behavioral health clinicians, social workers, and psychiatrists within school-based health centers offers the opportunity to increase collaboration between most of the relevant ASD treatment team members (Plax & Garwood, 2018). However, the workforce shortages experienced by child and adolescent psychiatry may limit the dissemination of these models.

Primary Components to Interprofessional Psychotropic Management

Safe and effective psychotropic prescribing involves several steps including obtaining diagnostic clarity, exchanging information, providing education, joint treatment planning, addressing barriers to adherence, and evaluating and monitoring medication effects to support successful titration over time. Each step offers numerous opportunities for interprofessional collaboration among treatment team members.

Supporting Diagnostic Clarity

Psychologists and other behavioral health clinicians are trained to evaluate and diagnose mental health disorders using psychometrically valid assessment tools and to incorporate historical, interview, observational, and collateral assessment data. This expertise is ideally suited to assist prescribing clinicians in providing diagnostic clarity around ASD as well as identification of comorbid diagnoses and impairing symptoms. However, comprehensive assessment should include assessment of multiple domains (educational, behavioral, social, speech, occupational, medical, etc.); and therefore, integrated interprofessional assessment teams ideally involve team members with expertise in each of these domains. Practically, however, this is often unrealistic in most settings. Instead, careful coordination across providers and gathering data from multiple sources to integrate into the evaluation is important.

Selecting the Appropriate Medication and Titration

Psychiatrists and developmental behavioral pediatricians are ideally suited for determining the most effective medications and dosage to manage comorbid symptoms. As previously mentioned, PCCs often report a lack of confidence in managing psychotropic medication; however, consultation and implementation support may allow for PCCs to increase their level of comfort and expertise. Increasingly, clinical pharmacists are found within primary care practices as essential members of the interdisciplinary team (Kozminski et al., 2011; Scott et al., 2011). Clinical pharmacists can add an additional layer of quality, safety, and accuracy by recommending appropriate therapy and dosages, identifying and addressing drug interactions and medication non-adherence, and managing therapy by titration and lab monitoring (Kozminski et al., 2011; Scott et al., 2011; Wongpakaran et al., 2017).

Providing Psychotropic Information to Families

Psychiatrists, developmental-behavioral pediatricians, and clinical pharmacists are all well-versed in providing education about psychotropic medications to families. Despite not having prescriptive authority in most U.S. states, the American Psychological Association (APA) has recommended three levels of Psychopharmacological Roles that psychologists may be positioned to undertake, depending upon their level of training (Smyer et al., 1993). At the first and most basic level, all psychologists can undertake a Level 1—*Psychotropic Information Providing* role—whereby they help inform treatment decision-making by providing information on psychotropic medication as one potential treatment modality as part of a comprehensive treatment plan (types, indications/contraindications, costs/benefits, and risk potential). Psychologists may commonly provide information that may be relevant to treatment decision-makers such as opinions relevant to pharmacotherapy without necessarily playing a formal role in decision-making. This can include pointing patients to vetted referral or information sources (e.g., handouts on evidence-based treatments including psychotropic medications), or discussing with patients how to address their concerns about the medication with a prescriber.

Similarly, clinical pharmacists often are not granted prescriptive authority in most U.S. States. However, clinical pharmacists are trained in the safe and efficacious use of medications, and complete extensive training in the delivery of complex medical information to patients and families using age-level appropriate language. In addition to having an essential role in the appropriate selection and monitoring of a psychotropic agent, clinical pharmacists can also effectively assist prescribers in the initial and follow-up education related to psychotropic agents and how they may interact with other medications given the frequently co-occurring medical needs of youth with ASD.

Joint Planning and Care Coordination

Although they may not be ultimately responsible for the decision that is made in these circumstances, psychologists often play a substantive role in the decision-making process that includes determining indications/contraindications for available treatment options, weighing treatment decisions in the context of risk-benefit analyses, planning treatment regimens that emphasize the "least intrusive" principle and sequencing options (benefits of first evaluating response to behavioral treatments before initiating psychotropic medications), and coordination of behavioral and pharmacological interventions as part of a comprehensive regimen. These roles include involving and engaging patients and families in treatment planning through shared decision-making and valuing and deferring to patient choice and autonomy. This is defined as a Level 2—*Collaborative Practice* role—and many psychologists are positioned to undertake this collaborative role by virtue of their training. Given a significant barrier to coordination is that many providers are required to meet face-to-face clinical productivity; relying on other team members who do not have the same requirements such as care navigators or sometimes medical social workers to arrange for care and communication can be helpful. Research on group-based decision-making and treatment planning in medical contexts suggests that team-based care can significantly improve outcomes (e.g., Sharma et al., 2016).

Addressing Barriers to Adherence

The importance of involving and engaging patients and families in the choice of potential initiation of psychotropic medications (as mentioned above) lies in the research showing that parents typically prefer behavioral treatment options over pharmacological options (Al-Haidar, 2008). Eliciting and clarifying attitudes and perspectives around the use of these medications is important as many individuals may lack an accurate understanding of what these medications are and how they work. They may overestimate or underestimate their risk of side/adverse effects, and/or may have had prior negative experiences with a particular medication either with themselves or their child or via friends, family, and media outlets. Psychologists can address perceptual obstacles that patients have toward psychotropic medications or other treatments such as stigma or misinformation that leads them to believe that a particular treatment is not a good option for their child. Psychologists and other behavioral health clinicians can also work closely with patients and families to address more concrete obstacles such as adherence difficulties or skill deficits related to medication use including difficulties with pill swallowing. Clinical pharmacists collaborate with providers to ensure medications are prescribed according to proper indication, dosage, and formulation and in alignment with evidence-based guidelines. Clinical pharmacists maintain a vast understanding of multiple formulations of drugs (e.g., chewable, liquid, and sprinkles), facilitate conversations and authorizations with insurance companies to ensure families have access to the most appropriate type and formulation of a medication, and are skilled in safe and effective ways to support the administration on the correct schedule. Additionally, pharmacists based in traditional dispensing community pharmacy locations can offer insight into filling trends and behaviors at the pharmacy. Medical social workers can help families navigate difficult social determinants of health including helping families problem-solve financial, housing, and transportation barriers. For families who struggle with adherence or behavioral interference with medication administration, letters can be written so that school nurses can administer medications at school.

Evaluation and Monitoring of Medication Effects

Multi-informant monitoring of medication effectiveness and side/adverse effect is best practice. Careful monitoring is important for children with ASD as they are more sensitive to medication and more likely to experience adverse effects than the general population (Aman, Farmer, Hollway, & Arnold, 2008; Towbin, 2003). While all areas of psychotropic prescribing can be supported by multiple professionals, evaluation and monitoring may be supported by the widest range of professionals for collaboration, particularly for those without prescribing privileges spend considerable time with patients in naturalistic settings where the impairment is occurring.

Children spend a majority of their waking time in school during the school year and are often tasked with many challenging situations wherein interfering symptoms are present. Thus, despite the barriers previously mentioned, schools remain an important area for evaluation and monitoring of psychotropic medications (Shaw et al., 2011). Approximately one out of four school psychologists report direct psychopharmacologic services such as monitoring behavioral response or side effects and most school psychologists report indirect support to children prescribed psychotropic medications such as behavioral management consultation, providing assessment data to prescribing physicians, and implementing adjunctive psychosocial treatment (Shahidullah & Carlson, 2014). DuPaul and Franklin (2019) outline several psychotropic-related roles for school psychologists that include consulting with physicians, teachers, and families to assess medication effects, assisting physicians and families to determine the optimal dosage of medication, assessing and supporting adherence, and facilitating the integration of all interventions provided (i.e., medical, behavioral, and educational).

School nurses are often knowledgeable about medications used in children with ASD and can serve as an important resource in the school setting to monitor and evaluate the effect medications and serve as a conduit between school and prescriber (Strunk, 2009). Partnerships between school nurses and nursing staff in the prescribing provider's clinic could also reduce the barriers that arise from differing language, ethics, and professional style.

Integrated primary care teams can also support the monitoring of psychotropic medication effectiveness. PCCs, clinical pharmacists, nursing staff, and integrated behavioral health providers on the team can work collaboratively to monitor symptoms, adverse effects, and impairment during well-child visits and routine sick care. Shahidullah, Hostutler, & Stancin (2018a) delineated a number of collaborative medication-related roles that integrated pediatric psychologists who can undertake in the support of prescribing clinicians (see Shahidullah et al., 2019, for a review of relevant ethical considerations for when psychologists undertake these medication-related roles). Clinical pharmacists are trained to conduct comprehensive medication reviews through medication therapy management (MTM), which includes the identification and classification of medication therapy problems such as adverse effects, efficacy, and duplication of therapy (American Pharmacists Association and the National Association of Chain Drug Stores Foundation [APhA], 2008). The pharmacists' patient care process, which integrated clinical pharmacists utilize in the clinic and community-based settings, is a collaborative tool that pharmacists use to optimize and monitor medications (Joint Commission of Pharmacy Practitioners [JCCP], 2014). Clinical pharmacists integrated into the primary care team can complete MTM to assist clinicians in proper management of medications for ASD. There has been less formal delineation of the collaborative medication-related roles that other behavioral health clinicians (e.g., social workers, licensed counselors, and licensed marriage and family therapists) are positioned to undertake.

Community-based providers outside of the school are also well-positioned to help monitor and guide psychotropic management of conditions. Treatment monitoring data collected by behavior therapists and speech and occupational therapists can also be integrated into medication response to assess improvements in impairment, frequency, and severity of interfering behaviors. Behavioral health providers are well-positioned to monitor side/adverse effects and to evaluate behavioral response to medication through progress monitoring, standardized rating scales, and observational data collected as part of behavioral interventions. This data monitoring, when shared with prescribing pediatric clinicians can be helpful in dosage titration/tapering and discontinuation/withdrawing phases of medication management.

While integrating this data across professions and settings is important in psychotropic medication management, it can be difficult to gather this data in an effective way. The use of electronic health records (EHRs) can provide secure access to documentation across providers and facilitate communication between families and medical providers through the use of secure messaging. Traditionally these functions have been available to providers practicing in the same organization, but increasingly EHRs are able to coordinate information across health systems for more comprehensive access to patient information. Clinical registries can help organize and retain the information collected across providers and settings as well as track the progress of patients through the systematic application of measurement-based care. In addition, online patient portals that allow tracking of data and secure communication across multiple professions and settings are increasingly being used to track response to psychotropic medications such as HealthTracker™ (Santosh et al., 2017) and the ADHD Care Assistant (Power et al., 2016).

Conclusion

While psychotropic medication use is relatively common in children with ASD, it is ideally but one component of a comprehensive treatment plan developed and supported through interprofessional care. Members of the interprofessional team may include school personnel, staff from community agencies, behavioral health specialists, pharmacists, and PCCs, in addition to the patient and family. Given the breadth of professionals and service sectors involved, multiple barriers to providing this type of care exist but can be overcome through effective communication and processes that facilitate efficient information exchange. Increasingly, innovative models of care are being developed to extend the knowledge and expertise of behavioral health specialists into the medical home to support PCCs in prescribing psychotropic medications using a team-based approach. Beneficial aspects of an interprofessional approach to psychotropic prescribing include assistance with diagnostic clarity, patient and family education, medication monitoring, and adherence.

References

Al-Haidar, F. A. (2008). Parental attitudes toward the prescription of psychotropic medications for their children. *Journal of Family and Community Medicine, 15,* 35–42.

Aman, M. G., Farmer, C. A., Hollway, J., & Arnold, L. E. (2008). Treatment of inattention, overactivity, and impulsiveness in autism spectrum disorders. *Child and Adolescent Psychiatric Clinics of North America, 17,* 713–738.

American Pharmacists Association and the National Association of Chain Drug Stores Foundation. (2008). Medication therapy management in pharmacy practice: core elements of an MTM service model (version 2.0). *Journal of the American Pharmacists Association,* 48, 341–353.

Brachlow, A. E., Ness, K. K., McPheeters, M. L., & Gurney, J. G. (2007). Comparison of indicators for a primary care medical home between children with autism or asthma and other special health care needs: National Survey of Children's Health. *Archives of Pediatrics and Adolescent Medicine, 161*(4), 399–405.

Carbone, P., Behl, D., Azor, V., & Murphy, N. (2010). The medical home for children with autism spectrum disorders: Parent and pediatrician perspectives. *Journal of Autism and Developmental Disorders, 40*(3), 317–324.

Carbone, P., Murphy, N., Norlin, C., Azor, V., Sheng, X., & Young, P. (2013). Parent and pediatrician perspectives regarding the primary care of children with autism spectrum disorders. *Journal of Autism and Developmental Disorders, 43,* 964–972.

DuPaul G. J., & Franklin M. K. (2019). Legal, Ethical, and Professional Issues Related to Use of Psychotropic Medications in School-Aged Populations. In J. Carlson & J. Barterian (Eds.), *School psychopharmacology. Pediatric school psychology*. Cham: Springer.

Frazier, T. W., Shattuck, P. T., Narendorf, S. C., Cooper, B. P., Wagner, M., & Spitznagel, E. L. (2011). Prevalence and correlates of psychotropic medication use in adolescents with an autism spectrum disorder with and without caregiver-reported attention-deficit/hyperactivity disorder. *Journal of Child and Adolescent Psychopharmacology, 21*(6), 571–579.

Gureasko-Moore, D., DuPaul, G. J., & Power, T. J. (2005). Stimulant treatment for ADHD: Medication monitoring practices of school psychologists. *School Psychology Review, 34,* 232–245.

Health Resources and Services Administration/National Center for Health Workforce Analysis; Substance Abuse and Mental Health Services Administration/Office of Policy, Planning, and Innovation. (2015). National Projections of Supply and Demand for Behavioral Health Practitioners: 2013–2025. Rockville, Maryland. Retrieved from https://www.mdedge.com/clinicalneurologynews/article/58501/health-policy/neurology-shortfall-worsen-2025

Heneghan, A., Garner, A. S., Storfer-Isser, A., Kortepeter, K., Stein, R. E., & Horwitz, S. M. (2008). Pediatricians' role in providing mental health care for children and adolescents: Do pediatricians and child and adolescent psychiatrists agree? *Journal of Developmental and Behavioral Pediatrics, 29,* 262–269.

Herman, K. C., Cho, E., Marriott, B. R., & Walker, L. Y. (2018). Bridging the gap in psychiatric care for children with a school-based psychiatry program. *School Mental Health, 10*(2), 181–189.

Individuals with Disabilities Education Act. (2004). 20 U.S.C. § 1400.

Joint Commission of Pharmacy Practitioners. (2014). Pharmacists' patient care process. https://jcpp.net/wp-content/uploads/2016/03/PatientCareProcess-with-supporting-organizations.pdf. Accessed 26 Jan 2020.

Katon, W., Von Korff, M., Lin, E., Walker, E., Simon, G. E., Bush, T., … & Russo, J. (1995). Collaborative management to achieve treatment guidelines: impact on depression in primary care. *JAMA, 273*(13), 1026–1031.

Koegel, L. K., Krasno, A. M., Taras, H., Koegel, R. L., & Frea, W. (2013). Is medication information for children with autism spectrum disorder monitored and coordinated across professionals? findings from a teacher survey. *School Mental Health, 5*(1), 48–57.

Kogan, M. D., Strickland, B. B., Blumberg, S. J., Singh, G. K., Perrin, J. M., & van Dyck, P. C. (2008). A national profile of the health care experiences and family impact of autism spectrum disorder among children in the United States, 2005–2006. *Pediatrics, 122*(6), e1149–e1158.

Kozminski, M., Busby, R., McGivney, M. S., Klatt, P. M., Hackett, S. R., & Merenstein, J. H. (2011). Pharmacist integration into the medical-home: Qualitative analysis. *Journal of the American Pharmacists Association, 51*(2), 173–183.

Kirsch, A. C., Huebner, A. R. S., Mehta, S. Q., Howie, F. R., Weaver, A. L., Myers, S. M., ….& Katusic, S. K. (2020). Association of comorbid mood and anxiety disorders with autism spectrum disorder. *JAMA Pediatrics, 174*, 63–70.

Logan, S. L., Nicholas, J. S., Carpenter, L. A., King, L. B., Garrett-Mayer, E., & Charles, J. M. (2012). High prescription drug use and associated costs among Medicaid-eligible children with autism spectrum disorders identified by a population-based surveillance network. *Annals of Epidemiology, 22*(1), 1–8.

Madden, J. M., Lakoma, M. D., Lynch, F. L., Rusinak, D., Owen-Smith, A. A., Coleman, K. J., … & Croen, L. A. (2018). Psychotropic medication use among insured children with autism spectrum disorder. *Journal of Autism and Developmental Disorders, 47*, 144–154.

Mazurek, M. O., Brown, R., Curran, A., & Sohl, K. (2017). ECHO autism: A new model for training primary care providers in best-practice care for children with autism. *Clinical Pediatrics, 56*(3), 247–256.

Meadows, T., Valleley, R., Haack, M. K., Thorson, R., & Evans, J. (2011). Physician "costs" in providing behavioral health in primary care. *Clinical Pediatrics, 50,* 447–455.

Myers, S. M., & Johnson, C. P. (2007). Management of children with autism spectrum disorders. *Pediatrics, 120*(5), 1162–1182.

Njoroge, W. F., Hostutler, C. A., Schwartz, B. S., & Mautone, J. A. (2016). Integrated behavioral health in pediatric primary care. *Current Psychiatry Reports, 18*(12), 106.

Plax, K., & Garwood, S. (2018). Integrating Behavioral Health into a School Based Health Center. *Pediatrics*, 141(1 MeetingAbstract), 187–187. https://doi.org/10.1542/peds.141.1_meetingabstract.187

Polaha, J., Dalton, W. T., & Allen, S. (2011). The prevalence of emotional and behavior problems in pediatric care serving rural children. *Journal of Pediatric Psychology, 36,* 652–660.

Power, T. J., DuPaul, G. J., Shapiro, E. S., & Kazak, A. E. (2003). Promoting children's health: Integrating health, school, family, and community systems. *Guilford.*

Power, T. J., Michel, J., Mayne, S., Miller, J., Blum, N. J., Grundmeier, R. W., … & Fiks, A. G. (2016). Coordinating systems of care using health information technology: Development of the ADHD care assistant. *Advances in School Mental Health Promotion*, *9*(3–4), 201–218.

Riley, A. R., Paternostro, J. K., Walker, B. L., & Wagner, D. V. (2019). The impact of behavioral health consultations on medical encounter duration in pediatric primary care: A retrospective match-controlled study. *Families, Systems, & Health, 37*(2), 162.

Ryan, J. B., Katsiyannis, A., Losinski, M., Reid, R., & Ellis, C. (2014). Review of state medication policies/guidelines regarding psychotropic medications in public schools. *Journal of Child and Family Studies*, *23*(4), 704–715.https://doi.org/10.1007/s10826-013-9805-3

Sarvet, B., Gold, J., Bostic, J. Q., Masek, B. J., Prince, J. B., Jeffers-Terry, M., et al. (2010). Improving access to mental health care for children: The Massachusetts Child Psychiatry Access Project. *Pediatrics, 126,* 1191–1200.

Santosh, P. J., Bell, L., Fiori, F., & Singh, J. (2017). Pediatric antipsychotic use and outcomes monitoring. *Journal of Child and Adolescent Psychopharmacology, 27*(6), 546–554.

Scott, M. A., Hitch, B., Ray, L., & Colvin, G. (2011). Integration of pharmacists into a patient-centered medical home. *Journal of the American Pharmacists Association, 51*(2), 161–166.

Section 504 of the Rehabilitation Act of 1973, 34. C.F.R. Part 104.

Shahidullah, J. D., & Carlson, J. S. (2014). Survey of Nationally Certified School Psychologists' roles and training in psychopharmacology. *Psychology in the Schools, 51,* 705–721.

Shahidullah, J., Hostutler, C. A., & Stancin, T. (2018a). Collaborative medication-related roles for pediatric primary care psychologists. *Clinical Practice in Pediatric Psychology, 6*(1), 61–72.

Shahidullah, J. D., Kettlewell, P. W., Palejwala, M. H., Forman, S. G., Billups, A., Anismatta, S. L., et al. (2018b). Behavioral health training in pediatric residency programs: a national survey of training directors. *Journal of Developmental and Behavioral Pediatrics, 39*(4), 292–302.

Shahidullah, J. D., Hostutler, C. A., & Forman, S. G. (2019). Ethical considerations in medication-related roles for pediatric primary care psychologists. *Clinical Practice in Pediatric Psychology, 7*(4), 405.

Sharma, V., Stranieri, A., Burstein, F., Warren, J., Daly, S., Patterson, L., … & Wolff, A. (2016). Group decision making in health care: A case study of multidisciplinary meetings. *Journal of Decision Systems*, *25*(sup1), 476–485.

Shaw, S. R., Glaser, S. E., & Ouimet, T. (2011). Developing the medical liaison role in school settings. *Journal of Educational and Psychological Consultation, 21,* 106–117.

Sohl, K., Mazurek, M. O., & Brown, R. (2017). ECHO autism: Using technology and mentorship to bridge gaps, increase access to care, and bring best practice autism care to primary care. *Clinical Pediatrics, 56,* 509–511.

Smyer, M. A., Balster, R. L., Egli, D., Johnson, D. L., Kilbey, M. M., Leith, N. J., et al. (1993). Summary of the report of the ad hoc task force on psychopharmacology of the American Psychological Association. *Professional Psychology: Research and Practice, 2,* 394–403.

Straus, J. H., & Sarvet, B. (2014). Behavioral health care for children: The Massachusetts Child Psychiatry Access Project. *Health Affairs, 33,* 2153–2161.

Strunk, J. A. (2009). School nurses' knowledge of autism spectrum disorders. *The Journal of School Nursing, 25*(6), 445–452.

Swiezy, N., Stuart, M., & Korzekwa, P. (2008). Bridging for success in autism: Training and collaboration across medical, educational, and community systems. *Child and Adolescent Psychiatric Clinics of North America, 17*(4), 907–922.

Towbin, K. E. (2003). Strategies for pharmacologic treatment of high functioning autism and Asperger syndrome. *Child and Adolescent Psychiatric Clinics of North America, 12,* 23–45.

Van Cleave, J., Holifield, C., Neumeyer, A. M., Perrin, J. M., Powers, E., Van, L., et al. (2018). Expanding the capacity of primary care to treat co-morbidities in children with autism spectrum disorder. *Journal of Autism and Developmental Disorders, 48*(12), 4222–4230.

Wegner, S. E., Humble, C. G., Feaganes, J., & Stiles, A. D. (2008). Estimated savings from paid telephone consultations between subspecialists and primary care physicians. *Pediatrics, 122,* e1136–e1140.

Wongpakaran, R., Suansanae, T., Tan-khum, T., Kraivichian, C., Ongarjsakulman, R., & Suthisisang, C. (2017). Impact of providing psychiatry specialty pharmacist intervention on reducing drug-related problems among children with autism spectrum disorder related to disruptive behavioural symptoms: A prospective randomized open-label study. *Journal of Clinical Pharmacy and Therapeutics, 42*(3), 329–336.

Telehealth Approaches to Care Coordination in Autism Spectrum Disorder

Dasha Solomon and Neelkamal Soares

Abstract This chapter examines the current literature regarding the use of telehealth, and its potential benefits and limitations for diagnosis, treatment, and coordination of care for children diagnosed with Autism Spectrum Disorder (ASD). Barriers to access drive the need to have telehealth as a modality for delivering evidence-based diagnostic and therapeutic processes, which can be impactful in improving developmental trajectories and functional outcomes. The chapter concludes with guidance for clinicians interested in leveraging telehealth, with directions elucidated to further advance the use of telehealth to support families with ASD. More recently, in light of Coronavirus disease 2019 (COVID-19) pandemic and social distancing guidelines and restrictions, this chapter highlights changes in telehealth policy and the use of telehealth for diagnosis and treatment of ASD as well as thoughts about future directions.

This chapter examines current literature regarding the use of telehealth, potential benefits and limitations for diagnosis, treatment, and coordination of care for Autism Spectrum Disorder (ASD). Telehealth may help to bridge the "detection gap" seen between urban and rural communities and expedite access to care during the crucial toddler years, when evidence-based treatments can be especially impactful in improving developmental trajectories and functional outcomes (Wagner et al., 2015; Warren et al., 2011). Children, adolescents, and adults with ASD present with many unique challenges but also have a number of strengths that may make them an especially good target audience for teletherapy interventions.

D. Solomon
Boston Children's Hospital, Harvard Medical School, Boston, MA, USA

N. Soares (✉)
Pediatric and Adolescent Medicine, Western Michigan University Homer Stryker M.D. School of Medicine, Kalamazoo, MI, USA
e-mail: neelkamal.soares@med.wmich.edu

M. B. McClain et al. (eds.), *Interprofessional Care Coordination for Pediatric Autism Spectrum Disorder*, https://doi.org/10.1007/978-3-030-46295-6_19

Access and ASD Services

Current prevalence of ASD is reported as 1 in 54 children in the United States (US) (Maenner, Shaw, Baio, et al., 2020), affecting individuals across all racial, ethnic, and socioeconomic groups equally. Early diagnosis can help parents connect with providers and resources in their community, as well as obtain genetic counseling (Shattuck et al., 2009). However, although parents often notice differences in their child's development between 15 and 22 months, ASD is typically diagnosed when a child is 3 years or older (Johnson & Myers, 2007; Zuckerman, Lindly, & Sinche, 2015), and in more rural communities, the average age of diagnosis is around age 7 (Shattuck et al., 2009). One possible reason is the paucity of qualified professionals: a recent survey of medical professionals who work with developmental disabilities across the US concluded that there are challenges in meeting the current service demands (initial diagnosis and ongoing care), resulting in long wait times for appointments (Bridgemohan et al., 2018). Others have also highlighted that overburdened providers, combined with a growing demand, often lead to wait times that can exceed 12 months for an initial diagnostic appointment and can be even longer in rural communities (Chiri & Warfield, 2012; Dawson & Bernier, 2013; Gordon-Lipkin, Foster, & Peacock, 2016; Siklos & Kerns, 2007). Ning et al. found that 84% of US counties did not have ASD diagnostic resources (Ning et al., 2019).

Delays in definitive diagnosis have significant downstream effects: in many areas, families who are waiting to be evaluated can typically only access more general services from early intervention providers or special education and thus may miss out on ASD-specific therapy, (Pierce et al., 2011; Stahmer & Mandell, 2007). These challenges are magnified for families from traditionally underserved populations such as those with lower income, racial minorities, families with less formal education, and for those who live in rural areas (Chlebowski, Robins, Barton, & Fein, 2013; Zwaigenbaum et al., 2015). Thus, there is a need for the implementation of telehealth as a possible solution (among others) to reaching a wider range of families to provide initial diagnosis as well as therapeutic interventions (Gordon-Lipkin et al., 2016).

Telehealth

Telehealth is defined broadly as the "use of electronic information and telecommunications technologies to support long-distance clinical health care, patient and professional health-related education, public health and health administration"(Office for the Advancement of Telehealth, n.d.). For the purposes of this chapter, we will only discuss real-time audio-video ("synchronous") models, even though telehealth can broadly encompass "asynchronous" exchanges (images, videos, online patient portals) and mobile health (smart device applications or "apps" and wearable technology), which is beyond the scope of this chapter. Also, while we acknowledge that ASD is diagnosed and managed by a variety of disciplines (psychology, medicine, behavior analysis, speech-language therapy, education, among others), there is more literature in the medical domain than the others, which is reflected in this chapter. Also, some disciplines prefer the term *telepractice* rather than telehealth to convey the idea that these services aren't exclusively used in healthcare settings. To maintain consistency with the terminology, the term telehealth will be used moving forward.

Technical Advances and Barriers

There has been increased interest and uptake of telehealth in the last decade, in part due to increased awareness, and reduction in technological barriers. Broadband deployment has been expanded by the Federal Communications Commission (FCC) with about 98% of the US having access to either fixed or mobile connectivity, though it is less in rural areas (FCC, 2018). With 95% of the US population owning a cell phone and 77% owning a smartphone (Pew Research Center, n.d.), telehealth usage has increased from 2011 to 2016, 643% overall (960% in rural areas and 629% in urban areas) (Fair Health Inc, 2018). Cost continues to be a barrier; software-based solutions can cost up to $3000 and hard-based solutions can range from $7000 to $30000, not including training of staff. A larger hurdle is the integration of telehealth solutions with electronic health records (EHRs). Despite widespread adoption of the latter, only a few telehealth solutions are achieving integration, and not to a high degree of bidirectionality (KLAS, 2018). There are concerns by providers and professional societies about telehealth disrupting the provider–patient relationship if conducted in an on-demand fashion (Committee on Pediatric Workforce, 2015). Another barrier for provider adoption is lack of comfort with an unfamiliar technology (Utidjian & Abramson, 2016), and fear of liability, though younger physicians are more willing to adopt telehealth compared to older physicians (American Well, 2019). Reimbursement for telehealth is often mentioned as the largest barrier to telehealth expansion (KLAS, 2017). It is not uniform, depending on the type of provider, the modality of telehealth being used, the insurance provider policy around telehealth, even the nature of the encounter (e.g., mental health versus medical). Not all states have "parity laws", i.e., equivalent reimbursement for telehealth as "in-person" care. Even states that require parity only require parity in covered services, not necessarily in reimbursement (Center for Connected Health Policy, 2019).

Rationale for Telehealth with Children with ASD

Telehealth has been used in clinical care for children and adolescents with developmental and behavioral concerns and disorders for several years. Telehealth is beginning to be viewed as an appropriate avenue of intervention given the limited supply of providers (and their general location in urban or suburban settings) and the nature of the encounter which relies on more observation and interviewing and less procedures (Soares & Langkamp, 2012). In fact, for certain situations, telehealth might even be considered superior to in-person encounters. In ASD, this could be due to the novelty of the modality and that the separation (physical and psychological) allows for more naturalistic observations (Pakyurek, Yellowlees, & Hilty, 2010). Since children and adolescents with ASD may not "travel well" to tertiary centers, the reduced burden of travel may also allow for more baseline/typical presentation and telehealth may also alleviate the geographic access barriers (Soares, Johnson, & Patidar, 2013). The remainder of this chapter will review the literature regarding telehealth and diagnosis and treatment, as well as the feasibility and practical implementation of telehealth in ASD. Additionally, given the complex neurodevelopmental profile of many with ASD, telehealth allows multiple specialty providers to work with an individual which may provide a greater level of interprofessional care and collaboration among professionals.

Telehealth and Diagnosis

The process of diagnosing ASD is often multi-modal and complex, due to the lack of a definitive biological marker/test, the variability in ASD presentation and the need to consider DSM-5 criteria, functional abilities, and co-occurring or confounding conditions (Dawson & Bernier, 2013; Filipek et al., 2000; Huerta & Lord, 2012). As such, it often requires an in-depth developmental history (or diagnostic interview), observation of a child's social communication and behavior (usually through semi-structured diagnostic instruments), and an assessment of cognitive, adaptive, language, and behavioral functioning (Filipek et al., 2000). The utilization of multiple data modes and sources improves the reliability of ASD diagnosis (Huerta & Lord, 2012). That said, the diagnostic process presents a challenge to telehealth as many of the validated psychological instruments used in ASD evaluations have not been translated into a telehealth format or rely on procedures that are hard to replicate at a distance. Many studies report the efficacy of telehealth evaluations use modified or adapted instruments and compare them against evaluation-as-usual instruments. For example, Reese and colleagues (Reese et al., 2013) administered a modified Autism Diagnostic Observation Schedule (ADOS) via video to children previously diagnosed with ASD or developmental delay to determine whether ASD symptoms could be observed using modified ADOS "presses". Results highlighted that autism assessment could be administered via telehealth with similar levels of usability and reliability as face-to-face assessments. However, an important limitation to note is that these participants already had a diagnosis of ASD, and thus stakes for an accurate diagnosis were not considered. Additionally, certain items on the ADOS-2 could not be administered remotely. Juárez and colleagues conducted a tele-evaluation with families of children with concerns of ASD, and 13% of participating providers did not feel comfortable making the diagnosis via telehealth and 20% of children diagnosed with ASD in-person were not diagnosed via telehealth (Juárez et al., 2018). Schutte and colleagues found that the ADOS-2 Module 4 (used with older adolescents and adults who exhibit fluent speech) could be viably delivered via telehealth as it relies more on conversation than the use of manipulatives to ascertain samples of reciprocal social behavior. Most participants found the platform was effective and user friendly, and allowed the diagnostician to capture patients' social communication and behavior (Schutte et al., 2015).

Results of these studies suggest a potential benefit of using telehealth to accurately diagnose ASD. However, these studies also highlight potential challenges in diagnosis via telehealth for children with more subtle presentations and less severe symptoms of ASD, where in-person assessment would be required. Additionally, some items on the ADOS-2 require manipulatives which can lead to truncating an evaluation to make it feasible (if no parent or staff is present at the originating site to facilitate). Additionally, other aspects of a complete diagnostic evaluation such as completing a physical checkup with a medical provider are also challenging via telehealth. Thus, telehealth may be used in diagnostic assessments of ASD, but standard protocols and preconceived notions about elements of an evaluation must be altered, while maintaining quality and evidence-based approaches (see chapter "Interdisciplinary Evaluation of Autism Spectrum Disorder" for more information about interdisciplinary evaluation).

Telehealth and Early Intensive Intervention

Early intensive behavioral intervention (EIBI) strategies based on the principles of Applied Behavioral Analysis (ABA) with parent psychoeducation are the most effective intervention in ASD (Makrygianni & Reed, 2010; Reichow, 2012; Reichow, Hume, Barton, & Boyd, 2018). Generally, the overarching goal of ABA, developed by Ivar Lovaas, is to increase behaviors that positively influence a child's learning and development, while decreasing behaviors that are interfering by changing immediate antecedents and consequences to behaviors (Smith & Eikeseth 2010). A study of five meta-analyses of EIBI indicated that ABA is effective in improving various areas of development and functioning for children with ASD including adaptive skills (i.e., activities of daily living), IQ, and language (Reichow et al., 2018). However, the availability of therapists and programs that offer ABA vary across the country and are more limited in more rural areas (Antezana, Scarpa, Valdespino, Albright, & Richey, 2017; Heflinger, Shaw, Higa-McMillan, Lunn, & Brannan, 2015). Even for communities that provide more options to obtain ABA therapy, there can often be lengthy waitlists to be matched with a provider. Thus, there is greater interest in exploring the feasibility of implementing telehealth-supported behavioral interventions. Ferguson et al. (2019) conducted a systematic literature review of 28 studies, and found that while telehealth can be used for both diagnosis and treatment for ASD, telehealth failed to meet criteria for being considered a true evidence-based treatment due to methodological issues in the studies. They accordingly suggested that more research was needed to determine whether telehealth is a truly efficacious treatment model. Of note, Discrete Trial Training (DTT), which is a highly researched and evidence-based treatment in ASD and functional/daily living skills training, was not included in the review. See chapters "Coordinating ABA Services" and "The Early Start Denver Model (ESDM)" for more information about ABA therapies.

Additional Therapies Via Telehealth

Given the complex neurodevelopmental profile of individuals with ASD individuals and their varied strengths and areas of need, as well as co-occurring conditions, not all clients may benefit from ABA therapies. Additional modalities such as cognitive-behavioral therapy (CBT) and speech-language therapy may be more applicable or helpful to a particular child, though these therapies can also be difficult to obtain, especially for families in rural areas.

CBT

Hepburn and colleagues conducted a case study on a manualized telehealth-based CBT treatment for individuals with co-occurring ASD and anxiety and found acceptability for most participants with some limitations around technical difficulties (Internet connectivity, sound quality), which could be troubleshot in advance (Hepburn, Blakeley-Smith, Wolff, & Reaven, 2016). However, there is very limited research examining potential telehealth CBT treatment for ASD and co-occurring mental health conditions such as depression and anxiety.

Speech and Language Therapy

Individuals with ASD often experience severe communication impairments (Simacek, Dimian, & McComas, 2017). A systematic review of the literature about speech and language therapy via telehealth (Sutherland, Trembath, & Roberts, 2018) concluded that families who received speech and language therapy via telehealth had equivalent outcomes to that of in-person treatment. Simacek et al. (2017) conducted a study evaluating the efficacy of providing communication intervention coaching for caregivers via telehealth. Results of their study demonstrated that all children met their communication goals and benefited from this modality of telehealth treatment). See chapter "Coordinating Speech-Language Pathology Services for Youth with Autism Spectrum Disorder" for more information about speech and language therapies.

Telepsychiatry

Telepsychiatry generally can be done with little variation from usual in-person care due to its emphasis on verbal and nonverbal communication and clinical observations. Over the last decade, increased use of telepsychiatry has resulted in the American Academy of Child and Adolescent Psychiatry (AACAP) to issue a practice parameter (American Academy of Child and Adolescent Psychiatry (AACAP) Committee on & Telepsychiatry and AACAP Committee on Quality Issues, 2017). Telepsychiatry can be delivered through either a traditional "direct care model", in which the psychiatrist assumes the role of medication management, or a "consultative model", in which the primary care provider (PCP) assumes the role of medication management with the psychiatrist providing guidance and consultation. A combination model "Collaborative-Care Model" involves both the PCP and psychiatrist as well as a local treatment team, including staff, case managers, and other providers (social workers, therapists) (Szeftel et al., 2011). However, there is yet no published literature on outcomes or comparative effectiveness of telepsychiatry in ASD. See chapter "Psychopharmacology of Autism Spectrum Disorder" for more information about psychopharmacology.

Overall, telehealth is emerging as a potential mode for both initial diagnosis as well as treatment for individuals with ASD and their families. Although more research is required, emerging themes of benefits and limitations have been highlighted. See Table 1 highlighting initial benefits and limitations to treatment of ASD via telehealth.

Professional Training

Training serves to increase the number of intervention professionals and ongoing professional training enables service providers to learn and keep themselves updated on evidence-based intervention techniques to implement with children and families in their communities. Vismara and colleagues conducted a study examining the efficacy of training Early Intervention providers live versus telehealth (Vismara, Young, Stahmer, Griffith, & Rogers, 2009) to learn direct treatment and parent coaching. They found no significant differences in therapists' skill level and reported satisfaction between those who participated in the live training versus telehealth. Similarly, Ruble and colleagues conducted a randomized controlled study of ASD looking at specific coaching to teachers in person and via web-based modality. Results showed that students did equally well in both groups (Ruble, McGrew, Toland, Dalrymple, & Jung, 2013).

Table 1 Benefits and limitations of telehealth in ASD

Benefits	Limitations
Can provide diagnosis and treatment options to a wider range of families who live in rural or underserved populations	Potential for technical difficulties
Can be a more cost-effective way to provide educational and therapeutic intervention compared to in-home therapies	Potential risk to maintaining confidentiality
May be a shorter wait time to be seen by a provider who is specialized in ASD treatment	Potential difficulty scheduling emergency sessions
Has shown to be effective in training therapists, teachers, and parents specialized in ASD therapeutic techniques which can be implemented at home and in the community	Longer wait time for prescriptions when electronic prescribing is not possible
Is generally received well from those who receive training and treatment	Difficulty providing supplementary written materials to families
Decreases the time children and families wait to access care which can lead to earlier initiation of interventions and more consistent therapy over the course of development	May make establishing rapport and trust with families more difficult when engaging through video rather than in person
May decrease the need to miss school or work	Wide variation in reimbursement for services provided via telehealth in the United States which may limit providers ability to provide care
Limits transportation requirement for families without transportation or for individuals with ASD who have difficulty with transition, being in a car, or clinic/hospital setting	More difficult to detect with more subtle presentations of ASD
Potential for multiple specialty providers to work with an individual which may provide a greater level of interprofessional care and collaboration.	Insurance policies often require one in person visit before establishing telehealth care

Parent Training

Parents and caregivers know their child best, and their involvement in interventions is important. They help professionals understand a child's unique areas of strength and challenges and can ensure consistent implementation of therapeutic techniques in the home and community settings. Researchers have investigated the use of telehealth to provide therapeutic intervention for parents of children with ASD. Lindgren and colleagues compared the effects of assessing and analyzing functions of challenging behavior and implementation of functional communication training in clinic-based telehealth, in-home therapy, and home-based telehealth to help parents manage difficult behaviors in children with ASD (Lindgren et al., 2016). They concluded that all three modalities led to a significant reduction of problem behavior (> 90%), and parent-rated acceptability was high for all groups. Interestingly, they also concluded that home-based telehealth delivered through videoconferencing was the most cost-effective way to provide treatment to families.

Research findings suggest that not only is telehealth a potential method to reach more families, but it is more cost-effective as well. Many studies (Heitzman-Powell, Buzhardt, Rusinko, & Miller, 2014; Ingersoll, Wainer, Berger, Pickard, & Bonter, 2016) have evaluated the efficacy of parent training (for families in rural areas with a wide variety of educational backgrounds) via telehealth and found it to be feasible and effective, though larger sample sizes would be needed to make a more definitive conclusion. For example, Heitzman-Powell et al. (2014) note that families from rural areas who completed their training spent less time and money traveling with the telehealth training model compared to in-person visits.

Guidance for Clinicians

For interdisciplinary clinicians interested in leveraging telehealth to serve families and children with ASD, there are several areas to be aware of and to address if telehealth for ASD is to become acceptable and sustainable in their communities.

Getting Started

Clinicians should view telehealth as a *modality* for delivering care instead of a separate form of care. The first step is for the clinician to recognize the geographic draw of patients/families and the burden of travel they endure to access traditional in-person services. Data from the EHR can be used for planning prospective community sites to deliver telehealth (Soares, Dewalle, & Marsh, 2017). Engaging community partners (local practices, outpatient centers) can help identify the originating sites, and community partnerships showcase collaborations with specialists in ASD and provide a closer-to-home option for families. Analyzing gaps in service is an important step in developing a business proposition for expanding telehealth, whether through the capture of new geographic and demographic constituencies or serving as a marketing opportunity to demonstrate family-centered community partnerships and thus increase market share. By reducing geographic barriers (an important contributor to no-show rates), organizations can capture revenue otherwise lost.

Clinicians interested in leveraging telehealth can engage in "pilot projects" with a limited subset of the population: geographically, specific diagnoses, specific visit types (e.g., return office visits only). It is important to understand what measures are used by systems, particularly around patient satisfaction, such as Press Ganey's recently developed two *Telemedicine for Medical Practice Surveys* (Press Ganey, n.d.), though there are no studies comparing satisfaction between telehealth and in-person visits.

Process and Workflow

Operationally, for systems to embrace telehealth, support from senior leadership is key to committing resources (equipment, personnel) to launch a program, and balancing the impact of a new program on existing "in person" delivery with regards to space, time, and resource allocation. There can also be concerns from staff around time/effort spent in training on telehealth, including division of roles/responsibilities between usual care and telehealth care, particularly in systems without designated roles for telehealth. Similar workflow concerns can arise with delivering telehealth providers as many protocols veer from their "usual practice" of patients in clinic rooms, such as the use of a designated room, workflow (including connectivity) that also is different from in-person care, and concerns around time spent/lost in setting up and completing the encounter. This can be counterbalanced by improved access and completed visits (through possibly reducing no-show rates).

Systems must work with clinicians to identify "champions" at every level (clinicians, staff) and empower them to identify areas of improvement through telehealth in their practice and that of their colleagues (Ellimoottil, An, Moyer, Sossong, & Hollander, 2018). Champions can energize colleagues by sharing results of pilot initiatives to show how telehealth aligns with the system's mission and strengthens existing initiatives (including improving access and the overall patient experience) (Ellimoottil et al., 2018).

Professional Education

Increasing the workforce in telehealth—clinicians and facilitators/coordinators at both the originating and distal sites—is an important step to address increasing demand to serve families challenged with ASD. There is an increasing number of training programs, educational modules, and hands-on practicum to teach staff to facilitate, evaluate, and advocate for telehealth in their organizations (Papanagnou, Sicks, & Hollander, 2015). Continuing education programming and rotational experiences with trainees should underscore professional practice standards, user factors including privacy, and fluency with telehealth technologies (modalities, security, operations) (Committee on Pediatric Workforce, 2015).

Clinicians and leaders can enhance their own knowledge and skills around telehealth through training and education. Networking and learning can be achieved at numerous national conferences such as the American Telemedicine Association (ATA) and Healthcare Information and Management Systems Society (HIMSS) annual meetings. There are many ATA resources such as practice guidelines and best practices on pediatrics (McSwain et al., 2017) and mental health (Myers et al., 2017). For clinicians desiring a higher level of skill, there are certificate courses in telehealth and even clinical informatics fellowships that provide training on a broad array of biomedical data, computational systems, and clinical process improvement.

Client Factors

Families and patients are generally satisfied with telehealth (Weinstein et al., 2014), in part due to improved access to care and reduced burden of travel. Millennials and Generation Xers are more likely than older patients to consider telehealth (Fronstin & Dretzka, 2017), particularly for follow-up visits (Donelan et al., 2019). It is important to maintain a perspective of family-centered care (Kuo et al., 2012), which includes delivering care in their communities to reduce the burden of job-related absence and cost of travel (Soares et al., 2013). Families appear to be ready to engage in telehealth; almost 80% of mothers want to learn more about telehealth for acute, non-emergency medical issues and 65% view it as convenient and not disruptive to school or daily routines (EmpowHER®, n.d.). Family and patient education using signage, patient detailing materials, and "show and tell" open houses can also help to increase awareness and demystify notions around telehealth.

Licensure and Reimbursement

Recent efforts to ease licensure burdens on providers are evident, notably the Interstate Medical Licensure Compact which provides an expedited pathway to licensure across multiple states. By the end of 2019, 29 states, District of Columbia and Guam are part of the compact (IMLC Commission, n.d.). Similarly, 12 states have signed on to the Psychology Interjurisdictional Compact (PSYPACT), developed by the Association of State and Provincial Psychology Boards (ASPPB), which will allow psychologists to avail expedited credentialing in the near future to use telehealth technology (The Association of State and Provincial Psychology Boards, n.d.). Under Medicare legislation, speech-language pathologists are not currently able to provide telehealth services (American Speech Language Hearing Association, n.d.).Reimbursement for ABA delivered via telehealth also varies by state, and, even if permitted, coverage may be limited (Frank, n.d.).

Most states do not have restrictions on Medicaid reimbursements when telehealth is used in rural areas; but Medicare regulations still have restrictions to the "originating site" being located in certain types of geographic areas (rural health professional shortage area or a county outside of a Metropolitan Statistical Area (Centers for Medicare & Medicaid Services, 2018). By the end of 2019, only 14 states (Center for Connected Health Policy, 2019) explicitly allow telehealth delivery in the home (but only under certain circumstances). While there is no sweeping requirement to have an in-person encounter prior to delivering telehealth, in some states, advanced practitioners, psychologists, and counselors must still see patients in person before providing telehealth. Ease in provider credentialing policies has also eased the burden on the prospective telehealth provider (Centers for Medicare & Medicaid Services, 2011).

Technology Factors

Technology options abound today for telehealth; with the basic needs for synchronous telehealth being a monitor/display, camera, speakers, microphone, and a connection portal (either hardware or software). Equipment varies in terms of size, available options, mobility (fixed versus mobile), with varying cost of actual equipment, maintenance, and upgrades. A prospective program has to identify equipment requirements that match with the specific program's need and operability within their institution's larger Information Technology (IT) infrastructure. Seeking consultation from institutional IT specialists as well as other content experts (like regional Telehealth Resource Centers) helps, but should always include the key stakeholders actually involved in encounters (staff, clinicians, and families). A videoconferencing platform must be compliant with the Health Insurance Portability and Accountability Act (HIPAA; Codified at 42 U.S.C. §1320d et seq. and §300gg; and 29 U.S.C. §1181 et seq., 1996), and security risks can be mitigated with end-to-end encryption and by using protections against malware and other security breaches.

Future Directions

With increasing consumer demand for efficient, accessible options for care delivery, and technology innovation yielding devices capable of such delivery, there will be a need to offer telehealth interventions and coordination for families and children with ASD to a greater extent than currently available. With no end in sight to health professional shortages and a continuing disparity in access for rural and underserved urban populations, an important family-centered direction is to permit telehealth delivery in the home. This allows for better access, particularly for families with transportation and childcare challenges, and observing the child in his/her naturalistic environment allows for more accurate data collection and more family-centered recommendations. Legislation underway in the US Congress includes the Mental Health Telemedicine Expansion Act (H.R. 6781), designed to increase access to mental health services through telehealth by allowing the patient's home to be an originating site (DelBene & Reed, 2018).

Access is the prime driver for telehealth in ASD, and clinicians and family advocates should share this perspective with policy makers, payers, and other individuals who can facilitate the sustainability of telehealth. An important effort is to continue to reduce licensure and regulatory barriers, and optimize reimbursement. Clinicians should become familiar with recent reimbursement codes around telehealth that have implications in ASD care coordination. (Center for Connected Health Policy, n.d.). Advocacy for payment is important since levels of private payer reimbursement continue to be low (Medicare Payment Advisory Commission [MedPAC], 2018).

Developing and extending the research-base for telehealth is an important endeavor for multiple reasons: it provides information for policy makers to base their decisions around reimbursement and regulations (Agboola, Hale, Masters, Kvedar, & Jethwani, 2014) and allows sharing of evidence-based strategies among the clinical and research community. Until recently, telehealth research had been heterogeneous with studies of mixed quality and varied outcomes, making it difficult to estimate pooled effects (Ekeland, Bowes, & Flottorp, 2012). In addition to the usual randomized, controlled trials (RCTs), new collaborative research methodologies and novel analytic techniques emphasizing patient outcomes, large-scale feasibility, and cost-effectiveness will be needed (Tuckson, Edmunds, & Hodgkins, 2017). There is sufficient evidence to support effectiveness around communication and counseling for patients with chronic conditions, and psychotherapy as part of behavioral health (Totten et al., 2016). Building on this research-base will be important to select outcomes with two viewpoints: (a) to replicate and/or compare rates and effect sizes of developmental and behavioral outcomes to traditional intervention studies (Fein et al., 2013); and (b) to identify meaningful outcomes (including their measurement) while maintaining an inclusive spectrum approach to ASD (Georgiades & Kasari, 2018).

Epilogue: The COVID-19 Effect

In early 2020, Coronavirus disease 2019 (COVID-19) erupted around the globe, and by mid-March 2020 the US declared a pandemic emergency. As a result, swift changes in regulations in favor of telehealth occurred; including reduced barriers to access (Centers for Medicare & Medicaid Services, 2020) such as waiving co-pays associated with telehealth visits, permitting delivery of care to the patient's home, permitting both new and established patients to receive telehealth, among others. At the same time, US Department of Health and Human Services expanded the use of public facing technologies which may not fully comply with the requirements of the HIPAA Rules, as long as conducted with the good faith provision of telehealth during the crisis (Department of Health & Human Services, 2020). This meant a lot of previously seldom used platforms for telehealth such as Apple FaceTime, Facebook Messenger, Google Hangouts, Zoom, or Skype could be used; however providers are still responsible to notify patients about potential privacy risks with these applications, and should use available encryption and privacy modes as much as possible.

COVID-19 social distancing restrictions are creating even longer wait times for families to receive an in-person evaluation as well as follow up care and intervention. Thus, clinicians and researchers are developing and beginning to implement new assessment tools as well as modify existing instruments in order to provide telehealth assessment and diagnosis of ASD. The Vanderbilt University team have developed assessment tools that can be administered via telehealth. A diagnostic measure, Telemedicine-based Autism Spectrum Disorder Assessment in Toddlers (TELE-ASD-PEDS), can be administered remotely either in a clinic or home setting by a qualified provider (with expertise in diagnosing ASD) observing via video

(Corona et al., 2020). While there is ongoing data collection and validation of the tools for use via telehealth, the group has shared the training and tools with clinicians for use during COVID-19. Additionally, many major psychometric testing companies are moving towards making available digital test administration and scoring for remote options.

While welcome, this has left clinicians scrambling to balance patient access vs. becoming familiar with new processes/technologies/delivery of standard instruments at a time when many are secluded at home, while some are furloughed or deployed to other critical areas of the healthcare or service delivery system. Although not published, certain ABA companies in the US are offering virtual therapy and intervention to families as well, and professional organizations from psychology to speech therapy are putting out guidance on telepractice delivery.

Although the duration of social distancing practices are unknown at this time and will depend on local public health guidance, the COVID-19 crisis has certainly advanced the use of telehealth. There will likely be an increase in telehealth moving forward even after restrictions have been lifted, and with more research and validation of novel tools, clinicians will hopefully be able to provide access to assessment and treatment to underserved populations.

References

Agboola, S., Hale, T. M., Masters, C., Kvedar, J., & Jethwani, K. (2014). "Real-world" practical evaluation strategies: A review of telehealth evaluation. *JMIR Research Protocols, 3,* e75.

American Academy of Child and Adolescent Psychiatry (AACAP) Committee on, & Telepsychiatry and AACAP Committee on Quality Issues. (2017). Clinical update: telepsychiatry with children and adolescents. *Journal of the American Academy of Child and Adolescent Psychiatry, 56,* 875–893.

American Speech Language Hearing Association. (n.d.). Reimbursement of telepractice services.

American Well. (2019). *Telehealth Index 2019 Physician Survey.*

Antezana, L., Scarpa, A., Valdespino, A., Albright, J., & Richey, J. A. (2017, April). Rural trends in diagnosis and services for autism spectrum disorder. *Frontiers in Psychology*, 8.

Bridgemohan, C., Bauer, N. S., Nielsen, B. A., DeBattista, A., Ruch-Ross, H. S., Paul, L. B., et al. (2018). A workforce survey on developmental-behavioral pediatrics. *Pediatrics, 141,* e20172164.

Center for Connected Health Policy. (n.d.). Retrieved September 15, 2019, from https://mailchi.mp/cchpca/big-changes-in-2019-for-medicare-telehealth-policy.

Center for Connected Health Policy. (2019). *State telehealth laws and medicaid program policies.*

Centers for Medicare & Medicaid Services. (2011). *Medicare and medicaid programs: Changes affecting hospital and critical access hospital conditions of participation: telemedicine credentialing and privileging.*

Centers for Medicare & Medicaid Services. (2018). *Information on medicare telehealth.*

Centers for Medicare & Medicaid Services. (2020). *Physicians and other clinicians: CMS flexibilities to fight COVID-19.*

Chiri, G., & Warfield, M. E. (2012). Unmet need and problems accessing core health care services for children with autism spectrum disorder. *Maternal and Child Health Journal, 16,* 1081–1091.

Chlebowski, C., Robins, D. L., Barton, M. L., & Fein, D. (2013). Large-scale use of the modified checklist for autism in low-risk toddlers *Pediatrics, 131.*

Committee on Pediatric Workforce. (2015). The use of telemedicine to address access and physician workforce shortages. *Pediatrics, 136,* 202–209.
Corona, L., Hine, J., Nicholson, A., Stone, C., Swanson, A., Wade, J., Wagner, L., Weitlauf, A., & Warren, Z. (2020). TELE-ASD-PEDS: A telemedicine-based ASD evaluation tool for toddlers and young children. Vanderbilt University Medical Center. https://vkc.vumc.org/vkc/triad/tele-asd-peds.
Dawson, G., & Bernier, R. (2013). A quarter century of progress on the early detection and treatment of autism spectrum disorder. *Development and Psychopathology, 25,* 1455–1472.
DelBene, S., & Reed, T. (2018). *Mental health telemedicine expansion act (HR 6781).*
Donelan, K., Barreto, E. A., Sossong, S., Michael, C., Estrada, J. J., Cohen, A. B., … Schwamm, L. H. (2019). Patient and clinician experiences with telehealth for patient follow-up care. *The American Journal of Managed Care, 25,* 40–44.
Ekeland, A. G., Bowes, A., & Flottorp, S. (2012). Methodologies for assessing telemedicine: A systematic review of reviews. *International Journal of Medical Informatics, 81,* 1–11.
Ellimoottil, C., An, L., Moyer, M., Sossong, S., & Hollander, J. E. (2018). Challenges and opportunities faced by large health systems implementing telehealth. *Health Affairs, 37,* 1955–1959.
EmpowHER®. (n.d.). Moms and health technology survey. Retrieved from http://www.empowher.com/healthy-technology/content/infographic-are-you-tech-savvy-mom-see-what-our-community-said.
Fair Health Inc. (2018). *FH Healthcare Indicators and FH medical price index: A new view of place of service trends and medical pricing.*
Federal Communications Commission. (2018). *Broadband deployment report 2018.*
Fein, D., Barton, M., Eigsti, I.-M., Kelley, E., Naigles, L., Schultz, R. T., … Tyson, K. (2013). Optimal outcome in individuals with a history of autism. *Journal of Child Psychology and Psychiatry, 54,* 195–205.
Filipek, P. A., Accardo, P. J., Ashwal, S., Baranek, G. T., Cook, E. H., Dawson, G., … Volkmar, F. R. (2000). Practice parameter: screening and diagnosis of autism: report of the Quality Standards Subcommittee of the American Academy of Neurology and the Child Neurology Society. *Neurology, 55,* 468–479.
Frank, H. (n.d.). Telehealth: ABA's new frontier. Retrieved from BSci21.org, https://bsci21.org/telehealth-abas-new-frontier/.
Fronstin, P., & Dretzka, E. (2017). *Consumer engagement in health care among millennials, baby boomers, and generation x: Findings from the 2017 consumer engagement in health care survey.*
Georgiades, S., & Kasari, C. (2018). Reframing optimal outcomes in autism. *JAMA Pediatrics, 172,* 716.
Gordon-Lipkin, E., Foster, J., & Peacock, G. (2016, October 1). Whittling down the wait time: Exploring models to minimize the delay from initial concern to diagnosis and treatment of autism spectrum disorder. *Pediatric Clinics of North America,* 63, 851–859.
Health Insurance Portability and Accountability Act. (1996). *Codified at 42 U.S.C. §1320d et seq. and §300gg; and 29 U.S.C. §1181 et seq.*
Heflinger, C. A., Shaw, V., Higa-McMillan, C., Lunn, L., & Brannan, A. M. (2015). Patterns of child mental health service delivery in a public system: Rural children and the role of rural residence. *Journal of Behavioral Health Services and Research, 42,* 292–309.
Heitzman-Powell, L. S., Buzhardt, J., Rusinko, L. C., & Miller, T. M. (2014). Formative evaluation of an ABA outreach training program for parents of children with autism in remote areas. *Focus on Autism and Other Developmental Disabilities, 29,* 23–38.
Hepburn, S. L., Blakeley-Smith, A., Wolff, B., & Reaven, J. A. (2016). Telehealth delivery of cognitive-behavioral intervention to youth with autism spectrum disorder and anxiety: A pilot study. *Autism, 20,* 207–218.
Huerta, M., & Lord, C. (2012). Diagnostic evaluation of autism spectrum disorders. *Pediatric Clinics of North America, 59,* 103–111.

IMLC Commission. (n.d.). Interstate medical licensure compact. Retrieved May 31, 2019, from https://imlcc.org/.

Ingersoll, B., Wainer, A. L., Berger, N. I., Pickard, K. E., & Bonter, N. (2016). Comparison of a self-directed and therapist-assisted telehealth parent-mediated intervention for children with ASD: A pilot RCT. *Journal of Autism and Developmental Disorders, 46,* 2275–2284.

Johnson, C. P., & Myers, S. M. (2007). Identification and evaluation of children with autism spectrum disorders: Guidance for the clinician in rendering pediatric care. *Pediatrics, 120,* 1183–1215.

Juárez, A. P., Weitlauf, A. S., Nicholson, A., Pasternak, A., Broderick, N., Hine, J., … Warren, Z. (2018). Early Identification of ASD Through telemedicine: Potential value for underserved populations. *Journal of Autism and Developmental Disorders*, *48*, 2601–2610.

KLAS. (2017). *Telehealth virtual care platforms 2017: An early look at the state oftelehealth.*

KLAS. (2018). *Telehealth virtual care platforms: Which telehealth vendors have the scalability customers need?*

Kuo, D. Z., Houtrow, A. J., Arango, P., Kuhlthau, K. A., Simmons, J. M., & Neff, J. M. (2012). Family-centered care: Current applications and future directions in pediatric health care. *Maternal and Child Health Journal, 16,* 297–305.

Lindgren, S., Wacker, D., Suess, A., Schieltz, K., Pelzel, K., Kopelman, T., … Waldron, D. (2016). Telehealth and autism: Treating challenging behavior at lower cost. *Pediatrics*, *137*, S167–S175.

Makrygianni, M. K., & Reed, P. (2010). October). A meta-analytic review of the effectiveness of behavioural early intervention programs for children with autistic spectrum disorders. *Research in Autism Spectrum Disorders, 4,* 577–593.

Maenner, M. J., Shaw, K. A., Baio, J., Washington, A., Patrick, M., DiRienzo. M., et al. (2020). Prevalence of autism spectrum disorder among children aged 8 years. *Autism and Developmental Disabilities Monitoring, 69*, 1–12. https://www.cdc.gov/mmwr/volumes/69/ss/ss6904a1.htm.

McSwain, S. D., Bernard, J., Burke, B. L., Cole, S. L., Dharmar, M., Hall-Barrow, J., … Yeager, B. (2017). American Telemedicine Association operating procedures for pediatric telehealth. *Telemedicine and E-Health*, *23*, 699–706.

Medicare Payment Advisory Commission (MedPAC). (2018). *Mandated report: Telehealth services and the Medicare program.* Retrieved from http://www.medpac.gov/docs/default-source/reports/mar18_medpac_ch16_sec.pdf?sfvrsn=0.

Myers, K., Nelson, E.-L., Rabinowitz, T., Hilty, D., Baker, D., Barnwell, S. S., … Bernard, J. (2017). American Telemedicine Association practice guidelines for telemental health with children and adolescents. *Telemedicine and E-Health*, *23*, 779–804.

Ning, M., Daniels, J., Schwartz, J., Dunlap, K., Washington, P., Kalantarian, H., … Wall, D. P. (2019). Identification and quantification of gaps in access to autism resources in the United States: An infodemiological study. *Journal of Medical Internet Research*, *21*, e13094.

Office for the Advancement of Telehealth. (n.d.). Retrieved May 28, 2019, from https://www.hrsa.gov/rural-health/telehealth/index.html.

Pakyurek, M., Yellowlees, P., & Hilty, D. (2010). The child and adolescent telepsychiatry consultation: Can it be a more effective clinical process for certain patients than conventional practice? *Telemedicine and E-Health, 16,* 289–292.

Papanagnou, D., Sicks, S., & Hollander, J. E. (2015). Training the next generation of care providers: Focus on telehealth. *Healthcare Transformation, 1,* 52–63.

Pew Research Center. (n.d.). Mobile Fact Sheet. Retrieved June 1, 2019, from 2018 website: https://www.pewinternet.org/fact-sheet/mobile/.

Pierce, K., Carter, C., Weinfeld, M., Desmond, J., Hazin, R., Bjork, R., & Gallagher, N. (2011). Detecting, studying, and treating autism early: The one-year well-baby check-up approach. *Journal of Pediatrics*, *159*.

Press Ganey. (n.d.). Telemedicine for medical practice surveys. Retrieved from https://www.pressganey.com/docs/default-source/default-document-library/telemedicine-for-medical-practice_faqs_040918.pdf?sfvrsn=0.

Reese, R. M., Jamison, R., Wendland, M., Fleming, K., Braun, M. J., Schuttler, J. O., et al. (2013). Evaluating interactive videoconferencing for assessing symptoms of Autism. *Telemedicine and E-Health, 19,* 671–677.
Reichow, B. (2012). Overview of meta-analyses on early intensive behavioral intervention for young children with autism spectrum disorders. *Journal of Autism and Developmental Disorders, 42,* 512–520.
Reichow, B., Hume, K., Barton, E. E., & Boyd, B. A. (2018, May 9). Early intensive behavioral intervention (EIBI) for young children with autism spectrum disorders (ASD). In: *Cochrane database of systematic reviews* (Vol. 2018). John Wiley and Sons Ltd.
Ruble, L. A., McGrew, J. H., Toland, M. D., Dalrymple, N. J., & Jung, L. A. (2013). A randomized controlled trial of COMPASS web-based and face-to-face teacher coaching in autism. *Journal of Consulting and Clinical Psychology, 81,* 566–572.
Schutte, J. L., McCue, M. P., Parmanto, B., McGonigle, J., Handen, B., Lewis, A., … Saptono, A. (2015). Usability and reliability of a remotely administered adult autism assessment, the autism diagnostic observation schedule (ADOS) module 4. *Telemedicine and E-Health, 21,* 176–184.
Shattuck, P. T., Durkin, M., Maenner, M., Newschaffer, C., Mandell, D. S., Wiggins, L., … Cuniff, C. (2009). Timing of identification among children with an autism spectrum disorder: Findings from a population-based surveillance study. *Journal of the American Academy of Child and Adolescent Psychiatry, 48,* 474–483.
Siklos, S., & Kerns, K. A. (2007). Assessing the diagnostic experiences of a small sample of parents of children with autism spectrum disorders. *Research in Developmental Disabilities, 28,* 9–22.
Simacek, J., Dimian, A. F., & McComas, J. J. (2017). Communication intervention for young children with severe neurodevelopmental disabilities via telehealth. *Journal of Autism and Developmental Disorders, 47,* 744–767.
Soares, N., Johnson, A. O., & Patidar, N. (2013). Geomapping telehealth access to developmental-behavioral pediatrics. *Telemedicine and E-Health, 19,* 585–590.
Soares, Neelkamal, Dewalle, J., & Marsh, B. (2017). Utilizing patient geographic information system data to plan telemedicine service locations. *Journal of the American Medical Informatics Association, 24,* 891–896.
Soares, N. S., & Langkamp, D. (2012). Telehealth in developmental-behavioral pediatrics. *Journal of Developmental and Behavioral Pediatrics, 33,* 656–665.
Stahmer, A. C., & Mandell, D. S. (2007). State infant/toddler program policies for eligibility and services provision for young children with autism. *Administration and Policy in Mental Health and Mental Health Services Research, 34,* 29–37.
Sutherland, R., Trembath, D., & Roberts, J. (2018). Telehealth and autism: A systematic search and review of the literature. *International Journal of Speech-Language Pathology, 20,* 324–336.
Szeftel, R., Mandelbaum, S., Sulman-Smith, H., Naqvi, S., Lawrence, L., Szeftel, Z., … Gross, L. (2011). Telepsychiatry for children with developmental disabilities: Applications for patient care and medical education. *Child and Adolescent Psychiatric Clinics of North America, 20,* 95–111.
The Association of State and Provincial Psychology Boards. (n.d.). *PSYPACT Legislative Updates.* Retrieved from https://www.asppb.net/mpage/legislative.
Totten, A., Womack, D., Eden, K., McDonagh, M., Griffin, J., Grusin, S., & Hersh, W. (2016). *Telehealth: mapping the evidence for patient outcomes from systematic reviews. Technical Brief No. 26.* Retrieved from www.effectivehealthcare.ahrq.gov/reports/final.cfm.
Tuckson, R. V., Edmunds, M., & Hodgkins, M. L. (2017). Telehealth. *New England Journal of Medicine, 377,* 1585–1592.
U.S. Department of Health & Human Services. (2020). *Notification of enforcement discretion for telehealth remote communications during the COVID-19 Nationwide public health emergency.*
Utidjian, L., & Abramson, E. (2016). Pediatric telehealth: opportunities and challenges. *Pediatric Clinics of North America, 63,* 367–378.
Vismara, L. A., Young, G. S., Stahmer, A. C., Griffith, E. M. M., & Rogers, S. J. (2009). Dissemination of evidence-based practice: can we train therapists from a distance? *Journal of Autism and Developmental Disorders, 39,* 1636–1651.

Wagner, S., Granpeesheh, D., Wetherby, A., Natowicz, M. R., Choueiri, R., Pierce, K., … Robins, D. (2015). Early intervention for children with autism spectrum disorder under 3 years of age: recommendations for practice and research. *Pediatrics, 136*, S60–S81.

Warren, Z., McPheeters, M. L., Sathe, N., Foss-Feig, J. H., Glasser, A., & Veenstra-VanderWeele, J. (2011). A systematic review of early intensive intervention for autism spectrum disorders. *Pediatrics, 127,* e1303–e1311.

Weinstein, R. S., Lopez, A. M., Joseph, B. A., Erps, K. A., Holcomb, M., Barker, G. P., et al. (2014). Telemedicine, telehealth, and mobile health applications that work: opportunities and barriers. *The American Journal of Medicine, 127,* 183–187.

Zuckerman, K. E., Lindly, O. J., & Sinche, B. K. (2015). Parental concerns, provider response, and timeliness of autism spectrum disorder diagnosis. *Journal of Pediatrics, 166,* 1431–1439.e1.

Zwaigenbaum, L., Bauman, M. L., Choueiri, R., Kasari, C., Carter, A., Granpeesheh, D., … Natowicz, M. R. (2015). Early intervention for children with autism spectrum disorder under 3 years of age: recommendations for practice and research. *Pediatrics, 136*, S60–S81.

ECHO Autism

Micah O. Mazurek, Christina Harkins, Michelle Menezes, and Kristin Sohl

Abstract Children and adults with autism spectrum disorder (ASD) have significant healthcare needs, from timely and accurate diagnosis, through ongoing care and support. However, shortages of healthcare providers with training in ASD, limited capacity at specialty centers, and geographic and socioeconomic barriers contribute to diagnostic delays and gaps in healthcare delivery. The ECHO Autism program seeks to address these challenges by leveraging videoconferencing technology to provide interdisciplinary training and mentorship to community-based providers in best-practice care for children and adults with ASD. This chapter provides an overview of the healthcare needs and barriers experienced by individuals with ASD, and describes applications and evidence supporting the use of the ECHO Autism model for increasing local expertise in best-practice autism care.

Individuals with autism spectrum disorder (ASD) face significant developmental, health, and mental health challenges across their life span. These challenges require timely, coordinated, and comprehensive healthcare services from initial diagnosis through ongoing support (Carbone, Farley, & Davis, 2010; Hyman & Johnson, 2012). However, children and adults with ASD experience significant healthcare gaps and barriers, and those from underserved populations face even greater disparities (Karpur, Lello, Frazier, Dixon, & Shih, 2019). The current healthcare system is not fully equipped to address the needs of individuals with ASD, with critical shortages of autism specialists across professional disciplines.

The Project Extension for Healthcare Outcomes (Project ECHO) model is an innovative solution that aims to enhance the capacity for best-practice care for common and complex conditions (Arora et al., 2011a). The ECHO model leverages technology and interdisciplinary teams to train and mentor community-based providers in evidence-based practices, thereby addressing significant barriers to healthcare access.

M. O. Mazurek (✉) · C. Harkins · M. Menezes
Department of Human Services, Curry School of Education and Human Development, University of Virginia, Charlottesville, VA, USA
e-mail: mazurekm@virginia.edu

K. Sohl
Department of Child Health, University of Missouri, Columbia, MO, USA

M. B. McClain et al. (eds.), *Interprofessional Care Coordination for Pediatric Autism Spectrum Disorder*, https://doi.org/10.1007/978-3-030-46295-6_20

This chapter will provide a brief overview of healthcare needs and barriers experienced by individuals with ASD, and will describe new applications of the ECHO model for increasing local expertise in best-practice autism care.

Healthcare Needs and Barriers for Children with ASD

Early Identification and Diagnosis

Individuals with ASD have significant healthcare needs across their life span, beginning with a critical need for timely and accurate identification. The earlier children are identified and can begin intervention, the greater are their developmental gains (MacDonald, Parry-Cruwys, Dupere, & Ahearn, 2014). Although behavioral signs of ASD can be detected in early toddlerhood and can reliably be diagnosed by 24 months of age (Webb & Jones, 2009; Zwaigenbaum et al., 2015), the average age of diagnosis remains between 4 and 7 years (Baio et al., 2018; Sheldrick, Maye, & Carter, 2017), leading to significant intervention delays.

Pediatricians and other pediatric primary care providers (PCPs) serve an important role in the diagnostic process, and the American Academy of Pediatrics (AAP) recommends that formal autism screening be administered for all children at 18- and 24-months of age (Johnson & Myers, 2007). However, pediatricians and other PCPs have difficulty implementing these recommendations (Carbone, Norlin, & Young, 2016; Self, Parham, & Rajagopalan, 2015). Physician surveys have indicated that less than 60% are administering standardized autism screening tools at well-child visits (Arunyanart et al., 2012; Gillis, 2009; Keil, Breunig, Fleischfresser, & Oftedahl, 2014), leading to missed or delayed diagnosis for many children.

Health and Mental Health Conditions

Autism is also frequently accompanied by a complex range of comorbid health and mental health conditions. Up to 95% of children with ASD experience one or more co-occurring conditions (Soke, Maenner, Christensen, Kurzius-Spencer, & Schieve, 2018). Some of the most common co-occurring medical conditions include epilepsy, sleep problems, gastrointestinal dysfunction, and immune dysfunction (Tye, Runicles, Whitehouse, & Alvares, 2019; see also chapter "Medical Comorbidities in Pediatric Autism Spectrum Disorder" of this volume). These problems can significantly impact overall health and quality of life, and can lead to impairments in overall functioning. Additionally, many of these symptoms appear to be interrelated and associated with mental health and behavioral difficulties (Aldinger, Lane, Veenstra-VanderWeele, & Levitt, 2015; Mazurek & Petroski, 2015; Mazurek et al., 2013).

Up to 70% of individuals with ASD have a comorbid psychiatric disorder (Simonoff et al., 2008), the most common of which include attention deficit/hyperactivity disorder (ADHD), anxiety disorders, and depressive disorders (Brookman-Frazee, Stadnick, Chlebowski, Baker-Ericzén, & Ganger, 2018; de Bruin, Ferdinand, Meester, de Nijs, & Verheij, 2007). The co-occurrence of these conditions can be associated with exacerbation of autism symptoms and worse overall outcomes (Chiang & Gau, 2016; Mattila et al., 2010; Sprenger et al., 2013).

Despite the almost universal presence of co-occurring conditions among children and adults with ASD, the screening and management of these problems can pose challenges to providers who have not received formal training in ASD (Carbone et al., 2016; Unigwe et al., 2017). The dynamic nature of symptoms, variability in symptom presentations, and communication difficulties associated with ASD contribute to challenges for both diagnosis and treatment of comorbid conditions. Additionally, it can be difficult to distinguish when observed behavioral symptoms may be better explained by another condition (Tye et al., 2019).

Barriers to Healthcare Access

Individuals with ASD face a number of healthcare barriers. Children with ASD experience worse access to care and greater unmet health needs than those with other complex conditions (Croen, Najjar, Ray, Lotspeich, & Bernal, 2006; Kogan et al., 2008). Families from racial and ethnic minority populations face even greater health disparities due to cultural and linguistic factors (Begeer, El Bouk, Boussaid, Terwogt, & Koot, 2009; Lin & Yu, 2015; Newacheck, Hung, & Wright, 2002; see also chapter "Clinical and School Identification and Intervention for Youth with ASD: Culturally and Linguistically Responsive Interdisciplinary Considerations" of this volume). Financial, geographic, and sociocultural factors further contribute to difficulties accessing health care for individuals in rural communities. Conversely, individuals in urban areas also face challenges accessing autism specialists due to limited capacity and excessive wait times (Bishop-Fitzpatrick & Kind, 2017; Tregnago & Cheak-Zamora, 2012). As adults with ASD age out of the pediatric health system, there are even fewer providers who have the training to adequately care for their unique health and mental health needs (Mandell, 2013; Raymaker et al., 2017).

Overall, there are a few healthcare providers with expertise and training in best-practice care for individuals ASD. Although PCPs are perfectly positioned within local communities to provide accessible and responsive health care, they often lack training and confidence in diagnosis and medical management of ASD (Carbone, Behl, Azor, & Murphy, 2010; Carbone et al., 2013). Thus, there is a critical need for innovative models to support the ability of healthcare providers to meet the needs of individuals with ASD in their own communities. As will be described in the sections that follow, Extension for Community Healthcare Outcomes (ECHO) is one such model that holds particular promise.

Project ECHO

Overview of the Framework

Project ECHO is a web-based guided practice model that connects PCPs in underserved areas to specialists at academic medical centers so that PCPs can deliver evidence-based care to patients with complex health conditions in their own communities (Arora et al., 2007, 2014). Originally developed at the University of New Mexico, Project ECHO began as a program to expand access to quality care for individuals with hepatitis C. In response to a critical shortage of specialists in New Mexico, Arora and colleagues began training PCPs in rural areas to provide best-practice care for patients with hepatitis C to reduce the need for specialist referrals and wait times for treatment (Arora et al., 2011a).

Project ECHO uses a "hub" and "spoke" framework to connect specialist teams ("hubs") at academic medical centers to clinicians ("spokes") in rural and underserved communities to increase their knowledge of difficult-to-treat conditions. The specialist teams and community providers participate in weekly videoconference sessions or ECHO clinics. Before each ECHO clinic, PCPs complete a case template (which excludes identifying patient information) to present to the specialists and other community providers. The majority of each virtual clinic is dedicated to case discussions, in which PCPs take turns sharing their cases and seeking input on the treatment plan. Each session also includes a short didactic presentation from the hub team focused on best-practice care (Arora et al., 2011a).

ECHO clinics are alternatively called "knowledge networks" because they bring together one team of interdisciplinary specialists and many community-based providers. The sharing of knowledge among specialists and PCPs creates a "learning loop" through which PCPs gain expertise in a complex health condition (Arora et al., 2010). Unlike traditional telemedicine in which the specialist assumes care of the patient, in the ECHO model, community providers retain responsibility for managing the patient under specialist guidance. Through participation in ECHO clinics and increased knowledge and confidence, the PCP becomes capable of treating complex patients independently of the specialist team (Arora et al., 2011a).

The ECHO model is based on established educational theories about learning and behavior change, including social cognitive theory (Bandura, 1986), situated learning theory (Vygotsky, 1980), and communities of practice (Lave & Wenger, 1991). According to social cognitive theory, for effective behavior change, individuals must have high self-efficacy (i.e., believe that they are capable of performing the behavior), and be reinforced for utilization of the behavior by persons perceived as important. The ECHO model enhances provider self-efficacy by increasing domain-specific knowledge through case-based learning, and providers are reinforced for effective patient care by positive feedback from trusted peers and specialists. ECHO's "knowledge networks" and "learning loops" are founded in situated learning theory, which posits that learning requires collaboration. This framework also creates a community of practice in which clinicians are building knowledge and gaining skills in treatment of patients with complex health conditions through guided practice and ongoing feedback from the specialist team and one another (Arora et al., 2010).

Overview of ECHO Research and Applications

Early studies indicated that participation in Project ECHO led to significant improvements in community provider knowledge, self-efficacy, and professional satisfaction (Arora et al., 2010). Notably, a prospective cohort study found that patients receiving care through a PCP enrolled in ECHO had similar outcomes to patients receiving care at a specialist hepatitis C clinic, demonstrating the effectiveness of the model in achieving high-quality care (Arora et al., 2011b). As the ECHO model has expanded to management of over 100 other complex mental and physical health conditions, evidence supporting its efficacy in improving provider knowledge and clinical skills has grown, with emerging evidence that participation in ECHO influences provider behavior and improves patient outcomes (Office of Health Policy, Office of the Assistant Secretary for Planning and Evaluation, 2019; Zhou, Crawford, Serhal, Kurdyak, & Sockalingam, 2016).

ECHO Autism

Based on the prior success of the Project ECHO model, the framework was adapted to enhance access to best-practice care for children with autism. The ECHO Autism model uses the "hub" and "spoke" framework to connect an interdisciplinary team of experts to community-based providers using HIPAA-compliant videoconferencing (Zoom). The program facilitates real-time interactions among participants and experts, enables sharing of resources, and provides a platform for teaching and collaborative case-based learning. Over time, ECHO Autism has been further adapted to meet the needs of professionals across disciplines. The following sections will describe the original model, more recent adaptations, and future directions.

ECHO Autism: Pediatric Primary Care

The ECHO Autism program was first launched in 2015 at the University of Missouri to improve knowledge, skills, and confidence among pediatricians and other PCPs in the identification of autism symptoms and in management of common co-occurring medical and psychiatric conditions in children with autism (Mazurek, Brown, Curran, & Sohl, 2017; Sohl, Mazurek, & Brown, 2017). The original hub team included a pediatrician, a clinical psychologist, a child and adolescent psychiatrist, a dietician, a social worker, and a parent of a child with ASD. This team developed a curriculum focused on screening and medical management of autism, with specific integration of evidence-based guidelines and algorithms (Buie et al., 2010; Furuta et al., 2012; Johnson & Myers, 2007; Maglione, Gans, Das, Timbie, & Kasari, 2012; Mahajan et al., 2012; Malow et al., 2012; Vasa et al., 2016). The resulting ECHO Autism program consists of regular 90- to 120-min ECHO Autism Clinics held twice per month. Each clinic follows a standard agenda, including introductions, a brief (15 min) didactic presentation, and one to two de-identified case presentations. Didactic topics include *What is Autism?, Screening and Next Steps, Supporting Families, Sleep Problems and Autism, Irritability & Agitation and Autism, Anxiety and Autism, ADHD and Autism, Constipation and Autism, Resources, Overview of ABA and Behavioral Strategies, Special Education Services,* and *Feeding Issues and Autism.* Copies of didactic materials, guidelines, and resources are made available through a secure online portal.

Consistent with the Project ECHO model (Arora et al., 2007), the majority of learning occurs within the context of case discussions. Cases are selected and presented by PCPs, and generally focus on autism screening and/or management of medical, behavioral, or psychosocial challenges in children with autism. The expert team and all participants have opportunities to discuss and ask questions, and the expert team provides evidence-based recommendations and guidance. PCPs are able to re-present cases during later sessions to receive feedback and ongoing coaching. Through this process, PCPs acquire new knowledge and skills through guided practice and collaborative learning while maintaining responsibility for the care of their own patients.

An initial 6-month pilot study was conducted with a sample of 14 PCPs practicing in rural and underserved areas (Mazurek et al., 2017). Measures of practice behavior and self-efficacy were administered at baseline and after participation in ECHO Autism program. The program greatly improved providers' confidence in their ability to effectively screen and identify autism symptoms, manage common co-occurring conditions, and support and assist families in accessing resources. Providers also reported increased use of autism screenings and autism-specific resources and toolkits. Based on these preliminary results, a large-scale multi-site study was more recently conducted to test the efficacy and effectiveness of the ECHO Autism program using a more rigorous study design. A modified stepped-wedge cluster randomized design study was implemented across ten ECHO Autism hub teams located at academic medical centers in the United States and Canada. Each site delivered the ECHO Autism curriculum to a target sample of 15 PCPs caring for underserved children. Assessments were conducted at four time points: baseline, mid-ECHO, post-ECHO, and follow-up (3 months after completion). In addition to measures of self-efficacy and satisfaction, direct assessments of knowledge and practice change were collected, including a knowledge test and chart reviews conducted by study staff. When the study is nearing completion, the results will provide important information about the effectiveness of the ECHO model in achieving practice change.

ECHO Autism STAT

The original ECHO Autism program aims to expedite access to early diagnosis and intervention by training PCPs in the administration of standardized general developmental and autism screening tools (Mazurek et al., 2017), as the systematic use of formal screening tools is an important component of the early identification process (Johnson & Myers, 2007). However, even children who are appropriately screened face barriers to diagnosis and early intervention. The wait time for diagnostic evaluations at academic medical centers or specialty clinics can range from 4 to 12 months or more, depending on the region (Austin et al., 2016; Bisgaier, Levinson, Cutts, & Rhodes, 2011; Jimenez, Martinez Alcaraz, Williams, & Strom, 2017). The ECHO Autism STAT model was developed to reduce these diagnostic delays by training community-based PCPs in both screening *and* diagnosis of young children at highest risk for autism (Mazurek, Curran, Burnette, & Sohl, 2019). ECHO Autism STAT builds upon and extends the original ECHO Autism program by combining ongoing virtual mentorship and practice with more in-depth diagnostic training, including hands-on training and practice with standardized tools. The program follows a multi-tiered approach to diagnostic evaluation, in which the tools and nature of the assessment are determined by symptom presentation and complexity (Missouri Autism Guidelines, 2010).

The program begins with an in-person training focused on autism assessment, including administration of the Screening Tool for Autism in Toddlers and Young Children (STAT). The STAT is a standardized play-based observational assessment tool that specifically targets behaviors most indicative of autism in children between the ages of 14 and 48 months (Stone, McMahon, & Henderson, 2008; Stone & Ousley, 2008). After this initial training, PCPs participate for 12 months in bimonthly 90-min ECHO Autism STAT sessions. Each session includes a brief didactic presentation and one PCP-presented case. In addition to the standard ECHO Autism curriculum, the expanded ECHO Autism STAT program includes specific emphasis on symptom identification, screening tools, diagnostic interviewing, differential diagnosis, and providing diagnostic feedback. In order to fully participate in the program, PCPs are required to achieve reliability in coding and administration of the STAT (including submission of videotaped recordings). Using a learning network approach, PCPs also engage in quality improvement methods to track and discuss strategies for administration of general developmental and autism-specific screening tools in their practices.

During the first 6 months of the program, case presentations focus on screening and management of symptoms. During the second 6 months, PCPs who have achieved STAT reliability are able to present cases for diagnostic consideration. For these diagnostic cases, PCPs follow a detailed ECHO Autism STAT diagnostic algorithm for assessment of children determined to be at-risk for autism following routine surveillance and/or formal screening. Instead of referring children elsewhere for diagnostic evaluation, PCPs administer the STAT and a semi-structured diagnostic interview for autism in their own practices. The results of this assessment are then presented for discussion during an ECHO Autism STAT session. During the session, cases are determined to either (1) meet criteria of a diagnosis of ASD, or (2) require referral for further evaluation due to subtle or complex symptom presentation. This risk-stratified process is designed to expedite access to diagnosis and intervention for children at highest risk for autism, while facilitating comprehensive assessments when warranted.

The ECHO Autism STAT program was initially tested in a sample of 18 PCPs practicing in underserved regions (Mazurek et al., 2019). Participants completed measures of practice behavior and self-efficacy at baseline and after completion of the 12-month program. De-identified case presentation forms were also examined. Participants demonstrated significant improvements in self-efficacy, increased their use of autism screening tools, and reported increased capacity for evaluating and caring for children with autism. A total of 47 cases were presented for diagnostic discussion; of those, 31 were diagnosed and 16 were referred for more comprehensive evaluation. Importantly, these children received streamlined care and expedited access to intervention and services within their communities, without the need for travel to diagnostic specialty centers. The ECHO Autism STAT program also has the potential for reducing diagnostic wait times at specialty centers by facilitating community-based diagnoses when possible, and reserving scarce specialty resources for children with more complex needs.

ECHO Autism Transition

Beyond the initial diagnosis and early intervention, individuals with ASD continue to require specialized care and support across their life span. In fact, their healthcare needs increase in complexity during the transition from adolescence to adulthood, with frequent worsening of co-occurring medical and psychiatric symptoms (Billstedt, Gillberg, & Gillberg, 2005; Davignon, Qian, Massolo, & Croen, 2018; Taylor & Seltzer, 2010). Unfortunately, the transition from pediatric to adult health care is particularly challenging for youth with ASD (Kuhlthau et al., 2016). Pediatric providers often struggle to transition their patients with ASD to adult healthcare providers, as there are few with adequate training in autism (Kuhlthau, Warfield, Hurson, Delahaye, & Crossman, 2015). As a result, youth with ASD experience significant unmet healthcare needs and receive fewer outpatient healthcare services as they age into adulthood (Nathenson & Zablotsky, 2017; Nicolaidis et al., 2013). Thus, training community-based PCPs to meet the needs of transition-age youth with ASD may help address these healthcare barriers.

The ECHO Autism Transition program was specifically developed to address the needs of transition-age youth and young adults with ASD (Mazurek et al., 2020). The program targets both pediatric and adult healthcare providers, and focuses on evidence-based healthcare strategies. Each 1-h session includes a brief didactic and a case presentation. The expert hub team includes an adult neurologist, an internal medicine-pediatrics physician, a clinical psychologist, a neurologist/sleep specialist, a parent advocate/transition specialist, and a young adult self-advocate with ASD. The initial 12-session curriculum included the following topics: *What is Autism?, Psychiatric Co-occurring Conditions, Medical Co-occurring Conditions, Behavior Management in Primary Care, Supporting Families through Transition to Adulthood, Healthcare Transition Planning, Life Skills Development, Supporting the Self Advocate, Guardianship, Special Education Transition to ADA, Housing and Community Supports for Adults with Autism, and Relationships and Sexuality in Autism.* The program has continued to evolve, with new didactic topics and resources being added to respond to the needs of participating PCPs.

An initial pilot study was conducted with a sample of 16 PCPs who participated in 12 weekly sessions over a 3-month period (Mazurek et al., 2020). Measures of self-efficacy, knowledge, and practice were administered at baseline and after completion of the program. Participants demonstrated significant improvements in self-efficacy regarding caring for youth and young adults with ASD and reported high satisfaction and practice improvements. However, there were no significant changes in knowledge or perceived barriers to caring for youth with ASD. The results suggest that the model may be promising for improving healthcare quality for transition-age youth with ASD, but that a more comprehensive solution may be needed to fully address the healthcare needs of this population. Additional research is currently underway to refine and enhance the scope of the program, particularly in meeting the specific needs of adult healthcare providers.

Case Study

"Alex Robinson" is a 2-year-old boy who lives with his parents and a baby sister in a small rural community. His mother stays at home with the children, and his father is a delivery driver for a local construction company. His parents have been concerned about his development for the past few months because he does not seem to be talking as much as other children his age. A friend of the family suggested that they contact a speech therapist who works in their community. Alex has been receiving speech therapy at a local clinic for the past 2 months. His speech therapist is concerned about his interactions with her and has observed that he has trouble moving from one task to another. He has made limited progress in therapy, and continues to have few words and some echolalia. The therapist mentions her concern to Mrs. Robinson, and suggests that she talk with Alex's doctor about his development. Mrs. Robinson makes an appointment with her family nurse practitioner. The nurse practitioner is also concerned about Alex's development, and makes a referral to a Developmental and Behavioral Pediatrics Clinic at the nearest academic medical center. The medical center is three hours away, and there is a 6-month wait for the next available appointment. Mrs. Robinson is very worried about Alex, but is concerned that she will not be able to afford the cost of the evaluation. Her husband uses the family car during the day and is not able to take off work, and she is afraid that she won't be able to secure transportation or a babysitter for her daughter.

At their next appointment, Mrs. Robinson discusses these issues with Alex's speech therapist. The therapist talks with Mrs. Robinson about the importance of identifying an accurate diagnosis so Alex can get the right treatment. Mrs. Robinson confides that she is really overwhelmed and not sure what to do next. She adds that Alex is starting to have significant problems with sleep and aggression, and these problems have become more and more challenging for her at home. The therapist suggests she see a local pediatrician, Dr. Flores, who is part of a new program called ECHO that connects local doctors with specialists at the academic medical center. Mrs. Robinson is relieved that a doctor in her community may be able to help and is willing to make an appointment. She also consents for the therapist to communicate with the pediatrician so she can share information prior to Alex's appointment.

When Dr. Flores meets Alex, she is immediately concerned. He has less than 10 words and makes very little eye contact. He engages in high-pitched squeals throughout the visit. She notes that he often flicks his fingers near his eyes and jumps up and down repeatedly when he sees a new object. She administers both the Ages and Stages Questionnaire 3rd Edition (ASQ-3) and the Modified Checklist for Autism in Toddlers (M-CHAT-R) with Follow-up Interview. The screening results indicate that Alex has significant communication delays and that he is at risk for autism. Dr. Flores schedules a follow-up appointment with Alex to conduct the STAT and to complete a diagnostic interview for autism with his mother. The interview and STAT are also strongly suggestive of an autism diagnosis. Dr. Flores shares some preliminary information about the evaluation with Mrs. Robinson and shares that she would like to discuss the results with the team of autism specialists through ECHO Autism. Mrs. Robinson is relieved to know that a team of professionals is supporting her son and Dr. Flores.

Two weeks later, Dr. Flores presents this case during an ECHO Autism STAT session. After joining the Zoom meeting from her office computer over the lunch hour, she is greeted by the interdisciplinary hub team. Many more familiar faces, including primary care physicians and nurse practitioners from other communities, join the videoconference. Dr. Flores uses a standard template to present de-identified results and information about Alex's development. As the case unfolds, the group learns about Alex's early language delays, social interaction difficulties, and repetitive behaviors. The group learns that his early health history was relatively uneventful, but that significant developmental and behavioral concerns emerged around 15 months of age. At that time, he began to have difficulty falling asleep and began to demonstrate picky eating and aggressive behavior. After Dr. Flores presents the initial case information and results of her evaluation, participants begin asking clarifying questions. Many of them recognize elements of this case in their own patients and are seeking more information to provide additional supports and recommendations.

After a hearty discussion, the specialty team engages in some clarifying questions and recommendations for Dr. Flores. The developmental pediatrician and clinical psychologist on the hub team discuss the red flags of autism presented during the case. They each "think out loud" about the behaviors observed during the STAT evaluation and the symptoms reported during the diagnostic interview. They discuss the diagnostic criteria and the components of a best-practice evaluation, and voice agreement with Dr. Flores that Alex meets criteria for a diagnosis of autism spectrum disorder. The team also discusses strategies for providing feedback and support to Alex's family.

The social worker on the hub team describes important community-based resources that may be useful to support this child and family. She notes that he has state-funded insurance and suggests a pathway to support his needs through this insurer. She also emphasizes the importance of enrolling in the state Early Intervention Program. She encourages Dr. Flores to have a conversation with Alex's mother about initiating an early intervention referral now and about planning for the transition to early childhood special education services in the near future. The parent expert also shares her lived experience and discusses the grief process that many parents feel when receiving a diagnosis. She recommends several parent-support guides and resources that may be helpful, including Autism Speaks Toolkits and Family 2 Family resources. She shares strategies for supporting this family through the feedback session and afterward.

For the remainder of the case discussion, the hub team focuses on supporting Dr. Flores in addressing other areas of concern. The child and adolescent psychiatrist and clinical psychologist discuss the importance of understanding the function of Alex's aggressive behavior in developing a treatment plan. They share information about early intervention and behavioral strategies that may be helpful to support Alex's communication and reduce his frustration and challenging behaviors. The psychiatrist notes that while medications are approved for irritability in children with autism, they would not be appropriate for this case. She also touches on sleep concerns and reinforces the need for consistent bedtime routines. She reminds Dr. Flores that the Autism Speaks Sleep Toolkit is a good resource for families, and shares a link to this resource. The conversation continues with the pediatric dietician discussing the potential for nutritional deficiencies in children with problem feeding and steps for further evaluation. She shares tips for improving food acceptance and also makes a targeted recommendation to connect with a local pediatric dietician through the Early Intervention Program.

At the end of the 90-min ECHO Autism STAT session, Dr. Flores has developed a clear idea regarding the next steps for Alex and his family. She and the other participants will also receive written recommendations outlining the tools and recommendations discussed during the session. Since Alex's diagnosis was verified through this process, he and his family will not need to travel or wait 6 months for an evaluation, and he will be able to access the appropriate services to support his health and development from trusted providers in his own community.

New Applications and Future Directions

The ECHO Autism model is an innovative way to share specialized knowledge and support clinicians and professionals who are practicing in remote and underserved areas. The health inequalities that exist for rural and underserved populations are exacerbated by limited access to services and best-practice care. ECHO Autism allows the movement of knowledge without the movement of patients, thereby maximizing provider time in the office while accelerating practice-based learning in a cost-efficient manner. The program strives to redesign the care system to reduce disparities and to enhance access to timely and evidence-based care for children and families. The ECHO Autism Primary Care programs (including ECHO Autism STAT and ECHO Autism Transition) partner with primary care providers to expertly identify autism and proactively support families through their journey. However, primary care is only one component of the broader care community. Interdisciplinary solutions are needed to fully support individuals with autism, their families, and their communities.

Access to evidence-based practice and well-trained professionals across care settings is critical to reducing lifetime costs and burden and maximizing quality of life for individuals with autism. The strategic vision for ECHO Autism programs is to create communities of learners across disciplines and settings in which specialty and community-based professionals can support one another in improving the system for people with autism. As the ECHO Autism program has grown, the scope has expanded to create new expert hub teams to mentor and support teachers, behavior analysts, crisis care teams, mental health professionals, adult healthcare providers, early intervention providers, and family advocates.

For example, in addition to supporting early diagnosis in primary care, the ECHO Autism model was recently expanded to facilitate more comprehensive diagnostic assessments in the community. The ECHO Autism Diagnostics program provides community-based psychologists with additional training and mentorship in best-practice strategies for autism diagnosis. The program includes hands-on training in the administration of gold-standard tools (including the Autism Diagnostic Observation Schedule, ADOS-2) (Lord et al., 2012), and an intensive diagnostic curriculum focused on differential diagnosis and other comprehensive assessment components. With this additional mentorship and support, these psychologists are able to complement the work of ECHO Autism STAT providers by offering more comprehensive assessment options for diagnosis and treatment planning for families in local communities.

Expanding the reach of the program to an even broader range of professionals, the ECHO Autism Crisis Care program strives to enhance communication across crisis care settings. Participants in this program include professionals from outpatient mental health, emergency departments, and inpatient units who are building a learning community to facilitate safe and proactive care for individuals with autism. The ECHO Autism model is also being piloted as a vehicle to accelerate training and implementation practice for the World Health Organization's Caregiver Skills Training. This novel use of ECHO Autism, in partnership with Autism Speaks and Easterseals, is intended to significantly increase access to high-quality caregiver support in low-resourced areas.

The ECHO framework of case-based learning and guided practice is applicable across many disciplines. With worldwide shortages of autism resources and specialists, there is a growing need for programs that equip local communities and providers with the knowledge they need to provide best-practice care. The ECHO Autism Collaborative includes over 25 national and 8 international programs utilizing the ECHO Autism model to reshape autism care delivery around the world. As the ECHO Autism Collaborative continues to expand, the intent is to increase coordination among and across programs to achieve prepared and activated communities that foster inclusion and maximize outcomes for individuals with autism and their families. ECHO Autism is open to professionals across disciplines who are interested in improving access to best-practice care for individuals with autism. More information about the program is available online at www.echoautism.org.

References

Aldinger, K. A., Lane, C. J., Veenstra-VanderWeele, J., & Levitt, P. (2015). Patterns of risk for multiple co-occurring medical conditions replicate across distinct cohorts of children with autism spectrum disorder. *Autism Research, 8,* 771–781.

Arora, S., Geppert, C. M. A., Kalishman, S., Dion, D., Pullara, F., Bjeletich, B., … Scaletti, J. V. (2007). Academic health center management of chronic diseases through knowledge networks: Project ECHO. *Academic Medicine : Journal of the Association of American Medical Colleges, 82*, 154–160.

Arora, S., Kalishman, S., Dion, D., Som, D., Thornton, K., Bankhurst, A., … Murata, G. (2011a). Partnering urban academic medical centers and rural primary care clinicians to provide complex chronic disease care. *Health Affairs, 30*, 1176–1184.

Arora, S., Thornton, K., Murata, G., Deming, P., Kalishman, S., Dion, D., … Qualls, C. (2011b). Outcomes of hepatitis C treatment by primary care providers. *The New England Journal of Medicine, 364*, 2199–2207.

Arora, S., Kalishman, S., Thornton, K., Dion, D., Murata, G., Deming, P., … Pak, W. (2010). Expanding access to hepatitis C virus treatment—Extension for Community Healthcare Outcomes (ECHO) project: Disruptive innovation in specialty care. *Hepatology, 52*, 1124–1133.

Arora, S., Thornton, K., Komaromy, M., Kalishman, S., Katzman, J., & Duhigg, D. (2014). Demonopolizing medical knowledge. *Academic Medicine, 89,* 30.

Arunyanart, W., Fenick, A., Ukritchon, S., Imjaijitt, W., Northrup, V., & Weitzman, C. (2012). Developmental and autism screening: A survey across six states. *Infants & Young Children, 25,* 175–187.

Austin, J., Manning-Courtney, P., Johnson, M. L., Weber, R., Johnson, H., Murray, D., … Murray, M. (2016). Improving access to care at autism treatment centers: A system analysis approach. *Pediatrics, 137*, S149–S157.

Baio, J., Wiggins, L., Christensen, D. L., Maenner, M. J., Daniels, J., Warren, Z., … White, T. (2018). Prevalence of autism spectrum disorder among children aged 8 years—Autism and developmental disabilities monitoring network, 11 sites, United States, 2014. *MMWR Surveillance Summaries, 67*, 1–23.

Bandura, A. (1986). *Social foundations of thought and action*. Englewood Cliffs, NJ: Prentice Hall.

Begeer, S., El Bouk, S., Boussaid, W., Terwogt, M. M., & Koot, H. M. (2009). Underdiagnosis and referral bias of autism in ethnic minorities. *Journal of Autism and Developmental Disorders, 39,* 142–148.

Billstedt, E., Gillberg, C., & Gillberg, C. (2005). Autism after adolescence: Population-based 13-to 22-year follow-up study of 120 individuals with autism diagnosed in childhood. *Journal of Autism and Developmental Disorders, 35,* 351–360.

Bisgaier, J., Levinson, D., Cutts, D. B., & Rhodes, K. V. (2011). Access to autism evaluation appointments with developmental-behavioral and neurodevelopmental subspecialists. *Archives of Pediatrics & Adolescent Medicine, 165,* 673–674.

Bishop-Fitzpatrick, L., & Kind, A. J. H. (2017). A scoping review of health disparities in autism spectrum disorder. *Journal of Autism and Developmental Disorders, 47,* 3380–3391.

Brookman-Frazee, L., Stadnick, N., Chlebowski, C., Baker-Ericzén, M., & Ganger, W. (2018). Characterizing psychiatric comorbidity in children with autism spectrum disorder receiving publicly funded mental health services. *Autism, 22,* 938–952.

Buie, T., Campbell, D. B., Fuchs, G. J., Furuta, G. T., Levy, J., VandeWater, J., … Beaudet, A. L. (2010). Evaluation, diagnosis, and treatment of gastrointestinal disorders in individuals with ASDs: A consensus report. *Pediatrics, 125,* S1–S18.

Carbone, P. S., Behl, D. D., Azor, V., & Murphy, N. A. (2010). The medical home for children with autism spectrum disorders: Parent and pediatrician perspectives. *Journal of Autism and Developmental Disorders, 40,* 317–324.

Carbone, P. S., Farley, M., & Davis, T. (2010). Primary care for children with autism. *American Family Physician, 81,* 453–460.

Carbone, P. S., Murphy, N. A., Norlin, C., Azor, V., Sheng, X., & Young, P. C. (2013). Parent and pediatrician perspectives regarding the primary care of children with autism spectrum disorders. *Journal of Autism and Developmental Disorders, 43*(4), 964–972.

Carbone, P. S., Norlin, C., & Young, P. C. (2016). Improving early identification and ongoing care of children with autism spectrum disorder. *Pediatrics, 137,* e20151850.

Chiang, H.-L., & Gau, S. S.-F. (2016). Comorbid psychiatric conditions as mediators to predict later social adjustment in youths with autism spectrum disorder. *Journal of Child Psychology and Psychiatry, 57,* 103–111.

Croen, L. A., Najjar, D. V., Ray, G. T., Lotspeich, L., & Bernal, P. (2006). A comparison of health care utilization and costs of children with and without autism spectrum disorders in a large group-model health plan. *Pediatrics, 118,* e1203–e1211.

Davignon, M. N., Qian, Y., Massolo, M., & Croen, L. A. (2018). Psychiatric and medical conditions in transition-aged individuals with ASD. *Pediatrics, 141,* S335–S345.

de Bruin, E. I., Ferdinand, R. F., Meester, S., de Nijs, P. F., & Verheij, F. (2007). High rates of psychiatric co-morbidity in PDD-NOS. *Journal of Autism and Developmental Disorders, 37,* 877–886.

Furuta, G. T., Williams, K., Kooros, K., Kaul, A., Panzer, R., Coury, D. L., & Fuchs, G. (2012). Management of constipation in children and adolescents with autism spectrum disorders. *Pediatrics, 130,* S98–S105.

Gillis, J. M. (2009). Screening practices of family physicians and pediatricians in 2 southern states. *Infants & Young Children, 22,* 321–331.

Hyman, S. L., & Johnson, J. K. (2012). Autism and pediatric practice: Toward a medical home. *Journal of Autism and Developmental Disorders, 42,* 1156–1164.

Jimenez, M. E., Martinez Alcaraz, E., Williams, J., & Strom, B. L. (2017). Access to developmental pediatrics evaluations for at-risk children. *Journal of Developmental and Behavioral Pediatrics, 38,* 228–232.

Johnson, C. P., & Myers, S. M. (2007). Identification and evaluation of children with autism spectrum disorders. *Pediatrics, 120,* 1183–1215.

Karpur, A., Lello, A., Frazier, T., Dixon, P. J., & Shih, A. J. (2019). Health disparities among children with autism spectrum disorders: Analysis of the National Survey of Children's Health 2016. *Journal of Autism and Developmental Disorders, 49,* 1652–1664.

Keil, A., Breunig, C., Fleischfresser, S., & Oftedahl, E. (2014). Promoting routine use of developmental and autism-specific screening tools by pediatric primary care clinicians. *WMJ, 113,* 227–231.

Kogan, M. D., Strickland, B. B., Blumberg, S. J., Singh, G. K., Perrin, J. M., & van Dyck, P. C. (2008). A national profile of the health care experiences and family impact of autism spectrum disorder among children in the United States, 2005–2006. *Pediatrics, 122,* e1149–e1158.

Kuhlthau, K. A., Delahaye, J., Erickson-Warfield, M., Shui, A., Crossman, M., & van der Weerd, E. (2016). Health care transition services for youth with autism spectrum disorders: Perspectives of caregivers. *Pediatrics, 137,* S158–S166.

Kuhlthau, K. A., Warfield, M. E., Hurson, J., Delahaye, J., & Crossman, M. K. (2015). Pediatric provider's perspectives on the transition to adult health care for youth with autism spectrum disorder: Current strategies and promising new directions. *Autism,* 262–271.

Lave, J., & Wenger, E. (1991). *Situated learning: Legitimate peripheral participation.* Cambridge, UK: Cambridge University Press.

Lin, S. C., & Yu, S. M. (2015). Disparities in healthcare access and utilization among children with autism spectrum disorder from immigrant non-English primary language households in the United States. *International Journal of MCH and AIDS, 3,* 159–167.

Lord, C., Rutter, M., DiLavore, P., Risi, S., Gotham, K., & Bishop, S. (2012). *Autism diagnostic observation schedule–2nd edition (ADOS-2).* Los Angeles, CA: Western Psychological Corporation.

MacDonald, R., Parry-Cruwys, D., Dupere, S., & Ahearn, W. (2014). Assessing progress and outcome of early intensive behavioral intervention for toddlers with autism. *Research in Developmental Disabilities, 35,* 3632–3644.

Maglione, M. A., Gans, D., Das, L., Timbie, J., & Kasari, C. (2012). Nonmedical interventions for children with ASD: Recommended guidelines and further research needs. *Pediatrics, 130,* S169–S178.

Mahajan, R., Bernal, M. P., Panzer, R., Whitaker, A., Roberts, W., Handen, B., … Veenstra-VanderWeele, J. (2012). Clinical practice pathways for evaluation and medication choice for attention-deficit/hyperactivity disorder symptoms in autism spectrum disorders. *Pediatrics, 130,* S125–S138.

Malow, B. A., Byars, K., Johnson, K., Weiss, S., Bernal, P., Goldman, S. E., … Glaze, D. G. (2012). A practice pathway for the identification, evaluation, and management of insomnia in children and adolescents with autism spectrum disorders. *Pediatrics, 130,* S106–S124.

Mandell, D. S. (2013). Adults with autism—A new minority. *Journal of General Internal Medicine, 28,* 751–752.

Mattila, M.-L., Hurtig, T., Haapsamo, H., Jussila, K., Kuusikko-Gauffin, S., Kielinen, M., … Moilanen, I. (2010). Comorbid psychiatric disorders associated with Asperger syndrome/high-functioning autism: A community- and clinic-based study. *Journal of Autism and Developmental Disorders, 40,* 1080–1093.

Mazurek, M. O., Brown, R., Curran, A., & Sohl, K. (2017). ECHO autism: A new model for training primary care providers in best-practice care for children with autism. *Clinical Pediatrics, 56,* 247–256.

Mazurek, M. O., Curran, A., Burnette, C., & Sohl, K. (2019). ECHO autism STAT: Accelerating early access to autism diagnosis. *Journal of Autism and Developmental Disorders, 49,* 127–137.

Mazurek, M. O., & Petroski, G. F. (2015). Sleep problems in children with autism spectrum disorder: Examining the contributions of sensory over-responsivity and anxiety. *Sleep Medicine, 16,* 270–279.

Mazurek, M. O., Stobbe, G., Loftin, R., Malow, B. A., Agrawal, M. M., Tapia, M., … Sohl, K. (2020). ECHO autism transition: Enhancing healthcare for adolescents and young adults with autism spectrum disorder. *Autism, 24,* 633-644.

Mazurek, M. O., Vasa, R. A., Kalb, L. G., Kanne, S. M., Rosenberg, D., Keefer, A., … Lowery, L. A. (2013). Anxiety, sensory over-responsivity, and gastrointestinal problems in children with autism spectrum disorders. *Journal of Abnormal Child Psychology, 41,* 165–176.

Missouri Autism Guidelines. (2010). *Autism spectrum disorders: Missouri best practice guidelines for screening, diagnosis, and assessment.* Missouri Autism Guidelines Initiative.

Nathenson, R. A., & Zablotsky, B. (2017). The transition to the adult health care system among youths with autism spectrum disorder. *Psychiatric Services, 68,* 735–738.

Newacheck, P. W., Hung, Y.-Y., & Wright, K. K. (2002). Racial and ethnic disparities in access to care for children with special health care needs. *Ambulatory Pediatrics, 2,* 247–254.

Nicolaidis, C., Raymaker, D., McDonald, K., Dern, S., Boisclair, W. C., Ashkenazy, E., & Baggs, A. (2013). Comparison of healthcare experiences in autistic and non-autistic adults: A cross-sectional online survey facilitated by an academic-community partnership. *Journal of General Internal Medicine, 28,* 761–769.

Office of Health Policy, Office of the Assistant Secretary for Planning and Evaluation (ASPE). (2019, February). *Current State of Technology-Enabled Collaborative Learning and Capacity Building Models. Report to Congress.* U.S. Department of Health and Human Services.

Raymaker, D. M., McDonald, K. E., Ashkenazy, E., Gerrity, M., Baggs, A. M., Kripke, C., … Nicolaidis, C. (2017). Barriers to healthcare: Instrument development and comparison between autistic adults and adults with and without other disabilities. *Autism, 21,* 972–984.

Self, T., Parham, D., & Rajagopalan, J. (2015). *Autism spectrum disorder early screening practices: A survey of physicians 36,* 195–207.

Sheldrick, R. C., Maye, M. P., & Carter, A. S. (2017). Age at first identification of autism spectrum disorder: An analysis of two US surveys. *Journal of the American Academy of Child and Adolescent Psychiatry, 56,* 313–320.

Simonoff, E., Pickles, A., Charman, T., Chandler, S., Loucas, T., & Baird, G. (2008). Psychiatric disorders in children with autism spectrum disorders: Prevalence, comorbidity, and associated factors in a population-derived sample. *Journal of the American Academy of Child and Adolescent Psychiatry, 47,* 921–929.

Sohl, K., Mazurek, M. O., & Brown, R. (2017). ECHO autism: Using technology and mentorship to bridge gaps, increase access to care, and bring best practice autism care to primary care. *Clinical Pediatrics, 56,* 509–511.

Soke, G. N., Maenner, M. J., Christensen, D., Kurzius-Spencer, M., & Schieve, L. A. (2018). Prevalence of co-occurring medical and behavioral conditions/symptoms among 4- and 8-year-old children with autism spectrum disorder in selected areas of the United States in 2010. *Journal of Autism and Developmental Disorders, 48,* 2663–2676.

Sprenger, L., Bühler, E., Poustka, L., Bach, C., Heinzel-Gutenbrunner, M., Kamp-Becker, I., & Bachmann, C. (2013). Impact of ADHD symptoms on autism spectrum disorder symptom severity. *Research in Developmental Disabilities, 34,* 3545–3552.

Stone, W. L., McMahon, C. R., & Henderson, L. M. (2008). Use of the screening tool for autism in two-year-olds (STAT) for children under 24 months: An exploratory study. *Autism, 12,* 557–573.

Stone, W. L., & Ousley, O. Y. (2008). *Screening tool for autism in toddlers and young children (STAT).* Vanderbilt University.

Taylor, J. L., & Seltzer, M. M. (2010). Changes in the autism behavioral phenotype during the transition to adulthood. *Journal of Autism and Developmental Disorders, 40,* 1431–1446.

Tregnago, M. K., & Cheak-Zamora, N. C. (2012). Systematic review of disparities in health care for individuals with autism spectrum disorders in the United States. *Research in Autism Spectrum Disorders, 6,* 1023–1031.

Tye, C., Runicles, A. K., Whitehouse, A. J. O., & Alvares, G. A. (2019). Characterizing the interplay between autism spectrum disorder and comorbid medical conditions: An integrative review. *Frontiers in Psychiatry, 9,* 751.

Unigwe, S., Buckley, C., Crane, L., Kenny, L., Remington, A., & Pellicano, E. (2017). GPs' confidence in caring for their patients on the autism spectrum: An online self-report study. *British Journal of General Practice, 67,* e445–e452.

Vasa, R. A., Mazurek, M. O., Mahajan, R., Bennett, A. E., Bernal, M. P., Nozzolillo, A. A., … Coury, D. L. (2016). Assessment and treatment of anxiety in youth with autism spectrum disorders. *Pediatrics, 137,* S115–S123.

Vygotsky, L. S. (1980). *Mind in society: The development of higher psychological processes.* Cambridge, MA: Harvard University Press.

Webb, S. J., & Jones, E. J. H. (2009). Early identification of autism: Early characteristics, onset of symptoms, and diagnostic stability. *Infants & Young Children, 22,* 100–118.

Zhou, C., Crawford, A., Serhal, E., Kurdyak, P., & Sockalingam, S. (2016). The impact of Project ECHO on participant and patient outcomes: A systematic review. *Academic Medicine, 91,* 1439–1461.

Zwaigenbaum, L., Bauman, M. L., Stone, W. L., Yirmiya, N., Estes, A., Hansen, R. L., … Wetherby, A. (2015). Early identification of autism spectrum disorder: Recommendations for practice and research. *Pediatrics*, *136*, S10–S40.

ASD, Trauma, and Coordinated Care

Samantha Fuld

Abstract This chapter explores issues related to trauma in youth with Autism Spectrum Disorder (ASD) and how trauma and its sequelae can be identified and addressed through interdisciplinary coordinated care. Foundational information on trauma-informed care (TIC) and intervention strategies are provided to help guide professionals and families in better understanding common experiences of trauma in youth with ASD and effective ways to offer support and promote healing.

Understanding Trauma in Youth with ASD

The Substance Abuse and Mental Health Services Administration (SAMHSA) defines trauma as an event, or a series of cumulative events that are "experienced by an individual as physically or emotionally harmful" (SAMHSA, 2014, p. 7) and which subsequently impact a person's biological, psychological, social, spiritual, or emotional well-being on an ongoing basis. This definition highlights trauma as subjective, and dependent on an individual's experience with distressing events. Due to the subjective nature of trauma, it is challenging to identify what type of event or experience may be considered traumatic.

An important development in understanding the impact of trauma has been the adverse childhood experience (ACE) studies (Felitti et al., 1998). This body of research has demonstrated a strong link between traumatic experiences in childhood and negative health outcomes (Anda et al., 2006; Edwards, Holden, Anda, & Felitti, 2003). This risk is cumulative, meaning that the more ACEs a child experiences, the higher their likelihood of developing multiple physical and psychological health problems including diabetes, cardiovascular disease, depression, and suicidality (Schilling, Aseltine & Gore, 2007). Berg, Shiu, Acharya, Stolbach, and Msall (2016) conducted a study examining rates of ACEs in children with ASD. Results indicated that a diagnosis of ASD is significantly associated with a higher probability of reporting one or more ACEs. Additionally, the number of children with ASD who

S. Fuld (✉)
School of Social Work, University of Maryland, Baltimore, MD, USA
e-mail: Samantha.Fuld@ssw.umaryland.edu

M. B. McClain et al. (eds.), *Interprofessional Care Coordination for Pediatric Autism Spectrum Disorder*, https://doi.org/10.1007/978-3-030-46295-6_21

were exposed to four or more ACEs was twice as high as neurotypical peers, substantially increasing their risk for negative health outcomes. Importantly, this research focused on situational indicators of trauma such as traumatic loss, poverty, family instability (domestic violence, substance abuse), and neighborhood violence which may not fully capture the breadth of experiences common to children with ASD that may be experienced as traumatic.

Kerns et al. (2015) point out that youth with ASD:

> Encounter a number of distinct daily stressors related to their diagnosis that may have untoward effects on their emotional functioning…such as social confusion, peer rejection, prevention or punishment of preferred behaviors (e.g. restricted, repetitive interests) and sensory sensitivity to daily stimuli (e.g. lights, loud sounds) (p. 3476).

Each of these stressors when experienced cumulatively over time have the potential to be experienced as traumatic. Furthermore, characteristics of ASD such as difficulties with novel experiences, socialization, frustration tolerance, and sensory integration can result in children with ASD perceiving such sensations and experiences as more stressful and potentially traumatic than typically developing children (Kerns et al., 2015). There is also a significant body of research to suggest that trauma in the form of adverse social experiences such as peer victimization is as much as four times higher among youth with ASD than their neurotypical peers (Cappadocia, Weiss & Pepler, 2012; Hoover & Kaufman, 2018; Zeedyk, Rodriguez, Tipton, Baker, & Blacher, 2014).

Myths and Misconceptions

The study of ACEs and trauma in ASD is a relatively new field of study. As a result, treatment frameworks that exist to help children with ASD meet behavioral goals and developmental benchmarks; however trauma-focused models for intervention that focus on mental health and well-being have yet to be fully researched and developed (Fuld, 2018). There are a few key myths that have likely contributed to the delay in acknowledging trauma as an important focus for research and practice to support youth with ASD. The first is an assumption that some core features of ASD including internal focus and lack of social awareness may protect youth with ASD from the subjective experience of trauma, particularly when the traumatic event is social or relational in nature. This is a misguided assumption. Studies have found that children with ASD experience high rates of social anxiety (Bellini, 2006; Wu et al., 2015). Many children with ASD notice and are quite distressed by social exclusion and the stigma associated with ASD (Humphrey & Lewis, 2008; Locke, Ishijima, Kasari, & London, 2010; Sebastian, Blakemore & Charman, 2009). There can also be a fear among providers that inquiring about traumatic experiences will cause the child to newly recognize that a traumatic experience has occurred, or retraumatize the child. In reality, inquiring about trauma, making space to talk about it, and offering support is critical in addressing the isolation that can be inherent in having to cope independently with the impact of trauma (The National Child Traumatic Stress Network, 2008).

Given the dearth of research in trauma-focused interventions for youth with ASD, there also may be an assumption that traditional models for youth who have experienced trauma are not effective for youth with ASD or that youth with ASD may not have the skills or capacity to participate. This is not a reason to deny youth with ASD access to trauma-informed care (TIC). In a review of diagnosis and treatment models for Post-Traumatic Stress Disorder (PTSD) in people with ASD, Rumball (2018) concluded that traditional trauma-informed treatment strategies for PTSD are applicable to people with ASD and likely to be effective. Modifications such as longer session-length and treatment time and the use of concrete language in explaining trauma and the treatment process were recommended to enhance effectiveness for people with ASD.

Challenges for Coordinated Care

There are several challenges to coordinating care as it relates to trauma in children with ASD. The first is a lack of knowledge about assessment and TIC in youth with ASD, which can make it challenging for families or care teams to find experienced providers and for providers looking to learn more about TIC to locate effective resources. As the experience of trauma is subjective, communication may also be a barrier. Some youth with ASD may not be able to effectively articulate that they have experienced trauma, even to those closest to them. Additionally, if the experience of trauma is communicated in a clinical care setting where confidentiality must be maintained, consent is required to share information about trauma with other members of a care team (school, community supports, etc.). Due to the sensitive nature of many traumatic experiences and fear of judgment or stigma, families may be hesitant to speak openly about these experiences with a broader care team.

Importantly, TIC for children requires significant family support. Depending on the type of trauma, families may be working through the challenges of the experience themselves or could be very distanced from it. Stavropoulos, Bolourian, and Blacher (2018) also point out that it can be challenging for parents to detect changes in behavior when children are young and changing regularly, and/or if the parents are coping with their own trauma. Thus, providers need to consider TIC resources to support the family in addition to the child.

Trauma-Informed Assessment

Effective assessment of individuals with ASD must include attention to stressful and traumatic life events and the impact of such experiences on a child's emotional well-being and sense of self (Berg et al., 2016). This includes not only distinct traumatic events such as those identified in the ACE studies, but also cumulative trauma associated with an individual's social struggles, communication difficulties, and sensory sensitivities (Kerns et al., 2015). Importantly, depending on an individual with ASD's abilities related to emotional processing and expression, additional time to get to know the individual and their communication style as well as to improve identification of emotions may be required prior to effective assessment (Sivaratnam, Newman, Tonge, & Rinehart, 2015).

Presentation and Differential Diagnosis

One challenge in identifying the existence of trauma in children with ASD is that it may present differently than in neurotypical children. Children with ASD may also have difficulty communicating the subjective experience of traumatic events or the cumulation of stressors that result in a trauma reaction. Kerns et al., (2015) points out that cumulative stress or trauma may present as an exacerbation of core symptoms of ASD including self-stimulating behaviors, ritualized or stereotypic behavior, scripting, fixation on topics connected to the trauma or topics of interest that serve as a distraction from the trauma, anxiety regarding future events, social withdrawal, difficulty with social boundaries, isolation, social anxiety, or shutting down. Likewise, symptoms of PTSD and other trauma-and-stressor-related disorders include social withdrawal or avoidance, flat affect, social anxiety, sensory sensitivity, difficulty with emotional regulation, irritability, and high reactivity (American Psychiatric Association, 2013). Stavropoulos et al. (2018) highlight five domains that are especially common in both ASD and post-traumatic stress response: lack of interest in peer relationships, lack of positive emotions or difficulty communicating emotional experiences, repetition, outbursts of anxiety, irritability or aggression, and difficulty sleeping.

Many of the symptoms of a post-traumatic stress reaction mirror common symptoms of ASD and thus can remain hidden from providers who are not attuned to the potential for stress-and trauma-related symptoms in the assessment process. In addition to symptoms of stress-and-trauma-related disorders, other types of mental health struggles can be precipitated by trauma including anxiety, aggression, difficulty with attention or concentration, suicidality, and self-injury, all of which occur in higher rates among individuals with ASD than the neurotypical population (Haruvi-Lamdan, Horesh, & Golan, 2018; Mannion, Brahm, & Leader, 2014; Storch et al., 2013).

Considerations in Conducting Trauma-Informed Assessment

While none of the abovementioned symptoms in and of themselves are conclusive in identifying trauma, the appearance or worsening of any of these symptoms indicates that trauma should be considered in the assessment process. Consideration of triggers, timeline, and progression of symptoms is important; however, this can be challenging to determine in instances of cumulative stress or trauma, particularly in the cumulation of stressful social experiences. Repetition of themes connected with potential stressors or traumatic events in play, verbalizations, or general interests can also be indicative that trauma has occurred or is impacting a child's well-being. Increases in repetition or focus on specific interests unrelated to stress or trauma can also represent efforts to cope with upsetting memories or intrusive thoughts by distracting oneself from these experiences.

Due to the variability in expressive communication associated with ASD, many studies of anxiety and trauma in children with ASD rely on caregivers or other types of observer reports. This is also likely the case in clinical and other settings where assessment may occur. However, Hoover and Romero (2019) point out that this is likely to miss important components of the diagnostic picture and there is evidence to suggest that children with ASD demonstrate greater self-awareness than we may assume. Whenever possible, collateral reports of symptoms, that is reporting from caregivers, teachers, service providers, and other observers, should be combined with a child's self-reporting (in whatever way the child communicates).

Hoover and Romero (2019) developed and piloted a web-based Interactive Trauma Scale for children with ASD. This scale, while not yet extensively studied, was effective in capturing self-reported trauma symptoms among children with ASD who had a known history of trauma exposure. Other scales for measuring trauma reactions in children have been used with children with ASD including the Schedule for Affective Disorders and Schizophrenia for School-Age Children-Present and Lifetime Version (K-SADS-PL) (Kaufman et al., 1997) and the Traumatic Events Screening Inventory for Children (TESI-C) (Ford et al., 2002). These assessment scales were not created to specifically capture the experience and impact of trauma in children with ASD but nonetheless may be useful.

Trauma-informed assessment should be active and ongoing when it is known that a traumatic event has occurred. However, given the prevalence of trauma in children with ASD, any professional working with children with ASD should be attuned to issues of trauma and cumulative stress as treatment implications are different if the underlying cause of a symptom is trauma. Ultimately, if it cannot be determined whether or not a child's symptoms are attributable to trauma, incorporating principles of TIC into their framework of supports and services is likely to be beneficial. These principles are helpful in creating an affirmative environment whether or not specific trauma has occurred.

Trauma-Informed Care and Intervention

Given the dearth of specific trauma-focused frameworks for youth with ASD, this section will present considerations based on the SAMHSA guidelines for trauma-informed approaches to practice and service delivery. These best-practice principles are broadly applicable across a variety of professional fields and settings. Given their applicability across different realms of care, these principles can offer guidance for a unified philosophy of care coordination across disciplines. Clinical treatment models are also discussed, recognizing that this is a developing area of research.

SAMSHA's Six Principles of a Trauma-Informed Approach

Safety. Safety when it comes to children with ASD has a dual meaning. When any person has experienced trauma, helping them regain a sense of safety and control is paramount to healing. Fostering safety often involves taking steps (1) to ensure that the event does not happen again, (2) in situations that may occur again, such as peer-victimization, ensure that the child has a concrete plan of action steps to take to exit the situation and seek help, (3) to enhance overall safety in all aspects of a child's life. The third may be especially challenging because some children with ASD may experience the world as an inherently unsafe place. It is challenging to live with ASD in a world that was not designed for neurologically diverse ways of being (Gates, 2019). In this case, enhancing safety may mean finding strategies that allow a child to function in ways that are most comfortable to them. Many behavior modification programs and expectations of school and vocational settings can be stressful. In all cases, but perhaps particularly when trauma has occurred, looking for ways to allow safety and comfort and build on strengths rather than focus on modification of maladaptive behavior may help intervene on a lack of safety of a child as a result of trauma.

Trustworthiness and Transparency. Children with ASD and their families who have experienced trauma may find it challenging to share their experience or seek help. Since trauma and its impacts are so often overlooked in youth with ASD, it is critical to spend time developing a relationship and fostering a sense of trust. Transparency is part of this process. There is often concern about what a child can understand and how much should be shared regarding the diagnosis and treatment process. A strength of people with ASD is often their transparency and it is important to echo this in a sensitive way.

Peer Support. A critical element of peer support is the opportunity to both share your story and hear the stories of others going through similar experiences who can share strategies for coping and healing. This brings about some challenges when applied to youth with ASD as for some, peer interactions can be a source of additional stress and offering support to others can also be difficult for some children with ASD. This is certainly not the case universally. Many children with ASD badly want to engage with peers, and creating opportunities for meaningful connection around challenging experiences can be healing in multiple ways. For those who may not be ready for that type of peer connection, there is still much that can be gained from hearing stories of others, whether through books, movies, or other types of narratives. The important question is *what type of social support would help this child feel a sense of hope and belonging*? Peer support is also critically important for families of youth with ASD who have experienced trauma.

Collaboration and Mutuality. The central theme of collaboration and mutuality are of particular importance given unequal power dynamics that often exist in professional settings. SAMSHA (2014) highlights the importance of shared decision-making and relationship development, which may be especially relevant to youth with ASD who are often accustomed to being in the role of *client, patient, student, or participant.* All children in our society lack power, but perhaps more so for children with ASD who interact with so many professional settings.

Empowerment, Voice, and Choice. Connected to collaboration and shifting power dynamics are the ideas of promoting empowerment and elevating the voice of youth who have experienced trauma. Goal setting is often driven by both caregivers and professionals, and when trauma is present it is critical that the child take on as much leadership as possible. They should be fully a part of and to the extent they're able, driving decisions made about goals, treatment, needed supports and services, and daily activities. Increasing someone's sense of control and self-esteem is a critical aspect of healing from trauma. Opportunities for advocacy to prevent similar experiences of trauma for themselves and their peers can also help to increase a child's self-esteem, which is an important part of the healing process.

Cultural, Historical and Gender Issues. It is important to be attuned to the impact of multiple forms of oppression on both youth with ASD who have experienced trauma and their families. We are likely to hold implicit biases as a result of living in a society where ableism is an inherent part of our culture. Likewise, children with ASD have often grown up in a society that fails to recognize the benefits of neurodiversity. Furthermore, other aspects of a child's identity such as their race, sex, gender identity, religion, socioeconomic status, and cultural background are known to impact the quality of services they receive (Bishop-Fitzpatrick, Dababnah, Baker-Ericzén, Smith, & Magaña, 2019). Central to TIC is creating an affirmative environment that recognizes the impact of stigma and actively works to counter it, supporting a person in expressing their authentic identity. Children with ASD may feel pushed to hide the aspects of their ASD that make them unique which in and of itself can be traumatic. Utilizing a capabilities perspective (Sen, 2005) and affirming the unique aspects of their identity can help to foster resilience in overcoming and moving forward from traumatic experiences.

Clinical Treatment Models

SAMSHA's six principles offer a general trauma-informed lens through which supports and services should be delivered and this chapter has aimed to frame these general principles in terms of how professionals can apply them to understanding and approaching the experience of trauma in youth with ASD. This framework is supportive and can create a healing environment, however, it is not a therapeutic framework. While clinical treatment frameworks for addressing trauma have not been extensively researched or adapted for children with ASD, there are several that offer promising approaches and given their current evidence base in trauma-informed treatment, may be good starting points for treatment.

Cognitive Behavior Therapy (CBT). CBT is widely used with children to treat a variety of struggles related to anxiety, anger, depression, and attention and has also been applied to treating symptoms of post-traumatic stress as a result of trauma (Crawley, Podell, Beidas, Braswell, & Kendall, 2010). Core components of CBT focus on problem-solving, reframing thoughts to increase accuracy, identifying and regulating emotions, learning coping and relaxation strategies, modeling or role-playing to practice new skills, and reinforcement of healthy behaviors (Beck, 2011). CBT models focused on trauma typically incorporate additional elements of education on trauma and common reactions to trauma, processing the trauma experience, working toward a helpful way of thinking about the traumatic event(s), and addressing behavioral changes that occurred as a result of the trauma. While CBT has not been studied specifically for youth with ASD who have experienced trauma, it is the primary recommended treatment modality for the treatment of post-traumatic stress symptoms for youth in the United Kingdom (National Institute for Health and Care Excellence [NICE], 2018). While also not related to trauma, several studies have explored adaptations to CBT to enhance its effectiveness for children with ASD and it has been utilized in a variety of clinical and school settings (Rotheram-Fuller & MacMullen, 2011). Combined, this evidence suggests that CBT may be a viable approach for youth with ASD who have experienced trauma.

Trauma-Focused Cognitive Behavior Therapy (TF-CBT). TF-CBT is a trauma-focused framework building on the principles of traditional CBT and applying them specifically to trauma. This model provides therapeutic intervention simultaneously for a child who has experienced trauma and a trusted caregiver who can support the child through the healing process (Cohen, Mannarino, Kliethermes, & Murray, 2012). It incorporates the following elements, which are often noted with the acronym PPRACTICE: (1) psycho-education, (2) parenting skills [to support a child who has experienced trauma], (3) relaxation skills, (4) affective/emotional identification and coping skills, (5) cognitive coping skills, (6) telling and processing the trauma narrative, (7) in-vivo practice to work through avoidance of trauma reminders, (8) conjoint child-caregiver sessions, and (9) enhancing safety and planning for the future. TF-CBT has a strong evidence base and is widely used with children who have experienced both single-event and cumulative trauma. Holstead and Dalton (2013) conducted a study of TF-CBT for children with intellectual disabilities (ID), about a third of whom also had ASD. That study did not find this model to be more effective than standard behavioral strategies, however, the authors did not feel evidence was strong enough to rule out TF-CBT as an effective treatment model for youth with ID and ASD. This study did not examine the effectiveness of TF-CBT in youth with ASD who did not have co-occurring ID.

Narrative and Narrative Exposure Therapies (NT and NET). Narrative therapies and a trauma-specific model called Narrative Exposure Therapy for children (KIDNET) focus on the development of a trauma narrative or a story of the traumatic event or events that have occurred. The development of the trauma narrative serves to get a child accustomed to retelling or thinking about the story so it becomes less emotionally overwhelming, help a child intellectually process and reframe the way they relate to the narrative and how it impacts their life, and if they are interested, use their story in advocacy efforts toward meaningful change. While not specifically focused on trauma, there is evidence to support narrative therapy as an effective treatment framework for children with ASD (Cashin, Browne, Bradbury, & Mulder, 2013). Importantly, when working with children, trauma narratives do not need to be a written or verbal telling of a story. Narratives can also be shared and processed through creative mechanisms such as drawing, drama, play, and music.

Creative Therapies. Several creative therapies such as animal-assisted therapeutic interventions (O'Haire, 2013), art therapies (Martin, 2009), music therapies, drama therapies, and affinity therapies (Suskind, 2016) which incorporate a person with ASD's specific interests as a central theme in the therapy process have been recommended as effective therapeutic supports for youth with ASD. The integration of creative therapies into trauma-focused interventions for children with ASD has not been researched but hold promise when considering adaptations to traditional frameworks which build on the strengths of neurodiverse features in children with ASD.

Interdisciplinary Roles in Coordinating Care

This section discusses specific roles for members of interdisciplinary care teams from a variety of settings to effectively coordinate and support youth with ASD and their families who experience trauma. Importantly, these roles often intersect, and responsibilities may not be as clearly defined as presented here. However, the discussions of each professional's role can offer good starting points for collaboration.

The Self-advocate

While the role of the young person who experienced trauma may differ somewhat based on their age, communication, and interest, their voice and choice should be the primary driver in collaboratively choosing the direction of care. It is incumbent upon members of the care team to make space for this and ensure that the young person has the tools and supportive environment (created through the integration of SAMSHA's principles) they need to take on this role.

Case Management

Knowledge of TIC is essential for a professional (or other supportive individual) in a case management role. Case managers are critical in identifying providers with knowledge of TIC and may need to advocate for the provision and insurance coverage of trauma-informed services. As case managers may be in the role of coordinating between interdisciplinary care team members, they also play a central role in ensuring that the team provides person-centered care encompassing empowerment, voice, and choice as well as collaboration and mutuality (with both family and the young person who experienced trauma).

Education

Professionals involved in the education system play a central role in creating an affirmative and trauma-sensitive learning environment. Resources such as those provided through the Trauma and Learning Policy Initiative (Cole, Eisner, Gregory, & Ristuccia, 2013) can offer guidance to school-based professionals in fostering a trauma-sensitive climate. School-based professionals are also likely to be in a position to observe and identify symptoms and behaviors that may be indicative of a trauma response and thus may be a primary point for initial referral for trauma-informed assessment and service provision. Importantly, the school environment is uniquely positioned to offer opportunities for peer support. School professionals with knowledge of youth's background, strengths, and relationships can facilitate this connection.

Clinical Care

All clinical care professionals are likely to be involved in assessment and psychoeducation related to the impact of trauma as well as offering options for treatment and support.

Mental Health Care. Mental health care for youth with ASD who have experienced trauma should include diagnostic assessments for trauma and stressor-related disorders, consideration of ways that trauma and/or stress may exacerbate other physical or psychological symptoms, and the treatment of trauma and stress-related symptoms. Psychotherapy is a necessary service for children experiencing the sequelae of trauma and should focus on processing the traumatic experience(s) and resulting narrative (stories) and/or cognitive schemas (ideas about safety, trust, etc.) that may have developed as a result of the trauma. Professionals providing psychotherapeutic services should work in concert with caregivers and other supportive individuals who are part of the care team to understand the child's trauma response and be able to effectively respond and offer support.

Psychiatry may also play a role in providing a trauma-informed assessment and determining differential diagnosis if it is unclear whether existing symptoms are related to trauma. Psychiatrists should work closely with clinicians providing psychotherapeutic services as these two disciplines are most effective when working in concert for assessment, differential diagnosis, and symptom relief. As clinicians providing psychotherapy often have more frequent contact with youth receiving services, they can provide valuable insight for psychiatrists making decisions as to whether medication may be an effective part of trauma-informed treatment. Importantly, psychiatrists serve a critical gate-keeping function as it relates to youth with ASD who have experienced trauma as many children are inappropriately referred for psychopharmacology when trauma is missed and symptoms are misinterpreted.

Medical Care. Medical professionals responsible for physical health and well-being also have an important role to play in trauma-informed assessment, differential diagnosis, and referral for trauma-related symptoms in youth with ASD. Primary care providers or other physicians may be the first point of contact for families when youth with ASD experience physical manifestations of trauma-related symptoms. It is imperative that healthcare professionals are attuned to the possibility of trauma contributing to physical symptomatology in order to provide appropriate referrals for mental/behavioral healthcare and other supportive services. Of course, physical symptoms should never be assumed to have a psychological basis without thorough examination and testing, however, trauma-informed assessment and services can begin concurrently with the investigation of physical symptoms. From a trauma-informed perspective, it is also critical that nurses, physicians, and any professional in the role of providing physical care fully communicate what a child should expect from examinations and when possible offer choices as to how examinations are conducted in order to offer transparency and enhance a child's sense of control.

Rehabilitation. Rehabilitative service professionals may be an important part of the care team as it relates to healing and recovery from trauma for youth with ASD. Speech-language therapy services can work to enhance communication skills and a child's ability to articulate events, thoughts, and feelings related to trauma. Increasing communication skills related to safety and asking for help can also be an important focus of speech-language therapy services. Occupational therapists also can support youth with ASD who have experienced trauma in developing skills for increasing safety. Additionally, occupational therapy can help to address sensory issues that are attributed to or exacerbated by trauma. Feelings and somatic experiences related to trauma can be an overwhelming sensory experience for anyone, particularly youth with ASD, so it is important that the sensory element of trauma is assessed and addressed. When physical therapy services are relevant, sensitivity to how trauma may impact the experience of physical touch or physical discomfort would be important considerations on the part of the provider to ensure that the child feels in control of their body.

Community and Community-Based Services

Community-based services that enhance skills for safety are important for both prevention and recovery from trauma. Additionally, community-based service providers may offer support with some of the behavioral exposure tasks associated with therapeutic intervention for avoidance associated with trauma. The community also has the potential to provide affirmation and peer or community support.

Family

The family plays a vital role in the care team when a child with ASD (and perhaps the family themselves) have experienced trauma. The family is so often in the role of advocating for services, and their presence may provide a sense of safety for the child. Ultimately, the family's role is one of collaboration with and support for their child which can be challenging, especially if trauma symptoms have exacerbated underlying difficulties with communication and emotional regulation. The family often has to manage a dual-role on the care team of both providing support and insight and needing support. Professionals in all roles should keep this duality in mind when collaborating with families and creating care plans that may involve additional responsibilities, stressors, or demands on the part of the family.

Conclusion

This chapter has provided a general overview of the causes and presentation of trauma in youth with ASD, considerations for assessment, TIC, treatment, and the role of interdisciplinary care providers in providing comprehensive trauma-informed supports and services across settings. There is still much we need to know about this field. Ultimately, care providers being aware of the prevalence and presentation of trauma in youth with ASD and understanding their role in helping to create a sense of safety and facilitate conditions for recovery can make a significant impact in the trajectory for youth with ASD who have experienced trauma.

References

American Psychiatric Association. (2013). *Diagnostic and statistical manual of mental health disorders* (5th ed.). Washington, DC: American Psychiatric Association.

Anda, R. F., Felitti, V. J., Bremner, J. D., Walker, J. D., Whitfield, C. H., Perry, B. D., … & Giles, W. H. (2006). The enduring effects of abuse and related adverse experiences in childhood. *European Archives of Psychiatry and Clinical Neuroscience, 256*(3), 174–186.

Beck, J. (2011). *Cognitive behavior therapy: Basics and beyond* (2nd ed.). New York, NY: Guilford Press.

Bellini, S. (2006). The development of social anxiety in adolescents with autism spectrum disorders. *Focus on Autism and Other Developmental Disabilities, 21*(3), 138–145.

Berg, K. L., Shiu, C. S., Acharya, K., Stolbach, B. C., & Msall, M. E. (2016). Disparities in adversity among children with autism spectrum disorder: A population-based study. *Developmental Medicine and Child Neurology, 58,* 1124–1131.

Bishop-Fitzpatrick, L., Dababnah, S., Baker-Ericzén, M. J., Smith, M. J., & Magaña, S. M. (2019). Autism spectrum disorder and the science of social work: A grand challenge for social work research. *Social Work in Mental Health, 17*(1), 73–92.

Cappadocia, M. C., Weiss, J. A., & Pepler, D. (2012). Bullying experiences among children and youth with autism spectrum disorders. *Journal of Autism and Developmental Disorders, 42*(2), 266–277.

Cashin, A., Browne, G., Bradbury, J., & Mulder, A. (2013). The effectiveness of narrative therapy with young people with autism. *Journal of Child and Adolescent Psychiatric Nursing, 26*(1), 32–41.

Cohen, J. A., Mannarino, A. P., Kliethermes, M., & Murray, L. A. (2012). Trauma-focused CBT for youth with complex trauma. *Child Abuse and Neglect, 36*(6), 528–541.

Cole, S. F., Eisner, A., Gregory, M., & Ristuccia, J. (2013). *Helping traumatized children learn: Creating and advocating for Trauma-sensitive schools.* Retrieved from https://traumasensitiveschools.org/tlpi-publications/.

Crawley, S. A., Podell, J. L., Beidas, R. S., Braswell, L., & Kendall, P. C. (2010). Cognitive-behavioral therapy with youth. In K. S. Dobson (Ed.), *Handbook of cognitive-behavioral therapies* (pp. 375–410). New York, NY: The Guildford Press.

Edwards, V. J., Holden, G. W., Anda, R. F., & Felitti, V. J. (2003). Relationship between multiple forms of childhood maltreatment and adult mental health: results from the adverse childhood experiences (ACE) study. *American Journal of Psychiatry, 160*(8), 1453–1460.

Felitti, V. J., Anda, R. F., Nordenberg, D., Williamson, D. F., Spitz, A. M., Edwards, V., … & Marks, J. S. (1998). Relationship of childhood abuse and household dysfunction to many of the leading causes of death in adults: The adverse childhood experiences (ACE) study. *American Journal of Preventive Medicine, 14*(4), 245–258.

Ford, J. D., Racusin, R., Rogers, K., Ellis, C., Schiffman, J., Ribbe, D., & Edwards, J. (2002). Traumatic Events Screening Inventory for Children (TESI-C) Version 8.4. *National Center for PTSD and Dartmouth Child Psychiatry Research Group.*

Fuld, S. (2018). Autism spectrum disorder: The impact of stressful and traumatic life events and implications for clinical practice. *Clinical Social Work Journal, 46*(3), 210–219.

Gates, G. (2019). *Trauma, stigma, and autism: Developing resilience and loosening the grip of shame*. Philadelphia, PA: Jessica Kingsley Publishers.

Haruvi-Lamdan, N., Horesh, D., & Golan, O. (2018). PTSD and autism spectrum disorder: Co-morbidity, gaps in research, and potential shared mechanisms. *Psychological Trauma: Theory, Research, Practice, and Policy, 10*(3), 290.

Holstead, J., & Dalton, J. (2013). Utilization of trauma-focused cognitive behavioral therapy (TF-CBT) for children with cognitive disabilities. *Journal of Public Child Welfare, 7*(5), 536–548.

Hoover, D. W., & Kaufman, J. (2018). Adverse childhood experiences in children with autism spectrum disorder. *Current Opinion in Psychiatry, 31*(2), 128–132.

Hoover, D. W., & Romero, E. M. (2019). The Interactive Trauma Scale: a web-based measure for children with autism. *Journal of Autism and Developmental Disorders*. Advance online publication.

Humphrey, N., & Lewis, S. (2008). 'Make me normal': The views and experiences of pupils on the autistic spectrum in mainstream secondary schools. *Autism, 12*(1), 23–46.

Kaufman, J., Birmaher, B., Brent, D., Rao, U. M. A., Flynn, C., Moreci, P., … & Ryan, N. (1997). Schedule for affective disorders and schizophrenia for school-age children-present and lifetime version (K-SADS-PL): Initial reliability and validity data. *Journal of the American Academy of Child & Adolescent Psychiatry, 36*(7), 980–988.

Kerns, C. M., Newschaffer, C. J., & Berkowitz, S. J. (2015). Traumatic childhood events and autism spectrum disorder. *Journal of Autism and Developmental Disorders, 45*(11), 3475–3486.

Locke, J., Ishijima, E. H., Kasari, C., & London, N. (2010). Loneliness, friendship quality and the social networks of adolescents with high-functioning autism in an inclusive school setting. *Journal of Research in Special Educational Needs, 10*(2), 74–81.

Mannion, A., Brahm, M., & Leader, G. (2014). Comorbid psychopathology in autism spectrum disorder. *Review Journal of Autism and Developmental Disorders, 1*(2), 124–134.

Martin, N. (2009). Art therapy and autism: Overview and recommendations. *Art Therapy, 26*(4), 187–190.

The National Child Traumatic Stress Network. (2008). *Child trauma toolkit for educators*. Retrieved from https://www.nctsn.org/sites/default/files/resources//child_trauma_toolkit_educators.pdf.

National Institute for Health and Care Excellence. (2018). *Post-traumatic stress disorder* (NICE Guideline No. 116). Retrieved from https://www.nice.org.uk/guidance/ng116/chapter/Recommendations#management-of-ptsd-in-children-young-people-and-adult.

O'Haire, M. E. (2013). Animal-assisted intervention for autism spectrum disorder: A systematic literature review. *Journal of Autism and Developmental Disorders, 43*(7), 1606–1622.

Rotheram-Fuller, E., & MacMullen, L. (2011). Cognitive-behavioral therapy for children with autism spectrum disorders. *Psychology in the Schools, 48*(3), 263–271.

Rumball, F. (2018). A systematic review of the assessment and treatment of posttraumatic stress disorder in individuals with autism spectrum disorders. *Review Journal of Autism and Developmental Disorders*, 1–31.

Schilling, E. A., Aseltine, R. H., & Gore, S. (2007). Adverse childhood experiences and mental health in young adults: A longitudinal survey. *BMC Public Health, 7*(1), 30.

Sebastian, C., Blakemore, S. J., & Charman, T. (2009). Reactions to ostracism in adolescents with autism spectrum conditions. *Journal of Autism and Developmental Disorders, 39*(8), 1122–1130.

Sen, A. (2005). Human rights and capabilities. *Journal of Human Development, 6*(2), 151–166.

Sivaratnam, C. S., Newman, L. K., Tonge, B. J., & Rinehart, N. J. (2015). Attachment and emotion processing in children with autism spectrum disorders: Neurobiological, neuroendocrine, and neurocognitive considerations. *Review Journal of Autism and Developmental Disorders, 2*(2), 222–242.

Stavropoulos, K., Bolourian, Y., & Blacher, J. (2018). Differential diagnosis of autism spectrum disorder and post traumatic stress disorder: Two clinical cases. *Journal of Clinical Medicine, 7*(4), 71–82.

Storch, E. A., Sulkowski, M. L., Nadeau, J., Lewin, A. B., Arnold, E. B., Mutch, P. J., … & Murphy, T. K. (2013). The phenomenology and clinical correlates of suicidal thoughts and behaviors in youth with autism spectrum disorders. *Journal of Autism and Developmental Disorders, 43*(10), 2450–2459.

Substance Abuse and Mental Health Services Administration. (2014). *SAMHSA's concept of trauma and guidance for a trauma-informed approach*. Rockville, MD: Substance Abuse and Mental Health Services Administration.

Suskind, R. (2016). *Life, animated: A story of sidekicks, heroes, and autism*. Glendale, CA: Kingswell.

Wu, C. L., An, C. P., Tseng, L. P., Chen, H. C., Chan, Y. C., Cho, S. L., et al. (2015). Fear of being laughed at with relation to parent attachment in individuals with autism. *Research in Autism Spectrum Disorders, 10,* 116–123.
Zeedyk, S. M., Rodriguez, G., Tipton, L. A., Baker, B. L., & Blacher, J. (2014). Bullying of youth with autism spectrum disorder, intellectual disability, or typical development: victim and parent perspectives. *Research in Autism Spectrum Disorders, 8*(9), 1173–1183.

Facilitating Social Inclusion of Individuals with Autism Spectrum Disorder

Tiffany Otero and Susan Copeland

Abstract As a result of characteristic deficits in social communication, individuals with Autism Spectrum Disorder (ASD) often struggle to engage in social interaction and form meaningful relationships with their peers. They face disproportionate levels of social exclusion when compared to their peers with and without disabilities. Through a comprehensive understanding of social competence, authors provide an integrated framework in which to base intervention, and utilize interdisciplinary practice to facilitate social inclusion of individuals with ASD. A brief review of factors impacting social inclusion and the current state of evidence-based practices that facilitate social competence and inclusion are provided. Finally, authors discuss examples for how readers might coordinate with professionals, family members, community members, and peers to promote social inclusion of individuals with ASD across time and settings.

Elijah sat quietly as I interviewed his parents. With eyes downcast, he shifted his gaze between me, his parents, and the napkin twisted between his fingers. "Does Elijah participate in any extracurricular activities?" "No," his parents responded, "we're taking a break right now. But he used to." It was a common response to an important question. Elijah had recently entered middle school. A time when many children his age begin to prioritize friendships over family relationships. However, as it is for many children with Autism Spectrum Disorder (ASD), Elijah struggled with the constant changes, transitions, and social demands. Despite therapies, intervention, and school-based supports, he came home exhausted, moody, and needing time to recharge. "Elijah," I asked, "when do you get together with friends?" He shrugged, "at lunch, sometimes." His parents chimed in, "he tends to sit alone unless his teachers make him talk to someone."

I addressed him again, "Are you lonely?" He hummed, "Hmmm, yeah. Kinda."

His experience is not uncommon. Due to characteristic deficits in social communication, individuals with ASD face greater levels of social rejection and lower levels

T. Otero (✉) · S. Copeland
Department of Special Education, University of New Mexico, Albuquerque, NM, USA
e-mail: oterot@unm.edu

M. B. McClain et al. (eds.), *Interprofessional Care Coordination for Pediatric Autism Spectrum Disorder*, https://doi.org/10.1007/978-3-030-46295-6_22

of peer acceptance than others their age, and are more likely to function on the periphery of the social network (Kasari, Locke, Gulsrud, & Rotheram-Fuller, 2011; Locke, Ishijima, Kasari, & London, 2010; Symes & Humphrey, 2010). When compared to those with intellectual disability, learning disability, and emotional disorders, adolescents and young adults with ASD face greater social isolation (Orsmond et al., 2013; Shattuck, Orsmond, Wagner, & Cooper, 2011). This social isolation is manifested in varied ways such as by never receiving phone calls, never seeing friends, and never being asked to go out to an activity. They also report increased feelings of loneliness and have few or no close friendships (Bauminger & Kasari, 2000; Kasari et al., 2011; Orsmond, Krauss, & Seltzer, 2004), and the ones who do form friendships rate them as being of poorer quality than the friendships reported by their typically developing peers (Calder, Hill, & Pellicano, 2013).

As I spoke to Elijah, I couldn't help but reflect on how social inclusion is established. For many of us, social inclusion results from the successful development of social competence. The development of social competence is a complex process that begins in infancy with attachment, and progresses to instrumental social learning (i.e., learning that communication with others helps to obtain goals), and finally experience-sharing (i.e., reciprocal) relationships (Gutstein & Whitney, 2002). Our initial inclusion in non-familial social settings is fueled first by our interests, circumstances, or ambitions. As children, our interests and circumstance might have led our parents to identify activities in which to involve us or to enroll us in particular care centers, schools, or instructional settings where we were surrounded by other peers. This involvement in activities led to social contacts. Through social contact and engagement, we learned new behaviors and ways of relating. Our social contacts expanded until our core group of friends were those who shared our interests, such as teammates, dance partners, bandmates, or group members. We also developed skills to form acquaintances across social circles. We formed tighter bonds that helped us to feel comfortable, protected, liked, and included. This process is how many of us remain socially included as adults. We meet others at work, within hobbies, and through mutual contacts. We enjoy relationships that vary in depth and purpose, but all of these help us to feel connected.

Conversely, individuals with ASD often have less access to peers throughout their lifetime and have smaller social networks (Kasari et al., 2011; Orsmond, Shattuck, Cooper, Sterzing, & Anderson, 2013), resulting in a cycle of circumstances wherein deficits in social communication result in fewer social opportunities to develop social skills, further increasing social impairment and isolation. While significant research efforts have been put toward the development of interventions to address social skill deficits, these interventions alone have not helped to address the problem of limited social inclusion. As a result, individuals with ASD continue to report increased levels of social rejection and low levels of acceptance (Symes & Humphrey, 2010), poorer academic achievement (Welsh, Parke, Widaman, & O'Neil, 2001), loneliness (Bauminger & Kasari, 2000), lower Quality of Life (Arias et al., 2018), and increased vulnerability to bullying (Sreckovic, Brunsting, & Able, 2014). Therefore, the purpose of this chapter is to provide a more comprehensive understanding of social competence and propose a framework to apply the use of evidence-based practices that facilitate social inclusion across settings for children, adolescents, and young adults with ASD. To achieve this, we define social competence and inclusion and present a brief review of factors impacting social inclusion and the current state of evidence-based practices that facilitate social competence and inclusion. Finally, we provide examples for how readers might coordinate with professionals, family members, community members, and peers to promote social inclusion of individuals with ASD.

Social Characteristics in ASD

Deficits in social communication are a core feature of the ASD diagnosis. However, the presentation of these deficits is varied and complex. According to the *Diagnostic and Statistical Manual of Mental Disorders* (5th ed.; DSM-5; American Psychiatric Association, 2013, p. 50), social communication deficits are manifested by impairment in: (a) social and emotional reciprocity; (b) understanding and use of nonverbal communicative behaviors; and (c) developing, maintaining, and understanding relationships. These deficits range along a spectrum of severity with some individuals displaying more overtly challenging social behaviors and having comorbid medical and developmental challenges (including intellectual impairment and/or language disorders) that further influence the severity of social communication deficits (please refer to chapter "Medical Comorbidities in Pediatric Autism Disorder" for more information). On the opposite end of the spectrum, individuals may have intact, or age-appropriate, cognitive and language skills, but still exhibit clinically significant deficits in social communication. Generally speaking, these deficits may include limited eye contact, difficulty expressing and understanding nonverbal communication, limited engagement with others, a tendency to be alone, poor emotional recognition, impaired Theory of Mind and executive functioning, and the inability to infer sociocultural constructs of interaction (Attwood, 2000; Carrington, Templeton, & Papinczak, 2003; Kroeger, Schultz, & Newsom, 2007; Lopata, Thomeer, Volker, Nida, & Lee, 2008; Ochs, Kremer-Sadlik, Sirota, & Solomon, 2004). For diagnostic purposes, individuals with ASD are identified along the spectrum according to the level of support they require in the domains of social communication and repetitive behaviors or restricted interests. These levels range from requiring "very substantial support" to "substantial support," to "support." In addition, individuals with ASD commonly exhibit difficulty in regulating emotions, and have restricted interests or repetitive behaviors that interfere with their functioning.

Furthermore, in addition to the variability of skills that individuals with ASD can possess, they also vary with regard to social preferences similar to individuals without ASD. Researchers have proposed a multi-factored model to explain this variability (Mundy, Henderson, Inge, & Coman, 2007). Initial Causal Processes (ICPs), or neurological deficits specific to autistic symptomatology, as well as the variability of social characteristics found in the typical population (e.g., introversion, extroversion, cultural differences) interact to form a unique presentation of ASD in each individual. In other words, preference for social engagement of individuals with ASD varies significantly based on the nature of their symptoms, social personality, and individual social/cultural factors.

Social Inclusion and Competence

For the purpose of this chapter, social inclusion is defined as the degree to which a person is engaged in age-appropriate social relationships with others that fosters a sense of belonging. It represents the outcome of the interaction between a person and his or her social environment. If the skills or goals of an individual are not well understood or well-matched to the social group, that person is at risk of marginalization, neglect, or stigmatization.

Thankfully, human beings are socially dynamic, meaning that we have the ability to interact with varied social groups to meet varied needs. Our social groups are not uniform, adhering to the same rules, norms, and customs. In fact, from one group to the next, there is a different set of norms, requiring a different set of skills that one must employ. A person who successfully integrates him or herself into many different social circles, and is, therefore, less likely to be socially excluded, is referred to as having a high level of social competence. Dodge and colleagues (Dodge, Pettit, McClaskey, Brown, & Gottman, 1986) defined social competence as an interaction between the environment and biologically determined characteristics. Rubin and Rose-Krasnor describe social competence as "the ability to achieve personal goals in social interaction while simultaneously maintaining positive relationships with others over time and across settings" (Rubin & Rose-Krasnor, 1992, p. 285). For example, a person with the goal to maintain positive family relationships will develop and employ skills such as expressions of affection, hospitality, and conflict resolution because these skills support and strengthen those bonds. Similarly, a child who values relationships with peers in a certain social circle will seek to understand and employ the behaviors and skills valuable to that group. In summary, social competence is an interactional process between individuals and their social environments that involves: (a) social cognition, (b) social behaviors, and (c) the norms and customs of the social group. Finally, what is often ignored in developing social interventions, but highlighted in the definition of social competence by Rubin and Rose-Krasnor (1992), is the importance of achieving personal goals.

Figure 1 models this integrated definition of social competence. At the center is the primary motivation behind all voluntary social interaction: the personal goal of the social agent. Goals are infinite, varied, and personal, and have a direct influence on the social settings in which the agent chooses to engage. Goals also dictate how the individual chooses to behave in these settings.

Operating in a feedback loop are environmental factors and personal factors. The environmental side (to the left) includes the social context and the normative value system. The social context refers to the literal environment in which the person is socially engaged. Examples may include settings such as school, home, store, faith communities, and are even further defined by event. Is the person at school in a classroom or an assembly? Is the person in a faith community attending a sermon or a concert? The normative value system refers to culturally defined patterns of social behavior and rules. For example, rules dictating personal space, tone of confrontation, regard for elders, etc., are defined by this value system. Together, the social context and the normative value system dictate the exact behaviors that result in successful social engagement. For children, or those developing social competence, time is also a key component of the context as the social context takes into account the developmental level of the peer group. Waters and Sroufe (1983) argued that the development of social competence hinges not only on the execution of behaviors that meet goals in the immediate setting, but also on behaviors that promote positive developmental outcomes later in life.

Individual characteristics include the individual's ability to understand social cues to successfully adapt to their social environment, or social cognition. Social cognition includes the receptive processes that allow a person to "read" a social environment for cues. These include looking for models, perspective-taking, empathy, and other cognitive social behaviors. This cognitive process, then, directly influences the behaviors exhibited by the individual. In order to be successful, behaviors have to be appropriate to the context and the value system. Well-developed social cognition and social behaviors allow a person to decipher social codes and behave accordingly in a fluent and accurate manner. As previously explained, a person's success is measured by the degree they are able to accomplish his or her goals in this environment. The ability to be highly adaptable across various contexts and maintain the delicate balance between the needs of the self and the needs of others is where children with ASD are at a particular disadvantage.

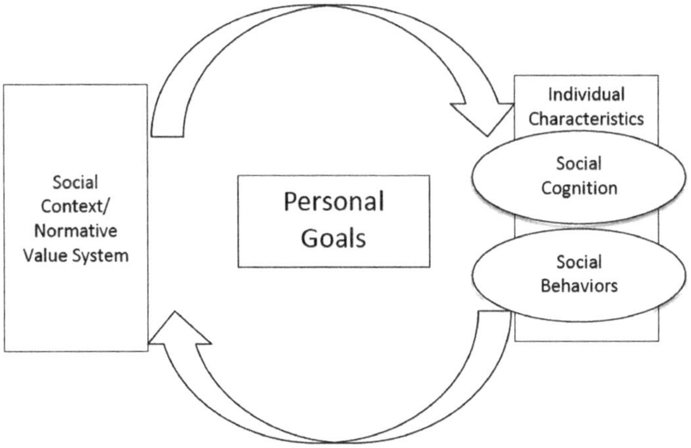

Fig. 1 Integrated model for social competence

Factors Impacting Social Inclusion of Individuals with ASD

Given the amount of variability in symptom presentation in ASD, it is difficult to use broad generalizations to describe the social involvement of all individuals with that diagnosis. Rather, there are several factors that impact the degree to which some individuals with ASD are socially integrated. Consistent with the components of the model presented in Fig. 1, these can be categorized as individual, or within-person characteristics, and contextual factors, including others in the social circle and setting.

Individual Factors

Regardless of the severity of the symptom presentation, having ASD places one at risk of social exclusion. When looking at inclusion of individuals with disabilities, broadly, Koller and colleagues (Koller, Pouesard, & Rummens, 2018) found that individuals with disabilities that impacted their behavior, social, or emotional skills tend to experience more social exclusion than those with specific physical disabilities (e.g., visual impairment, mobility limitations). Diamond and Tu (2009) found that peers make their decisions on whether to include someone with a disability based on the extent to which the disability may interfere with the chosen activity. Therefore, a child with ASD may be less likely to be included in a recreational setting highly dependent on reciprocal skills, but more likely to be included in a physical or team-based activity.

There are conflicting findings with regard to the impact that symptom severity and comorbid conditions have. Some studies report that those with higher cognitive abilities and adaptive skills are more likely to form meaningful social relationships than those who are more severely impacted (Farley et al., 2009; Howlin, 2000). Young adults with impairments in verbal communication skills were also more likely to be socially isolated (Orsmond et al., 2013). However, others have found that when individuals present with more overt symptoms, they receive more social support in the form of assistance and tolerance from others (Jones & Frederickson, 2010; Tuersley-Dixon & Frederickson, 2016). So, in some ways, the invisibility of the disability in those who are diagnostically identified as requiring only "support" (versus "substantial support" or "very substantial support") may actually function as a deterrent to social inclusion, as peers are less likely to tolerate and support an individual with ASD with intact cognitive and adaptive skills, but still presents with clinically significant social deficits.

Gender also impacts the degree to which individuals are socially included. In a study conducted in Spain on the Quality of Life (QoL) of individuals with Intellectual Disability (ID) and co-occurring ASD with ID, researchers found that respondents for male participants reported higher levels of social inclusion than females (Arias et al., 2018). When examined further, researchers found that it was not due to the severity of the presentation of symptoms among the sample of girls, but was related to the nature of female versus male social interactions. Males tend to engage in more action-based interaction through play, sports, or games. Females, on the other hand, tend to engage in more verbally mediated interaction, placing a greater demand on an area of deficit for girls with ASD.

As previously mentioned, individuals with ASD vary by tendencies of introversion and extroversion, in the same way that the typically developing population does. However, they also differ from typically developing individuals in the way they perceive friendship, and the need for it. In the literature, this variability is sometimes referred to as social motivation, and refers to how motivated one is to engage in social interaction and form relationships. In one particularly thorough study of perceptions of friendships shared by a group of children with ASD, the authors concluded that children with ASD may not want or need the same amount of social engagement that is desired by their typically developing peers (Calder et al., 2013). Therefore, some individuals with ASD may be satisfied with less social inclusion than one might assume given their age.

Contextual Factors

Peer attitudes toward others with ASD impact social engagement. In one study, Jones and Frederickson (2010) found that typically developing peers tended to rate children with ASD as significantly more shy, less cooperative, and more help-seeking than other students. Students in this study were also less likely to choose children with ASD as workmates. To address this perceived bias, researchers (Jones & Frederickson, 2010; Ochs, Kremer-Sadlik, Solomon, & Sirota, 2001) have found that that social inclusion of students with ASD may be facilitated when their social partners have an awareness about the characteristics of ASD. Based on associations identified through rating scales and observation, both sets of researchers found that when the diagnosis of ASD was known by the peers, they made more social allowances and provided more support for those with ASD.

It is possible that the presence of adults or other support providers reduces the possibility of contact with others, further inhibiting social inclusion. While additional adult support is often necessary for those with ASD in inclusive classrooms and social settings, the presence of an adult or support staff may actually hinder naturalistic social inclusion (as opposed to prearranged social interactions). For example, Kasari et al. (2011) found that children with ASD were generally less socially engaged during recess than their typically developing peers and that those with one-to-one adult support were even less likely than their peers with ASD without additional adult support to engage socially with their classmates. They also did not consistently engage with adult aides, so overall were even less likely to participate in any type of social interactions during recess. Young adults with ASD living with a parent were more likely than their peers with and without disabilities to never see friends (Orsmond et al., 2013). However, this finding should be considered in context, as individuals who have greater functional impairment and communication deficits are most likely to live with their parents in adulthood. Therefore, the factors related to the presentation of the disability, and not specifically the individual's living situation, could be more impactful to their social participation in adulthood.

Evidence-Based Practices (EBP) for Social Skills Development

Fortunately, researchers have successfully established evidence-based practices to address the multiple factors influencing social inclusion of individuals with ASD. Although there has been debate on what specific standards apply when determining what constitutes a practice as evidence-based (an EBP), in general these are interventions based on sound research, conducted with multiple groups of participants, that result in empirical evidence that supports their effectiveness in improving participant outcomes (Agran, Spooner, & Singer, 2017; Cook & Odom, 2013). Use of EBPs by teachers, therapists, and other service providers results in improved outcomes for individuals with disabilities (Cook & Odom, 2013). Indeed, federal laws related to provision of services for children and youth with disabilities, including those with ASD, mandate use of EBPs in service delivery (ESSA, 2015; IDEA, 2004 [Note: IDEA, 2004 used the term "scientifically-based" while ESSA uses the more current term "evidence-based"]).

Interest in developing EBPs related to social inclusion of individuals with ASD has grown steadily as researchers, practitioners, and families have recognized the critical importance of social skills for positive life outcomes (e.g., Reichow & Volkmar, 2010). Multiple research groups and national organizations such as the National Professional Development Center on ASD (NPDC; Wong et al., 2014) have conducted reviews of existing social intervention research seeking to establish EBPs to facilitate social inclusion of children and adults with ASD (Hughes et al., 2012; Reichow & Volkmar, 2010; Whalon, Conroy, Martinez, & Werch, 2015). In the sections below we will provide a description of evidence-based practices determined to support social inclusion of individuals with ASD across the age span. We will also highlight limitations to these practices and identify gaps in research and practice. This overview will be organized into practices that focus on building specific skills associated with social competence of individuals with ASD and practices that focus on teaching social partners of individuals with ASD skills to facilitate social inclusion or social skill development of their peers with ASD.

EBPs for Individual Social Skills Development

As mentioned previously, the social cognitive skills and social behaviors individuals use when interacting with others in their environments are one aspect of an integrated model of social competence (see Fig. 1). The majority of social skills taught through EBPs are related to increasing the frequency or quality of interactions with peers and others in the social environment. Most of the practices judged to be EBPs across all age groups have largely been derived from behavioral principles (e.g., prompting, reinforcement, imitation/modeling, self-management). In addition, naturalistic interventions (i.e., a group of practices that build on child motivation and interest within typical settings or activities), pivotal response training (i.e., teaching the foundational skills necessary for building more complex skills within typical routines and settings), video modeling (i.e., a group of practices that teach social skills by video recording the skill being performed correctly and having the individual view the video), visual supports (e.g., using words, photos, or icons, as cues to perform social behaviors), social narratives (i.e., individualized narratives describing a social situation and highlighting the cues and responses required for that situation), and technology-aided social skills instruction (e.g., using an electronic device to cue social responses) all have an established a research base supporting their use to teach or support social skills development (e.g., Wong et al., 2014). Cognitive-behavioral interventions (i.e., teaching individuals to monitor their thoughts and emotions and use specific strategies to alter their behavior) have shown promise with older children as has scripting (i.e., providing a written or verbal script for an individual to use that is specific for a particular social setting, such as playing a game) for older adolescents and young adults (Wong et al., 2014).

Limitations. Despite determination of a large number of EBPs supporting social skill development of individuals with ASD, several crucial limitations and gaps in knowledge and practice exist. One critical limitation of the research and practice in this area is that most EBPs are focused on teaching discrete skills (e.g., social initiation). While learning discrete social skills is necessary, it is not sufficient for developing social competence. In reality, as described in the previous sections, the process of building social relationships is complex, comprised of many skills that require both recognizing subtle social cues across varying settings and selecting and using multiple behaviors in response to these cues.

Moreover, there is a dearth of EBPs focused on social skill development of older adolescents and adults with ASD. The majority of research has focused on teaching young children with ASD (preschool and early elementary school-aged) skills to increase social interactions, yielding a larger number of EBPs identified for this age group (e.g., Reichow & Volkmar, 2010; Wong et al., 2014). There is a significant gap in social skills intervention research conducted with adults with ASD over the age of 30, despite growing documentation that social skills deficits persist into adulthood and are associated with social isolation and accompanying mental health issues (Howlin & Taylor, 2015). The lack of documented effective practices affects individuals' successful employment, ability to have satisfying intimate relationships, and full participation in their communities.

It is also important to highlight that the majority of social skills intervention research studies conducted with individuals with ASD has included individuals considered to have moderate to high functioning levels versus individuals with ASD who have cognitive impairment (e.g., ASD and intellectual disability [ID]) (e.g., Walton & Ingersoll, 2013; Wong et al., 2014). This gap leaves practitioners and families at a loss of how to effectively support social competence of a substantial number of individuals with ASD.

EBPs Focused on Social Partners

As the integrated model of social competence illustrates, the social context is an important component of competence and includes the particular environments an individual encounters and the social partners in those environments. Not surprisingly, the behaviors of social partners have been found to facilitate or inhibit social inclusion of those with ASD (Carter, Hughes, Copeland, & Breen, 2001). Recognizing this, researchers have developed a group of interventions that focus on the social partners encountered by individuals with ASD across home, school, and community settings. These interventions focus upon the normative value system and social context can balance the interaction, so the onus of improvement does not rest entirely upon the individual with a disability. Many of these practices fall under a broad category of peer-mediated interventions and typically include components such as providing information to peers about the characteristics of ASD and/or teaching them specific strategies to successfully engage their peers with ASD in social interactions or to teach their partners with ASD specific behavioral, academic, or social skills. This group of interventions has proved successful in increasing social engagement with both young children (Lee, Odom, & Loftin, 2007) and adolescents with ASD (Hochman, Carter, Bottema-Beutel, Harvey, & Gustafson, 2015) as well as increasing reciprocal conversational skills, and social interactions between peers with and without ASD outside of school contexts.

Limitations. As with individual social skill instruction, interventions focused on social partners have primarily been examined in children and adolescents rather than with adult populations. Adult relationships may differ in important ways from those of younger people so it is crucial that EBPs are investigated and identified for adults with ASD across the lifespan.

Some researchers and adolescents and adults with ASD have also criticized peer-mediated interventions facilitated by adults as sometimes intrusive and likely to increase stigma (Bottema-Beutel, Mullins, Harvey, Gustafson, & Carter, 2016). Engaging older adolescents and adults in determining their own social goals and participating in selecting intervention and support strategies with which they are comfortable is one way to ensure the social validity of social development strategies.

Interdisciplinary Coordination to Promote Social Inclusion

In light of these findings, it is evident that a comprehensive, multidisciplinary approach to intervention is necessary in order to adequately target the complexities of social inclusion for individuals with ASD. Therefore, in reference to Fig. 1, we propose an integrated model of intervention that targets both individual characteristics (e.g., personal goals and values, social cognitive skills, and social behaviors) and contextual factors (e.g., peer/adult interventions, consideration of social context). Within this person-centered model, members of the team include, but are not limited to, the individual, the individual's parents or other family members, their therapeutic and medical service providers (e.g., psychologists, behavior therapists, speech and language pathologists, occupational therapists, social workers), case managers, educators, and those with whom they would like to have social contact (e.g., circles of support that include peers). While coordinating schedules to have everyone meet is often impossible, communication can be enhanced through clear and concise articulation of goals so that each person can contribute his or her expertise to meet the individual's needs. For more information on coordinating services between providers, please refer to chapters "Partners in School: An Example of Care Coordination to Ensure Consistency of Evidence-Based Practices Across Home and School for Youth with Autism Spectrum Disorder (ASD)", "Coordinating ABA Services", "Coordinating Speech-Language Pathology Services for Youth with Autism Spectrum Disorder", and "Care Coordination in Primary Care".

Therefore, facilitation of social inclusion should begin with a careful assessment of the individual's goals, values, and interests. For many with ASD, their ability to form and articulate abstract concepts such as goals and values may be hindered by their disability; however, they often have very clearly defined interests that can operate as both indicators of potential social goals as well as motivation for social engagement. This initial assessment may answer the following questions: (a) What purpose does social interaction serve for this individual and what do they hope to obtain?, (b) What environment and with whom do they hope to engage?, and (c) What skills do they need to be successful? This initial assessment can be done by any interprofessional team member or provider who is facilitating intervention for the individual. For young children, or those with limited communication skills, efforts should be made to ensure enough collateral data are collected to pinpoint the goals and values of the individual and not just the preferences of those surrounding or working with the individual. To the greatest degree possible, the views and perspectives of the individuals with ASD should be central to the initial assessment with careful attention to the amount of social engagement the individual needs in order to feel included (Calder et al., 2014). For example, a child's teacher may wish for the child to interact with more peers at lunch. However, after assessing the child's needs and preferences, it is found that the child needs the time during lunch to socially disconnect and recharge for the school day, but may be more interested in engaging socially in an after school club. By considering these preferences and modifying supports accordingly, we can develop a system of intervention that is more ecologically and socially valid, targeted to the needs of the individual, and based on naturally occurring sources of motivation and reinforcement.

Once needs, preferences, and values are identified, intervention planning can begin. Using established evidence-based practices and the individual's preferences as a starting point, teachers, therapists, or other providers can work with the individual and family to identify the most appropriate combination of interventions that target both the environment and individual characteristics. For example, once a setting and potential peers have been identified, teachers or therapists may decide to provide peers with awareness training or select certain peers for formalized "peer buddy" training.

One issue with social skills interventions is that they often fail to generalize from the setting in which they are taught to the setting they are intended to be used (Bellini, Peters, Benner & Hopf, 2007; Rao, Beidel, & Murray, 2008). Therefore, when identifying targets for behavioral skills training of the child with ASD, it is important to identify the specific social skills that they will need to be successful in the setting they have chosen. This goes beyond just teaching an individual how to initiate a conversation and respond to questions simply because those are important parts of conversation. Rather, whomever will be developing or implementing the intervention (likely a therapist or team of therapists) should observe the social setting to gain an understand of how individuals interact in the setting. For example, a behavior analyst may choose to conduct a task analysis or take observational data to determine the topography (or "look") of the social behaviors required for that setting and develop appropriate operational definitions of needed skills. Peers may also be a valuable source of this information.

Finally, multiple team members should play a role in teaching skills to the individual. Behavior analysts, speech therapists, psychologists or other specialized providers, and trained peers can conduct the discrete skills training using established evidence-based practices. It is imperative that providers then work closely with parent or teachers, either through communication, observation, and training, to facilitate generalization of learned skills. For example, if a child is learning how to take turns with materials, parents can be coached on how to target and reinforce this skill on multiple opportunities in the time between teaching sessions. Similarly, teachers can support and maximize naturally occurring social situations that allow the child to use the targeted skill with peers and access naturalistic reinforcement. Peer-mediated or self-management approaches, that reduce reliance on adult presence, may be particularly helpful to adolescents and young adults in order to generalize skills while at the same time promoting their social inclusion and independence.

Conclusion

Social inclusion is what allows us to feel bonded, connected, and not alone. Some may argue it is a basic human need. For many individuals with ASD, the nature of their disability makes their inclusion in authentic and meaningful social relationships challenging. However, social inclusion is not easily intervened upon, because it is the outcome of several integrated parts working together. These include both individual characteristics and the environmental context. However, at the center, and perhaps the most important component, is the impetus for social engagement: the goals, desires, and values of the person seeking social inclusion.

Fortunately, advancements in research have led to the development of practices that help individuals with ASD develop social skills that support social inclusion and inform practices for peers and facilitators. However, these practices are often studied and developed in isolation from one another, resulting in applied practice that is grounded in sound but disparate theories and lacks integration. Furthermore, there is often emphasis placed on addressing someone's skill deficit, rather than focusing on the goals and interests of the individual as the starting point for interventions.

The Integrated Model for Social Competence (Fig. 1) introduced in this chapter provides a framework not only for the definition of social competence, but also how to structure intervention through a comprehensive approach that aims to promote social inclusion of individuals with ASD. Facilitation of social inclusion is a team effort, with the individual with ASD operating as the team captain. In this model, multidisciplinary collaboration is centered upon careful evaluation of the individual's needs and goals for social engagement. With common goals identified among collaborative interdisciplinary partners, multi teams can develop more targeted, efficient, and socially valid intervention packages that address the complex social needs of the individual. Individual team member can then each address the needs of the individual most fitting to their scope of practice, or role, by making appropriate environmental modifications, training aides and peers, teaching any necessary skills to the individual, and helping the individual to generalize across settings. It is through this approach that individuals with ASD can access skills that appeal to their needs, help them to be successful achieving their social goals, and promote their social inclusion.

References

American Psychiatric Association. (2013). Autism spectrum disorder. In *Diagnostic and statistical manual of mental disorders* (5th ed., pp. 50–59). Washington, DC: Author.

Agran, M., Spooner, F., & Singer, G. H. S. (2017). Evidence-based practices: The complexities of implementation. *Research and Practice for Persons with Severe Disabilities, 42,* 3–7.

Arias, V. B., Gómez, L. E., Morán, M. L., Alcedo, M. Á., Monsalve, A., & Fontanil, Y. (2018). Does quality of life differ for children with autism spectrum disorder and intellectual disability compared to peers without autism? *Journal of Autism and Developmental Disorders, 48,* 123–136.

Attwood, T. (2000). Strategies for improving the social integration of children with Asperger syndrome. *Autism, 4,* 85–100.

Bauminger, N., & Kasari, C. (2000). Loneliness and friendship in high-functioning children with autism. *Child Development, 71,* 447–456.

Bellini, S., Peters, J. K., Benner, L., & Hopf, A. (2007). A meta-analysis of school-based social skills interventions for children with autism spectrum disorders. *Remedial and Special Education, 28,* 153–162.

Bottema-Beutel, K., Mullins, T. S., Harvey, M. N., Gustafson, J. R., & Carter, E. W. (2016). Avoiding the "brick wall of awkward": Perspectives of youth with autism spectrum disorder on social-focused intervention practices. *Autism, 20,* 196–206.

Calder, L., Hill, V., & Pellicano, E. (2013). "Sometimes I want to play by myself": Understanding what friendship means to children with autism in mainstream primary schools. *Autism, 17,* 296–316.

Carrington, S., Templeton, E., & Papinczak, T. (2003). Adolescents with Asperger syndrome and perceptions of friendship. *Focus on Autism and Other Developmental Disabilities, 18,* 211–218.

Carter, E. W., Hughes, C., Copeland, S. R., & Breen, C. (2001). Differences between high school students who do and do not volunteer to participate in a peer interaction program. *Journal of the Association for Persons with Severe Handicaps, 26,* 229–239.

Cook, B. G., & Odom, S. L. (2013). Evidence-based practices and implementation science in special education. *Exceptional Children, 79,* 135–144.

Diamond, K., & Tu, H. (2009). Relations between classroom context, physical disability and preschool children's inclusion decisions. *Journal of Applied Developmental Psychology, 30,* 75–81.

Dodge, K. A., Pettit, G. S., McClaskey, C. L., Brown, M. M., & Gottman, J. (1986). Social competence in children. *Monographs of the Society for Research in Child Development, 51,* i–85.

Every Student Succeeds Act of 2015 (ESSA), Pub. L. No. 114-95 § 114 Stat. 1177 (2015–2016).

Farley, M. A., McMahon, W. M., Fombonne, E., Jenson, W. R., Miller, J., Gardner, M., & Coon. H. (2009). Twenty-year outcome for individuals with autism and average or near-average cognitive abilities. *Autism Research, 2,* 109–118.

Gutstein, S. E., & Whitney, T. (2002). Asperger syndrome and the development of social competence. *Focus on Autism and Other Developmental Disabilities, 17,* 161–171.

Hochman, J. M., Carter, E. W., Bottema-Beutel, K., Harvey, M. N., & Gustafson, J. R. (2015). Efficacy of peer networks to increase social connections among high school students with and without autism spectrum disorder. *Exceptional Children, 82,* 96–116.

Howlin, P. (2000). Outcome in adult life for more able individuals with autism or Asperger syndrome. *Autism, 4,* 63–83.

Howlin, P., & Taylor, J. L. (2015). Addressing the need for high quality research on autism in adulthood. *Autism, 19,* 771–773.

Hughes, C., Kaplan, L., Bernstein, R., Boykin, M., Reilly, C., Brigham, N., … Harvey, M. (2012). Increasing social interaction skills of secondary school students with autism and/or intellectual disability: A review of interventions. *Research and Practice for Persons with Severe Disabilities, 37,* 288–307.

Individuals with Disabilities Education Act (IDEA), 20 U.S.C. § 1400 (2004).

Jones, A. P., & Frederickson, N. (2010). Multi-informant predictors of social inclusion for students with autism spectrum disorders attending mainstream school. *Journal of Autism and Developmental Disorders, 40,* 1094–1103.

Kasari, C., Locke, J., Gulsrud, A., & Rotheram-Fuller, E. (2011). Social networks and friendships at school: Comparing children with and without ASD. *Journal of Autism and Developmental Disorders, 41,* 533–544.

Koller, D., Pouesard, M. Le, & Rummens, J. A. (2018). Defining social inclusion for children with disabilities: A critical literature review. *Children and Society, 32,* 1–13.

Kroeger, K. A., Schultz, J. R., & Newsom, C. (2007). A comparison of two group-delivered social skills programs for young children with autism. *Journal of Autism and Developmental Disorders, 37,* 808–817.

Lee, S. H., Odom, S. L., & Loftin, R. (2007). Social engagement with peers and stereotypic behavior of children with autism. *Journal of Positive Behavior Interventions, 9,* 67–79.

Locke, J., Ishijima, E. H., Kasari, C., & London, N. (2010). Loneliness, friendship quality, and the social networks of adolescents with high-functioning autism in an inclusive school setting. *Journal of Research in Special Educational Needs, 10,* 74–81.

Lopata, C., Thomeer, M. L., Volker, M. A., Nida, R. E., & Lee, G. K. (2008). Effectiveness of a manualized summer social treatment program for high-functioning children with autism spectrum disorders. *Journal of Autism and Developmental Disorders, 38,* 890–904.

Mundy, P. C., Henderson, H. A., Inge, A. P., & Coman, D. C. (2007). The modifier model of autism and social development in higher functioning children. *Research and Practice for Persons with Severe Disabilities, 32,* 124–139.

Ochs, E., Kremer-Sadlik, T., Sirota, K. G., & Solomon, O. (2004). Autism and the social world: An anthropological perspective. *Discourse Studies, 6,* 147–183.

Ochs, E., Kremer-Sadlik, T., Solomon, O., & Sirota, K. G. (2001). Inclusion as social practice: Views of children with autism. *Social Development, 10,* 399–419.

Orsmond, G. I., Krauss, M. W., & Seltzer, M. M. (2004). Peer relationships and social and recreational activities among adolescents and adults with autism. *Journal of Autism and Developmental Disorders, 34,* 245–256.

Orsmond, G. I., Shattuck, P. T., Cooper, B. P., Sterzing, P. R., & Anderson, K. A. (2013). Social participation among young adults with an autism spectrum disorder. *Journal of Autism and Developmental Disorders, 43,* 2710–2719.

Rao, P. A., Beidel, D. C., & Murray, M. J. (2008). Social skills interventions for children with Asperger's syndrome or high-functioning autism: A review and recommendations. *Journal of Autism & Developmental Disorders, 38,* 353–361.

Reichow, B., & Volkmar, F. R. (2010). Social skills interventions for individuals with autism: Evaluation for evidence-based practices within a best evidence synthesis framework. *Journal of Autism and Developmental Disorders, 40,* 149–166.

Rubin, K. H., & Rose-Krasnor, L. (1992). Interpersonal problem solving and social competence in children. In V. B. Van Hasselt & M. Hersen (Eds.), *Perspectives in developmental psychology. Handbook of social development: A lifespan perspective* (pp. 283–323). New York, NY, US: Plenum Press.

Shattuck, P. T., Orsmond, G. I., Wagner, M., & Cooper, B. P. (2011). Participation in social activities among adolescents with an autism spectrum disorder. *PLoS ONE, 6,* e27176.

Sreckovic, M. A., Brunsting, N. C., & Able, H. (2014). Victimization of students with autism spectrum disorder: A review of prevalence and risk factors. *Research in Autism Spectrum Disorders, 8,* 1155–1172.

Symes, W., & Humphrey, N. (2010). Peer-group indicators of social inclusion among pupils with autistic spectrum disorders (ASD) in mainstream secondary schools: A comparative study. *School Psychology International, 31,* 478–494.

Tuersley-Dixon, L., & Frederickson, N. (2016). Social inclusion of children with complex needs in mainstream: Does visibility and severity of disability matter? *International Journal of Developmental Disabilities, 62,* 89–97.

Walton, K. M., & Ingersoll, B. R. (2013). Improving social skills in adolescents and adults with autism and severe to profound intellectual disability: A review of the literature. *Journal of Autism and Developmental Disorders, 43,* 594–615.

Waters, E., & Sroufe, L. A. (1983). Social competence as a developmental construction. *Developmental Review, 3,* 79–97.

Welsh, M., Parke, R. D., Widaman, K., & O'Neil, R. (2001). Linkages between children's social and academic competence: A longitudinal analysis. *Journal of School Psychology, 39,* 463–482.

Whalon, K. J., Conroy, M. A., Martinez, J. R., & Werch, B. L. (2015). School-based peer-related social competence interventions for children with autism spectrum disorder: A meta-analysis and descriptive review of single case research design sudies. *Journal of Autism and Developmental Disorders, 45,* 1513–1531.

Wong, C., Odom, S. L., Hume, K. Cox, A. W., Fettig, A., Kucharczyk, S., … Schultz, T. R. (2014). *Evidence-based practices for children, youth, and young adults with autism spectrum disorder.* Chapel Hill: The University of North Carolina, Frank Porter Graham Child Development Institute, Autism Evidence-Based Practice Review Group.

The Early Start Denver Model (ESDM)

Jill Howard and Geraldine Dawson

Abstract The Early Start Denver Model (ESDM; Rogers and Dawson in The Early Start Denver Model for Young Children with Autism: Promoting Language, Learning, and Engagement. Guilford Press, New York, 2010) is an evidence-based early intervention designed to promote developmental and social communication skills in young children with autism spectrum disorder between the ages of 12 and 60 months. The ESDM is characterized as a Naturalistic Developmental Behavioral Intervention (NDBI; Schreibman et al. in Naturalistic Developmental Behavioral Interventions: Empirically validated treatments for autism spectrum disorder. J Autism Dev Disord 45(8):2411–2428, 2015), indicating that it shares commonalities with a number of similar types of early interventions including delivery in natural contexts, shared control between the child and clinician, and use of behavioral principles/natural contingencies. The ESDM is particularly well suited for an interdisciplinary approach to care for young children on the autism spectrum given that it promotes the development of an interdisciplinary treatment team, benefits from collaboration across disciplines, and values the input of varied perspectives. Several other ways in which the ESDM approach provides a range of opportunities to collaborate and coordinate interdisciplinary care are described throughout the chapter.

The Early Start Denver Model (ESDM; Rogers & Dawson, 2010) is an evidence-based early intervention for young children with Autism Spectrum Disorder (ASD) between the ages of 12 and 60 months, which was developed by Geraldine Dawson and Sally Rogers. The intervention is based on principles of Applied Behavior Analysis (ABA) and incorporates a strong developmental focus. The treatment approach is largely play-based and emphasizes relationship-building and communication, with treatment objectives spanning several developmental domains delivered in a naturalistic format. The ESDM was developed as a downward extension of the Denver

J. Howard (✉) · G. Dawson
Department of Psychiatry and Behavioral Sciences, Duke Center for Autism and Brain Development, Duke University School of Medicine, Durham, NC, USA
e-mail: jill.howard@duke.edu

M. B. McClain et al. (eds.), *Interprofessional Care Coordination for Pediatric Autism Spectrum Disorder*, https://doi.org/10.1007/978-3-030-46295-6_23

Model, originally designed for preschoolers with ASD between 24 and 60 months (Rogers, Hall, Osaki, Reaven, & Herbison, 2000; Rogers, Herbison, Lewis, Pantone, & Reis, 1986). Several aspects of the ESDM make the program well suited for an interdisciplinary approach, to be discussed in greater detail throughout this chapter.

History/Background of ESDM

In addition to origins stemming from the Denver Model, the ESDM is also informed by Pivotal Response Training (PRT; Koegel & Koegel, 1988; Schreibman & Pierce, 1993), Rogers and Pennington's (1991) model relating early social capacities to interpersonal development in individuals with autism, and Dawson and colleagues' (2004) model characterizing autism as a disorder of social motivation. Foundations in these models ensure that the ESDM incorporates relationship-building as a platform for developing social communication skills, using engaging dyadic exchanges within play routines, and considering all aspects of a child's development. Treatment goals emphasize imitation and affective sharing. Further, these foundational models focus on enhancing a child's social attention and motivation through shifting the value associated with social rewards, and on allowing for child choice and following the child's lead.

ESDM in the Context of Naturalistic Developmental Behavioral Interventions (NDBIs)

The ESDM falls under the umbrella of Naturalistic Developmental Behavioral Interventions (NDBIs; Schreibman et al., 2015), which is a group of early interventions that share key characteristics. NDBIs combine applied behavioral and developmental sciences. Among their common principles are delivery in natural contexts (e.g., the child's natural environment, or structured in a way that promotes generalization to the child's natural environment), shared control between the child and clinician, natural contingencies/reinforcers, and use of a range of behavioral principles to promote developmental skill acquisition. In addition, some of the evidence-based features of these interventions include a solid basis in applied behavior analysis, clear procedures which are well-defined in intervention manuals, a means for assessing fidelity of implementation in a standardized manner, individually tailored treatment goals, regular assessment of treatment progress, and child-led teaching. Teaching opportunities are embedded within both object and social play activities, using techniques of modeling and imitation to teach new skills. A strong base of research supports the efficacy of NDBIs in producing positive outcomes for children with ASD. In addition to the ESDM, interventions that fall under the umbrella of NDBIs include PRT, Joint Attention Symbolic Play Engagement and Regulation (JASPER; Kaale, Smith, & Sponheim, 2012; Kasari, Freeman, & Paparella, 2006), and Social Communication/Emotional Regulation/Transactional Support (SCERTS; Prizant, Wetherby, Rubin, & Laurent, 2003), among others.

Modalities of ESDM Delivery

ESDM can be delivered in a number of different ways, including therapist-delivered (i.e., therapist working 1:1 with child), parent coaching (i.e., coach provides in-the-moment feedback to the parent on ways of interacting with the child that support social-communicative development, in the context of live activities during session), group (e.g., preschool and daycare settings), and telehealth (i.e., remote delivery via technology-based platform; see chapter "Telehealth Approaches to Care Coordination in Autism Spectrum Disorder" for an overview of other approaches to telehealth). Further, efforts are underway that seek to make the ESDM more accessible to culturally and linguistically diverse populations, including in low resource settings, that require an extensive understanding of what adaptations are necessary to support a successful intervention program. Currently, the ESDM therapist manual (Rogers & Dawson, 2010) is available worldwide in 16 languages.

Principles of ESDM

The ESDM draws from both transactional (Sameroff, 2009) and constructionist (Piaget, 1963) models of child development. As such, the cycle of the interactive relationship between child and caregiver is viewed as critical, involving exchanging emotions, and responding to the other's temperament, thereby affecting behavior in both directions. Additionally, the basis in the constructionist model suggests that children actively shape their own social world through participation in motor, sensory, and socially interactive experiences.

The ESDM primarily aims to promote the child's social initiative and social engagement through affectively rich interactions, where multiple treatment objectives are targeted simultaneously rather than in a sequential manner. Data collection is essential in monitoring treatment progress and making modifications to the treatment plan as needed. Further, the intervention spans and targets a range of developmental domains, as shown below:

Receptive communication
Expressive communication
Joint attention behaviors
Social skills
Imitation
Cognition
Play
Fine motor
Gross motor
Behavior
Personal independence

Key principles of the ESDM are well represented in the criteria for fidelity of implementation, as they indicate expectations for successful delivery of the intervention. These criteria lie at the core of an ESDM intervention program and describe characteristics of a successful interaction between the child and either the therapist (if therapist-delivered) or parent (if delivered via parent coaching). Fidelity of implementation is systematically tracked using a detailed coding system, and for the purposes of simply describing key principles, criteria are as follows:

Management of child attention
Antecedent-Behavior-Consequence (ABC) format—quality of behavioral teaching
Instructional techniques application
Adult ability to modulate child affect and arousal
Management of unwanted behaviors
Quality of dyadic engagement
Adult optimization of child motivation for participating in the activity
Adult use of positive affect
Adult sensitivity and responsivity to child communicative cues
Multiple and varied communicative opportunities occur in the activity
Appropriateness of adult language for child's language level
Joint activity structure and elaboration
Transitions between activities

In addition to these overarching key principles, some additional principles apply uniquely to specific delivery modalities. For example, in group-delivered ESDM, peer interactions are meant to serve as the predominant mechanism for teaching. In this setting, children with ASD who might initially attend minimally to their peer group are supported in practicing parallel play and imitation as attention to peers increases over time. Having double sets of toys available, and facilitating face-to-face positioning, serve to support these aims. Additionally, in this setting children with ASD gain experience with transitioning between activities and participating in both small and larger group activities.

For parent-delivered ESDM, the interactions between the clinician and parent are of key importance. Rather than the coach serving in an "expert" role, the dyad is meant to be viewed as a partnership, where the parent has valuable expertise pertaining to his or her child to contribute to the intervention. The sessions are typically low intensity (i.e., one 60- to 90-min session per week) and the course of treatment can be relatively short (e.g., 12 weeks), although longer term coaching relationships are also possible. Parents are encouraged to spend time outside of session practicing strategies taught in session, by embedding practice into typical daily routines (e.g., mealtime, bathtime, playtime). During session, parent coaches employ a cycle of a parent–child activity (including live coaching) and discussion/reflection with the parent following the activity to generate changes in the parent's behavior, which are intended to promote change in the child's behavior. In reflection, the coach works actively to describe (rather than judge) the parent's and child's behavior, and to communicate support and respect for the parent. Ultimately, developing parental self-efficacy is a key goal, such that parents are not reliant on the coach to facilitate growth in their child.

Research Support for the ESDM

The ESDM has been empirically tested in a number of different trials, which have evaluated different modes of delivery (therapist- and caregiver-delivered). Research has demonstrated significant improvements in children's developmental and adaptive skills, particularly following an intensive, long-term (i.e., two years) course of treatment. Emerging research has begun to investigate the effect of delivery via telehealth and group settings, as well as international applications of the ESDM since it was developed and has primarily been tested in the United States.

A number of Randomized Controlled Trials (RCTs) have evaluated the efficacy of the ESDM. Dawson and colleagues (2010) compared outcomes in 18–30-month-old children with ASD who received either intensive ESDM (delivered via therapist, alongside simultaneous parent coaching) for 2 years, or referrals to community providers for treatment as usual within the community. Results revealed that children in the ESDM group demonstrated significant improvements in IQ (i.e., cognitive functioning) and adaptive behavior, and were significantly more likely to have had their diagnosis reclassified to a more moderate presentation (i.e., pervasive developmental disorder—not otherwise specified), when compared to the community treatment group. Analysis of the IQ outcomes indicated that the positive effects were primarily related to gains in receptive and expressive language, rather than nonverbal IQ. Follow-up analyses from this study reflected the ability of the ESDM to produce normalized patterns of children's brain activity relative to the community intervention group (Dawson et al., 2012). Specifically, the ESDM group and typical children showed increased cortical activation (decreased α power and increased θ power) when viewing faces, whereas the community intervention group showed the opposite pattern (greater cortical activation when viewing objects). Greater cortical activation while viewing faces was associated with improved social behavior. The sample of children who participated in the 2010 trial was assessed at age 6 years, 2 years after the intervention ended, across multiple domains of functioning by clinicians naive to previous intervention group status (Estes et al., 2015). The ESDM group, on average, maintained gains made in early intervention during the 2-year follow-up period in overall intellectual ability, adaptive behavior, symptom severity, and challenging behavior. No group differences in core autism symptoms were found immediately post-treatment; however, 2 years later, the ESDM group demonstrated improved core autism symptoms and adaptive behavior as compared with the community-intervention-as-usual group. An economic analysis was then conducted to determine the effect of the ESDM on health care service use and costs in this sample (Cidav et al., 2017). In the post-intervention period, compared with children who had earlier received treatment as usual in community settings, children in the ESDM group used fewer hours of ABA, occupational/physical therapy, and speech therapy services, resulting in significant cost savings in the amount of about $19,000 per year per child.

Subsequently, a multi-site, single-blind, randomized trial evaluating the efficacy of ESDM with 118 children with ASD between the ages of 14 and 24 months was published (Rogers et al., 2019). Children were randomly assigned to receive either ESDM (3 months of weekly parent coaching, followed by 24 months of therapist-delivered treatment in homes or daycare settings for an average of 15 h per week, while parents continued to receive 4 h of coaching per month) or community intervention for a period of 27 months. In light of the 2010 RCT which showed positive effects for language, the primary outcome was receptive and expressive language based on the Mullen Scales of Early Learning. Results revealed a significant treatment effect on receptive and expressive language skills for the ESDM group. Both the ESDM and community group showed similar significant gains in overall developmental quotient and adaptive behavior. Overall, results partially replicated the findings of Dawson and colleagues (2010).

In addition to these RCTs, several other studies have investigated lower-intensity ESDM delivered via parent coaching and other modalities. Rogers and colleagues (2012) conducted an RCT with 98 toddlers at risk for ASD (ages 14–24 months) and their families. Specifically, the study examined the efficacy of parent coaching in ESDM over 12 weeks of low-intensity intervention, compared to community treatment as usual. Significant and roughly equal gains were observed in both groups; however, children in the treatment as usual group required a significantly greater number of hours of intervention to generate comparable outcomes to that of the ESDM group. Current research is being conducted to examine how to make ESDM parent coaching most effective as a low intensity (and thus less costly) form of intervention.

Vismara and colleagues investigated ESDM parent coaching delivered via telehealth (Vismara et al., 2018). Parents of children with ASD were randomized to receive either 1.5 h per week of parent training delivered via telehealth, plus access to ESDM online learning resources, or 1.5 h per month of parent training delivered via telehealth, plus access to non-ESDM online learning resources; study participation spanned a period of 12 weeks. Following intervention, those in the ESDM parent training group showed greater gains in parent fidelity and program satisfaction relative to those in the control group. With regard to child outcomes, communication skills improved in both groups. Vismara and colleagues highlighted the feasibility of this modality of delivery while noting that more research is needed to better understand the potential positive effects of this treatment for improving outcomes in young children with ASD.

Vivanti and colleagues (2014) have spearheaded efforts to adapt the ESDM to a group-based setting, specifically a group-based community childcare. While children with ASD in both the ESDM group (15–25 h per week of ESDM over 12 months, in a group childcare setting) and active control group (who received a different intervention in a similar setting) gained cognitive, adaptive, and social skills, those in the ESDM group showed a relatively greater rate of development and greater gains in receptive language skills. Finally, Zhou and colleagues (2018) conducted a non-randomized controlled trial in China with toddlers with ASD between the ages of 1.5 and 2.5 years. The intervention consisted of 26 weeks of high-intensity parent coaching, compared to the control group of community treatment as usual. Following intervention, children in the ESDM group showed greater improvement in language development, social affect, and parent-reported social communication and symbolic play. Further, parents in the ESDM group reported experiencing significantly reduced parenting stress relative to those in the community treatment as usual group.

The evidence base for the ESDM continues to expand, investigating novel modalities of delivery, applications to diverse cultures, long-term follow-up, and other important approaches including treating infants showing early signs of ASD. Future research seeks to more clearly identify active ingredients of the ESDM intervention, determine optimal levels of training and supervision necessary to support an effective intervention program, compare variations of dosage and teaching style, and examine enhancements offered to the ESDM through technologically assisted modifications. Continued long-term follow-up studies will reveal how intervention in the early years contributes to later outcomes, allowing for further examination of the cost offset generated by high-quality early intervention for ASD.

Interdisciplinary Care Within Early Intervention

Common Disciplines/Types of Interventions Serving Very Young Children

For very young children on the autism spectrum, some commonly recommended treatments include ABA, speech therapy, occupational therapy, developmental preschool, and medical/psychiatric intervention, in the event of co-occurring concerns or diagnoses. Each child has unique needs that necessitate a different set of recommended treatments. A comprehensive diagnostic evaluation for ASD (typically conducted by a psychologist or developmental pediatrician, involving gold-standard tools for characterizing ASD, developmental history, and a cognitive/developmental assessment; see chapter "Interdisciplinary Evaluation of Autism Spectrum Disorder" for more details on interdisciplinary evaluation of ASD) may identify what treatments would be beneficial, or what additional follow-up testing would be warranted.

Examples of Collaboration Across Disciplines

While ASD is characterized by deficits in social communication and social interaction and the presence of restricted and repetitive behaviors and interests, associated difficulties are common, including motor and speech-language deficits, difficulties with learning and attention, co-occurring medical conditions (e.g., problems with sleep, feeding, seizures), and behavioral challenges (e.g., self-injury, aggression). Thus, it is wise to coordinate care across disciplines in order to most effectively serve the child and family. Additionally, when considering the early intervention period, most locations in the United States experience a transition in care when the child turns 3 years old, and services generally provided through the state early intervention program discontinue as the child becomes eligible for services through the public school system (i.e., developmental preschool programs, which commonly provide speech language therapy, occupational therapy, and other supports; chapter "Transition to Early Schooling for Children with ASD" provides an overview of the transition to early schooling). In order to facilitate a smooth transition and to continue to advance progress toward goals, collaboration across disciplines and teams remains critical.

How an ESDM Therapist Collaborates with Other Disciplines

ESDM is by nature a model well suited to collaboration across disciplines. The ESDM, including the ESDM curriculum, was created by an interdisciplinary team comprised of clinical and developmental psychologists, occupational therapists, and speech-language therapists. The ESDM therapist manual promotes the formation of an interdisciplinary treatment team, with both a designated team leader and parents at the center (Rogers & Dawson, 2010). The ESDM therapist is not meant to function independently or in isolation, and is ideally part of an interdisciplinary treatment team, where disciplines work together to develop and deliver the intervention plan. In doing such, the importance of effective and consistent communication cannot be understated. Two common ways of supporting effective communication include the use of a treatment notebook (consisting of individual daily data sheets and progress notes for each clinician delivering treatment) and regular team meetings focused on addressing the specific needs of the child and ensuring that the treatment goals and strategies are aligned and synergistic.

Several aspects of the ESDM make it a good fit for coordination of care across disciplines, and there are many ways in which an ESDM therapist might collaborate with other disciplines. First, professionals from a range of fields may be qualified to become trained as ESDM therapists. Training requirements mandate an advanced degree, but do not necessitate training in any particular specialty. For example, backgrounds of ESDM therapists include special education, psychology, psychiatry, speech-language therapy, occupational therapy, and behavior analysis. Thus, when communicating with fellow ESDM therapists either for peer supervision, discussions around reliability, or other topics, it is likely that one would collaborate with individuals from outside one's own discipline. Additionally, since the ESDM targets skills from across a range of developmental domains, it becomes important to consider perspectives of those who may have relatively greater expertise in particular areas. For example, a speech-language therapist may be more comfortable addressing items/questions related to the Receptive and Expressive Communication domains, while an occupational therapist may have greater familiarity with the Personal Independence items. Participation in peer supervision with others trained in the ESDM facilitates an excellent opportunity for care informed by an interdisciplinary perspective.

Second, while a child's ESDM therapist is working toward improving skills across domains, it may additionally be appropriate to communicate with the child's other therapists. For example, multiple therapists using similar language and teaching techniques increase consistency, positively contributing to a child's ability to acquire the target skills. The child's other therapists may also be a valuable source of information regarding the child's skills, both during the curriculum assessment (administered with the ESDM Curriculum Checklist for Young Children with Autism; Rogers & Dawson, 2009) when the ESDM therapist is formally addressing the child's current skillset, as well as during treatment, to have an outsider's prospective on progress, effective strategies, etc. An ESDM therapist might use information previously gathered from a recent comprehensive diagnostic evaluation, or from recent treatment progress notes, when scoring the curriculum assessment, as final codes are generated from a combination of observed behavior, parent report, and other/teacher report. An outside therapist may also provide feedback on whether improvements observed during ESDM sessions appear to have generalized to other settings.

An ESDM therapist might coordinate care with clinicians from other disciplines to develop a consistent response to challenging or disruptive behavior. For example, in the case of a child who demonstrates severe headbanging, an ESDM therapist might first request permission from the child's caregiver(s) to rule out the possibility of a medical explanation for this behavior, possibly by consulting with the child's pediatrician and/or neurologist. Next, the therapist might request to involve the child's ABA therapist, speech-language pathologist, and occupational therapist in an effort to determine (1) whether the function of the behavior has been determined, (2) how communication delays may be impacting the child's behavior and whether alternative communication strategies have been employed, and (3) if there are sensory techniques that would be appropriate to use in session.

A scenario in which it may be appropriate to lean more on other members of the child's treatment team is when the child's progress fails to advancc as expected. A detailed decision tree denotes appropriate steps to take should this occur, including modification to teaching approaches in order to increase the likelihood of successful learning (Rogers & Dawson, 2010). For example, modifications entail a hierarchy of steps starting with the addition of reinforcers, then increasing structure, and finally incorporation of visual supports. The final step of adding visual supports suggests enhancements including adding visual symbols/icons to receptive language tasks, using a Treatment and Education of Autistic and Related Communication-Handicapped Children (TEACCH; Mesibov, Shea, & Schopler, 2004)-style work system for teaching tasks involving sequencing, and adding picture exchange systems to support more effective communication (e.g., Picture Exchange Communication System (PECS); Bondy & Frost, 1994).

The Structured Teaching approach of TEACCH posits four important components, including structuring the environment appropriately to the needs of the individual, using visual strengths to support relatively weaker areas, using special interests as motivation, and supporting spontaneous functional communication (Mesibov & Shea, 2010). Many of these tenets may sound similar to the ESDM, although the ESDM does not typically include visual supports unless deemed necessary due to lack of progress, after consulting the decision tree (Rogers & Dawson, 2010). PECS is a form of augmentative and alternative communication aimed at enhancing communication by first teaching children to exchange pictures with a communication partner to request desired items (Bondy & Frost, 1994). Subsequently, the system progresses to more advanced forms of picture exchange communication. This can be an impactful addition to the ESDM when progress is slow and when children are affected by significant difficulties with communication. When the ESDM decision tree indicates the need to consider supports such as TEACCH or PECS strategies, it would be sensible to collaborate with a therapist with expertise in these systems to ensure they generate maximal benefit.

The objectives and steps generated from the ESDM curriculum assessment are commonly shared with other therapists in order to communicate a child's current skill level and treatment plan. A completed curriculum assessment identifies the approximate age range where the child's skills fall across all domains, and this information is used to develop treatment objectives broken down by small steps. Through sharing this information with other therapists, the treatment team can coordinate goals and priorities, and ensure consistency across therapies where possible. This alignment and reduction of competing goals may also help to facilitate parent understanding and engagement in home practice.

As described, the ESDM approach provides a multitude of opportunities to collaborate and coordinate care with other disciplines. Since the ESDM targets development across a range of domains (e.g., receptive communication, expressive communication, social skills, play, motor, personal independence), it is an intervention ripe for drawing upon the expertise of those beyond the therapist's own discipline. Further, individuals who seek training in the ESDM are not required to have a background in a particular discipline, which is indicative of the intervention model's appreciation for a diverse range of perspectives. An ESDM treatment program benefits from two-way communication with other clinicians who may interact with the child, including but not limited to speech-language pathologists, occupational therapists, psychologists, and physicians. Additionally, even when caregivers are not directly involved in the intervention (i.e., when delivered through modalities other than parent coaching) frequent communication with caregivers is critical to successful implementation, and the development of a good treatment plan relies on input from caregivers. The ESDM represents an example of an intervention model particularly well suited for interdisciplinary care coordination in order to optimize efficiency and effectiveness of treatment and to generate best possible outcomes for very young children on the autism spectrum.

References

Bondy, A. S., & Frost, L. A. (1994). The picture exchange communication system. *Focus on Autistic Behavior, 9*, 1–19.

Cidav, Z., Munson, J., Estes, A., Dawson, G, Rogers, S. J., & Mandell, D. (2017). Cost offset associated with Early Start Denver Model for children with autism. *Journal of the American Academy of Child and Adolescent Psychiatry, 56*(9), 777–783.

Dawson, G., Jones, E. J. H., Merkle, K., Venema, K., Lowy, R., Faja, S., … Webb, S. J. (2012). Early behavioral intervention is associated with normalized brain activity in young children with autism. *Journal of the American Academy of Child and Adolescent Psychiatry, 51*(11), 1150–1159.

Dawson, G., Rogers, S. J., Munson, J., Smith, M., Winter, J., Greenson, J., … Varley, J. (2010). Randomized, controlled trial of an intervention for toddlers with autism: The Early Start Denver Model. *Pediatrics, 125*(1), e17–e23.

Dawson, G., Toth, K., Abbott, R., Osterling, J., Munson, J., Estes, A., & Liaw, J. (2004). Defining the early social attention impairments in autism: Social orienting, joint attention, and responses to emotions. *Developmental Psychology, 40*(2), 271–283.

Estes, A., Munson, J., Rogers, S. J., Greenson, J., Winter, J., & Dawson, G. (2015). Long-term outcomes of early intervention in 6-year old children with autism spectrum disorder. *Journal of the American Academy of Child and Adolescent Psychiatry, 54*(7), 580–587.

Kaale, A., Smith, L., & Sponheim, E. (2012). A randomized controlled trial of preschool based joint attention intervention for children with autism. *Journal of Child Psychology and Psychiatry, 53*(1), 97–105.

Kasari, C., Freeman, S., & Paparella, T. (2006). Joint attention and symbolic play in young children with autism: A randomized controlled intervention study. *Journal of Child Psychology and Psychiatry, 47*(6), 611–620.

Koegel, R., & Koegel, L. K. (1988). Generalized responsivity and pivotal behavior. In R. H. Horner, G. Dunlap, & R. L. Koegel (Eds.), *Generalization and maintenance: Lifestyle changes in applied settings* (pp. 41–66). Baltimore: Brookes.

Mesibov, G. B., & Shea, V. (2010). The TEACCH program in the era of evidence-based practice. *Journal of Autism and Developmental Disorders, 40*(5), 570–579.

Mesibov, G. B., Shea, V., & Schopler, E. (2004). *The TEACCH approach to autism spectrum disorders*. New York: Springer Publishers.

Piaget, J. (1963). *The origins of intelligence in children*. New York: Norton.

Prizant, B. M., Wetherby, A. M., Rubin, E., & Laurent, A. (2003). The SCERTS model: A transactional, family-centered approach to enhancing communication and socioemotional abilities of children with autism spectrum disorder. *Infants & Young Children, 16*(4), 296–316.

Rogers, S. J., & Dawson, G. (2009). *Early Start Denver Model curriculum checklist for young children with autism*. New York: Guilford Press.

Rogers, S. J., & Dawson, G. (2010). *The Early Start Denver Model for young children with autism: Promoting language, learning, and engagement*. New York: Guilford Press.

Rogers, S. J., Estes, A., Lord, C., Vismara, L., Winter, J., Fitzpatrick, A., … Dawson, G. (2012). Effects of a brief Early Start Denver Model (ESDM)-based parent intervention on toddlers at risk for autism spectrum disorders: A randomized controlled trial. *Journal of the American Academy of Child and Adolescent Psychiatry, 51*(10), 1052–1065.

Rogers, S. J., Estes, A., Lord, C., Munson, J., Rocha, M., Winter, J., … Talbott, M. (2019). A multisite randomized controlled two-phase trial of the Early Start Denver Model compared to treatment as usual. *Journal of the American Academy of Child and Adolescent Psychiatry, 58*(9), 853–865.

Rogers, S. J., Hall, T., Osaki, D., Reaven, J., & Herbison, J. (2000). The Denver model: A comprehensive, integrated educational approach to young children with autism and their families. In S. L. Harris & J. S. Handleman (Eds.), *Preschool education programs for children with autism* (2nd ed., pp. 95–134). Austin, TX: Pro-Ed.

Rogers, S. J., Herbison, J., Lewis, H., Pantone, J., & Reis, K. (1986). An approach for enhancing the symbolic, communicative, and interpersonal functioning of young children with autism and severe emotional handicaps. *Journal of the Division of Early Childhood, 10*, 135–148.

Rogers, S. J., & Pennington, B. F. (1991). A theoretical approach to the deficits in infantile autism. *Development and Psychopathology, 3*, 137–162.

Sameroff, A. (Ed.) (2009). *The transactional model of development: How children and contexts shape each other*. Washington, DC: American Psychological Association.

Schreibman, L., Dawson, G., Stahmer, A. C., Landa, R., Rogers, S. J., McGee, G. G., … Halladay, A. (2015). Naturalistic developmental behavioral interventions: Empirically validated treatments for autism spectrum disorder. *Journal of Autism and Developmental Disorders, 45*(8), 2411–2428.

Schreibman, L., & Pierce, K. L. (1993). Achieving greater generalization of treatment effects in children with autism: Pivotal response training and self-management. *Clinical Psychologist, 46*(4), 184–191.

Vismara, L. A., McCormick, C. E. B., Wagner, A. L., Monlux, K., Nadhan, A., & Young, G. Y. (2018). Telehealth parent training in the Early Start Denver Model: Results from a randomized controlled study. *Focus on Autism and Other Developmental Disabilities, 33*(2), 67–79.

Vivanti, G., Paynter, J., Duncan, E., Fothergill, H., Dissanayake, C., Rogers, S. J., & Victorian ASELCC Team (2014). Effectiveness and feasibility of the Early Start Denver Model implemented in a group-based community childcare setting. *Journal of Autism and Developmental Disorders, 44*(12), 3140–3153.

Zhou, B., Xu, Q., Li, H., Zhang, Y., Wang, Y., Rogers, S. J., & Xu, X. (2018). Effects of parent-implemented Early Start Denver Model intervention on Chinese toddlers with autism spectrum disorder: A non-randomized controlled trial. *Autism Research, 11*, 654–666.

Interprofessional Education and Training

Maryellen Brunson McClain, Cassity R. Haverkamp, Judith Holt, Gretchen Gimpel Peacock, and Sarah Winter

Abstract Working in interprofessional teams is best practice in providing services to individuals with Autism Spectrum Disorder (ASD). In order to provide quality Interprofessional Care (IPC) for individuals with ASD and their families, associated healthcare professionals need a foundation for practice based in interprofessional training. This training can be achieved through Interprofessional Education (IPE). This chapter, which is divided into three sections, focuses on IPE and training with an emphasis on ASD. Section 1, *Teamwork in Interprofessional Care and Education*, addresses team science, how to effectively work in groups, and the link between IPC and service provision for individuals with ASD. Section 2, *The Details of IPE*, addresses the who, what, where, when, and why of IPE and outlines its various components. Section 3, *A Detailed Example of an IPE Program*, discusses the federally funded Leadership Education in Neurodevelopmental and Related Disabilities (LEND) program, including exploring relevant historical information and a specific example of one LEND program. The chapter concludes with a brief conclusion and recommendations.

Teamwork in Interprofessional Care and Education

As the prevalence of autism spectrum disorder (ASD) has increased (Maenner et al., 2020), professionals from multiple disciplines are needed to evaluate, diagnose, and support children with ASD. Interprofessional assessment teams are necessary to identify ASD and determine specific intervention and support needs (Beatson, 2006; Prelock, Beatson, Bitner, Broder, & Ducker, 2003). Many children with ASD have

M. B. McClain (✉) · C. R. Haverkamp · G. G. Peacock
Department of Psychology, Utah State University, Logan, UT, USA
e-mail: maryellen.mcclainverdoes@usu.edu

J. Holt
Utah State University, Logan, UT, USA

S. Winter
Department of Pediatrics, University of Utah, Salt Lake City, UT, USA

M. B. McClain et al. (eds.), *Interprofessional Care Coordination for Pediatric Autism Spectrum Disorder*, https://doi.org/10.1007/978-3-030-46295-6_24

several intervention needs often including, but not limited to, speech-language therapy, physical and occupational therapy, mental health services, special education, and specialized medical supports. Interprofessional collaboration among providers is critical in ensuring that children with ASD receive appropriate services (Banach & Couse, 2012; Beverly & Wooster, 2018; Ji, Sun, Yi, & Tang, 2014; Loutzenhiser & Hadjistavropoulos, 2008; Prelock, Potvin, & Savard, 2017). See chapter "Medical Comorbidities in Pediatric Autism Spectrum Disorder" for more information on ASD and co-occurring concerns that result in a higher need for interprofessional care (IPC).

Professionals who interact with children with ASD and their families should be interconnected and coordinating their evaluation and support services. Professionals who integrate and coordinate their care avoid poor patient care and communication, duplication of services, and inefficient services (Stange et al., 2009). In order to provide quality IPC for individuals who have ASD, healthcare professionals need a solid foundation for practice based on interprofessional training. Research shows that interprofessional teams can be highly effective in meeting the needs of children with ASD and their families (Banach & Couse, 2012; Fiscella & McDaniel, 2018; Rosen et al., 2018; Self & Parham, 2016).

The Benefits of Working in Teams

Research on team dynamics provides evidence as to why working in teams and providing interprofessional team training is beneficial. When training in a team setting, team members can reach agreement on respective roles and are able to share knowledge, skills, best practices, and enhance their overall team performance (Driskell, Salas, & Driskell, 2018; Fiscella & McDaniel, 2018). When healthcare providers are trained in an interprofessional setting and learn effective care coordination, clinical or medical errors may be avoided (Rosen et al., 2018). When practitioners are not trained within an interprofessional setting, they may lack some of these important team elements and may only approach cases from their specific discipline rather than from a holistic perspective. Some of the most important pieces of successful teams include a shared mission, creating goals and monitoring their progress, and formulating alternative strategies when unexpected difficulties arise (Driskell et al., 2018; Lacerenza, Marlow, Tannenbaum, & Salas, 2018).

Effective teams also practice conflict management, provide support and encouragement, and produce a positive environment for work relations (Driskell et al., 2018). In a medical setting, members of healthcare teams must coordinate care between professionals, listen effectively to colleagues, and speak up for their respective disciplines (Rosen et al., 2018). These are guidelines professionals can learn and practice in a training setting, whether it be pre-service or in-service training. These general healthcare-based team-building strategies can be readily applied to training in working with children with ASD in interprofessional settings.

Interprofessional Education (IPE) for ASD

Within the area of ASD, IPE and IPC teams for ASD assessment and intervention are best practices (Prelock et al., 2003; Prior et al., 2011). Within the ASD screening and diagnostic process, using an interprofessional team is faster and more cost effective than a typical evaluation by a psychologist without sacrificing diagnostic precision (Ahlers et al., 2019). Providing efficient and cost-effective care is important within the field of ASD, as it is not only best practice, but it can reduce wait times for services, a large concern for this population (Gordon-Lipkin, Foster, & Peacock, 2016). Within IPE for ASD assessment training, best practices include focusing on family-centered care, cultural competence, and using a strengths perspective (Prelock et al., 2003). For intervention, research-based applied behavior analysis interventions for children with ASD often include an integrated and interprofessional team across home, school, medical, and community organizations (Swiezy, Stuart, & Korzekwa, 2008).

Best practice guidelines for ASD evaluations and intervention within an interprofessional context are also often tied to insurance requirements. Nearly every state (46 states and the District of Columbia) includes some form of insurance mandates for ASD evaluations and services (American Speech-Language-Hearing Association, 2019). Most states also include what type of services are covered and who can provide them, which usually includes professionals in many fields. Minnesota law (2013) specifically requires large-group insurance companies to cover interprofessional assessment for ASD. Of the 14 states within the Autism and Developmental Disabilities Monitoring (ADDM) network sites, most require insurers to cover applied behavior analysis services and allied health services (typically occupational therapy, physical therapy, and speech-language services) and about half require behavioral therapy coverage (Douglas, Benevides, & Carretta, 2017). Federally and state-funded Medicaid for the diagnosis and service management of ASD also may have requirements related to interprofessional teams. For instance, Utah Medicaid (2019) states that a diagnostic evaluation for ASD ideally includes an interprofessional team approach. In fact, an interprofessional team must be employed on a case if ASD-specific screeners and parent questionnaires will be used in place of an ASD diagnostic evaluation instrument (e.g., Autism Diagnostic Observation Schedule-2, Autism Diagnostic Interview-Revised) and the team members must have prior advanced training in ASD. Outside of insurance, some states provide funding for other interdisciplinary teams for ASD. Alaska has created state-funded interdisciplinary teams for the early detection of ASD, Arkansas offers interdisciplinary training in ASD through their IDEA Part C services, and Hawai'i has state funding to facilitate care coordination and holistic services for children with ASD (L&M Policy Research, 2014). Likewise, there are many state and federally funded services for children with ASD that include interdisciplinary evaluations and early intervention (Autism Speaks, 2019; L&M Policy Research, 2014).

Beyond state and federal funding and state law for insurance companies, several professional accreditation bodies now require interprofessional training as part of their standards. For instance, the Accreditation Council for Graduate Medical Education (ACGME, 2018), Liaison Committee on Medical Education (LCME, 2019), the Accreditation Commission for Education in Nursing (ACEN, 2017), and the Accreditation Council on Pharmacy Education (ACPE, 2016) are all accrediting bodies in the medical field that require interprofessional education. Accreditation bodies outside of the medical field and in related healthcare fields also include statements about interprofessional care within training programs. The American Psychological Association (APA, 2018), the Association for Behavior Analysis International Accreditation Board (ABAI, 2019), the Accreditation Council for Occupational Therapy Education (ACOTE, 2013), The American Speech-Language-Hearing Association (ASHA, 2019), and the Commission for Accreditation in Physical Therapy Education (CAPTE, 2016) are accreditation bodies that all include a requirement for interprofessional training.

The Details of IPE

Developing skills required for effective IPC requires training and education. This training, known as Interprofessional Education (IPE), can occur during one's pre-service training and throughout one's career via professional development. According to the World Health Organization (WHO), IPE is "two or more professionals learning about, from and with each other, to enable effective collaboration and improve health outcomes" (WHO, 2010, p. 10). Considering the increase in IPC for individuals with complex conditions, such as ASD, and the importance of delivering high-quality IPC, there is a need for pre-service trainees and practitioners to participate in IPE to ensure high quality and effective care.

What Is the Purpose of IPE and Who Are the Trainers?

Participation in IPE should result in trainees further developing their own professional identity while simultaneously becoming knowledgeable about the roles of, and valuing, other professional disciplines (Bridges, Davidson, Odegard, Maki, & Tomkowiak, 2011). IPE should also allow trainees to cultivate the necessary attitudes, skills, and knowledge to effectively engage in IPC (Freeth et al., 2005). Trainers in IPE should represent various disciplines and careers; researchers, educators, and clinicians all play an important role in IPE as they bring unique perspectives in how to promote interprofessional engagement. Furthermore, self-advocates, parents, and families should be meaningfully involved as they add a critical viewpoint and promote patient-centered care.

When Should IPE Occur?

Interprofessional training is not a one-time event or even something that happens at only one point in a person's training. Interprofessional training should begin early in a student's training program—ideally toward the beginning—so that the students can understand how their discipline fits in with other disciplines in providing the best possible care to clients. It is also important that students be exposed early to the concept and principles of interprofessional training so that their buy-in is maximized. Waiting too long to expose students to an interprofessional model may result in students who are too entrenched in their own discipline to clearly see and appreciate the values and input from other professionals. Initial exposure may be rather modest as students are spending much of their time learning about their own discipline. A developmental approach in which more interprofessional exposure/training happens as more discipline-specific knowledge and skills are obtained may be the best way to conceptualize interprofessional training. It is also important to recognize that interprofessional training is not just for students. Just as professionals engage in continuing education in their own discipline, continuing education regarding interprofessional practices is also important.

Where Should IPE Occur?

It is important to structure IPE opportunities so that trainees have both didactic and applied experiences in understanding how to work effectively with individuals from a variety of disciplines and backgrounds. Discussion of interprofessional training will most likely be embedded in coursework. Incorporating IPE in coursework for pre-service healthcare trainees is recommended (Bressler & Perisco, 2016) and effective. For example, students who participated in an online IPE training course and a day-long ASD conference showed significantly improved attitudes toward other disciplines and in their interprofessional competencies specific to communication and teamwork (Beverly & Wooster, 2018).

As described in a document from the Health Professions Accreditors Collaborative (2019), "deliberate design" of learning activities in which students from different professions engage in learning experiences together are important in successful interprofessional training. In placing students together, they can learn from each other, both directly and through observation of how different disciplines respond to questions and scenarios in class. This in-class work can set the stage for joint learning experiences in applied settings. The Health Professions Accreditors Collaborative (2019) provides a framework in which longitudinal integration of both professional and interprofessional health competencies are developed. This includes professional socialization, learning (in classroom and clinical activities), and professional/team identity all developing over time to promote a dual identity development in which individuals can then contribute to their professional expertise in team settings to promote effective services for clients.

For most pre-professionals, however, it is during applied clinical experiences (e.g., practicum, internship) that the most meaningful learning will occur. For example, Howell, Whittman, and Bundy (2012) found that occupational therapy and psychology graduate students who participated in an IPE experience focused on the implementation of social skills interventions for children with ASD developed a stronger understanding of their professional identity and scope of practice, developed an appreciation and understanding of the perspective of other disciplines, valued communication and its role in effective teamwork and patient care, and realized the importance of handling interprofessional conflict and disagreements effectively. A similar study found that interprofessional trainees who participated in a university-based autism interprofessional diagnostic team showed no difference from pre- to post-test (with scores being high at both times) on a measure of interprofessional learning. However, informal qualitative data suggest students developed new knowledge, found the experience exciting, and encouraged self-reflection regarding their professional role (Self & Parham, 2016).

As trainees engage in applied experiences, it is important that they learn not only their discipline-specific skills but also how to work effectively with team members. Particularly given the nature of ASD, with diagnostic symptoms crossing professional disciplines (e.g., psychology, speech, occupational therapy) understanding of these multiple disciplines in terms of what each contributes to the assessment and service management of individuals with ASD is important. In the context of applied experiences, it is important to build in learning opportunities in which trainees are interacting in meaningful ways with other professionals. Observing the work of other professionals, asking questions about this approach, and discussing patients in a team context in which individuals across disciplines demonstrate respect and appreciation for each other's work is important.

IPE training model examples. There are several ways in which IPE, both embedded in coursework and/or as applied experiences, can be implemented. Bridges et al. (2011) reviewed three IPE training models from Rosalind Franklin University of Medicine and Science (RFUMS), University of Florida, and the University of Washington. RFUMS has a 1 credit hour pass/fail course on Interprofessional Healthcare Teams. The 8-month course includes didactic, clinical, and service-learning components. The University of Florida offers a two-semester that required Interdisciplinary Family Health (IFH) course for many students across several disciplines. Similarly, their course also incorporates clinical and service-learning as well as course assignments and small group work. The University of Washington started the Center for Health Sciences Interprofessional Education (CHSIE) to streamline teaching, research, and professional activates across their health professional schools. Through the CHSIE, more than 50 IPE courses are offered. Service-learning and clinical opportunities are also offered. For more detailed information about these three exemplar IPE programs, including program competencies, objectives, and components, as well as general resources and recommendations for successful IPEs, see the Bridges et al. (2011) article.

In addition to determining a training model, experiences and opportunities to incorporate IPC within IPE is important. Trainers of IPE have various options, such as indirect approaches (e.g., facilitating interaction), modeling professional respect, setting up observations and/or participation of real-life clinical IPC experiences, and utilizing seminar/didactic sessions relevant to IPC. For those in more isolated settings, utilizing technology and online methods, such as the Team-Based Learning Collaborative (http://www.teambasedlearning.org) or ECHO Autism (see chapter "ECHO Autism") is encouraged. In a systematic review, Fox et al. (2017) reported on 33 studies that evaluated effective methods to teach interprofessional teamwork skills to health professional students. There was notable variability in designs across studies: 19 used pre-post (without a control group) designs, 6 used pre- or post-test designs, and 2 were qualitative. Only five were randomized control trials. There was also a range in teaching methods utilized, length of IPE, and the IPE context. Methods included contextual simulation, simulated patients, experiential training, and active learning groups (e.g., online learning, workshops, discussion, role-playing scenarios). Length of IPE ranged from one session to multiple years. IPE contexts included hospitals/clinics, simulation centers, and hospice/palliative care centers. The researchers were unable to make claims about specific teaching methods that were more effective than others; however, it was noted that all studies reported positive outcomes associated with participating in IPE, regardless of teaching methods, context, or IPE length.

IPE Program Evaluation

Regardless of the structure of IPE, program evaluation is important as it guides and influences future iterations and promotes effectiveness. Leaders of IPE programs should create meaningful learning outcomes that directly link their measurement strategies. There is variability in how IPE programs incorporate and evaluate measurement outcomes. A systematic review conducted by Thistlewaite and Moran (2010) indicated learning objectives that emphasize teamwork, collaboration, discipline roles and responsibilities, patient-centered care, and knowledge of interprofessional teamwork to be among the most commonly incorporated IPE learning outcomes. Some IPE programs have learning objectives that fall under broader competencies—examples include common competencies (relevant for all professionals), complementary competencies (discipline specific), and collaborative competencies (for interprofessional collaboration; Thistlewaite & Moran, 2010). The Interprofessional Educational Collaborative (IPEC, 2016) has defined also four core competencies: (1) Values/Ethics for Interprofessional Practice, (2) Role/Responsibilities, (3) Interprofessional Communication, and (4) Teams and Teamwork. Although the content of learning objectives may be similar across IPE programs, how they are measured may differ depending on a program's framework. For example, some IPE programs may last throughout a trainee's pre-service training while others may be limited to a semester or a day. Regarding specific assessment techniques, outcomes often include attitudes and behaviors and are assessed through both quantitative and qualitative means (Fox et al., 2017). Quantitative methods can include standardized self-report rating forms, such as the Attitudes Toward Health Care Teams' Scale (Hyer et al., 2000) or the Readiness for Interprofessional Learning Scale (McFayden et al., 2005), or through specific questions created by IPE leadership. Open-ended survey questions, focus groups, or self-reflection pieces may be used to qualitatively determine program effectiveness. Leaders should define their learning objectives and associated outcomes and adequately assess how to measure them given their IPE framework.

Detailed Example of an IPE Program

Preparing personnel to provide interprofessional diagnostic assessments and services for children with ASD has been a formidable challenge for many decades. Even as professionals struggled to better understand the complexities of ASD, families advocated for availability of highly qualified professionals to provide the services and supports their children needed. Historically, children with ASD were often classified as having an Intellectual Disability (ID) and early national efforts focused on children with Intellectual or Developmental Disabilities (DD). Although the current heightened visibility of the increasing prevalence of ASD has certainly brought many of these issues to the forefront, national efforts to prepare personnel and provide services which began in the 1950s and 1960s. One outcome of these efforts was the creation of the Leadership Education in Neurodevelopmental and related Disabilities (LEND) programs, which are funded competitively through the Maternal and Child Health Bureau in the Health Resources and Services Administration (HRSA). Currently, the Autism CARES Act is the primary source of funding for the LEND programs.

What is LEND?

Generally located at medical schools or teaching hospitals and often co-located with University Centers for Excellence in Developmental Disabilities (UCEDDs), LEND programs promote education, early detection, and intervention in ASD. LEND program trainees participate in academic, clinical, leadership and community opportunities and receive training in cultural and linguistic competence using a family-centered approach. All training is delivered within an interprofessional context. LENDs are located in 44 US states, with an additional six states and three territories reached through program partnerships.

While each LEND program is unique, with its own focus and expertise, they all provide interprofessional training, have faculty and trainees in a wide range of health-related disciplines, and include parents, family members, or adults with disabilities as paid program participants. They also share the following objectives:

1. "Advance the knowledge and skills of all child health professionals to improve health care delivery systems for children with developmental disabilities.
2. Provide high-quality interdisciplinary education that emphasizes the integration of services from state and local agencies and organizations, private providers, and communities.
3. Provide health professionals with skills that foster community-based partnerships.
4. Promote innovative practices to enhance cultural competency, family-centered care, and interdisciplinary partnerships (Association of University Centers on Disabilities, 2011)."

For additional information regarding the objectives of LEND we direct readers to the following websites: (1) https://mchb.hrsa.gov/training/documents/fs/factsheet-LEND.pdf and (2) https://www.aucd.org/template/page.cfm?id=473.

LEND trainees. LEND trainees are selected from a number of health-related disciplines. These disciplines include medicine, dentistry, nursing, genetics, psychology, nutrition, social work, audiology, speech and language pathology, public health, and special education. Other disciplines may also be included. The trainees must be enrolled in a graduate program or be practicing professionals who want to enhance their knowledge and skills regarding children with ASD/DD and interprofessional practice. LEND programs are often most beneficial for doctoral students in their third year or beyond of training, post-doctorates, or practicing professionals. It is sometimes challenging for students who are still early in their discipline-specific training to competently represent their discipline in interprofessional discussions and activities. Trainees must also be willing to learn about and work with other disciplines in an interprofessional manner. Additional trainees are recruited/selected who are parents, or adult-self advocates, or community members with an interest in the field of disabilities.

LEND faculty. LEND faculty are generally tenure-track or clinical faculty from their home discipline or clinicians at a collaborating clinic or hospital. The faculty represent health-related and other relevant disciplines. They work in interprofessional teams to support the LEND program.

LEND Training Program. Each LEND program designs its own curriculum which includes didactic, clinical, leadership, and research experiences to prepare trainees to provide services and supports to children with ASD and their families. The curriculum is based on the competencies developed by the MCHB. These competencies were developed around the framework of self, others, and wider community. These include an emphasis on the self, others, family-professional partnerships, and the wider community (MCHB, 2018).

The interprofessional training program generally extends over one academic year and trainees must complete at least 300 clock hours to be considered long-term trainees. The LEND program is designed to address the unique learning objectives of the trainees and all trainees have an individualized training/leadership plan. These plans are developed with the trainee and the faculty advisor and set the outcomes for the LEND experience.

The role of family members of children with ASD and self-advocates is also critical within the LEND programs. LEND programs include family members and self-advocates as faculty, trainees, consultants, advisors, mentors, and instructors. Due to the overall program focus on preparing professionals to provide interprofessional services that are family-centered with families and children as full partners, the active roles of families and self-advocates are embedded in all aspects of the program. This unique aspect engages trainees in better understanding their role with families and children and enhances their ability to form meaningful productive parent-professional partnerships.

Research experiences are also an integral part of LEND although there is wide variance on how this component is addressed. In some programs, trainees are expected to conduct individual or team-based research projects or support ongoing faculty-mentored projects. Research may also be part of clinical activities or addressing issues in community agencies. Products from the research may include peer-reviewed articles, virtual materials, posters and presentations at state and national conferences, and reports.

LEND programs are highly individualized based on their location, history, and needs of their community and state. However, all programs are expected to provide well-designed experiences for trainees from a variety of disciplines in settings and with children with ASD and related disabilities who have varying challenges and require highly specialized services and supports. Trainees have the opportunity to interact, learn from, and be mentored by interprofessional faculty. Trainees also work with their peers in diagnosing and providing interventions for children with ASD, understanding and addressing both family and system challenges.

Snapshot of a LEND Program

Funded in 2001, The Utah Regional Leadership Education in Neurodevelopmental Disabilities (URLEND) program is the largest LEND program based on geography and encompasses 10 sites across five states (Utah, Idaho, Montana, North Dakota, and Wyoming). URLEND is co-directed by a neurodevelopmental pediatrician and a psychologist with 21 faculty representing 16 disciplines and enrolls about 35 trainees annually. URLEND has a general track and the Autism Enhanced (AE) track (for trainees who have completed the general track and desire more specialized training in ASD). URLEND relies heavily on distance technology to implement its program and keep faculty and trainees connected. Currently, URLEND utilizes ZOOM® and Canvas® as the platforms for program activities. A brief description of the URLEND activities follows.

Didactic Component

URLEND trainees participate in didactic seminars throughout the training year. Didactic experiences include pre-orientation tasks, completion of a 2-day orientation, and participation in weekly 4-hour seminars. Didactic components are interactive and cover topics relevant to interprofessional work with individuals with ASD and DD and the systems that support them.

Clinical Component

A broad array of clinical activities is available to URLEND trainees with experiences ranging from observation to full team membership. The clinical settings range from hospital outpatient clinics to home-based early intervention programs. The populations served range in age from 3 months to 25 years with at least 70% of the sites seeing primarily children with either ASD or related neurodevelopmental disorders. Sites include specialty clinics (e.g., Prader-Willi, spina bifida, craniofacial, genetics), post-secondary programs for individuals with disabilities, and recreational programs for individuals with disabilities.

In addition to more traditional clinical activities, URLEND trainees also participate in Parent Directed Consultations (PDC) and the Family Mentorship Program (FMP). The PDC is designed to provide experiences for trainees to work with families and trainees from other disciplines to problem solve in an interprofessional process. The consultation takes place at a site in any of the five participating states and trainees and families participate via ZOOM® with the other sites. Participating parents are asked to provide background information regarding their child and current concerns which is shared with all of the URLEND faculty and trainees. Depending upon the issues and questions generated by the parents, a team of trainees is formed to specifically address these concerns. PDCs emphasize a consultative approach and families identify the primary issues to be addressed. These experiences provide a rich learning opportunity for the trainees.

During the year, each trainee is matched with a family in the FMP. Its purpose is to support trainees in gaining insight into and appreciation of the perspectives of families who have children with special health care needs. Trainees are matched to a mentor family and journal entries, reflection papers, and discussions are utilized to capture the trainees' experiences.

Leadership Component

URLEND trainees are involved in several leadership activities, which include the completion of leadership readings and discussions, a leadership project completed within an interprofessional group, and involvement in a community cultural experience. Leadership readings and discussions are designed to engage the trainees in a better understanding of their leadership styles and leader roles and functions as well as participate in leadership opportunities. Trainees are assigned to a leadership project group that includes 3–5 trainees. Leadership Projects are designed to provide opportunities to practice and strengthen leadership skills, especially those outlined in the MCH Leadership Competencies. The Leadership Project is a major component of URLEND and each project results in a product that is shared with the URLEND group and in many cases the broader MCH community. Each year at least half of the projects have an ASD emphasis. Recent leadership project topics include Evidenced-Based Apps for Children with ASD; Training and Support for Early Identification of Autism in Early Intervention Systems; Genetic Testing in Children with Autism Spectrum Disorder; and Teaching Women, Infant, and Children (WIC) Clients about Healthy Child Development with the "Learn the Signs. Act Early" Program. The community cultural experiences, also conducted in interprofessional groups, provide the trainees an opportunity to engage with culturally diverse groups in their states. Although specific activities vary across states, as one example, trainees develop, prepare, and present information to Spanish-speaking families at local health clinic and school district. The topics of the training are identified by the participating families.

Conclusion

Over the past 15–20 years, an increasing number of experts and researchers have shown that providing team-based interprofessional diagnostic and interventional services is best practice for individuals with ASD. With increasing prevalence of ASD, attention has been given to how best to diagnose and intervene. IPC has been shown to be efficient, cost effective, and highly effective in meeting the needs of children with ASD and their families. Members of the team need to have advanced skills in their own discipline as well as being knowledgeable about the roles, and valuing the skills, of other professional disciplines. Increasingly, best practice guidelines involving IPC for evaluations and interventions are tied to insurance requirements with most states now having specific mandates for ASD evaluations and services, which include what types of services are covered and who can provide those services.

In order to adequately prepare professionals for this work, it is essential to provide IPE. Leaders in graduate education must address this skillset in the curriculum with careful planning for evaluating the trainees' competence in IPC. Standardized self-report rating forms exist for this purpose if desired. Many professional accreditation bodies require interprofessional training as part of their standards. Within IPE for ASD assessment training, best practices include focusing on family-centered care, cultural competence, and using a strengths perspective. Ideally this type of training would be introduced early in training through the evolution of becoming aware of interprofessional teams and the benefits of this type of care, then acquiring the knowledge of the theoretical construct of IPC and ultimately, having applied clinical experiences in which IPC is delivered. A variety of methods for delivering IPE include but are not limited to role play, simulations, teleECHO case-based discussions, and participating in real-life clinical experiences.

To acquire expertise in interprofessional care in ASD, many professionals have chosen to engage in LEND programs. For less intensive experiences, several universities have offered semester-long coursework on interprofessional healthcare teams. Partnering with parents and individuals with ASD is rewarding work but takes the sophisticated skills required of interprofessional care to do it well. Training for this work should include specific skill-directed training that includes IPE.

References

Accreditation Commission for Education in Nursing. (2017). *ACEN 2017 accreditation manual: Section III, 2017 standards & criteria*. Retrieved from http://www.acenursing.net/manuals/SC2017.pdf.

Accreditation Council for Graduate Medical Education. (2018). *ACGME common program requirements (residency)*. Retrieved from https://www.acgme.org/Portals/0/PFAssets/ProgramRequirements/CPRResidency2019.pdf.

Accreditation Council for Occupational Therapy Education. (2018). *2018 Accreditation Council for Occupational Therapy Education (ACOTE) standards and interpretive guide*. Retrieved from https://www.aota.org/~/media/Corporate/Files/EducationCareers/Accredit/StandardsReview/2018-ACOTE-Standards-Interpretive-Guide.pdf.

Accreditation Council on Pharmacy Education. (2016). *Accreditation standards and key elements for the professional program in pharmacy leading to the Doctor of Pharmacy degree*. Retrieved from https://www.acpe-accredit.org/pdf/Standards2016FINAL.pdf.

Ahlers, K., Gabrielsen, T. P., Ellzey, A., Brady, A., Litchford, A., Fox, J., … Carbone, P. S. (2019). A pilot project using pediatricians as initial diagnosticians in multidisciplinary autism evaluations for young children. *Journal of Developmental and Behavioral Pediatrics, 40*, 1–11.

American Psychological Association. (2019). Office of program consultation and accreditation. Retrieved from https://www.apa.org/ed/accreditation/?tab=3.

American Speech-Language-Hearing Association: Council on Academic Accreditation. (2019). *Standards for accreditation of graduate education programs in audiology and speech-language pathology*. Retrieved from https://caa.asha.org/wp-content/uploads/Accreditation-Standards-for-Graduate-Programs.pdf.

American Speech-Language-Hearing Association. (2019). State insurance mandates for autism spectrum disorder. Retrieved from https://www.asha.org/Advocacy/state/States-Specific-Autism-Mandates/.

Association for Behavior Analysis International Accreditation Board. (2019). *Accreditation handbook*. Retrieved from https://accreditation.abainternational.org/media/110571/abai_accreditation_board_accreditation_handbook_20190214.pdf.

Association of University Centers on Disabilities. (2011). About LEND. Retrieved from https://www.aucd.org//template/page.cfm?id=473.

Autism Speaks. (2019). State early intervention information. Retrieved from https://www.autismspeaks.org/state-early-intervention-information.

Baio, J., Wiggins, L., Christensen, D. L., Maenner, M. J., Daniels, J., Warren, Z., … Dowling, N. F. (2018). Prevalence of Autism Spectrum Disorder among children aged 8 years – Autism and developmental disabilities monitoring network, 11 sites, United States, 2014. *Morbidity and Mortality Weekly Report Surveillance Summaries, 67*, 1–23.

Banach, M., & Couse, L. J. (2012). Interdisciplinary co-facilitation of support groups for parents of children with autism: An opportunity for professional preparation. *Social Work with Groups, 35,* 313–329.

Beatson, J. E. (2006). Preparing speech-language pathologists as family-centered practitioners in assessment and program planning for children with autism spectrum disorder. *Seminars in Speech and Language, 27,* 1–9.

Beverly, B. L., & Wooster, D. (2018). An interprofessional education initiative for allied health students preparing to serve individuals with autism spectrum disorders. *Interprofessional Practice and Education, 47,* 90–95.

Bressler, T., & Perisco, L. (2016). Interprofessional education: Partnerships in the educational proc. *Nurse Education in Practice, 16,* 144–147.

Bridges, D. R., Davidson, R. A., Odegard, P. S., Maki, I. V., & Tomkowiak, J. (2011). Interprofessional collaboration: Three best practice models of interprofessional education. *Medical Education Online, 16,* 6035.

Commission for Accreditation in Physical Therapy Education. (2016). *Standards and required elements for accreditation of physical therapist education programs.* Retrieved from http://www.capteonline.org/uploadedFiles/CAPTEorg/About_CAPTE/Resources/Accreditation_Handbook/CAPTE_PTStandardsEvidence.pdf.

Division of Medicaid and Health Financing. (2019). *Utah medicaid provider manual: Autism spectrum disorder related services for EPSDT eligible individuals.* Retrieved from https://medicaid.utah.gov/Documents/manuals/pdfs/Medicaid%20Provider%20Manuals/Autism%20Spectrum%20Disorder%20Services/AutismSpectrumDisorder3–19.pdf.

Douglas, M. D., Benevides, T. W., & Carretta, H. (2017). Analyzing state autism private insurance mandates for allied health services: A pilot study. *OTJR: Occupation. Participation and Health, 37,* 218–226. https://doi.org/10.1177/1539449217730355.

Driskell, J. E., Salas, E., & Driskell, T. (2018). Foundations of teamwork and collaboration. *American Psychologist, 73,* 334–348.

Fiscella, K., & McDaniel, S. H. (2018). The complexity, diversity, and science of primary care teams. *American Psychologist, 73,* 451–467.

Fox, L., Onders, R., Hermansen-Kobulnicky, C. J., Nguyen, T., Myran, L., Linn, B., et al. (2017). Teaching interprofessional teamwork skills to health professional students: A scoping review. *Journal of Interprofessional Care, 32,* 127–135.

Freeth, D., Hammick, M., Reeves, S., Koppel, I., & Barr, H. (2005). Effective interprofessional education: Development, delivery and evaluation. In H. Barr (Ed.), *Promoting partnership for health series.* Malden, MA: Blackwell Publishing.

Gordon-Lipkin, E., Foster, J., & Peacock, G. (2016). Whittling down the wait time: Exploring models to minimize the delay from initial concern to diagnosis and treatment of autism spectrum disorder. *Pediatric Clinics of North America, 63,* 851–859.

Collaborative, Health Professions Accreditors. (2019). *Guidance on developing quality interprofessional education for the health professions.* Chicago, IL: Health Professions Accreditors Collaborative.

Health Resources and Services Administration: Maternal and Child Health Bureau. (2018). *Maternal and child health leadership competencies: Version 4.0.* Rockville, MD: Author.

Health Resources and Services Administration: Maternal and Child Health Bureau. (2019). *Leadership Education in Neurodevelopmental and Related Disabilities (LEND) fact sheet.* Rockville, MD: Author.

Howell, D. M., Wittman, P., & Bundy, M. B. (2012). Interprofessional clinical education for occupational therapy and psychology students: A social skills training program for children with autism spectrum disorders. *Journal of Interprofessional Care, 26,* 49–55.

Hyer, K., Fairchild, S., Abraham, I., Mezey, M., & Fulmer, T. (2000). Measuring attitudes related to interdisciplinary training: Revisiting the Heinemann, Schmitt and Farrell 'Attitudes Toward Health Care Teams' Scale. *Journal of Interprofessional Care, 14,* 249–258.

Interprofessional Education Collaborative. (2016). *Core competencies for interprofessional collaborative practice: 2016 update*. Washington, DC: Interprofessional Education Collaborative.

Ji, B., Sun, M., Yi, R., & Tang, S. (2014). Multidisciplinary parent education for caregivers of children with autism spectrum disorders. *Archives of Psychiatric Nursing, 28,* 319–326.

L&M Policy Research, LLC. (2014). *Autism spectrum disorders (ASD): State of the states of services and supports for people with ASD*. Washington, DC: Author.

Lacerenza, C. N., Marlow, S. L., Tannenbaum, S. I., & Salas, E. (2018). Team development interventions: Evidence-based approaches for improving teamwork. *American Psychologist, 73,* 517–531.

Liaison Committee on Medical Education. (2019). *Functions and structure of a medical school: Standards for accreditation of medical education programs leading to the MD degree*. Retrieved from https://www.aamc.org/services/first-for-financial-aid-officers/lcme-accreditation.

Loutzenhiser, L., & Hadjistavropoulos, H. (2008). Enhancing interprofessional patient-centered practice for children with autism spectrum disorders: A pilot project with pre-licensure health students. *Journal of Interprofessional Care, 22,* 429–431.

Maenner, M. J., Shaw, K. A., Baio, J., Washington, A., Patrick, M. & Dietz, P. M. (2020). Prevalence of autism spectrum disorder among children aged 8 years—autism and developmental disabilities monitoring network, 11 Sites, United States, 2016. *MMWR. Surveillance Summaries, 69*(4), 1–12.

McFayden, A. K., Webster, V., Strachan, K., Figgins, E., Brown, H., & McKechnie, J. (2005). The Readiness for Interprofessional Learning Scale: A possible more stable sub-scale model for the original version of RIPLS. *Journal of Interprofessional Care, 19,* 595–603.

Minnesota Session Laws. (2013). Regular Session, Minn. Stat. §62A-3094.

Prelock, P. A., Beatson, J., Bitner, B., Broder, C., & Ducker, A. (2003). Interdisciplinary assessment of young children with autism spectrum disorder. *Language, Speech, and Hearing Services in Schools, 34,* 194–202.

Prelock, P. A., Potvin, M., & Savard, L. (2017). Interprofessional education and practice: A family-centered approach to autism. *Seminars in Speech and Language, 38,* 360–367.

Prior, M., Roberts, J. M. A., Rodger, S., Williams, K., Dodd, S., Ridley, G., et al. (2011). *A review of the research to identify the most effective models of practice in early intervention for children with autism spectrum disorders*. Australia: The Australian Society for Autism Research.

Rosen, M. A., DiazGranados, D., Dietz, A. S., Benishek, L. E., Thompson, D., Pronovost, P. J., et al. (2018). Teamwork in healthcare: Key discoveries enabling safer, high-quality care. *American Psychologist, 73,* 433–450.

Self, T. L., & Parham, D. F. (2016). Students' self-perceptions of interprofessional education following participation on a diagnostic team for autism spectrum disorder. *Journal of Interprofessional Care, 30,* 682–684.

Stange, G., Fowler, R., Jary, C., Dalton, B., Stewart, S., & Gabbay, E. (2009). Integrated care and optimal management of pulmonary arterial hypertension. *Journal of Multidisciplinary Healthcare, 2,* 67–78. https://doi.org/10.2147/JMDH.S3085.

Swiezy, N., Stuart, M., & Korzekwa, P. (2008). Bridging for success in autism: Training and collaboration across medical, educational, and community systems. *Child and Adolescent Psychiatric Clinics of North America, 17,* 907–922.

Thistlewaite, J., & Moran, M. (2010). Learning outcomes for interprofessional education (IPE): Literature review and synthesis. *Journal of Interprofessional Care, 24,* 503–513.

World Health Organization. (2010). *Framework for action on interprofessional education and collaborative practice*. Geneva, Switzerland: Author.

Psychopharmacology of Autism Spectrum Disorder

Sirin Ozdemir, Christopher J. Keary, Gagan Joshi, Atilla T. Ceranoglu, and Christopher J. McDougle

Abstract Increasingly, pharmacologic agents are used in treatment for children with ASD for related behaviors. This chapter describes trends in psychopharmacology related to ASD and the evidence base for its use in treatment. For each common medication group, mechanisms of action, possible symptom targets, adverse effects, and research base are discussed. The chapter then ends with recommendations for practitioners.

The use of pharmacologic agents as part of the treatment approach in children with autism spectrum disorder (ASD) has increased substantially in recent decades (Aman, Lam, & Van Bourgondien, 2005; Coury et al., 2012). Despite the lack of pharmacological treatment options for the core symptoms of ASD (persistent deficits in social communication and restricted, repetitive patterns of behaviors, interests, or activities), children with ASD are prescribed considerably more psychotropic medications compared to typically developing children. This is likely related to the high prevalence of psychotropic medication use for non-core, associated symptoms of autism and psychiatric co-morbidities. Apart from risperidone and aripiprazole, atypical antipsychotics which are approved by the US Food and Drug Administration [FDA] specifically for irritability, psychotropic drugs are used off-label in youth with ASD. The use of psychotropic agents in this population is often symptom-based as opposed to disease modifying which often results in high rates of polypharmacy. One study looking at the prevalence and prescribing patterns of psychotropic medications among 33,565 children with ASD determined that 64% were taking at least

S. Ozdemir (✉)
Department of Psychiatry, Harvard Medical School, Massachusetts General Hospital, Boston, MA, USA
e-mail: STAPAN@mgh.harvard.edu

C. J. Keary · C. J. McDougle
Department of Psychiatry, Harvard Medical School, Lurie Center for Autism, Massachusetts General Hospital, Boston, MA, USA

G. Joshi · A. T. Ceranoglu
Department of Psychiatry, Bressler Clinical and Research Program for Autism Spectrum Disorders, Harvard Medical School, Massachusetts General Hospital, Boston, MA, USA

M. B. McClain et al. (eds.), *Interprofessional Care Coordination for Pediatric Autism Spectrum Disorder*, https://doi.org/10.1007/978-3-030-46295-6_25

one psychotropic medication and 35% had evidence of polypharmacy (Spencer et al., 2013).

Determining the primary target symptom, choosing the right medication and monitoring adverse effects in individuals with ASD can be difficult owing to their challenges in identifying and communicating their physical sensations and emotional state. In addition, co-occurring behavioral symptoms related to ASD can be more difficult to treat as children with ASD are generally more sensitive to the dosages of medications and more likely to have adverse effects than typically developing children. Therefore, psychotropic agents should be started at lower doses and titrated up more slowly in this population than in youth without ASD.

To date, no medication has been shown to consistently improve the core symptoms of ASD. However, the use of psychiatric medications can be considered if the child's emotional and behavioral challenges interfere with their ability to access other non-drug therapeutic options. Pharmacologic treatment should be initiated only after educational and behavioral interventions are exhausted, co-morbid medical illness is ruled out, and psychosocial/environmental stressors are considered (McGuire et al., 2016). Because the etiology of the presenting problem or "chief complaint" is often multifactorial, successful treatment of children with ASD should include a broad differential diagnostic approach, evaluation by providers from multiple disciplines, and the use of numerous treatment modalities depending on the best evidence for treatment of specific target symptoms.

Medications for children with ASD ideally should be prescribed by specialists with training and experience working with this population and their families (e.g., developmental-behavioral pediatricians, child psychiatrists, child neurologists). However, given the limited number of providers with experience treating ASD and related conditions, access to such specialists is not always an option. Due to the increasing prevalence of ASD and the limited number of specialized clinicians, it is becoming apparent that primary care physicians will likely be needed to play a larger role in the care and management of this patient population. As pediatricians and family practitioners assume more first-line treatment of youth with ASD, ongoing consultation with a developmental-behavioral pediatrician, child psychiatrist, child neurologist, or another mental health professional with expertise in ASD may be necessary and welcome.

In this chapter, we present current evidence regarding the pharmacotherapy of associated symptom targets in ASD, review the common adverse effects of the medications used, and provide a rational approach to pharmacological management with the use of treatment algorithms.

ADHD Medications

Psychostimulants

Methylphenidate (MPH).
Mechanism of action. Psychostimulant medications hypothetically increase the availability of dopamine (DA) and norepinephrine (NE) in the prefrontal cortex by blocking the reuptake of both DA and NE into presynaptic neurons.

Potential treatment targets. Symptoms of inattention, hyperactivity, and impulsivity are common in children with ASD and these symptoms are often severe enough to meet the diagnostic criteria for attention-deficit/hyperactivity disorder (ADHD) (Frazier et al., 2001). Psychostimulants are considered first-line agents for the treatment of ADHD in typically developing school-aged children (ages 6–17 years) (Greenhill et al., 2002; Subcommittee on Attention-Deficit/Hyperactivity et al., 2011). To date, the best-studied psychostimulant in children and adolescents with ASD and co-morbid ADHD is methylphenidate (MPH).

Review of research findings. Randomized controlled trials (RCTs) and meta-analyses indicate that psychostimulants improve symptoms in approximately 70% of typically developing latency age children with ADHD (MTA, 1999). Some preliminary studies suggested that stimulants were mostly ineffective and associated with increased adverse effects in patients with autism (Aman, 1982; Campbell, 1975; Stigler, Desmond, Posey, Wiegand, & McDougle, 2004a). However, four-crossover studies with a total of 113 subjects indicated that short-term treatment with MPH may be effective in children with ASD who can tolerate the medication (Handen, Johnson, & Lubetsky, 2000; Pearson et al., 2013; Quintana et al., 1995; Research Units on Pediatric Psychopharmacology Autism Network, 2005).

A double-blind, placebo-controlled, crossover study of MPH (0.3 and 0.6 mg/kg/day, each dose administered for 7 days) found a positive response, based upon a 50% decrease on the Conners Hyperactivity Index, in eight out of 11 of children (62%) with autism (ages 5–11 years) (Handen et al., 2000). Adverse effects, more common at the 0.6 mg/kg/day dosage, included social withdrawal and irritability. Another double-blind crossover study conducted in 10 children with autism, aged 7–11 years, comparing MPH to placebo found a modest but statistically significant improvement in ADHD symptoms with MPH (Quintana et al., 1995). No statistically significant adverse effects were reported on either the 10 or 20 mg dosage of MPH. The most commonly reported adverse effects included insomnia, irritability, and decreased appetite. The largest RCT of a psychostimulant in subjects with ASD thus far was completed by the RUPP Autism Network (Research Units on Pediatric Psychopharmacology Autism Network, 2005). This study involved 72 children and adolescents, aged 5–14 years, with target symptoms of moderate to severe hyperactivity. Low to moderate doses of MPH were compared to placebo in a cross-over design. During a 7-day test-dose period, six out of 72 children exited the study due to adverse effects (primarily irritability). During the 4-week double-blind, crossover period, 66 subjects were randomized to three dosage levels of MPH (0.125, 0.25, 0.50 mg/kg/dose) or placebo. Forty-nine percent of children were responders to MPH versus 18% given placebo, with response defined as a ≥25% decrease in ADHD symptoms from baseline on the Hyperactivity (H) subscale of the Aberrant Behavior Checklist (ABC), and a Clinical Global Impressions-Improvement (CGI-I) rating of "much improved" or "very much improved." The effect sizes ranged from 0.20 to 0.54, depending upon dosage, with greater improvement at higher doses. Eighteen percent of the subjects dropped out of the study due to inability to tolerate the drug (primarily irritability).

Clinical implementation and monitoring parameters. Although the response rate to MPH may be lower in ASD compared to typically developing children with ADHD alone, the data from trials in ASD suggest that stimulants, especially MPH, may at times be helpful in this population. The treatment success may be limited by a lower rate of response and a higher risk of adverse effects in ASD than in ADHD alone; however, stimulants have the benefit of rapid onset of action, such that treatment response can be determined relatively quickly, making them a reasonable treatment option for ADHD in children with ASD.

Adverse effects that need close monitoring include decreased appetite; weight loss; insomnia; increased irritability, agitation and hyperactivity; exacerbation/development of tics; and psychosis (rarely). A comprehensive cardiovascular history and examination should be completed, and baseline height, weight, blood pressure, and heart rate should be established. Adolescent patients should be assessed for substance use due to the risk of misuse and diversion of stimulants (Wilens et al., 2008). Because of the increased risk of adverse effects and variable treatment response, stimulants should be started at a low dose and titrated slowly in small increments.

Mixed amphetamine salts.

Mechanism of action. Amphetamines are non-catecholamine, sympathomimetic amines that promote release of DA and NE from the presynaptic nerve terminals. A secondary mechanism may include their ability to block the reuptake of catecholamines by competitive inhibition.

Potential treatment targets. See "Potential treatment targets" in MPH section.

Review of research findings. To date, there have been no RCTs of stimulants for treatment of co-morbid ADHD in youth with ASD other than MPH. Preliminary studies with D-amphetamine and levoamphetamine (Campbell et al., 1972, 1976) found limited benefit in young children with ASD, along with increased irritability and heightened stereotypic behavior.

Clinical implementation. If MPH is not well tolerated or only a partial response is attained, a second trial of a stimulant from the amphetamine class could be considered as suggested in the "Practice Parameter for the Assessment and Treatment of Children and Adolescents With ADHD" (Pliszka & AACAP Work Group on Quality Issues, 2007).

Non-stimulants

Alpha-2-Adrenergic agonists.

Mechanism of action. Clonidine and guanfacine are classified as central presynaptic α_2-adrenergic agonists that primarily act at the level of the locus coeruleus, located in the brainstem, facilitating both NE and DA neurotransmission. It is by this mechanism that α_2 agonists are primarily thought to improve the impulsivity and hyperactivity seen in ADHD. Clonidine is a relatively non-selective agonist at α_2 receptors that has affinity for all three subtypes of α_2 receptors (α_{2A}, $\alpha_{2B,}$ *and* α_{2C}) that are responsible for the sedating effects of the drug. Guanfacine is a selective α_{2A}-adrenergic receptor agonist. Clonidine also has indirect effects on serotonin (5-HT) receptors, and is known to increase gamma aminobutyric acid (GABA) levels, which can be effective for improving symptoms in other behavioral disorders, as well (Wang et al., 2007).

Potential treatment targets. Both clonidine and guanfacine are FDA-approved for the treatment of ADHD in children and adolescents between 6 and 17 years of age. In individuals with ASD, hyperarousal in response to environmental triggers is quite common (Toichi & Kamio, 2003). Aggression and self-injurious behavior, in which the adrenergic system may play an etiological role, maybe behavioral manifestations resulting from this environmental over-stimulation (King, 2000). That α_2 adrenergic agonists facilitate NE and DA neurotransmission in the prefrontal cortex, may contribute to the improvement in symptoms of inattention, hyperactivity, and impulsivity in children with ASD (Posey et al., 2004b).

Review of research findings. Two small crossover trials evaluated clonidine in patients with ASD, aged 5–33 years and 5–11 years, respectively. Decreased irritability, stereotypy, hyperactivity, inappropriate speech, and oppositional behavior were observed in both studies (Fankhauser, Karumanchi, German, Yates, & Karumanchi, 1992; Jaselskis, Cook, Fletcher, & Leventhal, 1992). One double-blind, placebo-controlled, crossover trial of clonidine was conducted in eight boys with ASD (mean age, 8.1 years) who demonstrated symptoms of inattention, impulsivity, and hyperactivity, and had not tolerated or responded to other pharmacologic treatments including stimulants and antipsychotics (Jaselskis et al., 1992). Clonidine had modest effects on irritability and hyperactivity in some of the children as suggested by teacher and parent ratings. However, there were no treatment-associated differences found on clinician ratings. Common side effects included hypotension, sedation, and irritability. The investigators were uncertain whether, in part, symptom reduction could be attributed to the sedative effects of the drug. A second RCT investigated the efficacy and safety of transdermal clonidine for hyperarousal in nine males (ages 5–33 years) with ASD (Fankhauser et al., 1992). Subjects received either clonidine approximately 0.005 mg/kg/day or placebo administered via a weekly transdermal patch. Significant improvement in social relationships and overall behavior was noted and the most commonly reported side effects were sedation and fatigue.

A small RCT of guanfacine was completed in 11 children with hyperactivity and intellectual disability (ID) and/or ASD. Forty-five percent of study participants had a significant reduction of hyperactivity with the drug. The most common adverse effects included increased irritability and drowsiness (Handen, Sahl, & Hardan, 2008). A prospective open-label trial of guanfacine was conducted in 25 children (aged 5–14 years) with ASD whose hyperactive symptoms had not responded to MPH (Scahill et al., 2006). Forty-eight percent of the subjects responded to guanfacine at total daily doses of 1–3 mg. Three subjects exited the study due to decreased frustration tolerance and tearfulness. In an 8-week multicenter RCT, extended-release guanfacine was compared with placebo in 62 children with ASD, and significant symptoms of ADHD (Scahill et al., 2015). The guanfacine group showed greater declines in scores on the ABC-H subscale compared to the placebo group (43.6 vs. 13.2%) and a higher response rate on the CGI-I scale (50 vs. 9.4%). Four guanfacine-treated subjects and four placebo subjects exited the study before the end of week 8. Common side effects included drowsiness, fatigue, and decreased appetite. Blood pressure declined during the first four weeks in guanfacine-treated subjects, but returned close to baseline levels by week 8. Heart rate showed a similar pattern of decline but remained lower than baseline at study endpoint. A retrospective analysis of open-label guanfacine in 80 children and adolescents with ASD found treatment to be effective in 19 of 80 subjects. Subjects without co-morbid ID had a greater response rate (9 of 24 subjects; 37.5%) compared to those with ID (10 of 56 subjects; 17.9%) (Posey et al., 2004b). Adverse effects of guanfacine included sedation, constipation, irritability, and aggression; significant changes in blood pressure or heart rate did not occur.

Clinical implementation and monitoring parameters. Alpha-2 agonists have been used as adjunctive or alternative agents to stimulant drugs for decades in typically developing children and adolescents with ADHD. Stimulants, especially MPH, have data supporting their use for this symptom cluster in children with ASD as well; however, the lower response rate and increased risk of adverse effects in this population may limit their use. Alpha-2 agonists may be a reasonable and safer first-line choice, especially given their proven efficacy and tolerability.

Alpha-2 agonists are typically well-tolerated, aside from possible adverse effects of sedation and hypotension. Other less common side effects include rebound hypertension if the medication is discontinued abruptly, dizziness, dry mouth, increased irritability, aggression and self-injury, sleep disturbance, decreased appetite, headache, and nocturnal enuresis. Constipation can also occur which is important to monitor considering the heightened co-morbidity of gastrointestinal (GI) disorders in children with ASD. It is important to counsel caregivers about the medicationsnarrow window of therapeutic safety with α_2 agonists and the risk of significant harm from these medications if taken in excess. Children treated with α_2 agonists should have their heart rate and blood pressure monitored at each clinic visit. Electrocardiogram (ECG) monitoring should be considered in patients with a significant history of cardiovascular problems or who are taking other medications affecting cardiac conduction.

Atomoxetine.

***Mechanism of action*.** Atomoxetine is a potent selective NE reuptake inhibitor with prominent effects in the prefrontal cortex, with minimal affinity for other neurotransporters and neuroreceptors, indicated for use in patients with ADHD (Garnock-Jones & Keating, 2009).

***Potential treatment targets*.** Atomoxetine is FDA-approved for the treatment of ADHD in children and adolescents aged 6–18 years as well as adults. In addition to stimulants and α_2 agonists, there is evidence to support the use of atomoxetine for the treatment of ADHD symptoms in children with ASD.

***Review of research findings*.** In a 3-site, 10-week, double-blind, 2 × 2 trial of atomoxetine and parent training in children with ASD and ADHD symptoms, aged 5–14 years, 128 participants were randomized to atomoxetine, atomoxetine + parent training, placebo + parent training, or placebo. The dosage of atomoxetine was titrated up to 1.8 mg/kg/day and then maintained for 4 additional weeks. Atomoxetine alone and atomoxetine with parent training were superior to placebo and parent training with placebo in decreasing ADHD symptoms. Atomoxetine (both alone and combined with parent training) was also associated with a significant decrease in measures of noncompliance. Atomoxetine was associated with decreased appetite but was otherwise well-tolerated (Handen et al., 2015).

In an RCT of 97 children with ASD and ADHD, aged 6–17 years, atomoxetine moderately improved ADHD symptoms and was well-tolerated. Among the atomoxetine group, improvement was greater for hyperactivity-impulsivity symptoms than those of inattention (Harfterkamp et al., 2012). However, a significant difference in the rate of treatment response between drug and the placebo was not found on the CGI-I. The most common adverse effects were nausea, decreased appetite, fatigue, and early morning awakening (reported in 81.3% of atomoxetine patients and 65.3% of placebo patients). No improvement was observed in social interaction. There was, however, some degree of improvement on the ABC subscales for Inappropriate Speech and Stereotypic Behavior, and on the Children's Social Behavior Questionnaire (CSBQ) subscale of Fear of and Resistance to Changes. Eighty-eight subjects were followed for an additional 20 weeks in an open-label extension phase (Harfterkamp et al., 2014). No serious adverse effects occurred during this phase and subjects continued to demonstrate improvement in ADHD symptoms, as well as adverse effects.

Another small 6-week RCT in 16 children with ASD and ADHD, aged 5–15 years, at doses of 1.2–1.4 mg/kg per day, and not exceeding a total dose of 100 mg per day, identified some improvement in symptoms of hyperactivity compared with placebo (Arnold et al., 2006). However, as in the MPH trial by the RUPP Autism Network, the overall effect size for atomoxetine in children with ASD and symptoms of ADHD was smaller than for children with ADHD only. One subject was re-hospitalized for recurrent violent episodes on the drug. Otherwise, the adverse events were tolerable.

This study was small and allowed concomitant administration of other psychotropic medications, placing limitations on its generalizability.

Clinical implementation and monitoring parameters. Methylphenidate, α_2 agonists, and atomoxetine appear to have fairly similar rates of response (45–55%) for the treatment of ADHD symptoms in youth with ASD. However, the placebo-controlled effect sizes for ADHD symptoms seem to be greater for atomoxetine than for the alternative medications. A potential advantage of atomoxetine over stimulants includes having less of an impact on appetite, weight, irritability, and sleep. The potential disadvantages of atomoxetine include longer lasting adverse effects because of a longer half-life, slowing of growth (but less than with stimulants), and adverse GI effects (Aman et al., 2014). Other potential adverse effects of atomoxetine include fatigue, sleep problems, mood swings, dizziness, appetite suppression, and a rare but potentially serious side effect, hepatotoxicity. Also in 2005, the FDA required manufacturers of atomoxetine to include a black box warning regarding a possible increase in suicidal ideation which warrants regular risk assessment in patients taking this drug.

Other Medications for Treatment of Hyperactivity and Inattention

Many studies have demonstrated the benefit of antipsychotic medications for symptoms of hyperactivity and inattention in children with ASD. The benefit of risperidone for hyperactivity in ASD has consistently been supported by open-label and RCTs (Barnard, Young, Pearson, Geddes, & O'Brien, 2002; Hazell, 2007; McCracken et al., 2002). However, due to significant concerns 2007 about adverse effects, the potential benefits of antipsychotics for symptoms of ADHD should be carefully weighed against the prominent risks. In the absence of significant aggression or irritable behavior, the use of antipsychotics should be reserved until the options described in detail above have been found to be ineffective or intolerable for treating symptoms of ADHD in youth with ASD.

Antidepressant and Antianxiety Medications

Selective Serotonin Reuptake Inhibitors (SSRIs)

Mechanism of action. Selective serotonin reuptake inhibitors increase the extracellular level of 5-HT in the synaptic cleft available to bind to postsynaptic receptors by limiting its reuptake into presynaptic neurons. By this mechanism, SSRIs reduce many of the symptoms associated with various conditions including depression, anxiety disorders, and obsessive-compulsive disorder (OCD).

Potential treatment targets. Serotonin-enhancing medications and other agents with strong affinity for serotonin receptors (e.g. atypical antipsychotics) are commonly used in patients with ASD, partly due to their efficacy in the treatment of anxiety disorders and OCD (Fatemi, Realmuto, Khan, & Thuras, 1998; Hollander, Kaplan, Cartwright, & Reichman, 2000; King et al., 2009). Furthermore, there is some evidence linking ASD to alterations in 5-HT function (McDougle et al., 1996a, 1996b). Researchers hypothesized that SSRIs might be effective for restricted, repetitive behaviors (RRBs) associated with ASD, as such symptoms share certain aspects of the phenomenology of the obsessions and compulsions that occur in OCD that are known to respond to SSRIs. For a variety of reasons, SSRIs became a commonly prescribed medication for individuals with ASD (Mandell et al., 2008). Although many case reports and uncontrolled studies describe their benefits, in general, their efficacy has not been confirmed in large-scale RCTs. Rigorous studies have been conducted in youth with ASD especially for fluoxetine, citalopram, and fluvoxamine among the SSRIs. There are no published RCTs of sertraline, paroxetine, or escitalopram in ASD, but several open-label studies and case reports have been published which found improvement in several symptom domains, including anxiety and RRBs (Branford, Bhaumik, & Naik, 1998; McDougle et al., 1998a).

Review of research findings.

Fluvoxamine. Fluvoxamine is FDA-approved for use in youth with OCD (aged 8–17 years). In an RCT involving 34 children, fluvoxamine (mean dose, 106.9 mg/day) was ineffective and poorly tolerated in youth with ASD (McDougle, Kresch, & Posey, 2000). Fourteen of the subjects experienced adverse effects, including aggression, behavioral activation, and insomnia. A 10-week open-label study of 18 children with ASD found only a 20% rate of response to low-dose fluvoxamine (1.5 mg/kg/day) (Martin, Koenig, Anderson, & Scahill, 2003). Three children exited the study due to behavioral activation. A 12-week RCT examined the relationship between response to fluvoxamine and the serotonin transporter gene promoter region polymorphism (5-HTTLPR). Fluvoxamine treatment (the dose was gradually titrated up to 3 mg/kg/day and maintained for 6 weeks) was clinically effective in 10 of 18 (56%) subjects with 28% showing an excellent drug response as measured by the CGI. In addition, the global effectiveness of fluvoxamine was more significant in subjects with the short allele of 5-HTTLPR compared to the long allele. The drug was generally well-tolerated (Sugie et al., 2005). The somewhat higher rate of response in this study was in part related to the investigators decision to consider subjects that were only "minimally improved" as "treatment responders." In the above-mentioned studies, the common adverse effects included aggression, insomnia, increased rituals, anxiety, anorexia, increased appetite, irritability, decreased concentration, and increased impulsivity. In contrast, another RCT found fluvoxamine to be effective in the treatment of repetitive and maladaptive behaviors in eight out of 15 *adults* with ASD as measured by the CGI-I (McDougle et al., 1996b). The drug was well-tolerated, with few reported side effects including nausea and sedation. In this study of adults with ASD, the dosage of fluvoxamine ranged from 50 to 300 mg/day (mean dose, 276.7 mg/day). The difference in the rate of response to fluvoxamine between youth and adults with ASD is somewhat striking. Fluvoxamine appears to be better tolerated in adults with ASD than in children. It is possible that developmental factors in 5-HT function contribute to the significant difference in efficacy and tolerability of fluvoxamine between youth and adults with ASD.

Fluoxetine. Fluoxetine is approved for the treatment of major depressive disorder (MDD) and OCD in youths (aged 8–17 years and 7–17 years, respectively). The Study of Fluoxetine in Autism (SOFIA) (Herscu et al., 2019), the largest RCT of an SSRI in youth with autism so far, found fluoxetine to be ineffective for the treatment of RRBs in children with autism. In this study, 158 children with ASD received fluoxetine (mean dose, 11.8 mg/day) for 14 weeks. No significant difference was noted between drug and placebo in change scores on the Children's Yale-Brown Obsessive-Compulsive Scale (C-YBOCS) and the proportion of responders was similar (fluoxetine: 36%, placebo: 41%). High rates of behavioral activation were reported for both the fluoxetine and placebo groups. Prior to this, three small placebo-controlled, crossover and two open-label trials of fluoxetine suggested that the drug may be effective for RRBs in individuals with ASD (Buchsbaum et al., 2001; DeLong, Ritch, & Burch, 2002; Fatemi et al., 1998; Hollander et al., 2005, 2012).

One of these RCTs, an 8-week study of 39 children and adolescents with ASD, concluded that liquid fluoxetine was superior to placebo in decreasing RRBs in children and adolescents with ASD, with minimal adverse effects (Hollander et al., 2005). No improvement in speech or social interaction was noted. Another of the RCTs of fluoxetine, this one involving higher-functioning *adults* with ASD by Hollander and colleagues (2012), showed a reduction in compulsive behavior and general improvement in obsessive-compulsive symptoms, with minimal adverse effects. In summary, results from studies of fluoxetine in ASD are similar to those of fluvoxamine where the drug appears to be more efficacious and better tolerated in adults than children and adolescents.

Sertraline. Sertraline is approved for the treatment of OCD in children and adolescents between the ages of 6 and 17 years. There has been no RCT of sertraline for the treatment of ASD. However, based on the results of two open-label trials, sertraline may be moderately effective and relatively well-tolerated in the management of repetitive, self-injurious, and aggressive behaviors in adults with ASD (Hellings, Kelley, Gabrielli, Kilgore, & Shah, 1996; McDougle et al., 1998a). There is minimal data in children with ASD from which to draw definitive conclusions, although adverse effects may be greater with sertraline in this population compared to adults. One case series of nine children (aged 6–12 years) with ASD receiving 25–50 mg/day of sertraline for two to eight weeks, reported improvement in insistence on sameness, anxiety, and irritability, although 33% of subjects had a loss of initial treatment response after a few months (Steingard, Zimnitzky, DeMaso, Bauman, & Bucci, 1997). In a 12-week, open-label study of 42 adults with ASD (McDougle et al., 1998a), sertraline was found to be effective in reducing aggression and repetitive behaviors. Subjects with lower-functioning autism and pervasive developmental disorder (PDD) not otherwise specified (NOS) showed significantly more improvement than those with Asperger's disorder. This difference in response was attributed to the higher-functioning subjects being less symptomatic at baseline. Three subjects exited the study due to worsening agitation and anxiety.

Paroxetine. Paroxetine is rarely considered as a first-line antidepressant among other SSRIs for children due to its side effect profile, including strong anticholinergic properties and the potential for sedation and orthostatic hypotension. Studies of paroxetine in children with ASD are limited to case reports and one open-label trial. Two case reports of patients with ASD have noted decreased irritability with paroxetine (Posey, Litwiller, Koburn, & McDougle, 1999; Snead, Boon, & Presberg, 1994). In an open-label study among 15 adults with ID with or without a concomitant diagnosis of ASD, paroxetine led to reduced aggression after one month but not at the four-month follow-up (Davanzo, Belin, Widawski, & King, 1998).

Citalopram. Two retrospective open-label studies of citalopram in youth with ASD found modest improvement in a range of symptoms, including RRBs, aggression, anxiety, and irritability. The dosages of citalopram ranged from 5 to 40 mg/day and the drug was well-tolerated with minimal adverse effects. In contrast to these positive preliminary findings, a large 12-week, RCT of citalopram (mean dosage, 16.5 ± 6.5 mg/day) conducted in 149 children (age range, 5–17 years) with ASD (King et al., 2009) found the drug to be ineffective for RRBs. In addition, citalopram caused more adverse events, particularly increased energy level and impulsivity, decreased concentration, hyperactivity, stereotypy, and insomnia. Based on the current evidence, citalopram has limited efficacy in the treatment of RRBs in children with ASD and is more likely to cause adverse effects.

Escitalopram. Escitalopram is an SSRI and the S-enantiomer of citalopram. It has minimal effects on NE or DA receptors. Escitalopram is approved for the treatment of MDD in adolescents between the ages of 12 and 17 years. An open-label trial of escitalopram in 28 children and adolescents with ASD between the ages of 6 and 17 years reported improvement in irritability, lethargy, stereotypy, hyperactivity, and inappropriate speech (Owley et al., 2005). A wide range of dose response was noted, with some patients showing significant improvement at a dosage of 2.5 mg/day, while others could not tolerate 10 mg/day.

Clinical implementation. In contrast to the preliminary evidence from small controlled studies (Fukuda, Sugie, Ito, & Sugie, 2001; Hollander et al., 2005), results of two large RCTs of citalopram and fluoxetine showed no statistical separation from placebo (Herscu et al., 2019; King et al., 2009) for the treatment of RRBs in children and adolescents with ASD. A recent meta-analysis of nine RCTs (five studies included only children and four studies included only adults) with a total of 320 participants taking serotonin reuptake inhibitors (SRIs), including SSRIs and particular tricyclic antidepressants, reported that the limited benefit of SRIs for RRBs was no longer present after adjustment for publication bias (Williams, Brignell, Randall, Silove, & Hazell, 2013). Studies also suggest that children with ASD may be more sensitive to SSRI-related adverse effects compared to adults, even when conservative dosing of SSRIs in children with ASD is followed (Posey, Erickson, Stigler, & McDougle, 2006). Although SSRIs are often prescribed for children with ASD as the initial medication for RRBs, it is important for providers to understand that the published literature from RCTs of this class of medication in youth with ASD does not support this approach. If clinicians consider prescribing SSRIs for children with ASD, it is important that they inform parents about their off-label use, discuss the potential risks and adverse effects, and discuss alternative pharmacological and non-pharmacological treatment options. Prescribers should clearly define the target symptoms and continuously monitor whether such symptoms have improved with the medication while keeping the possibility of placebo response and adverse effects in mind. All children being treated with antidepressants for any indication should be followed closely for clinical worsening, suicidality, and behavioral changes, especially during the first few months of treatment, and at times of dose adjustments. If the side effects outweigh the benefits or there is limited response to the medication of choice, discontinuing the ineffective agent before adding on new medications is essential to avoid polypharmacy. Common adverse effects that need monitoring with SSRIs include behavioral activation, agitation, change in appetite, headaches, anxiety, insomnia, GI upset, and drowsiness. The black box warning of increased suicidal ideation should also be monitored at each visit. The SSRIs fluvoxamine and fluoxetine may be more efficacious and better tolerated in *adults* versus children and adolescents with ASD.

Serotonin-Norepinephrine Reuptake Inhibitors (SNRIs)

Among the SNRIs only venlafaxine has been investigated in individuals with ASD.

Mechanism of action. Venlafaxine is an SNRI that inhibits the reuptake of 5-HT and also has a biphasic dose-dependent response on NE neurons. It functions like an SSRI at low doses (37.5 mg/day) and as a dual mechanism agent affecting 5-HT and NE at doses above 225 mg/day (Harvey, Rudolph, & Preskorn, 2000; Kelsey, 1996).

Review of research findings. There has been no RCT of venlafaxine in individuals with ASD. In an open-label, retrospective review of 10 individuals with ASD (aged 3–21 years) treated with venlafaxine (mean dose, 24.4 mg/day) six patients were responders with improvement noted in RRBs, social deficits, communication, inattention, and hyperactivity. One case report noted increased aggressive behavior when low-dose venlafaxine was added to the treatment regimen of an adolescent female with ASD who was taking olanzapine 10 mg/day (Marshall et al., 2003).

Clinical implementation. Findings in studies with venlafaxine in individuals with ASD have been inconsistent, therefore further evidence is required for its use in the treatment of children with ASD.

Tricyclic Antidepressants (TCAs)

Mechanism of action. Most TCAs inhibit both 5-HT and NE reuptake to variable degrees. Some TCAs have greater potency for 5-HT reuptake whereas others are more selective for NE reuptake inhibition. Clomipramine is a non-selective SRI with prominent anticholinergic effects. It potently inhibits 5-HT reuptake and also blocks the reuptake of NE and DA (Greist, Jefferson, Kobak, Katzelnick, & Serlin, 1995).

Potential treatment targets. Clomipramine is FDA-approved for the treatment of youths (aged 10–17 years) and adults with OCD. Clomipramine has been used to treat RRBs in children with ASD based in part upon its efficacy for the treatment of OCD in the general population, as demonstrated in controlled trials ("Clomipramine in the treatment of patients with obsessive-compulsive disorder. The Clomipramine Collaborative Study Group," 1991). However, the results of studies of clomipramine in children with ASD have been inconsistent at best, with evidence of significant adverse effects (Gordon, State, Nelson, Hamburger, & Rapoport, 1993; Hurwitz, Blackmore, Hazell, Williams, & Woolfenden, 2012; Remington, Sloman, Konstantareas, Parker, & Gow, 2001).

Review of research findings. A small RCT comparing clomipramine (mean dose, 152 ± 56 mg/day), desipramine (mean dose, 127 ± 52 mg/day), and placebo in 28 children (mean age, 9.6 years) with ASD found clomipramine to be superior to desipramine (a relatively selective NE reuptake inhibitor) and placebo for improving RRBs (Gordon et al., 1993). Clomipramine was also associated with decreased anger and ritualized behaviors. The reported adverse events included cardiac QTc interval prolon-gation, grand mal seizure, and tachycardia. Increased irritability and aggression were reported in eight of the 12 subjects receiving desipramine. Another RCT involving 31 children with ASD compared clomipramine, the typical antipsychotic haloperidol and placebo, and found no significant difference between clomipramine and placebo on the ABC, including the Stereotypy subscale. Twice as many subjects receiving clomipramine as haloperidol exited the study for reasons related to both side effects and lack of efficacy (Remington et al., 2001).

Clinical implementation. Findings from studies of TCAs for behavioral symptoms associated with ASD suggest that these drugs are poorly tolerated despite a minor degree of efficacy. Tricyclic antidepressants are broad-spectrum drugs in that they interact with many neurotransmitter systems, which is the basis for both their antidepressant properties and adverse effects. Blocking histamine, cholinergic and alpha-adrenergic receptors can cause sedation, increased appetite, dry mouth, constipation, diaphoresis, cardiac conduction abnormalities, and a decreased threshold for seizures. This class of medication can also be lethal in overdose. Overall, TCAs have insufficient supportive evidence to be recommended in the treatment of children with ASD.

Monoamine Oxidase Inhibitors (MAOIs)

MAOIs increase endogenous concentrations of NE, 5-HT and DA through inhibition of the enzyme monoamine oxidase which is responsible for the breakdown of these neurotransmitters. There have been no studies of MAOIs in the treatment of individuals with ASD (Fig. 1).

DRUG	STUDY	DEMOGRAPHICS	DOSE	DESIGN	SIDE EFFECTS	OUTCOMES
ALPHA-2-ADRENERGIC AGONISTS						
Clonidine	Jaselskis et al., 1992	8 children, 5–13 years old	0.15–0.20 mg divided TID	7 weeks, crossover	Hypotension, drowsiness	Statistically and clinically relevant decrease in ABC Irritability subscale score
Clonidine (transdermal patch)	Fankhauser et al. 1992	9 individuals, 5-33 years old	0.16 – 0.48 mg/d	4 weeks, crossover	Sedation, fatigue	Improvement in overall behaviors
Guanfacine	Handen et al., 2008	11 children with ASD, 5-9 years old	1–3 mg divided TID	6 weeks, crossover design	Drowsiness, irritability	45% improved with a 50% decrease in ABC Hyperactivity subscale score
Guanfacine ER	Scahill et al., 2015	62 children, 5-14 years old	1–4 mg/d	8 weeks, parallel	Drowsiness, decreased energy, sleep disturbance	Drug > placebo for improving hyperactivity and global functioning
STIMULANTS						
Methylphenidate	RUPP, 2005	58 children, 5–14 years old	7.5–50 mg per day divided TID	4 weeks, crossover	Decreased appetite, insomnia, irritability, emotionality	49% response to drug for hyperactivity versus 15.5% to placebo
Methylphenidate	Handen et al., 2000	13 children, 5–11 years old	0.3–0.6 mg per kg per dose, BID-TID	3 weeks, crossover	Social withdrawal, irritability	8 of 13 children with a 50% decrease in hyperactivity on the Teacher Conners Hyperactivity Index
Methylphenidate	Quintana et al., 1995	10 children, 7–11 years old	10–20 mg BID	4 weeks, crossover	Irritability, decreased appetite, insomnia	Drug > placebo for reducing ABC Hyperactivity subscale score
SELECTIVE NOREPINEPHRINE REUPTAKE INHIBITORS						
Atomoxetine	Arnold et al., 2006	16 children, 5–15 years old	20–100 mg divided BID (mean 44 mg/day)	6 weeks, crossover	Upper gastrointestinal (GI) side effects, fatigue, racing heart	57% response rate to drug vs. 25% to placebo
Atomoxetine	Harfterkamp et al., 2012	97 children, 6-17 years old	1.2 mg/kg/day	8 weeks, parallel	Nausea, anorexia, fatigue, early awakening	Significant difference between drug and placebo on the ADHD-R; no difference on CGI-I

Fig. 1 Table of selected RCTs

Atomoxetine and Parent Training	Handen et al., 2015	128 children, 5-14 years old	1.8 mg/kg/day	10 weeks, crossover	Upper GI side effects	ATX, ATX+PT and placebo+PT were each superior to placebo (effect sizes 0.57–0.98) on SNAP-IV rating scale
SELECTIVE SEROTONIN REUPTAKE INHIBITORS						
Fluoxetine	Hollander et al., 2005	39 children and adolescents, 5-16 years old	2.5–20 mg/day	8 weeks, crossover	The drug was well-tolerated	Drug was superior to placebo for improving repetitive behavior
Fluoxetine	Herscu et al., 2019	158 children and adolescents, 5-17 years old	2, 9, or 18 mg/day	14 weeks, parallel	Insomnia, diarrhea, vomiting. High rates of activation were reported in both drug and placebo groups	No drug vs. placebo difference for improving restricted, repetitive behaviors
Fluvoxamine	McDougle et al., 2000	34 children and adolescents, 8–17 years old	Mean dose, 106.9 mg/day	12 weeks, parallel	Aggression, behavioral activation, and insomnia	The drug was minimally effective and poorly tolerated
Fluvoxamine	Sugie et. al, 2005	18 children and adolescents, 3-8 years old	The dose was titrated up to 3mg/kg/day	12 weeks, parallel	The drug was well-tolerated	Drug superior to placebo. The results categorized CGI-I= "minimally improved" as treatment responders
Citalopram	King et al., 2009	149 children and adolescents, 5-17 years old	Mean dose, 16.5 mg/day	12 weeks, parallel	increased energy, impulsivity, decreased concentration, hyperactivity, stereotypy, insomnia	No drug vs. placebo difference for improving restricted, repetitive behaviors
ANTIPSYCHOTICS						
Risperidone	McCracken et al., 2002	101 children and adolescents, 5–17 years old	0.5–3.5 mg/d	8 weeks, parallel	Weight gain, increased appetite, fatigue, drowsiness, dizziness, drooling, tremor, constipation	Drug superior to placebo for improving irritability, stereotypy, and hyperactivity, but not social-communication
Risperidone	Shea et al. 2004	79 children and adolescents, 5–12 years old	0.01–0.06 mg/kg/day	8 weeks, parallel	Somnolence, weight gain, increased pulse rate and systolic blood pressure	Drug superior to placebo for improving irritability, hyperactivity, inappropriate speech, lethargy/social withdrawal, and stereotypic behavior

Fig. 1 (continued)

Risperidone	Kent et al. 2013	96 children and adolescents, 5–17 years old	0.125 or 0.175 mg/day vs 1.25 or 1.75 mg/day vs placebo	6 weeks, parallel	Sedation, and increased appetite (more frequently in high dose group)	High-dose drug superior to placebo for improving irritability and global functioning, but not low-dose
Aripiprazole	Marcus et al. 2009	218 children and adolescents, 6–17 years old	5, 10, or 15 mg/day fixed doses	8 weeks, parallel	Sedation, drooling, EPS, weight gain	Drug superior to placebo for improving irritability, self-injurious behavior, hyperactivity, and stereotypy
Haloperidol	Anderson et al., 1989	45 children, 2–7 years old	0.25–4 mg/day	12 weeks, crossover	None noteworthy	Drug superior to placebo for improving behavioral symptoms but not discrimination learning
Olanzapine	Hollander et al., 2006b	11 children and adolescents, 6–14 years old	7.5–12.5 mg/day	8 weeks, crossover	Weight gain, increased appetite, sedation	Drug superior to placebo for improving global functioning
Lurasidone	Loebel et al., 2016	150 children and adolescents, 6–17 years old	3 arms: 20 mg/d, 60 mg/d, placebo	6 weeks, parallel	Vomiting, somnolence Modest increases in weight and selected metabolic parameters, only with lurasidone 60 mg/day	No drug vs. placebo difference for improving irritability Drug superior to placebo for improving global functioning, but only at the 20 mg/day dosage
ANTICONVULSANTS						
Valproate	Hellings et al., 2005	30 individuals, 6–20 years old	20 mg/kg/day blood level 70–100 mcg/mL	8 weeks, parallel	Increased appetite, skin rash, increased serum ammonia level	No drug vs. placebo difference for improving irritability and aggression
Valproate	Hollander et al., (2010)	27 children and adolescents, 5–17 years old	Mean blood level of 89.8 mcg/mL	12 weeks, parallel	Skin rash, irritability	Drug superior to placebo for improving irritability
Lamotrigine	Belsito et al., 2001	28 children and adolescents, 3–11 years old	Mean dose, 5 mg/kg/day	18 weeks, parallel	Insomnia, increased stereotypies, aggression, echolalia	No drug vs. placebo difference on ABC-I or CGI-I
Levetiracetam	Wasserman et al.	20 children and adolescents, 5–17	20–30 mg/kg/day	10 weeks, parallel	Aggression, agitation	No drug vs. placebo difference on ABC-I

Fig. 1 (continued)

	2006	years old				
OTHER AGENTS						
Buspirone	Chugani et al., 2016	166 children, 2-6 years old	2 mg BID vs 5 mg BID vs. placebo	3 arms, 24 weeks, parallel	The drug was well-tolerated	No drug vs. placebo difference for improving symptoms of autism; drug superior to placebo for improving repetitive behaviors, but only at the 2.5 mg BID dosage
Memantine ER	Aman et al., 2017	121 children and adolescents, 6–12 years old	3–15 mg/day	12 weeks, parallel+48 weeks open-label	Two serious AEs deemed unrelated to the drug (lobar pneumonia and affective disorder)	No drug vs. placebo difference in improving social interaction and communication
Naltrexone	Campbell et al., 1993	41 children, 2–7 years old	0.5–1 mg/kg/day	3 weeks, parallel	The drug was well-tolerated	Drug superior to placebo for improving hyperactivity
Naltrexone	Willemsen- Swinkels et al., 1996	23 children, 3–7 years old	1 mg/kg/day	4 weeks, crossover	The drug was well-tolerated	No change in ABC scores following single-dose or long-term naltrexone treatment
D-Cycloserine	Minshawi et al., 2016	67 children and adolescents, 5–11 years old	50 mg given weekly before social skill training group	10 weeks, parallel	The drug was well-tolerated	No drug vs. placebo difference for improving social functioning

Fig. 1 (continued)

Other Medications (Mirtazapine, Bupropion, β-Adrenergic Blockers, Buspirone)

Mirtazapine. Mirtazapine is a tetracyclic antidepressant and presynaptic α_2-adrenoreceptor antagonist. It is also a potent antagonist of 5-HT_2, 5-HT_3, and H_1 histamine receptors, and a moderate peripheral $alpha_1$-adrenergic and muscarinic receptor antagonist. The most common side effects of mirtazapine are sedation, appetite increase, and weight gain. There has been no published RCT of mirtazapine in individuals with ASD. However, there are a number of case reports documenting the effectiveness of mirtazapine in the treatment of anxiety and compulsive behaviors in this population (Albertini, Polito, Sara, Di Gennaro, & Onorati, 2006; Coskun, Karakoc, Kircelli, & Mukaddes, 2009; Nguyen & Murphy, 2001). In an open-label study of 26 children and young adults (ages 3-23 years) with ASD receiving mirtazapine (7.5–45 mg/day), 35% of participants were responders as measured by the CGI-I, with reduced aggression, self-injury, irritability, hyperactivity, anxiety, insomnia, and depression. The medication was not effective for impaired social relatedness or communication (Posey, Guenin, Kohn, Swiezy, & McDougle, 2001). A retrospective study looking at the effectiveness and safety of mirtazapine for excessive masturbation and other inappropriate sexual behaviors in 10 youths with ASD, aged 5–16 years (Coskun et al., 2009) found that eight of 10 patients were responders on the CGI-I. Overall, the drug was well-tolerated in both trials and the common adverse effects included increased appetite, weight gain, sedation, and irritability.

Bupropion. Bupropion is an aminoketone antidepressant that is FDA-approved for the treatment of depression and smoking cessation in adults. Bupropion is a relatively weak reuptake inhibitor of NE and DA that does not inhibit monoamine oxidase or the reuptake of 5-HT. Randomized controlled trials suggest that bupropion may be effective for the treatment of ADHD in children and adults (Barrickman et al., 1995; Conners et al., 1996; Wilens et al., 2001). To date, bupropion has not been studied for the treatment of interfering symptoms in individuals with ASD. Bupropion can lower the seizure threshold; therefore, it is contraindicated in individuals with bulimia/anorexia nervosa, seizure disorders, and patients undergoing abrupt discontinuation of ethanol or sedatives.

β-Adrenergic blockers. Non-selective β-adrenergic blockers (propranolol, nadolol) competitively block the response to β_1- and β_2-adrenergic stimulation which leads to anxiolytic effects by decreasing NE neurotransmission. An open-label trial of propranolol or nadolol (mean dosage, 225 mg/day over 14.2 months) in eight hospitalized adults with ASD found improvement in social skills in six patients, improvement in speech in four patients, and reduced aggression in a number of patients (Ratey et al., 1987). In this study, seven patients were taking concomitant antipsychotic medications. For five patients, the dosage of antipsychotic was able to be reduced and for one patient the antipsychotic was discontinued. The authors suggested that the improvement in interfering symptoms could be due to a decreased state of hyperarousal. A recent pilot, double-blind, single-dose psychopharmacological challenge study with propranolol evaluated the immediate effects of the drug on conversational reciprocity in 20 adults with ASD without ID and found significant improvement as measured by the General Social Outcome Measure Conversational Reciprocity task (GSOM-CR) (Zamzow RM, effects of propranolol on conversational reciprocity). Subjects received a single dose of propranolol or placebo in two sessions. After the drug was administered, subjects completed a conversational reciprocity task by engaging in a short conversation with a clinician. Autonomic activity and anxiety were also measured before and after propranolol administration. The improvement in performance on the conversational reciprocity task total and nonverbal communication domain scores with the drug was statistically significant compared to placebo. Additionally, the investigators examined whether baseline autonomic activity and/or anxiety altered the response to propranolol and found that neither autonomic activity nor anxiety was associated with the drug response. The medication was well-tolerated in both studies described above, each of which involved the use of propranolol in adults. Therefore, further evidence is needed for the use of β-adrenergic blockers in children with ASD.

Buspirone. Buspirone is a novel anxiolytic which acts as a 5-HT_{1A} receptor partial agonist and a weak dopamine D_2 receptor antagonist. It is FDA-approved for the treatment of generalized anxiety disorder, as well as the short-term symptomatic relief of anxiety. Buspirone has a better side effect profile compared to other anxiolytic medications and there is no associated risk of physical dependence or withdrawal due to its lack of effect on GABA receptors. Despite a number of case reports and small open-label studies reporting on the effectiveness of buspirone in patients with ASD, larger open-label studies have reported conflicting findings. An open-label study of buspirone (dosage range, 30–60 mg/day) in 26 adults with ID, including nine patients with ASD, found the drug to be ineffective in reducing aggression and self-injury (King & Davanzo, 1996). In another open-label study, 22 children (aged 6–17 years) with ASD were treated with buspirone (15–45 mg/day) for 6–8 weeks (Buitelaar, van der Gaag, & van der Hoeven, 1998). Sixteen of the subjects were designated responders on the CGI-I. Side effects included orofacial-lingual dyskinesia in one subject which remitted after the drug was discontinued. An 8-week RCT in 40 children with ASD comparing buspirone + risperidone and placebo + risperidone reported that the combination of buspirone with risperidone was more effective than risperidone alone in the treatment of irritability. Thirteen of 16 subjects in the buspirone group were classified as responders compared with 7 of 18 subjects in the placebo group. The most common adverse effects in the buspirone group included increased appetite, drowsiness, and fatigue (Ghanizadeh & Ayoobzadehshirazi, 2015). A recent retrospective chart review of 31 children and adolescents with high-functioning ASD (aged 8–17 years) treated with buspirone (mean dose, 41.61 ± 24.10 mg/day; average duration of treatment, 272 ± 125 days) found that 58% of the subjects had significant improvement and 29% had mild improvement in anxiety symptoms (CGI-I scores ≤ 2 and 3, respectively). Buspirone was well-tolerated in this study with no significant adverse events reported, with the exception of two subjects who demonstrated behavioral activation and mood lability (Ceranoglu et al., 2019).

A large RCT evaluated the safety and efficacy of low-dose buspirone (2.5 or 5 mg twice a day for 24 weeks) for the treatment of core symptoms of ASD in

166 children (aged 2–6 years) with ASD. The drug was no better than placebo for improving the Autism Diagnostic Observation Scale (ADOS) Composite Total Score (the primary outcome measure), and only the low-dose (2.5 mg) group resulted in a significant reduction of RRBs as measured by the ADOS Restricted and Repetitive Behavior score. Behavioral activation was reported as a side effect; however, there was no statistically significant difference between the drug and placebo groups in the occurrence of this adverse event (Chugani et al., 2016).

Benzodiazepines (BZDs)

Benzodiazepines act as positive allosteric modulators at the $GABA_A$ receptor which enhances the inhibitory effect of GABA on neuronal excitability, resulting in sedative, hypnotic, anxiolytic, anticonvulsant, and muscle relaxant properties. So far there have been only case studies reporting the use of BZDs in the treatment of individuals with ASD. In one case report, lorazepam (1 mg/day) reduced catatonic symptoms in an 11-year-old boy with ASD (Bozkurt & Mukaddes, 2010) while in another lorazepam (1.5 mg/day, increased to 4 mg/day) had no effect on aggressive behavior in a 24-year-old male with ASD and ID (Allison, Basile, & MacDonald, 1991). Marrosu, Marrosu, Rachel, & Biggio (1987) reported paradoxical responses (increased anxiety and aggression) after administration of diazepam 10 mg intramuscular (i.m.) to seven children with autism. Benzodiazepines are favored options for acute and maintenance treatment of catatonia in individuals with ASD (Sienaert, Dhossche, Vancampfort, De Hert, & Gazdag, 2014); however, the increased risk of adverse and paradoxical effects limit its use as a standard treatment for anxiety in patients with ASD.

Antipsychotics

Mechanism of Action

The majority of the first (typical) and second (atypical) generation antipsychotics (FGAs and SGAs, respectively) are potent D_2 receptor antagonists. In addition, second-generation antipsychotics have a greater affinity for 5-HT2 receptors which potentially lowers the propensity to cause extrapyramidal symptoms (EPS), including tardive dyskinesia (TD). However, SGAs are associated with greater weight gain, and metabolic and endocrine adverse effects, compared to FGAs.

Potential Treatment Targets

There are a number of published studies examining the effects of typical antipsychotics in youth with ASD. Haloperidol was studied extensively owing to its better adverse effect profile compared to less potent FGAs (Anderson et al., 1989; Campbell et al., 1978; Cohen et al., 1980). Haloperidol's potent D_2-receptor antagonism, however, led to increased rates of acute EPS and TD (Campbell et al., 1997), which directed researchers toward studying the efficacy and safety of the SGAs in the treatment of ASD. So far, there has been strong evidence for the efficacy of SGAs, such as risperidone and aripiprazole, for reducing irritability, stereotypy, and hyperactivity in children with ASD (Ji & Findling, 2015). Risperidone and aripiprazole are approved by the FDA for the treatment of irritability in children with ASD (aged 5–16 years and 6–17 years, respectively). Reports on the use of the FGAs (haloperidol), as well as the SGAs, including clozapine, risperidone, olanzapine, quetiapine, ziprasidone, aripiprazole, and paliperidone, in ASD are reviewed in this section.

First-Generation (Typical) Antipsychotics (FGAs)

Review of research findings.
Haloperidol. Haloperidol is a potent D_2-receptor blocker and the most extensively studied antipsychotic in RCTs in the treatment of individuals with ASD. Haloperidol was found to significantly improve social withdrawal and stereotypies, as measured by the Children's Psychiatric Rating Scale (CPRS), in a 12-week RCT investigating haloperidol and behavioral therapy in 40 children (aged 2–7 years) with ASD (Campbell et al., 1978). A 14-week RCT of haloperidol in 40 children (aged 2–7 years) with ASD replicated these findings with significant improvement with haloperidol in CPRS and CGI scores (Anderson et al., 1984). This study also determined that haloperidol was associated with improved learning. Haloperidol has also been shown to be effective in the long-term treatment of maladaptive behaviors in children with ASD, with the greatest response occurring in those with prominent symptoms of irritability, angry and labile effect, and uncooperativeness. A 6-month RCT of haloperidol in 60 children (aged 2–8 years) with ASD (Perry et al., 1989) found that haloperidol remained effective at the end of 6 months of treatment as measured by the CPRS. Further studies found similar results for symptom improvement, but also reported a high frequency of TD and withdrawal dyskinesias (Campbell et al., 1997). Doses used in the above-mentioned studies ranged from 0.25 mg to 4 mg per day. The most commonly observed side effects included sedation, irritability, and acute dystonic reactions. The risk of developing dyskinesias increased in subjects with a higher cumulative dose of haloperidol (Campbell et al., 1997).

Clinical implementation. Studies in youth with ASD have suggested that haloperidol is superior to placebo in the short- and long-term for reducing stereotypies and social withdrawal. However, the increased risk of dyskinesias with long-term treatment limits the use of FGAs. Moreover, it remains unclear if improvements in core features of ASD (stereotypies, social withdrawal) are a direct result of haloperidol or a downstream result of treating co-occurring behavioral issues (hyperactivity or irritability). Thus, haloperidol should only be considered in the treatment of children with ASD if the patient does not respond to or is unable to tolerate the adverse effects associated with SGAs.

Second-Generation (Atypical) Antipsychotics (SGAs)

Review of research findings

Clozapine. Clozapine is the first atypical antipsychotic to be released in the United States. Studies in children and adults with ASD report good tolerability and efficacy in the treatment of severe aggression and irritability, although controlled trials are lacking. The use of clozapine is limited by the increased risk of agranulocytosis, the need for frequent venipuncture for monitoring blood counts and the potential to lower the seizure threshold. As an example, a retrospective analysis of six individuals with ASD (aged 14–34 years) found that clozapine was associated with decreased aggression and a reduction in the number and dosage of concomitantly administered psychotropics for behavioral management (Beherec et al., 2011). The clozapine dosage in these patients ranged from 200 to 475 mg per day. The drug was well-tolerated, and common adverse effects included weight gain and constipation. One subject had tachycardia and another developed metabolic syndrome.

Risperidone. The efficacy and tolerability of risperidone in youth with ASD and co-occurring irritability had been established by two large RCTs conducted by the RUPP Autism Network (McCracken et al., 2002) and Shea et al. (2004) prior to the drug's FDA approval. Several open-label studies also demonstrated the effectiveness of risperidone for core and associated symptoms of ASD (Findling, Maxwell, & Wiznitzer, 1997; Masi, Cosenza, Mucci, & Brovedani, 2001; McDougle et al., 1997; Nicolson, Awad, & Sloman, 1998).

The first RCT of risperidone in youths with ASD was conducted by the RUPP Autism Network (McCracken et al., 2002). In this 8-week study, 101 youths (mean age, 8.8 years) with target symptoms of irritability, aggression, or self-injury were randomly assigned to risperidone (mean dosage of 1.8 mg/day) or placebo. Sixty-nine percent (34/49) of the risperidone-treated subjects were deemed responders as measured by the ABC-Irritability (I) subscale (57% vs. 14% reduction in scores with risperidone and placebo, respectively). Adverse effects of the drug included an average weight gain of 2.7 kg, as compared with 0.8 kg with placebo, and increased appetite, sedation, drooling, and dizziness. Further analyses of these data found risperidone to be more efficacious than placebo for reducing interfering RRBs (McDougle et al., 2005). Subsequently, the results of an open-label extension study of risperidone were published. The effects of risperidone (mean dosage, 2 mg/day) were maintained in 83% of the 63 subjects who entered the 16-week open-label continuation phase, and compared to placebo, the drug prolonged the time to relapse during the following 8-week placebo-controlled discontinuation phase (McDougle et al., 2005). In a subsequent study, the investigators determined that the combination of parent management training and risperidone led to greater improvements in the ABC-I subscale and CGI-I scores compared to risperidone alone (Aman et al., 2009). In an 8-week RCT of risperidone in 79 youths with ASD (aged 5–12 years), it was determined that 69.2% of subjects treated with risperidone (mean dosage, 1.2 mg/day) responded versus 39.5% of the placebo group as rated by the ABC-I subscale (the primary outcome measure). The risperidone-treated group showed a significantly greater reduction of scores on the ABC-I subscale (64 vs. 31%). Risperidone was also significantly more efficacious than placebo on the other ABC subscales, including hyperactivity, inappropriate speech, lethargy/social withdrawal, and stereotypy subscales, as well as on the CGI-I (87.2 vs. 39.5%, respectively). Overall, risperidone was well-tolerated with sedation being the most common reported adverse effect. Weight gain, tachycardia, and increased systolic blood pressure were also reported (Shea et al., 2004). Kent et al. examined the efficacy and side effect profile of a "low" and "high" dosage of risperidone in a 6-week RCT in 79 youths with ASD (aged 5–17 years). The study found that, compared to placebo, "high" doses of risperidone (1.25 or 1.75 mg/day, based on weight) improved irritability and global functioning; however, the drug was not efficacious at "low" doses (0.125 or 0.175 mg/day, based on weight) (Kent, Hough, Singh, Karcher, & Pandina, 2013).

In a 12-week RCT in 31 adults (mean age, 28.1 years) with ASD, 8 out of 14 (57%) subjects randomized to risperidone (mean dosage, 2.9 mg/d) were deemed responders as measured by the CGI-I, versus none in the placebo group (McDougle et al., 1998b). Risperidone was effective in reducing RRBs as well as aggression. No significant difference between risperidone and placebo was reported on scales measuring social relatedness to people and communication. The most common adverse effect was transient sedation; weight gain was reported in only 2 out of 14 subjects in the risperidone group.

Olanzapine. Olanzapine has been found to improve symptoms associated with ASD in one small RCT, several open-label trials and case reports. The use of olanzapine, however, is limited in this population due to the increased risk of significant weight gain and metabolic side effects (Hollander et al., 2006b; Malone, Cater, Sheikh, Choudhury, & Delaney, 2001; Potenza, Holmes, Kanes, & McDougle, 1999). One small 8-week RCT evaluated olanzapine (mean dosage, 10 mg/day) in 11 children aged 6–14 years with ASD. Fifty percent (3/6) of the subjects in the olanzapine group were rated as responders versus 20% (1/5) in the placebo group based on the CGI-I. Adverse effects included sedation and weight gain (olanzapine 3.4 ± 2.2 kg; placebo 0.68 ± 0.68 kg) and no subjects experienced dyskinesias or EPS (Hollander et al., 2006b).

An open-label study of olanzapine in youth with ASD (aged 6–17 years) reported improvement in irritability, lethargy, stereotyped behavior, hyperactivity, and inappropriate or excessive speech (Kemner, Willemsen-Swinkels, de Jonge, Tuynman-Qua, & van Engeland, 2002). Another open-label study in eight individuals with

ASD (aged 5–42 years) found a 75% response rate with significant improvement in hyperactivity, irritability social relatedness, affectual reactions, sensory responses, language usage, self-injury, aggression, anxiety, and depression, but no changes in RRBs (Potenza et al., 1999). Olanzapine was administered to 10 males with Asperger's disorder (age 10–15 years) in another open-label trial. Significant differences were observed between baseline and completion scores of internalizing and externalizing behaviors on the Child Behavior Checklist, with a 90% rate of clinical response (Milin et al., 2006). In these open-label studies, dosages ranged from 2.5 to 20 mg/day and the most common adverse effects were weight gain, increased appetite, and fatigue.

Quetiapine. There are no published RCTs of quetiapine in youth with ASD and the currently published data consists of small open-label trials and retrospective chart reviews with varying findings. Quetiapine was poorly tolerated and generally ineffective in the open-label studies published to date (Findling et al., 2004; Martin, Koenig, Scahill, & Bregman, 1999). There was a moderate degree of response in the two retrospective chart reviews of quetiapine with the first reporting a 40% response rate among 20 subjects with ASD (aged 5–28 years) receiving a mean dosage of 248.7 mg per day for a mean duration of 59.8 weeks (Corson, Barkenbus, Posey, Stigler, & McDougle, 2004). Fifty percent of the patients reported adverse effects and 15% subsequently discontinued the treatment. The other retrospective review of 10 participants with ASD (aged 5–19 years) found a 60% response rate with subjects receiving a mean dose of quetiapine of 477 mg per day. Improvement was reported in symptoms of conduct, inattention, and hyperactivity (Hardan, Jou, & Handen, 2005). In these studies of quetiapine, the most common adverse effects included weight gain, sedation, behavioral activation, akathisia, and a possible seizure event. Controlled trials of quetiapine are needed to more accurately determine its efficacy, safety profile and appropriate dosing in the treatment of individuals with ASD.

Ziprasidone. Ziprasidone is both a D2 and 5-HT2 receptor antagonist, that also blocks the reuptake of 5-HT and NE, a mechanism that is unique among the SGAs (Reilly & Kirk, 2007). In addition, ziprasidone is not typically associated with significant weight gain (Meyer et al., 2008). One safety concern with ziprasidone is that it may cause prolongation of the corrected QT (QTc) interval which may lead to ventricular arrhythmia in severe cases. A potential benefit of ziprasidone is that it has a lower risk of drug–drug interactions, as the majority of its clearance is mediated by aldehyde oxidase, a liver enzyme which is not involved in the metabolism of other drugs. To date, there has been no published RCT of ziprasidone in youth with ASD. An open-label study in 12 individuals (aged 8–20 years) with ASD reported a 50% clinical response with ziprasidone (mean dosage of 59.2 mg per day over a duration of at least 6 weeks) as measured by the CGI-I. Two patients with co-morbid bipolar disorder were rated as "much worse." Transient sedation was the most commonly reported adverse effect. The mean weight change was −5.8 lb and there was no report of adverse cardiovascular effects (McDougle, Kem, & Posey, 2002). Another open-label study in 12 youths with ASD (age 12–18 years) revealed a 75% clinical response rate with ziprasidone (dosage range, 20–160 mg/day) as determined by the CGI-I. Dystonic reactions occurred in two subjects and mild-to-moderate sedation, as well as a clinically insignificant QTc prolongation by a mean of 14.7 ms, were reported (Malone, Delaney, Hyman, & Cater, 2007).

Aripiprazole. Aripiprazole was approved by the FDA for the treatment of irritability in children and adolescents with ASD between the ages of 6 and 17 years following two large RCTs that determined its efficacy in reducing irritability, hyperactivity, and stereotypies (Marcus et al., 2009; Owen et al., 2009). Prior to the RCTs, open-label trials in youth with ASD found clinical benefit for the treatment of significant irritability (Stigler, Posey, & McDougle, 2004b). A retrospective chart review, however, revealed a poorer response in the management of aggression, hyperactivity, impulsivity, and self-injury (Valicenti-McDermott & Demb, 2006). An 8-week fixed-dose (5, 10, or 15 mg/day or placebo) trial of aripiprazole in 218 children and adolescents with ASD (aged 6–17 years) found all dosages to be superior to placebo on the primary outcome measure, mean change on the ABC-I subscale from baseline to endpoint. Sedation and fatigue were the most commonly reported adverse effects. Weight gain was significantly higher at each dose of the drug when compared to placebo (Marcus et al., 2009). Another 8-week RCT in 98 youths with ASD (aged 6–17 years) demonstrated significant improvement in irritability with aripiprazole using a flexible dose schedule (2–15 mg/day) as measured on the CGI-I and ABC-I subscale. Weight gain, drooling, tremor, vomiting, and sedation were the most common adverse effects reported (Owen et al., 2009). Another more recent RCT from Japan evaluated 92 youths with ASD and found that aripiprazole improved irritability, hyperactivity, and global functioning, and was well-tolerated (Ichikawa et al., 2017).

The long-term safety and tolerability of aripiprazole (dosage range, 2–15 mg/day) for irritability was examined in a 52-week open-label study of youth with ASD (aged 6–17 years) treated with flexibly dosed aripiprazole (mean daily dose, 10.6 mg/d) (Marcus et al., 2011). The study included responders from the studies by Marcus et al. (Marcus et al., 2009) and Owen et al. (Owen et al., 2009) as well as de novo subjects. Three hundred and thirty subjects entered the treatment phase, and 60% (199 subjects) completed 52 weeks of treatment. Continued treatment with aripiprazole maintained the clinical response, as measured by the ABC-I subscale and the CGI-I. Common adverse effects included increased appetite, weight gain, and vomiting (Marcus et al., 2011). The authors concluded that long-term treatment with aripiprazole was well-tolerated and effective in reducing symptoms of irritability in children and adolescents with ASD between 6 and 17 years of age. In multicenter study of aripiprazole discontinuation, 85 of 157 (54%) subjects, who were deemed responders to 12 weeks of aripiprazole, were randomly assigned to ongoing aripiprazole for 16 additional weeks (mean dose, 9.7 mg/day) or placebo. The time to relapse did not differ between groups during this 16-week study phase (Findling et al., 2014). The hazard ratio (HR = 0.57) and number needed to treat (NNT = 6) suggested that some patients may benefit from maintenance treatment. Upper respiratory tract infection, constipation, and movement disorder were the most commonly reported long-term adverse effects (Findling et al., 2014). An 8-week RCT comparing the efficacy of aripiprazole versus risperidone in 59 youths with ASD found no significant difference between groups on the primary outcome measure (ABC-I subscale scores) or on adverse effects, including appetite increase and weight gain (Ghanizadeh, Sahraeizadeh, & Berk, 2014).

Paliperidone. An open-label study of paliperidone in 25 subjects with ASD (aged 12–21 years) reported 21 subjects (84%) as responders based on the CGI-I and ABC-I subscale scores. The dosage of paliperidone ranged from 3 to 12 mg per day, and mild-to-moderate EPS, weight gain (2.2 ± 2.6 kg) and sedation were reported as common adverse effects (Stigler, Mullett, Erickson, Posey, & McDougle, 2012). The mean serum prolactin level increased from 5.3 to 41.4 ng/mL without any reported clinical symptoms associated with hyperprolactinemia. There have also been several case reports on the successful treatment of irritability and aggression in patients with ASD using paliperidone palmitate (depot i.m. formulation). Current evidence suggests that paliperidone may be effective in individuals with ASD, although RCTs are needed.

Lurasidone. A 6-week RCT evaluated the short-term efficacy and safety of lurasidone for irritability in 150 children with ASD (aged 6–17 years). The subjects were randomized to three fixed-dose groups (lurasidone 20 mg/day, 60 mg/day, and placebo). Lurasidone was no better than placebo for reducing irritability at either dosage. Reported adverse effects included vomiting and somnolence. In addition, modest changes were reported in weight and metabolic parameters. Although lurasidone was no better than placebo for improving irritability, CGI-I scores showed greater improvement with the 20 mg/day dose compared to placebo (Loebel et al., 2016). However, at the higher dose of lurasidone (60 mg/day), CGI-I scores were no better than with placebo.

Clinical Implementation

- Risperidone and aripiprazole are the only antipsychotics approved by the FDA for the treatment of irritability in youth with ASD aged 5–16 years and 6–17 years, respectively. The results of multiple large RCTs strongly support the use of risperidone and aripiprazole to treat irritability in this population.
- The number of controlled trials of other SGAs is limited in individuals with ASD.
- Haloperidol has been shown to be efficacious for the short- and long-term treatment of maladaptive behaviors associated with ASD. However, the use of haloperidol is limited in the treatment of youth with ASD due to the risks of EPS and TD.
- Olanzapine was found to be moderately efficacious for irritability and other symptoms associated with ASD, but the adverse effects of significant weight gain and sedation limit its use.
- Overall, only minimal improvement in irritability has been found with quetiapine in ASD, and adverse events of sedation, weight gain, and aggression have been common.
- A RCT of lurasidone for irritability in ASD found no significant benefit over placebo.

- Ziprasidone may improve irritability in youth with ASD with less weight gain and fewer metabolic side effects compared to other SGAs, but the evidence has been limited to small open-label trials.
- The efficacy of the large majority of SGAs for the maintenance treatment of irritability in youth with ASD has not been thoroughly investigated, therefore clinical re-evaluation of the need for continued treatment with these agents is essential.

Monitoring. Most antipsychotic medications have been associated with significant adverse effects; hence, they should be used cautiously by clinicians as part of a broader multidisciplinary treatment approach in patients with ASD. The use of antipsychotics is associated with the risk of several serious adverse effects that warrant routine monitoring including metabolic effects (weight gain, hyperlipidemia, hyperglycemia, and hypertension), manifestations of EPS (dystonia, akathisia, parkinsonism, and TD), and hyperprolactinemia.

Metabolic syndrome. The consensus recommendations (American Diabetes, American Psychiatric, American Association of Clinical, & North American Association for the Study of Obesity, 2004) for monitoring the metabolic effects of atypical antipsychotic agents include assessments at baseline, 4 weeks, 8 weeks, 12 weeks, quarterly, annually, and then every 5 years for factors including the patient's medical/family history, weight (BMI), waist circumference, blood pressure, fasting plasma glucose, and fasting lipid profile. It is recommended that a fasting plasma glucose level (at baseline, then 12 weeks, then annually) and a fasting lipid profile (at baseline, then 12 weeks, then every 5 years if normal) be obtained. The RCTs of pharmacological interventions for weight gain related to the use of antipsychotics in patients with serious mental illness suggest that metformin and topiramate may be effective for reducing antipsychotic-induced weight gain in some patients (Crowley, Howe, & McDougle, 2015).

Extrapyramidal symptoms. Second-generation antipsychotics have a decreased risk of movement disorders in comparison with the FGAs; however, these events do occur in patients being treated with these agents. Patients should be evaluated for acute EPS until the medication dose has been stable for at least two weeks. Once the medication dose has been established, the monitoring frequency of EPS should be determined by the patient's sensitivity to develop EPS and the EPS liability of the antipsychotic drug being administered.

Hyperprolactinemia. Second-generation antipsychotics can cause hyperprolactinemia except for aripiprazole which can decrease prolactin levels. Hyperprolactinemia may cause galactorrhea, menstrual irregularities in women, sexual dysfunction in men, and osteoporosis if it impairs the production of sex hormones. Before starting treatment with an antipsychotic and annually thereafter, all patients should be assessed for symptoms associated with elevated prolactin levels. Plasma prolactin level should be measured if clinically indicated, and, if the level is determined to be elevated, a workup to find the cause should be initiated (e.g., pituitary prolactinoma).

Other parameters. Depending on the choice of agent, monitoring liver functions, complete blood count with differential (clozapine), and ECG (thioridazine, ziprasidone, pimozide, and mesoridazine) may be required. A QTc interval persistently greater than 500 ms is a substantial risk factor for the development of torsade de pointes, a ventricular arrhythmia that can cause syncope and may progress to ventricular fibrillation and sudden death. It is recommended that a baseline ECG be obtained for patients who are prescribed ziprasidone with known heart disease, a personal history of syncope or a family history of sudden death at an early age (<40 years). Patients with these cardiac risk factors should also not be prescribed thioridazine, pimozide, or mesoridazine. Providers who treat patients with clozapine should be aware of the signs and symptoms of myocarditis (unexplained fatigue, dyspnea, tachypnea, palpitations, fever, chest pain, and other signs or symptoms or ECG findings of heart failure).

Anticonvulsants (Valproic Acid, Levetiracetam, Oxcarbazepine, Lamotrigine, Topiramate)

Mechanisms of Action

The exact mechanism of action for most anticonvulsants is unknown. Currently, three primary mechanisms are recognized, including increased GABA-mediated inhibitory neurotransmission, modulation of voltage-gated ion channels, and decreased glutamate-mediated excitatory neurotransmission that prevents hyperexcitability of neurons. Anticonvulsants are FDA-approved for the treatment of epilepsy. In addition, certain anticonvulsants also have FDA approval for the treatment of bipolar disorder and neuropathic pain.

Potential Treatment Targets

There has been emerging evidence in the past decade suggesting that ASD may be associated with an imbalance between the excitatory neurotransmitter, glutamate, and the inhibitory neurotransmitter, GABA, which is often referred to as the excitatory/inhibitory (E/I) imbalance theory (Pizzarelli & Cherubini, 2011). Electroencephalogram (EEG) abnormalities are common in individuals with ASD, even without evidence of clinical seizures (Spence & Schneider, 2009). Although the clinical importance of EEG abnormalities in this population remains unclear (Hartley-McAndrew & Weinstock, 2010), researchers have hypothesized that abnormal EEG activity may be contributing to the mood and behavioral symptoms seen in individuals with ASD, and that treatment with anticonvulsants may decrease these symptoms.

Review of Research Findings

Valproic acid (divalproex sodium). The use of valproic acid (VPA) in the treatment of patients with ASD is supported by some open-label studies and RCTs, but not others (Hellings et al., 2005; Hollander et al., 2006a, 2010; Hollander, Dolgoff-Kaspar, Cartwright, Rawitt, & Novotny, 2001). An 8-week, RCT in 30 subjects with ASD (aged 6–20 years) and significant aggressive behavior investigated the efficacy and safety of VPA (mean blood level, 77.8 μg/mL at the endpoint of the trial) (Hellings et al., 2005). In this study, no significant differences were observed between the two treatment groups in improvement of irritability as measured by the ABC-I subscale, or global symptoms as measured by the CGI-I. Rash, which remitted after drug discontinuation, cognitive slowing, slurred speech, and elevated serum ammonia were reported adverse effects while taking VPA.

Hollander et al. compared VPA and placebo in the treatment of RRBs and irritability/agitation, respectively, in two RCTs (Hollander et al., 2006a, 2010). In the first study, which was conducted in 13 subjects with ASD (aged 5–17 years), treatment with VPA (mean trough level of 58.2 ± 21.6 μg/mL) was associated with a significant reduction in RRBs as measured by the C-YBOCS with a large effect size. The second study was conducted in 27 youths (aged 5–15 years) with ASD and irritability/agitation (Hollander et al., 2010). In the VPA group, 62.5% of subjects responded to the drug versus 9% in the placebo group. The responders had a mean VPA blood level of 89.8 μg/mL while non-responders had a level of 64.3 μg/mL. Irritability, insomnia, headache, and weight gain were reported as common adverse effects.

Levetiracetam. In an open-label trial, levetiracetam was associated with statistically significant improvement in emotional lability, inattention, hyperactivity, and aggression in six of 10 boys, between the ages of 4 and 10 years (Rugino & Samsock, 2002). The only RCT of levetiracetam to date, conducted in 20 subjects with ASD (aged 5–17 years), found no significant differences between the drug (mean dose of 862.5 mg/day for 10 weeks) and placebo groups on affective instability, irritability, RRBs, impulsivity or hyperactivity as measured by the CGI-I, C-YBOCS, and ABC-I subscale (Wasserman et al., 2006). The drug was overall well-tolerated, with mild adverse effects of agitation, aggression, and hyperactivity.

Oxcarbazepine. A retrospective case series of oxcarbazepine for irritability was conducted in 30 individuals with ASD (age 5–21 years). The majority of patients were being treated with concomitant psychotropic medications (range 0–4) for behavioral symptoms. Fourteen patients (47%) responded to oxcarbazepine based on a CGI-I score of "much improved." Ten patients (33%) showed improvement in the CGI-Severity score and seven patients (23%) reported adverse effects, including worsening irritability and seizure events leading to drug discontinuation (Douglas et al., 2013). In conclusion, it is hard to determine whether oxcarbazepine is beneficial for treating irritability/agitation associated with ASD without a placebo group. In addition, the relatively high rate of adverse effects reported suggests that it should be used judiciously in ASD.

Lamotrigine. Only one small RCT of lamotrigine has been published in youth with ASD (Belsito, Law, Kirk, Landa, & Zimmerman, 2001). In this 12-week study, 28 subjects (aged 3–11 years) were randomized to lamotrigine or placebo (mean dosage, 5.0 mg/kg/day). The results showed no significant difference between groups in the treatment of the core and associated symptoms of ASD as measured by the ABC, the Vineland Adaptive Behavior scales, the Pre-Linguistic Autism Diagnostic Observation Scale (PL-ADOS), and the Childhood Autism Rating Scale (CARS). Insomnia and hyperactivity were the most common side effects reported. There is currently insufficient evidence to support the use of lamotrigine in ASD, although the potential favorable effects as a mood stabilizer are still to be evaluated.

Topiramate. Topiramate has been investigated in a case series of youth with ASD and in a randomized add-on trial. Ten youths with ASD (aged 8–19 years) who were treated with antipsychotics received topiramate (1–3 mg/kg/day) for excessive weight gain, given its potential for reducing body weight. Eight subjects were on concomitant risperidone, one subject was taking pimozide and one subject was temporarily not on any antipsychotic. Four patients showed variable degrees of weight reduction (the maximum weight loss was 5 kg) and two subjects showed a weight increase. Adverse behavioral effects, including psychomotor agitation, hyperactivity, and irritability were reported in three subjects who subsequently stopped the trial (Canitano, 2005). In an 8-week RCT, 40 subjects (aged 4–12 years) with ASD were randomized to topiramate (100 mg/day for weight ≤30 kg and 200 mg/day for weight >30 kg) or placebo. All subjects were concurrently started on risperidone (2 mg/day for weight ≤40 kg and 3 mg/day for weight >40 kg). The topiramate treated group showed significantly greater improvement in ABC subscale scores for Irritability, Stereotypy, and Hyperactivity in comparison to the placebo group. Given that topiramate was administered as an adjunctive treatment, it is difficult to determine its effectiveness as a monotherapy (Rezaei et al., 2010).

Clinical Implementation

Anticonvulsants have been used broadly in ASD as mood stabilizers and to attenuate associated behavioral disorders; however, only a limited number of open-label and RCTs have been conducted in youth with ASD. The evidence available at present suggests that VPA may reduce RRBs and irritability in individuals with ASD; however, the number of controlled studies is somewhat limited. Patients receiving VPA should be monitored for serum drug levels to ensure that levels remain within the therapeutic range. Symptoms of VPA toxicity, including nausea, vomiting, ataxia, tremor, dizziness, headache, confusion, and somnolence, should also be followed closely. Hepatotoxicity is a possible serious adverse effect associated with the drug, warranting periodic liver function tests, especially during the first six months of treatment. Pancreatitis is another rare but serious complication. In addition, because of the risk of thrombocytopenia, checking baseline CBC with platelets and monitoring at periodic intervals should be considered for patients receiving VPA.

Lithium

Mechanism of Action

Lithium is approved by the FDA for the treatment of manic episodes and maintenance treatment of bipolar disorder in patients ≥7 years of age. Lithium's effect on reducing suicidal behavior and suicidal ideation has also been well-documented since the 1970s (Lewitzka et al., 2015). Although lithium has been widely used for its mood stabilizing properties, the exact mechanism of action is unknown. Traditionally, lithium is thought to decrease excitatory (DA and glutamate) and increase inhibitory GABA neurotransmission at the neuronal level. At the intracellular and molecular levels, lithium is thought to alter the second messenger systems that operate within neurons, which ultimately alter neurotransmission and promote neuroprotection (Malhi, Tanious, Das, Coulston, & Berk, 2013).

Potential Treatment Targets

Maladaptive behaviors are common in individuals with ASD and these behaviors may occur abruptly without any identifiable antecedent in the setting of a dysregulated mood state. Lithium has been one of the mood stabilizers used in the treatment of mood dysregulation and related symptoms in children and adolescents with ASD.

Review of Research Findings

To date, there has been no RCT of lithium in the treatment of ASD. A retrospective chart review of 30 individuals with ASD (mean age, 13.6 years) hospitalized on an inpatient psychiatry unit, and treated with lithium was conducted. Forty-three percent of subjects treated with lithium for mood disorder and/or irritability, were rated as "much improved" or "very much improved" on the CGI-I. The investigators reported that the subjects who had mania or elevated mood with no response to prior treatment with atypical antipsychotics showed the greatest improvement (Siegel et al., 2014). A high rate of adverse effects (47%) was reported, with the most common being vomiting, tremor, fatigue, irritability, and enuresis. In a case study of two patients with ASD and a mutation of the SHANK3 gene, who exhibited regression and symptoms of catatonia and were unimproved with antipsychotics, benzodiazepines, other mood stabilizers, antidepressants, and methylphenidate, a remarkable reversal of their symptoms was observed upon treatment with lithium (Serret et al., 2015). A retrospective chart review investigating the use of lithium in 19 individuals with ASD (mean age 22 years and 1 month) for the treatment of maladaptive behaviors reported that 14 (73.7%) of the subjects experienced "improvement" as rated on the

CGI-I after lithium was added to their treatment regimen. Having co-morbid ADHD was associated with a positive response. The mean dose of lithium was 5.3 mg/kg and the mean blood level at the most effective lithium dose was 0.6 ± 0.3 mmol/L. About 90% of the subjects with a serum lithium level above 0.6 mmol/L were rated as "improved" on the CGI-I. Eight subjects reported adverse effects and three of them discontinued the trial. The most common side effects reported were fatigue and tremor (Mintz & Hollenberg, 2019).

Clinical Implementation

Lithium should be further investigated in controlled trials targeting ASD-related aggression and mood dysregulation. Current evidence suggests that lithium may be effective in reducing maladaptive behaviors and mood symptoms in individuals with ASD; however, adverse effects with lithium are common and may be a limiting factor. Potential risks of lithium treatment include impaired thyroid and renal function warranting regular monitoring (Scahill, Farkas, & Hamrin, 2001). In addition, baseline ECGs are recommended in order to monitor for ECG changes including T-wave inversion and arrhythmias. Lithium levels must be routinely monitored and since lithium has a relatively narrow therapeutic range (0.6–1.2 μg/mL), it is essential to watch for signs and symptoms of lithium toxicity (lethargy, nausea, vomiting, diarrhea, tremor, weakness, and seizures) during treatment. Another concern is the significant risk of major congenital anomalies with prenatal exposure to lithium, especially cardiovascular malformations such as Ebstein's anomaly. Therefore, a baseline beta-hCG pregnancy test for all females not known to be sterile is necessary prior to administration of lithium.

Sleep Medications

Children with ASD have significantly higher rates of abnormal patterns of sleep, such as sleep-onset disturbances, nighttime awakenings, restlessness, and decreased sleep duration compared to typically developing children (Valicenti-McDermott et al., 2019). Sleep-related problems are likely the result of complex interactions between biological, psychological, and social/environmental factors and they are highly associated with worsening of maladaptive behaviors in children with neurodevelopmental disorders (Schreck, Mulick, & Smith, 2004). Abnormalities in melatonin, 5-HT, or GABA neurotransmission are considered among the possible biological etiologies of sleep disturbance in these individuals (Richdale & Schreck, 2009). Currently, there is no FDA-approved treatment for sleep disturbances in ASD, although certain agents like melatonin have been widely used in this population. Among the sleep-enhancing agents, melatonin is the only one that has been subjected to RCTs for the treatment of sleep impairment in youth with ASD.

According to the childhood insomnia treatment guidelines, it is important to establish appropriate sleep hygiene and utilize behavioral interventions prior to considering pharmacologic treatment. In addition, taking a detailed sleep history and screening for possible obstructive sleep apnea and other sleep disorders should be part of the assessment of sleep problems in children with ASD.

Several RCTs, observational and open-label studies have been conducted, showing benefits of melatonin for disturbed sleep onset and sleep maintenance in children with ASD (Andersen, Kaczmarska, McGrew, & Malow, 2008; Rossignol & Frye, 2011). In a meta-analysis of five RCTs with a total of 57 children with ASD, melatonin was reported to improve sleep duration by 73 min and reduce sleep onset latency by 66 min compared with placebo without any significant improvement in the number of nighttime awakenings (Rossignol & Frye, 2011). The dosage of melatonin ranged from 0.75 to 10 mg/day, and the duration of treatment ranged from 14 days to 6 months. Results from a recent large 13-week RCT in 125 youths between the ages of 2 and 17.5 years (96.8% with ASD, 3.2% with Smith–Magenis syndrome [SMS]) found that pediatric appropriate prolonged-release melatonin mini-tablets (PedPRM) (starting dose, 2 mg; titrated up to 5 mg per day) not only improved total sleep time (mean increase, 57.5 min) and sleep latency (mean decrease, 39.6 min), but also improved overall sleep disturbances (Gringras, Nir, Breddy, Frydman-Marom, & Findling, 2017). Although the adverse effects of melatonin were extremely rare, difficulty waking, daytime sleepiness, and enuresis were reported in certain studies (Giannotti, Cortesi, Cerquiglini, & Bernabei, 2006; Paavonen, Nieminen-von Wendt, Vanhala, Aronen, & von Wendt, 2003).

An observational study of clonidine in 19 children with ASD for the treatment of insomnia, and/or hyperactivity, inattention, mood disorder, and aggressive behaviors found the drug to be effective for reducing sleep latency and nighttime awakenings (Ming, Gordon, Kang, & Wagner, 2008). The dose of oral tablets was gradually advanced to 0.1 mg at bedtime and seven children were prescribed a transdermal clonidine patch at a dose of 0.1 mg per day. Five children discontinued the patch and switched to oral tablets due to skin irritation and/or hypersensitivity. Overall, clonidine was well tolerated in this study.

Trazodone is an antidepressant that inhibits the reuptake of 5-HT, causes adrenoreceptor sub-sensitivity, antagonizes 5-HT_{2A} receptors, and also blocks histamine and α_1-adrenergic receptors. Studies suggest that administration of trazodone 50–100 mg at bedtime may help with insomnia in the general population. Although RCTs of trazodone for sleep disturbances in ASD have not been conducted, this medication is often used for this purpose. Trazodone has also been used for other behavioral symptoms in ASD. In a case study of a 17-year-old male with ASD and ID whose behavioral symptoms did not respond to other medications, trazodone resulted in reduced aggression and self-injurious behavior. The most effective dose was 150 mg/day in divided doses. Another case study described a 13-year-old male with ASD and ID who developed priapism after taking trazodone 100 mg daily for 5 months. The priapism resolved after trazodone was discontinued (Gedye, 1991; Kem, Posey, &

McDougle, 2002). Although priapism is a rare side effect, it should always be discussed with patients and their family members because it can progress to a medical emergency.

When given 30 min before bedtime, melatonin, clonidine, and trazodone may be effective for reducing sleep latency and increasing sleep duration in children with ASD. In addition, for children who have medications with sedative properties prescribed for other indications, the timing of administration can be altered to take advantage of the sedative effects. It may be appropriate to also check ferritin levels in patients with ASD, as one open-label study suggested that iron supplementation may be beneficial for improving restless sleep in children with ASD who have decreased serum ferritin levels (Dosman et al., 2007).

Proposed Treatment Options for Social Impairment in Autism Spectrum Disorder

Researchers who study pharmacologic treatment options for the core symptoms of ASD have used various approaches, including targeting neuronal circuits proposed to subserve the social brain by altering the function of certain neurotransmitters, or targeting CNS-related physiological or non-CNS-related systematic abnormalities affecting overall functioning of the brain (Frye, 2018). Currently, there are no pharmacologic treatments that have been consistently shown to improve the social impairment associated with ASD. Although some medication trials (certain SSRIs and antipsychotics) have resulted in some improvement in social impairment, this has not been confirmed in large-scale RCTs. So far, pharmacologic agents that have shown some but inconsistent benefit for the treatment of social impairment in individuals with ASD include oxytocin, D-cycloserine, and cognitive enhancers used to treat Alzheimer's dementia (e.g., galantamine, memantine, and rivastigmine) (Chez, Aimonovitch, Buchanan, Mrazek, & Tremb, 2004; Erickson et al., 2007; Huffman, Sutcliffe, Tanner, & Feldman, 2011; Nicolson, Craven-Thuss, & Smith, 2006).

Oxytocin. Oxytocin is currently one of the most actively investigated drugs for the treatment of core symptoms of ASD. Following studies of the role of oxytocin in social cognition, many researchers examined its possible role in the pathophysiology and treatment of social impairment in ASD. Several of these studies suggested that oxytocin may improve emotional recognition (Anagnostou et al., 2012; Guastella et al., 2010; Hollander et al., 2007), eye gaze (Andari et al., 2010; Domes, Kumbier, Heinrichs, & Herpertz, 2014), social judgment (Gordon et al., 2013; Watanabe et al., 2014), mentalizing abilities (Aoki et al., 2014; Ocakoglu, Kose, Ozbaran, & Onay, 2018), and RRBs of individuals with ASD (Hollander et al., 2003). In contrast, a number of studies found no statistically significant change in social or RRBs with oxytocin (Dadds et al., 2014; Quintana et al., 2017; Yamasue et al., 2018).

A recent meta-analysis that included 16 RCTs (total number of 520 subjects) investigating the safety and efficacy of oxytocin for the treatment of core symptoms in ASD reported mixed findings and indicated that overall oxytocin had a small effect on social function and RRBs compared with placebo; however, the difference was not statistically significant (Wang, Wang, Rong, He, & Yang, 2019). The authors suggested that this could be attributed to RCTs having significant variations in the characteristics of participants (age, gender, IQ); primary outcome measures; route, dosage, and duration of drug administration; as well as variability in the OXTR gene which may potentially influence oxytocin's effects on the core symptoms of ASD (Alvares, Quintana, & Whitehouse, 2017; Guoynes et al., 2018; Watanabe et al., 2017). The majority of studies included in the meta-analysis reported mild adverse effects including fatigue, shakiness, nausea, and irritability. Serious adverse effects reported included hyperactivity and aggression in one study (Yatawara, Einfeld, Hickie, Davenport, & Guastella, 2016), and seizures in two subjects in another study (Munesue et al., 2016). However, it is unlikely that the seizures were associated with oxytocin since one subject forgot to administer the anticonvulsant medication prior to the seizure and the other subject experienced seizures during both the oxytocin and placebo phases of the trial. Because ASD is a highly heterogeneous neurodevelopmental disorder, therefore, to overcome the limitations of studies to date, further RCTs with larger cohorts should be conducted to determine the safety and efficacy of oxytocin for the treatment of social impairment in individuals with ASD.

Secretin. In 1998, Horvath et al. proposed secretin (a GI peptide) as a possible treatment for ASD after they observed improvement in the core symptoms in an open-label trial in three patients. Following this report, secretin was extensively studied in 16 RCTs including over 900 children with ASD (Williams, Wray, & Wheeler, 2005) making it one of the most widely studied potential treatments for ASD. However, none of the reports found secretin effective for treatment of the core symptoms of ASD. Considering these results, secretin is not recommended for the treatment of ASD.

Naltrexone. Results from preclinical studies indicated that "autistic symptoms" were observed in animals treated with opiates (Panksepp, Najam, & Soares, 1979). Some empirical evidence also suggested that self-injurious behaviors might be mediated by the endogenous opioid system (Sandman, 1988). Subsequently, naltrexone, an opioid receptor antagonist, has been studied and a number of case reports, open-label trials, and RCTs for self-injury and core and associated symptoms of ASD have been published (Elchaar, Maisch, Augusto, & Wehring, 2006). Several RCTs were conducted with naltrexone targeting the core symptoms of ASD, associated symptoms of hyperactivity and irritability, and discrimination learning in children with ASD (Campbell et al., 1990; Feldman, Kolmen, & Gonzaga, 1999; Willemsen-Swinkels, Buitelaar, Weijnen, & van Engeland, 1995b). The largest RCT, which included 41 youths with ASD, reported a significant improvement in hyperactivity, which has been the most consistent positive finding in studies of naltrexone in ASD so far (Campbell et al., 1990). Collectively, the evidence has suggested that naltrexone is ineffective for the treatment of social deficits in individuals with ASD (Farmer, Thurm, & Grant, 2013; Huffman et al., 2011).

A recent review of the literature on the use of naltrexone for the treatment of self-injurious behavior (SIB) reported that short-term treatment reduced the frequency of

SIB in individuals with ID. In this report, 27 articles involving 86 subjects (35% had ASD) with self-injury were reviewed. Overall, 80% of the subjects were reported to show improvement with naltrexone (dose range, 12.5–200 mg/day) (Symons, Thompson, & Rodriguez, 2004). However, findings in individuals with ASD have been mixed. While two of the studies looking at the short- and long-term effects of naltrexone reported no significant benefit in reducing the frequency and duration of SIB in subjects with ASD, another report described benefit in two females with ASD (Smith, Gupta, & Smith, 1995; Willemsen-Swinkels, Buitelaar, Nijhof, & van England, 1995a; Zingarelli et al., 1992). In summary, it appears that naltrexone may be modestly effective for reducing hyperactivity and impulsivity in youth with ASD, but ineffective for the core symptoms of ASD or discrimination learning (Feldman et al., 1999; Kolmen, Feldman, Handen, & Janosky, 1995; Willemsen-Swinkels et al., 1995b). The conflicting findings regarding the efficacy of naltrexone in reducing SIB in ASD warrant further investigation before its use can be recommended as a routine treatment for this purpose.

Memantine. Preliminary studies suggested that abnormal functioning of NMDA-receptors or altered glutamate metabolism may play a role in the pathophysiology of ASD. Memantine, an N-methyl-D-aspartate (NMDA) receptor antagonist, FDA-approved for the treatment of Alzheimer's disease, has been studied for the core symptoms of ASD and so far the findings have been mixed. An open-label case series of memantine (mean dosage, 12.7 mg/day) in 151 youths (aged 2–26 years) with ASD reported significant improvement in language, socialization and to a lesser degree stereotypies over 21 months of treatment (Chez et al., 2007). Eighty-two percent of the participants continued the drug, although 14.5% reported adverse effects including worsened behavior. An 8-week, open-label study of memantine in 14 subjects (aged 3–12 years) with ASD deemed four subjects as responders as demonstrated by some improvement on the ABC subscales of Hyperactivity, Lethargy/Social Withdrawal, and Irritability, as well as on a memory test (Owley et al., 2006). Reported adverse effects included hyperactivity, which led to discontinuation of the study by two subjects. A retrospective open-label study of memantine (mean dosage, 10.1 mg/day) in 18 youths (aged 6–19 years) with ASD reported a response rate of 61% for symptoms of social withdrawal and inattention (Erickson et al., 2007). Seven patients had adverse effects including increased irritability, seizure frequency, and sedation and four subjects discontinued the study. Another open-label trial of memantine (dosage range, 15–20 mg/day) was conducted in 18 adults (mean age, 28 ± 9.5 years) with high-functioning ASD. The investigators reported that at the study end point, 83% of the subjects had a significant reduction in ASD symptom severity as measured on the CGI-I (a score of "much" or "very much" improved) and one-third of the subjects demonstrated a >30% reduction on an informant-rated Social Responsiveness Scale for adults (SRS-A). In addition, memantine was also associated with statistically significant improvement in ADHD, anxiety, and general psychopathology scores as determined by clinician-rated measures. Memantine treatment was well-tolerated and not associated with any serious adverse effects (Joshi et al., 2016). A 12-week RCT followed by a 48-week open-label extension phase looked at the safety and efficacy of memantine ER in 121 children (aged

6–12 years) with ASD. During the first phase of the study, maximum memantine dosages were determined by body weight of the individual and ranged from 3 to 15 mg/day. The second phase of the study focused on randomization of subjects to drug or placebo and assessing the safety and efficacy of memantine. By the endpoint of the trial, there was a statistically significant increase (improvement) in SRS scores in each group; however, no statistically significant difference was observed between groups. One hundred and four children completed the 12-week trial (placebo: 82.0%; memantine: 90.0%) and 102 subjects participated in the 48-week open-label extension phase. Improvement in the primary outcome measure (the SRS) was maintained for the duration of the extension phase of the trial. Mild-to-moderate adverse effects and two serious adverse events, both of which were deemed unrelated to the drug, were reported (Aman et al., 2017).

Results from studies of memantine in children with ASD have not been consistent in demonstrating clinical efficacy. However, the evidence suggests that memantine may be beneficial for the treatment of symptoms associated with ASD in high-functioning adults. Additional RCTs are warranted to confirm the efficacy and safety of memantine before it can be recommended as a standard treatment option in ASD.

D-cycloserine. D-cycloserine, an antibiotic used to treat tuberculosis, has been extensively studied in neuropsychiatric diseases based upon its proposed mechanism as a partial NMDA-agonist. A prospective, single-blinded trial of D-cycloserine in 10 participants (aged 5–27 years) with ASD, investigated the short-term clinical benefits on social impairment (Posey et al., 2004a). The drug (administered at 0.7, 1.4, and 2.8 mg/kg/day for 2 weeks each) was associated with statistically significant improvement on the CGI-I and the Lethargy/Social Withdrawal subscale of the ABC with the highest dose leading to a 60% reduction in symptom severity. Two subjects discontinued the drug due to a transient motor tic and worsening echolalia, respectively. A 10-week, RCT of low-dose (50 mg) D-cycloserine was conducted in 67 children (aged 5–11 years) with ASD, without accompanying ID (Minshawi et al., 2016). Participants were randomized to receive one dose per week of D-cycloserine or placebo and the drug was administered 30 min prior to a weekly social skills group training session. There was no significant short-term improvement on the primary outcome measure, the SRS, or any of the secondary outcome measures. However, an overall significant improvement in SRS total raw score was observed from baseline to the end of treatment for all participants with ASD. 10-week RCT targeting stereotypies was conducted in 20 subjects (aged 14–25 years) with ASD, with participants randomized to either weekly or daily administration of 50 mg of D-cycloserine. The dosages of concomitant psychiatric medications were maintained until the end of the trial. The investigators reported a 37% decrease in ABC Stereotypy subscale scores. Scores on the SRS and the Lethargy/Social Withdrawal subscale of the ABC also improved significantly. Giving the drug on a weekly or daily basis did not affect the clinical response. Overall the drug was well-tolerated (Urbano et al., 2014).

Vasopressin. Vasopressin is a neuropeptide that is closely related to oxytocin, which is considered to have a regulatory role in social cognition and has recently emerged as a therapeutic target for core symptoms of ASD. A 12-week Phase-2 trial investigated the safety and efficacy of balovaptan (an oral selective vasopressin V1a receptor antagonist) in 223 adult males with ASD. The study reported no improvement in the primary outcome measure (SRS-2 score); however, improvement in adaptive behaviors as measured by the Vineland-II scale was noted (Bolognani et al., 2019). Following this study, a 4-week RCT studied the effects of intranasal vasopressin (dosage range, 24–32 International Units (IU) administered daily for 12 weeks) in 30 children (6–13 years) with ASD. In addition to improvements in the primary outcome measure (SRS-2 score) the drug was associated with a reduction in anxiety symptoms and RRBs (Parker et al., 2019). Both studies above reported that the drug was safe and well tolerated.

Folinic acid (Folate). Folate is a water-soluble vitamin which is essential for critical metabolic processes like redox metabolism and methylation. Abnormalities in folate metabolism, as well as genetic polymorphisms of the key enzymes in the folate pathway have been linked to ASD (Frye & James, 2014; Vahabzadeh & McDougle, 2013). Some studies suggested that folate supplementation during conception and the prenatal period could lower the risk of ASD in the offspring (Steenweg-de Graaff et al., 2017; Suren et al., 2013). In a recent 12-week RCT, high-dose folinic acid (2 mg/kg per day) was administered to 48 youths (mean age, 7 years 4 months) with ASD and language impairment. Subjects were subtyped by glutathione and folate receptor-α autoantibody (FRAA) status and folinic acid administration was associated with significant improvement in verbal communication (the primary outcome measure), as measured by an ability-appropriate standardized instrument, particularly in those subjects who were positive for FRAAs. The investigators suggested that folinic acid may improve verbal communication, especially in patients who are positive for FRAAs (Frye et al., 2018).

Summary and Recommendations

- Psychopharmacology should be considered as one component of a broader, comprehensive multimodal treatment approach in the management of maladaptive behaviors associated with ASD.
- Medications should be prescribed to reduce maladaptive behaviors, and augment other behavioral, social, and educational interventions.
- Pharmacotherapy of ASD should be based on a target symptom approach. The most commonly targeted symptom domains in ASD include irritability and aggression; hyperactivity and inattention; restricted, repetitive interests, behaviors and activities and sleep disturbance.
- For mild aggression or self-injury in youth, consider prescribing an α_2-adrenergic agonist. For those with more severe symptoms, consider prescribing an atypical antipsychotic. Risperidone and aripiprazole are the FDA-approved treatments for irritability and/or aggression in children and adolescents with ASD.
- Prepubertal children treated with selective serotonin reuptake inhibitors (SSRIs) may have increased rates of behavioral activation and irritability compared to post-pubertal adolescents and adults with ASD.

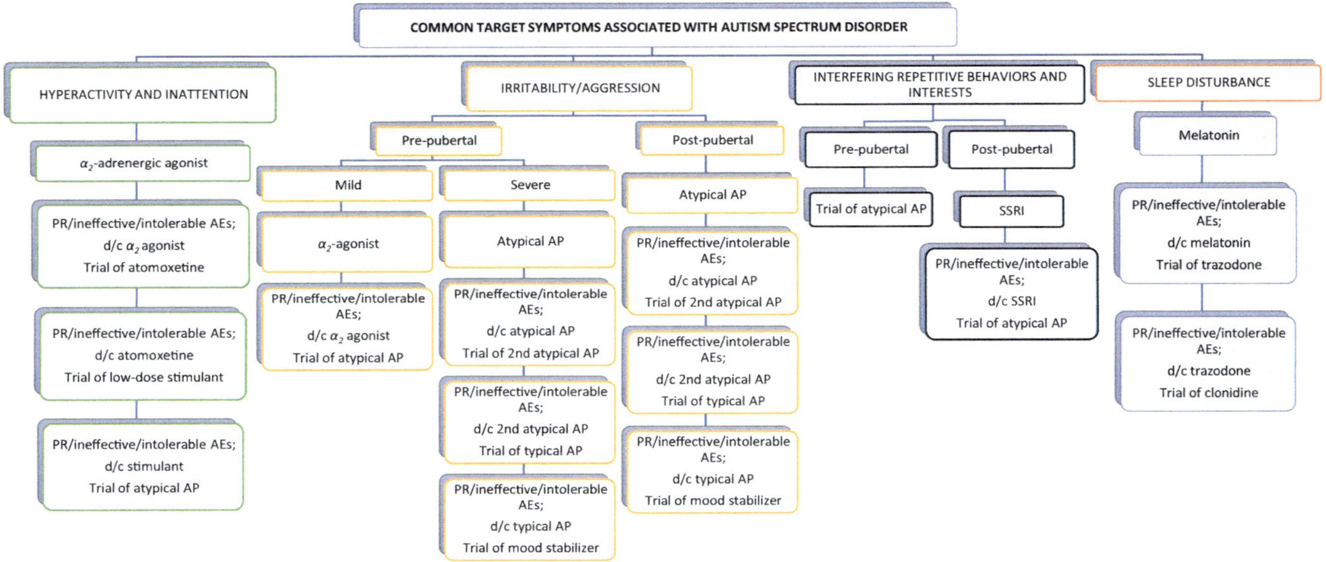

Fig. 2 Pharmacotherapy of common target symptom domains in ASD, including hyperactivity and inattention; irritability and aggression; interfering restricted, repetitive behaviors and interests and sleep disturbance. PR = partial response; d/c = discontinue; AE = adverse effect; AP = antipsychotic; SSRI = selective serotonin reuptake inhibitor

- For hyperactivity and inattention, psychostimulants may be beneficial but appear to be less efficacious and associated with more adverse effects compared to typically developing children with ADHD. Therefore, considering a trial of guanfacine or atomoxetine before a stimulant may be more appropriate.
- Consider buspirone prior to an SSRI or serotonin-norepinephrine reuptake inhibitor for the treatment of anxiety in individuals with ASD (Fig. 2).

Acknowledgments This work was supported in part by the Commonwealth of Massachusetts Department of Mental Health and Developmental Services and by the Nancy Lurie Marks family Foundation.

References

A 14-month randomized clinical trial of treatment strategies for attention-deficit/hyperactivity disorder. The MTA Cooperative Group. Multimodal Treatment Study of Children with ADHD. (1999). *Archives of General Psychiatry, 56*(12), 1073–1086.

Albertini, G., Polito, E., Sara, M., Di Gennaro, G., & Onorati, P. (2006). Compulsive masturbation in infantile autism treated by mirtazapine. *Pediatric Neurology, 34*(5), 417–418.

Allison, D. B., Basile, V. C., & MacDonald, R. B. (1991). Brief report: comparative effects of antecedent exercise and lorazepam on the aggressive behavior of an autistic man. *Journal of Autism and Developmental Disorders, 21*(1), 89–94.

Alvares, G. A., Quintana, D. S., & Whitehouse, A. J. (2017). Beyond the hype and hope: Critical considerations for intranasal oxytocin research in autism spectrum disorder. *Autism Research, 10*(1), 25–41.

Aman, M. G. (1982). Stimulant drug effects in developmental disorders and hyperactivity–toward a resolution of disparate findings. *Journal of Autism and Developmental Disorders, 12*(4), 385–398.

Aman, M. G., Findling, R. L., Hardan, A. Y., Hendren, R. L., Melmed, R. D., Kehinde-Nelson, O., et al. (2017). Safety and efficacy of memantine in children with autism: randomized, placebo-controlled study and open-label extension. *Journal of Child and Adolescent zPsychopharmacology, 27*(5), 403–412.

Aman, M. G., Lam, K. S., & Van Bourgondien, M. E. (2005). Medication patterns in patients with autism: temporal, regional, and demographic influences. *Journal of Child and Adolescent Psychopharmacology, 15*(1), 116–126.

Aman, M. G., McDougle, C. J., Scahill, L., Handen, B., Arnold, L. E., Johnson, C., Research Units on Pediatric Psychopharmacology Autism, N. (2009). Medication and parent training in children with pervasive developmental disorders and serious behavior problems: results from a randomized clinical trial. *Journal of the American Academy of Child and Adolescent Psychiatry, 48*(12), 1142–1154.

Aman, M. G., Smith, T., Arnold, L. E., Corbett-Dick, P., Tumuluru, R., Hollway, J. A., et al. (2014). A review of atomoxetine effects in young people with developmental disabilities. *Research in Developmental Disabilities, 35*(6), 1412–1424.

American Diabetes Association, American Psychiatric Association, American Association of Clinical Endocrinologists & North American Association for the Study of Obesity. (2004). Consensus development conference on antipsychotic drugs and obesity and diabetes. *Journal of Clinical Psychiatry, 65*(2), 267–272.

Anagnostou, E., Soorya, L., Chaplin, W., Bartz, J., Halpern, D., Wasserman, S., et al. (2012). Intranasal oxytocin versus placebo in the treatment of adults with autism spectrum disorders: a randomized controlled trial. *Molecular Autism, 3*(1), 16.

Andari, E., Duhamel, J. R., Zalla, T., Herbrecht, E., Leboyer, M., & Sirigu, A. (2010). Promoting social behavior with oxytocin in high-functioning autism spectrum disorders. *Proceedings of the National Academy of Sciences, 107*(9), 4389–4394.

Andersen, I. M., Kaczmarska, J., McGrew, S. G., & Malow, B. A. (2008). Melatonin for insomnia in children with autism spectrum disorders. *Journal of Child Neurology, 23*(5), 482–485.

Anderson, L. T., Campbell, M., Adams, P., Small, A. M., Perry, R., & Shell, J. (1989). The effects of haloperidol on discrimination learning and behavioral symptoms in autistic children. *Journal of Autism and Developmental Disorders, 19*(2), 227–239.

Anderson, L. T., Campbell, M., Grega, D. M., Perry, R., Small, A. M., & Green, W. H. (1984). Haloperidol in the treatment of infantile autism: effects on learning and behavioral symptoms. *American Journal of Psychiatry, 141*(10), 1195–1202.

Aoki, Y., Yahata, N., Watanabe, T., Takano, Y., Kawakubo, Y., Kuwabara, H., et al. (2014). Oxytocin improves behavioural and neural deficits in inferring others' social emotions in autism. *Brain, 137*(Pt 11), 3073–3086.

Arnold, L. E., Aman, M. G., Cook, A. M., Witwer, A. N., Hall, K. L., Thompson, S., et al. (2006). Atomoxetine for hyperactivity in autism spectrum disorders: placebo-controlled crossover pilot trial. *Journal of the American Academy of Child and Adolescent Psychiatry, 45*(10), 1196–1205.

Barnard, L., Young, A. H., Pearson, J., Geddes, J., & O'Brien, G. (2002). A systematic review of the use of atypical antipsychotics in autism. *Journal of Psychopharmacology, 16*(1), 93–101.

Barrickman, L. L., Perry, P. J., Allen, A. J., Kuperman, S., Arndt, S. V., Herrmann, K. J., et al. (1995). Bupropion versus methylphenidate in the treatment of attention-deficit hyperactivity disorder. *Journal of the American Academy of Child and Adolescent Psychiatry, 34*(5), 649–657.

Beherec, L., Lambrey, S., Quilici, G., Rosier, A., Falissard, B., & Guillin, O. (2011). Retrospective review of clozapine in the treatment of patients with autism spectrum disorder and severe disruptive behaviors. *Journal of Clinical Psychopharmacology, 31*(3), 341–344.

Belsito, K. M., Law, P. A., Kirk, K. S., Landa, R. J., & Zimmerman, A. W. (2001). Lamotrigine therapy for autistic disorder: A randomized, double-blind, placebo-controlled trial. *Journal of Autism and Developmental Disorders, 31*(2), 175–181.

Bolognani, F., Del Valle Rubido, M., Squassante, L., Wandel, C., Derks, M., Murtagh, L., … Fontoura, P. (2019). A phase 2 clinical trial of a vasopressin V1a receptor antagonist shows improved adaptive behaviors in men with autism spectrum disorder. *Science Translational Medicine, 11*(491).

Bozkurt, H., & Mukaddes, N. M. (2010). Catatonia in a child with autistic disorder. *Turkish Journal of Pediatrics, 52*(4), 435–438.

Branford, D., Bhaumik, S., & Naik, B. (1998). Selective serotonin re-uptake inhibitors for the treatment of perseverative and maladaptive behaviours of people with intellectual disability. *Journal of Intellectual Disabilities Research, 42*(Pt 4), 301–306.

Buchsbaum, M. S., Hollander, E., Haznedar, M. M., Tang, C., Spiegel-Cohen, J., Wei, T. C., et al. (2001). Effect of fluoxetine on regional cerebral metabolism in autistic spectrum disorders: a pilot study. *International Journal of Neuropsychopharmacology, 4*(2), 119–125.

Buitelaar, J. K., van der Gaag, R. J., & van der Hoeven, J. (1998). Buspirone in the management of anxiety and irritability in children with pervasive developmental disorders: results of an open-label study. *Journal of Clinical Psychiatry, 59*(2), 56–59.

Campbell, M. (1975). Pharmacotherapy in early infantile autism. *Biological Psychiatry, 10*(4), 399–423.

Campbell, M., Anderson, L. T., Meier, M., Cohen, I. L., Small, A. M., Samit, C., et al. (1978). A comparison of haloperidol and behavior therapy and their interaction in autistic children. *Journal of the American Academy of Child Psychiatry, 17*(4), 640–655.

Campbell, M., Anderson, L. T., Small, A. M., Locascio, J. J., Lynch, N. S., & Choroco, M. C. (1990). Naltrexone in autistic children: A double-blind and placebo-controlled study. *Psychopharmacoly Bulletin, 26*(1), 130–135.

Campbell, M., Armenteros, J. L., Malone, R. P., Adams, P. B., Eisenberg, Z. W., & Overall, J. E. (1997). Neuroleptic-related dyskinesias in autistic children: A prospective, longitudinal study. *Journal of the American Academy of Child and Adolescent Psychiatry, 36*(6), 835–843.

Campbell, M., Fish, B., David, R., Shapiro, T., Collins, P., & Koh, C. (1972). Response to triiodothyronine and dextroamphetamine: a study of preschool schizophrenic children. *Journal of Autism and Childhood Schizophrenia, 2*(4), 343–358.

Campbell, M., Small, A. M., Collins, P. J., Friedman, E., David, R., & Genieser, N. (1976). Levodopa and levoamphetamine: a crossover study in young schizophrenic children. *Current Therapeutic Research, Clinical & Experimental, 19*(1), 70–86.

Canitano, R. (2005). Clinical experience with Topiramate to counteract neuroleptic induced weight gain in 10 individuals with autistic spectrum disorders. *Brain Development, 27*(3), 228–232.

Ceranoglu, T. A., Wozniak, J., Fried, R., Galdo, M., Hoskova, B., DeLeon Fong, M., et al. (2019). A retrospective chart review of buspirone for the treatment of anxiety in psychiatrically referred youth with high-functioning autism spectrum disorder. *Journal of Child and Adolescent Psychopharmacology, 29*(1), 28–33. https://doi.org/10.1089/cap.2018.0021.

Chez, M. G., Aimonovitch, M., Buchanan, T., Mrazek, S., & Tremb, R. J. (2004). Treating autistic spectrum disorders in children: utility of the cholinesterase inhibitor rivastigmine tartrate. *Journal of Child Neurology, 19*(3), 165–169.

Chez, M. G., Burton, Q., Dowling, T., Chang, M., Khanna, P., & Kramer, C. (2007). Memantine as adjunctive therapy in children diagnosed with autistic spectrum disorders: an observation of initial clinical response and maintenance tolerability. *Journal of Child Neurology, 22*(5), 574–579.

Chugani, D. C., Chugani, H. T., Wiznitzer, M., Parikh, S., Evans, P. A., Hansen, R. L., ... Autism Center of Excellence, N. (2016). Efficacy of low-dose buspirone for restricted and repetitive behavior in young children with autism spectrum disorder: A randomized trial. *Journal of Pediatrics, 170*, 45–53 e41–44.

Cohen, I. L., Campbell, M., Posner, D., Small, A. M., Triebel, D., & Anderson, L. T. (1980). Behavioral effects of haloperidol in young autistic children. An objective analysis using a within-subjects reversal design. *Journal of the American Academy of Child Psychiatry, 19*(4), 665–677.

Conners, C. K., Casat, C. D., Gualtieri, C. T., Weller, E., Reader, M., Reiss, A., et al. (1996). Bupropion hydrochloride in attention deficit disorder with hyperactivity. *Journal of the American Academy of Child and Adolescent Psychiatry, 35*(10), 1314–1321.

Corson, A. H., Barkenbus, J. E., Posey, D. J., Stigler, K. A., & McDougle, C. J. (2004). A retrospective analysis of quetiapine in the treatment of pervasive developmental disorders. *Journal of Clinical Psychiatry, 65*(11), 1531–1536.

Coskun, M., Karakoc, S., Kircelli, F., & Mukaddes, N. M. (2009). Effectiveness of mirtazapine in the treatment of inappropriate sexual behaviors in individuals with autistic disorder. *Journal of Child and Adolescent Psychopharmacology, 19*(2), 203–206.

Coury, D. L., Anagnostou, E., Manning-Courtney, P., Reynolds, A., Cole, L., McCoy, R., et al. (2012). Use of psychotropic medication in children and adolescents with autism spectrum disorders. *Pediatrics, 130*(Suppl 2), S69–76.

Crowley, B., Howe, Y. J., & McDougle, C. J. (2015). Topiramate for weight loss in two young adult women with autism spectrum disorder. *Journal of Child and Adolescent Psychopharmacology, 25*(2), 183–185.

Dadds, M. R., MacDonald, E., Cauchi, A., Williams, K., Levy, F., & Brennan, J. (2014). Nasal oxytocin for social deficits in childhood autism: a randomized controlled trial. *Journal of Autism and Developmental Disorders, 44*(3), 521–531.

Davanzo, P. A., Belin, T. R., Widawski, M. H., & King, B. H. (1998). Paroxetine treatment of aggression and self-injury in persons with mental retardation. *American Journal of Mental Retardation, 102*(5), 427–437.

DeLong, G. R., Ritch, C. R., & Burch, S. (2002). Fluoxetine response in children with autistic spectrum disorders: correlation with familial major affective disorder and intellectual achievement. *Developmental Medicine and Child Neurology, 44*(10), 652–659.

Domes, G., Kumbier, E., Heinrichs, M., & Herpertz, S. C. (2014). Oxytocin promotes facial emotion recognition and amygdala reactivity in adults with asperger syndrome. *Neuropsychopharmacology, 39*(3), 698–706.

Dosman, C. F., Brian, J. A., Drmic, I. E., Senthilselvan, A., Harford, M. M., Smith, R. W., et al. (2007). Children with autism: effect of iron supplementation on sleep and ferritin. *Pediatric Neurology, 36*(3), 152–158.

Douglas, J. F., Sanders, K. B., Benneyworth, M. H., Smith, J. L., Dejean, V. M., McGrew, S. G., et al. (2013). Brief report: Retrospective case series of oxcarbazepine for irritability/agitation symptoms in autism spectrum disorder. *Journal of Autism and Developmental Disorders, 43*(5), 1243–1247.

Elchaar, G. M., Maisch, N. M., Augusto, L. M., & Wehring, H. J. (2006). Efficacy and safety of naltrexone use in pediatric patients with autistic disorder. *Annals of Pharmacotherapy, 40*(6), 1086–1095.

Erickson, C. A., Posey, D. J., Stigler, K. A., Mullett, J., Katschke, A. R., & McDougle, C. J. (2007). A retrospective study of memantine in children and adolescents with pervasive developmental disorders. *Psychopharmacology (Berl), 191*(1), 141–147.

Fankhauser, M. P., Karumanchi, V. C., German, M. L., Yates, A., & Karumanchi, S. D. (1992). A double-blind, placebo-controlled study of the efficacy of transdermal clonidine in autism. *Journal of Clinical Psychiatry, 53*(3), 77–82.

Farmer, C., Thurm, A., & Grant, P. (2013). Pharmacotherapy for the core symptoms in autistic disorder: current status of the research. *Drugs, 73*(4), 303–314.

Fatemi, S. H., Realmuto, G. M., Khan, L., & Thuras, P. (1998). Fluoxetine in treatment of adolescent patients with autism: a longitudinal open trial. *Journal of Autism and Developmental Disorders, 28*(4), 303–307.

Feldman, H. M., Kolmen, B. K., & Gonzaga, A. M. (1999). Naltrexone and communication skills in young children with autism. *Journal of the American Academy of Child and Adolescent Psychiatry, 38*(5), 587–593.

Findling, R. L., Mankoski, R., Timko, K., Lears, K., McCartney, T., McQuade, R. D., et al. (2014). A randomized controlled trial investigating the safety and efficacy of aripiprazole in the long-term maintenance treatment of pediatric patients with irritability associated with autistic disorder. *Journal of Clinical Psychiatry, 75*(1), 22–30.

Findling, R. L., Maxwell, K., & Wiznitzer, M. (1997). An open clinical trial of risperidone monotherapy in young children with autistic disorder. *Psychopharmacology Bulletin, 33*(1), 155–159.

Findling, R. L., McNamara, N. K., Gracious, B. L., O'Riordan, M. A., Reed, M. D., Demeter, C., et al. (2004). Quetiapine in nine youths with autistic disorder. *Journal of Child and Adolescent Psychopharmacology, 14*(2), 287–294.

Frazier, J. A., Biederman, J., Bellordre, C. A., Garfield, S. B., Geller, D. A., Coffey, B. J., et al. (2001). Should the diagnosis of attention-deficit/hyperactivity disorder be considered in children with pervasive developmental disorder? *Journal of Attention Disorders, 4*(4), 203–211.

Frye, R. E. (2018). Social skills deficits in autism spectrum disorder: Potential biological origins and progress in developing therapeutic agents. *CNS Drugs, 32*(8), 713–734.

Frye, R. E., & James, S. J. (2014). Metabolic pathology of autism in relation to redox metabolism. *Biomarkers in Medicine, 8*(3), 321–330.

Frye, R. E., Slattery, J., Delhey, L., Furgerson, B., Strickland, T., Tippett, M., et al. (2018). Folinic acid improves verbal communication in children with autism and language impairment: a randomized double-blind placebo-controlled trial. *Molecular Psychiatry, 23*(2), 247–256.

Fukuda, T., Sugie, H., Ito, M., & Sugie, Y. (2001). Clinical evaluation of treatment with fluvoxamine, a selective serotonin reuptake inhibitor in children with autistic disorder. *No To Hattatsu, 33*(4), 314–318.

Garnock-Jones, K. P., & Keating, G. M. (2009). Atomoxetine: A review of its use in attention-deficit hyperactivity disorder in children and adolescents. *Paediatric Drugs, 11*(3), 203–226.

Gedye, A. (1991). Trazodone reduced aggressive and self-injurious movements in a mentally handicapped male patient with autism. *Journal of Clinical Psychopharmacology, 11*(4), 275–276.

Ghanizadeh, A., & Ayoobzadehshirazi, A. (2015). A randomized double-blind placebo-controlled clinical trial of adjuvant buspirone for irritability in autism. *Pediatric Neurology, 52*(1), 77–81.

Ghanizadeh, A., Sahraeizadeh, A., & Berk, M. (2014). A head-to-head comparison of aripiprazole and risperidone for safety and treating autistic disorders, a randomized double blind clinical trial. *Child Psychiatry and Human Development, 45*(2), 185–192.

Giannotti, F., Cortesi, F., Cerquiglini, A., & Bernabei, P. (2006). An open-label study of controlled-release melatonin in treatment of sleep disorders in children with autism. *Journal of Autism and Developmental Disorders, 36*(6), 741–752.

Gordon, C. T., State, R. C., Nelson, J. E., Hamburger, S. D., & Rapoport, J. L. (1993). A double-blind comparison of clomipramine, desipramine, and placebo in the treatment of autistic disorder. *Archives of General Psychiatry, 50*(6), 441–447.

Gordon, I., Vander Wyk, B. C., Bennett, R. H., Cordeaux, C., Lucas, M. V., Eilbott, J. A., et al. (2013). Oxytocin enhances brain function in children with autism. *Proceedings of the National Academy of Sciences, 110*(52), 20953–20958.

Greenhill, L. L., Pliszka, S., Dulcan, M. K., Bernet, W., Arnold, V., Beitchman, J., et al. (2002). Practice parameter for the use of stimulant medications in the treatment of children, adolescents, and adults. *Journal of the American Academy of Child and Adolescent Psychiatry, 41*(2 Suppl), 26S–49S.

Greist, J. H., Jefferson, J. W., Kobak, K. A., Katzelnick, D. J., & Serlin, R. C. (1995). Efficacy and tolerability of serotonin transport inhibitors in obsessive-compulsive disorder. A meta-analysis. *Archives of General Psychiatry, 52*(1), 53–60.

Gringras, P., Nir, T., Breddy, J., Frydman-Marom, A., & Findling, R. L. (2017). Efficacy and safety of pediatric prolonged-release melatonin for insomnia in children with autism spectrum disorder. *Journal of the American Academy of Child and Adolescent Psychiatry, 56*(11), 948–957 e944.

Guastella, A. J., Einfeld, S. L., Gray, K. M., Rinehart, N. J., Tonge, B. J., Lambert, T. J., et al. (2010). Intranasal oxytocin improves emotion recognition for youth with autism spectrum disorders. *Biological Psychiatry, 67*(7), 692–694.

Guoynes, C. D., Simmons, T. C., Downing, G. M., Jacob, S., Solomon, M., & Bales, K. L. (2018). Chronic intranasal oxytocin has dose-dependent effects on central oxytocin and vasopressin systems in prairie voles (Microtus ochrogaster). *Neuroscience, 369,* 292–302.

Handen, B. L., Aman, M. G., Arnold, L. E., Hyman, S. L., Tumuluru, R. V., Lecavalier, L., et al. (2015). Atomoxetine, parent training, and their combination in children with autism spectrum disorder and attention-deficit/hyperactivity disorder. *Journal of the American Academy of Child and Adolescent Psychiatry, 54*(11), 905–915.

Handen, B. L., Johnson, C. R., & Lubetsky, M. (2000). Efficacy of methylphenidate among children with autism and symptoms of attention-deficit hyperactivity disorder. *Journal of Autism and Developmental Disorders, 30*(3), 245–255.

Handen, B. L., Sahl, R., & Hardan, A. Y. (2008). Guanfacine in children with autism and/or intellectual disabilities. *Journal of Developmental and Behavioral Pediatrics, 29*(4), 303–308.

Hardan, A. Y., Jou, R. J., & Handen, B. L. (2005). Retrospective study of quetiapine in children and adolescents with pervasive developmental disorders. *Journal of Autism and Developmental Disorders, 35*(3), 387–391.

Harfterkamp, M., Buitelaar, J. K., Minderaa, R. B., van de Loo-Neus, G., van der Gaag, R. J., & Hoekstra, P. J. (2014). Atomoxetine in autism spectrum disorder: no effects on social functioning; some beneficial effects on stereotyped behaviors, inappropriate speech, and fear of change. *Journal of Child and Adolescent Psychopharmacology, 24*(9), 481–485.

Harfterkamp, M., van de Loo-Neus, G., Minderaa, R. B., van der Gaag, R. J., Escobar, R., Schacht, A., et al. (2012). A randomized double-blind study of atomoxetine versus placebo for attention-deficit/hyperactivity disorder symptoms in children with autism spectrum disorder. *Journal of the American Academy of Child and Adolescent Psychiatry, 51*(7), 733–741.

Hartley-McAndrew, M., & Weinstock, A. (2010). Autism Spectrum Disorder: Correlation between aberrant behaviors. EEG abnormalities and seizures. *Neurol Int, 2*(1), e10.

Harvey, A. T., Rudolph, R. L., & Preskorn, S. H. (2000). Evidence of the dual mechanisms of action of venlafaxine. *Archives of General Psychiatry, 57*(5), 503–509.

Hazell, P. (2007). Drug therapy for attention-deficit/hyperactivity disorder-like symptoms in autistic disorder. *Journal of Paediatric and Child Health, 43*(1–2), 19–24.

Hellings, J. A., Kelley, L. A., Gabrielli, W. F., Kilgore, E., & Shah, P. (1996). Sertraline response in adults with mental retardation and autistic disorder. *Journal of Clinical Psychiatry, 57*(8), 333–336.

Hellings, J. A., Weckbaugh, M., Nickel, E. J., Cain, S. E., Zarcone, J. R., Reese, R. M., et al. (2005). A double-blind, placebo-controlled study of valproate for aggression in youth with pervasive developmental disorders. *Journal of Child and Adolescent Psychopharmacology, 15*(4), 682–692.

Herscu, P., Handen, B. L., Arnold, L. E., Snape, M. F., Bregman, J. D., Ginsberg, L., ... Autism Speaks Autism Clinical Trials, N. (2019). The SOFIA Study: Negative multi-center study of low dose fluoxetine on repetitive behaviors in children and adolescents with autistic disorder. *Journal of Autism and Developmental Disorders*.

Hollander, E., Bartz, J., Chaplin, W., Phillips, A., Sumner, J., Soorya, L., et al. (2007). Oxytocin increases retention of social cognition in autism. *Biological Psychiatry, 61*(4), 498–503.

Hollander, E., Chaplin, W., Soorya, L., Wasserman, S., Novotny, S., Rusoff, J., et al. (2010). Divalproex sodium vs placebo for the treatment of irritability in children and adolescents with autism spectrum disorders. *Neuropsychopharmacology, 35*(4), 990–998.

Hollander, E., Dolgoff-Kaspar, R., Cartwright, C., Rawitt, R., & Novotny, S. (2001). An open trial of divalproex sodium in autism spectrum disorders. *Journal of Clinical Psychiatry, 62*(7), 530–534.

Hollander, E., Kaplan, A., Cartwright, C., & Reichman, D. (2000). Venlafaxine in children, adolescents, and young adults with autism spectrum disorders: an open retrospective clinical report. *Journal of Child Neurology, 15*(2), 132–135.

Hollander, E., Novotny, S., Hanratty, M., Yaffe, R., DeCaria, C. M., Aronowitz, B. R., et al. (2003). Oxytocin infusion reduces repetitive behaviors in adults with autistic and Asperger's disorders. *Neuropsychopharmacology, 28*(1), 193–198.

Hollander, E., Phillips, A., Chaplin, W., Zagursky, K., Novotny, S., Wasserman, S., et al. (2005). A placebo controlled crossover trial of liquid fluoxetine on repetitive behaviors in childhood and adolescent autism. *Neuropsychopharmacology, 30*(3), 582–589.

Hollander, E., Soorya, L., Chaplin, W., Anagnostou, E., Taylor, B. P., Ferretti, C. J., et al. (2012). A double-blind placebo-controlled trial of fluoxetine for repetitive behaviors and global severity in adult autism spectrum disorders. *American Journal of Psychiatry, 169*(3), 292–299.

Hollander, E., Soorya, L., Wasserman, S., Esposito, K., Chaplin, W., & Anagnostou, E. (2006a). Divalproex sodium vs. placebo in the treatment of repetitive behaviours in autism spectrum disorder. *International Journal of Neuropsychopharmacology, 9*(2), 209–213.

Hollander, E., Wasserman, S., Swanson, E. N., Chaplin, W., Schapiro, M. L., Zagursky, K., et al. (2006b). A double-blind placebo-controlled pilot study of olanzapine in childhood/adolescent pervasive developmental disorder. *Journal of Child and Adolescent Psychopharmacology, 16*(5), 541–548.

Horvath, K., Stefanatos, G., Sokolski, K. N., Wachtel, R., Nabors, L., & Tildon, J. T. (1998). Improved social and language skills after secretin administration in patients with autistic spectrum disorders. *Journal of the Association for Academic Minority Physicians, 9*(1), 9–15.

Huffman, L. C., Sutcliffe, T. L., Tanner, I. S., & Feldman, H. M. (2011). Management of symptoms in children with autism spectrum disorders: a comprehensive review of pharmacologic and complementary-alternative medicine treatments. *Journal of Developmental and Behavioral Pediatrics, 32*(1), 56–68.

Hurwitz, R., Blackmore, R., Hazell, P., Williams, K., & Woolfenden, S. (2012). Tricyclic antidepressants for autism spectrum disorders (ASD) in children and adolescents. *Cochrane Database Systematic Reviews,* (3), CD008372.

Ichikawa, H., Mikami, K., Okada, T., Yamashita, Y., Ishizaki, Y., Tomoda, A., et al. (2017). Aripiprazole in the treatment of irritability in children and adolescents with autism spectrum disorder in Japan: A Randomized, Double-blind, Placebo-controlled Study. *Child Psychiatry and Human Development, 48*(5), 796–806.

Jaselskis, C. A., Cook, E. H., Jr., Fletcher, K. E., & Leventhal, B. L. (1992). Clonidine treatment of hyperactive and impulsive children with autistic disorder. *Journal of Clinical Psychopharmacology, 12*(5), 322–327.

Ji, N., & Findling, R. L. (2015). An update on pharmacotherapy for autism spectrum disorder in children and adolescents. *Current Opinion in Psychiatry, 28*(2), 91–101.

Joshi, G., Wozniak, J., Faraone, S. V., Fried, R., Chan, J., Furtak, S., et al. (2016). A prospective open-label trial of memantine hydrochloride for the treatment of social deficits in intellectually capable adults with autism spectrum disorder. *Journal of Clinical Psychopharmacology, 36*(3), 262–271.

Kelsey, J. E. (1996). Dose-response relationship with venlafaxine. *Journal of Clinical Psychopharmacology, 16*(3 Suppl 2), 21S-26S; discussion 26S-28S.

Kem, D. L., Posey, D. J., & McDougle, C. J. (2002). Priapism associated with trazodone in an adolescent with autism. *Journal of the American Academy of Child and Adolescent Psychiatry, 41*(7), 758.

Kemner, C., Willemsen-Swinkels, S. H., de Jonge, M., Tuynman-Qua, H., & van Engeland, H. (2002). Open-label study of olanzapine in children with pervasive developmental disorder. *Journal of Clinical Psychopharmacology, 22*(5), 455–460.

Kent, J. M., Hough, D., Singh, J., Karcher, K., & Pandina, G. (2013). An open-label extension study of the safety and efficacy of risperidone in children and adolescents with autistic disorder. *Journal of Child and Adolescent Psychopharmacology, 23*(10), 676–686.

King, B. H. (2000). Pharmacological treatment of mood disturbances, aggression, and self-injury in persons with pervasive developmental disorders. *Journal of Autism and Developmental Disorders, 30*(5), 439–445.

King, B. H., & Davanzo, P. A. (1996). Buspirone treatment of aggression and self-injury in autistic and nonautistic persons with severe mental retardation. *Developmental Brain Dysfunction, 90*(1), 22–31.

King, B. H., Hollander, E., Sikich, L., McCracken, J. T., Scahill, L., Bregman, J. D., et al. (2009). Lack of efficacy of citalopram in children with autism spectrum disorders and high levels of repetitive behavior: citalopram ineffective in children with autism. *Archives of General Psychiatry, 66*(6), 583–590.

Kolmen, B. K., Feldman, H. M., Handen, B. L., & Janosky, J. E. (1995). Naltrexone in young autistic children: a double-blind, placebo-controlled crossover study. *Journal of the American Academy of Child and Adolescent Psychiatry, 34*(2), 223–231.

Lewitzka, U., Severus, E., Bauer, R., Ritter, P., Muller-Oerlinghausen, B., & Bauer, M. (2015). The suicide prevention effect of lithium: More than 20 years of evidence-a narrative review. *International Journal of Bipolar Disorder, 3*(1), 32.

Loebel, A., Brams, M., Goldman, R. S., Silva, R., Hernandez, D., Deng, L., et al. (2016). Lurasidone for the treatment of irritability associated with autistic disorder. *Journal of Autism and Developmental Disorders, 46*(4), 1153–1163.

Malhi, G. S., Tanious, M., Das, P., Coulston, C. M., & Berk, M. (2013). Potential mechanisms of action of lithium in bipolar disorder. Current understanding. *CNS Drugs, 27*(2), 135–153.

Malone, R. P., Cater, J., Sheikh, R. M., Choudhury, M. S., & Delaney, M. A. (2001). Olanzapine versus haloperidol in children with autistic disorder: An open pilot study. *Journal of the American Academy of Child and Adolescent Psychiatry, 40*(8), 887–894.

Malone, R. P., Delaney, M. A., Hyman, S. B., & Cater, J. R. (2007). Ziprasidone in adolescents with autism: An open-label pilot study. *Journal of Child and Adolescent Psychopharmacology, 17*(6), 779–790.

Mandell, D. S., Morales, K. H., Marcus, S. C., Stahmer, A. C., Doshi, J., & Polsky, D. E. (2008). Psychotropic medication use among Medicaid-enrolled children with autism spectrum disorders. *Pediatrics, 121*(3), e441–448.

Marcus, R. N., Owen, R., Kamen, L., Manos, G., McQuade, R. D., Carson, W. H., et al. (2009). A placebo-controlled, fixed-dose study of aripiprazole in children and adolescents with irritability associated with autistic disorder. *Journal of the American Academy of Child and Adolescent Psychiatry, 48*(11), 1110–1119.

Marcus, R. N., Owen, R., Manos, G., Mankoski, R., Kamen, L., McQuade, R. D., et al. (2011). Safety and tolerability of aripiprazole for irritability in pediatric patients with autistic disorder: A 52-week, open-label, multicenter study. *Journal of Clinical Psychiatry, 72*(9), 1270–1276.

Marrosu, F., Marrosu, G., Rachel, M. G., & Biggio, G. (1987). Paradoxical reactions elicited by diazepam in children with classic autism. *Functional Neurology, 2*(3), 355–361.

Marshall, B. L., Napolitano, D. A., McAdam, D. B., Dunleavy, I. J., Tessing, J. L., & Varrell, J. (2003). Venlafaxine and increased aggression in a female with autism. *Journal of the American Academy of Child and Adolescent Psychiatry, 42*(4), 383–384.

Martin, A., Koenig, K., Anderson, G. M., & Scahill, L. (2003). Low-dose fluvoxamine treatment of children and adolescents with pervasive developmental disorders: A prospective, open-label study. *Journal of Autism and Developmental Disorders, 33*(1), 77–85.

Martin, A., Koenig, K., Scahill, L., & Bregman, J. (1999). Open-label quetiapine in the treatment of children and adolescents with autistic disorder. *Journal of Child and Adolescent Psychopharmacology, 9*(2), 99–107.

Masi, G., Cosenza, A., Mucci, M., & Brovedani, P. (2001). Open trial of risperidone in 24 young children with pervasive developmental disorders. *Journal of the American Academy of Child and Adolescent Psychiatry, 40*(10), 1206–1214.

McCracken, J. T., McGough, J., Shah, B., Cronin, P., Hong, D., Aman, M. G., … Research Units on Pediatric Psychopharmacology Autism. (2002). Risperidone in children with autism and serious behavioral problems. *New England Journal of Medicine, 347*(5), 314–321.

McDougle, C. J., Brodkin, E. S., Naylor, S. T., Carlson, D. C., Cohen, D. J., & Price, L. H. (1998a). Sertraline in adults with pervasive developmental disorders: A prospective open-label investigation. *Journal of Clinical Psychopharmacology, 18*(1), 62–66.

McDougle, C. J., Holmes, J. P., Carlson, D. C., Pelton, G. H., Cohen, D. J., & Price, L. H. (1998b). A double-blind, placebo-controlled study of risperidone in adults with autistic disorder and other pervasive developmental disorders. *Archives of General Psychiatry, 55*(7), 633–641.

McDougle, C. J., Holmes, J. P., Bronson, M. R., Anderson, G. M., Volkmar, F. R., Price, L. H., et al. (1997). Risperidone treatment of children and adolescents with pervasive developmental disorders: A prospective open-label study. *Journal of the American Academy of Child and Adolescent Psychiatry, 36*(5), 685–693.

McDougle, C. J., Kem, D. L., & Posey, D. J. (2002). Case series: Use of ziprasidone for maladaptive symptoms in youths with autism. *Journal of the American Academy of Child and Adolescent Psychiatry, 41*(8), 921–927.

McDougle, C. J., Kresch, L. E., & Posey, D. J. (2000). Repetitive thoughts and behavior in pervasive developmental disorders: Treatment with serotonin reuptake inhibitors. *Journal of Autism and Developmental Disorders, 30*(5), 427–435.

McDougle, C. J., Naylor, S. T., Cohen, D. J., Aghajanian, G. K., Heninger, G. R., & Price, L. H. (1996a). Effects of tryptophan depletion in drug-free adults with autistic disorder. *Archives of General Psychiatry, 53*(11), 993–1000.

McDougle, C. J., Naylor, S. T., Cohen, D. J., Volkmar, F. R., Heninger, G. R., & Price, L. H. (1996b). A double-blind, placebo-controlled study of fluvoxamine in adults with autistic disorder. *Archives of General Psychiatry, 53*(11), 1001–1008.

McDougle, C. J., Scahill, L., Aman, M. G., McCracken, J. T., Tierney, E., Davies, M., et al. (2005). Risperidone for the core symptom domains of autism: Results from the study by the autism network of the research units on pediatric psychopharmacology. *American Journal of Psychiatry, 162*(6), 1142–1148.

McGuire, K., Fung, L. K., Hagopian, L., Vasa, R. A., Mahajan, R., Bernal, P., et al. (2016). Irritability and problem behavior in autism spectrum disorder: A practice pathway for pediatric primary care. *Pediatrics, 137*(Suppl 2), S136–148.

Meyer, J. M., Davis, V. G., Goff, D. C., McEvoy, J. P., Nasrallah, H. A., Davis, S. M., … Lieberman, J. A. (2008). Change in metabolic syndrome parameters with antipsychotic treatment in the CATIE Schizophrenia Trial: Prospective data from phase 1. *Schizophrenia Research, 101*(0), 273–286.

Milin, R., Simeon, J. G., Batth, S., Thatte, S., Dare, G. J., & Walker, S. (2006). An open trial of olanzapine in children and adolescents with Asperger disorder. *Journal of Clinical Psychopharmacology, 26*(1), 90–92.

Ming, X., Gordon, E., Kang, N., & Wagner, G. C. (2008). Use of clonidine in children with autism spectrum disorders. *Brain Development, 30*(7), 454–460.

Minshawi, N. F., Wink, L. K., Shaffer, R., Plawecki, M. H., Posey, D. J., Liu, H., et al. (2016). A randomized, placebo-controlled trial of D-cycloserine for the enhancement of social skills training in autism spectrum disorders. *Molecular Autism, 7,* 2.

Mintz, M., & Hollenberg, E. (2019). Revisiting lithium: Utility for behavioral stabilization in adolescents and adults with autism spectrum disorder. *Psychopharmacology Bulletin, 49*(2), 28–40.

Munesue, T., Nakamura, H., Kikuchi, M., Miura, Y., Takeuchi, N., Anme, T., et al. (2016). Oxytocin for male subjects with autism spectrum disorder and comorbid intellectual disabilities: A randomized pilot study. *Front Psychiatry, 7,* 2.

Nguyen, M., & Murphy, T. (2001). Mirtazapine for excessive masturbation in an adolescent with autism. *Journal of the American Academy of Child and Adolescent Psychiatry, 40*(8), 868–869.

Nicolson, R., Awad, G., & Sloman, L. (1998). An open trial of risperidone in young autistic children. *Journal of the American Academy of Child and Adolescent Psychiatry, 37*(4), 372–376.

Nicolson, R., Craven-Thuss, B., & Smith, J. (2006). A prospective, open-label trial of galantamine in autistic disorder. *Journal of Child and Adolescent Psychopharmacology, 16*(5), 621–629.

Ocakoglu, F. T., Kose, S., Ozbaran, B., & Onay, H. (2018). The oxytocin receptor gene polymorphism -rs237902- is associated with the severity of autism spectrum disorder: A pilot study. *Asian Journal of Psychiatry, 31,* 142–149.

Owen, R., Sikich, L., Marcus, R. N., Corey-Lisle, P., Manos, G., McQuade, R. D., et al. (2009). Aripiprazole in the treatment of irritability in children and adolescents with autistic disorder. *Pediatrics, 124*(6), 1533–1540.

Owley, T., Salt, J., Guter, S., Grieve, A., Walton, L., Ayuyao, N., et al. (2006). A prospective, open-label trial of memantine in the treatment of cognitive, behavioral, and memory dysfunction in pervasive developmental disorders. *Journal of Child and Adolescent Psychopharmacology, 16*(5), 517–524.

Owley, T., Walton, L., Salt, J., Guter, S. J., Jr., Winnega, M., Leventhal, B. L., et al. (2005). An open-label trial of escitalopram in pervasive developmental disorders. *Journal of the American Academy of Child and Adolescent Psychiatry, 44*(4), 343–348.

Paavonen, E. J., Nieminen-von Wendt, T., Vanhala, R., Aronen, E. T., & von Wendt, L. (2003). Effectiveness of melatonin in the treatment of sleep disturbances in children with Asperger disorder. *Journal of Child and Adolescent Psychopharmacology, 13*(1), 83–95.

Panksepp, J., Najam, N., & Soares, F. (1979). Morphine reduces social cohesion in rats. *Pharmacology and Biochemical Behavior, 11*(2), 131–134.

Parker, K. J., Oztan, O., Libove, R. A., Mohsin, N., Karhson, D. S., Sumiyoshi, R. D., … Hardan, A. Y. (2019). A randomized placebo-controlled pilot trial shows that intranasal vasopressin improves social deficits in children with autism. *Science and Translational Medicine, 11*(491).

Pearson, D. A., Santos, C. W., Aman, M. G., Arnold, L. E., Casat, C. D., Mansour, R., et al. (2013). Effects of extended release methylphenidate treatment on ratings of attention-deficit/hyperactivity disorder (ADHD) and associated behavior in children with autism spectrum disorders and ADHD symptoms. *Journal of Child and Adolescent Psychopharmacology, 23*(5), 337–351.

Perry, R., Campbell, M., Adams, P., Lynch, N., Spencer, E. K., Curren, E. L., et al. (1989). Long-term efficacy of haloperidol in autistic children: continuous versus discontinuous drug administration. *Journal of the American Academy of Child and Adolescent Psychiatry, 28*(1), 87–92.

Pizzarelli, R., & Cherubini, E. (2011). Alterations of GABAergic signaling in autism spectrum disorders. *Neural Plastisity, 2011,* 297153.

Pliszka, S., & AACAP Work Group on Quality Issues. (2007). Practice parameter for the assessment and treatment of children and adolescents with attention-deficit/hyperactivity disorder. *Journal of the American Academy of Child and Adolescent Psychiatry, 46*(7), 894–921.

Posey, D. J., Erickson, C. A., Stigler, K. A., & McDougle, C. J. (2006). The use of selective serotonin reuptake inhibitors in autism and related disorders. *Journal of Child and Adolescent Psychopharmacology, 16*(1–2), 181–186.

Posey, D. J., Guenin, K. D., Kohn, A. E., Swiezy, N. B., & McDougle, C. J. (2001). A naturalistic open-label study of mirtazapine in autistic and other pervasive developmental disorders. *Journal of Child and Adolescent Psychopharmacology, 11*(3), 267–277.

Posey, D. J., Kem, D. L., Swiezy, N. B., Sweeten, T. L., Wiegand, R. E., & McDougle, C. J. (2004a). A pilot study of D-cycloserine in subjects with autistic disorder. *American Journal of Psychiatry, 161*(11), 2115–2117.

Posey, D. J., Puntney, J. I., Sasher, T. M., Kem, D. L., & McDougle, C. J. (2004b). Guanfacine treatment of hyperactivity and inattention in pervasive developmental disorders: A retrospective analysis of 80 cases. *Journal of Child and Adolescent Psychopharmacology, 14*(2), 233–241.

Posey, D. J., Litwiller, M., Koburn, A., & McDougle, C. J. (1999). Paroxetine in autism. *Journal of the American Academy of Child and Adolescent Psychiatry, 38*(2), 111–112.

Potenza, M. N., Holmes, J. P., Kanes, S. J., & McDougle, C. J. (1999). Olanzapine treatment of children, adolescents, and adults with pervasive developmental disorders: An open-label pilot study. *Journal of Clinical Psychopharmacology, 19*(1), 37–44.

Quintana, H., Birmaher, B., Stedge, D., Lennon, S., Freed, J., Bridge, J., et al. (1995). Use of methylphenidate in the treatment of children with autistic disorder. *Journal of Autism and Developmental Disorders, 25*(3), 283–294.

Quintana, D. S., Westlye, L. T., Hope, S., Naerland, T., Elvsashagen, T., Dorum, E., et al. (2017). Dose-dependent social-cognitive effects of intranasal oxytocin delivered with novel breath powered device in adults with autism spectrum disorder: a randomized placebo-controlled double-blind crossover trial. *Translational Psychiatry, 7*(5), e1136.

Ratey, J. J., Bemporad, J., Sorgi, P., Bick, P., Polakoff, S., O'Driscoll, G., et al. (1987). Open trial effects of beta-blockers on speech and social behaviors in 8 autistic adults. *Journal of Autism and Developmental Disorders, 17*(3), 439–446.

Reilly, T. H., & Kirk, M. A. (2007). Atypical antipsychotics and newer antidepressants. *Emergency Medicine Clinics of North America, 25*(2), 477–497; abstract x.

Remington, G., Sloman, L., Konstantareas, M., Parker, K., & Gow, R. (2001). Clomipramine versus haloperidol in the treatment of autistic disorder: A double-blind, placebo-controlled, crossover study. *Journal of Clinical Psychopharmacology, 21*(4), 440–444.

Research Units on Pediatric Psychopharmacology Autism, N. (2005). Randomized, controlled, crossover trial of methylphenidate in pervasive developmental disorders with hyperactivity. *Archives of General Psychiatry, 62*(11), 1266–1274.

Rezaei, V., Mohammadi, M. R., Ghanizadeh, A., Sahraian, A., Tabrizi, M., Rezazadeh, S. A., et al. (2010). Double-blind, placebo-controlled trial of risperidone plus topiramate in children with autistic disorder. *Progress in Neuropsychopharmacology Biological Psychiatry, 34*(7), 1269–1272.

Richdale, A. L., & Schreck, K. A. (2009). Sleep problems in autism spectrum disorders: Prevalence, nature, & possible biopsychosocial aetiologies. *Sleep Medicine Review, 13*(6), 403–411.

Rossignol, D. A., & Frye, R. E. (2011). Melatonin in autism spectrum disorders: a systematic review and meta-analysis. *Developmental Medicine and Child Neurology, 53*(9), 783–792.

Rugino, T. A., & Samsock, T. C. (2002). Levetiracetam in autistic children: An open-label study. *Journal of Developmental and Behavioral Pediatrics, 23*(4), 225–230.

Sandman, C. A. (1988). Beta endorphin dysregulation in autistic and self injurious behaviour: A neurodevelopmental hypothesis. *Synapse (New York, N.Y.), 2*, 193–199.

Scahill, L., Aman, M. G., McDougle, C. J., McCracken, J. T., Tierney, E., Dziura, J., et al. (2006). A prospective open trial of guanfacine in children with pervasive developmental disorders. *Journal of Child and Adolescent Psychopharmacology, 16*(5), 589–598.

Scahill, L., Farkas, L., & Hamrin, V. (2001). Lithium in children and adolescents. *Journal of Child and Adolescent Psychiatric Nursing, 14*(2), 89–93.

Scahill, L., McCracken, J. T., King, B. H., Rockhill, C., Shah, B., Politte, L., … Research Units on Pediatric Psychopharmacology Autism, N. (2015). Extended-release guanfacine for hyperactivity in children with autism spectrum disorder. *American Journal of Psychiatry, 172*(12), 1197-1206.

Schreck, K. A., Mulick, J. A., & Smith, A. F. (2004). Sleep problems as possible predictors of intensified symptoms of autism. *Research in Developmental Disabilities, 25*(1), 57–66.

Serret, S., Thummler, S., Dor, E., Vesperini, S., Santos, A., & Askenazy, F. (2015). Lithium as a rescue therapy for regression and catatonia features in two SHANK3 patients with autism spectrum disorder: case reports. *BMC Psychiatry, 15*, 107.

Shea, S., Turgay, A., Carroll, A., Schulz, M., Orlik, H., Smith, I., et al. (2004). Risperidone in the treatment of disruptive behavioral symptoms in children with autistic and other pervasive developmental disorders. *Pediatrics, 114*(5), e634–641.

Siegel, M., Beresford, C. A., Bunker, M., Verdi, M., Vishnevetsky, D., Karlsson, C., et al. (2014). Preliminary investigation of lithium for mood disorder symptoms in children and adolescents with autism spectrum disorder. *Journal of Child and Adolescent Psychopharmacology, 24*(7), 399–402.

Sienaert, P., Dhossche, D. M., Vancampfort, D., De Hert, M., & Gazdag, G. (2014). A clinical review of the treatment of catatonia. *Frontiers in Psychiatry, 5*, 181.

Smith, S. G., Gupta, K., & Smith, S. H. (1995). Effects of naltrexone on self-injury, stereotypy, and social behavior of adults with developmental disabilities. *Journal of Developmental and Physical Disabilities, 7*(2), 137–146.

Snead, R. W., Boon, F., & Presberg, J. (1994). Paroxetine for self-injurious behavior. *Journal of the American Academy of Child and Adolescent Psychiatry, 33*(6), 909–910.

Spence, S. J., & Schneider, M. T. (2009). The role of epilepsy and epileptiform EEGs in autism spectrum disorders. *Pediatric Research, 65*(6), 599–606.

Spencer, D., Marshall, J., Post, B., Kulakodlu, M., Newschaffer, C., Dennen, T., et al. (2013). Psychotropic medication use and polypharmacy in children with autism spectrum disorders. *Pediatrics, 132*(5), 833–840.

Steenweg-de Graaff, J., Roza, S. J., Walstra, A. N., El Marroun, H., Steegers, E. A. P., Jaddoe, V. W. V., et al. (2017). Associations of maternal folic acid supplementation and folate concentrations during pregnancy with foetal and child head growth: The Generation R Study. *European Journal of Nutrition, 56*(1), 65–75.

Steingard, R. J., Zimnitzky, B., DeMaso, D. R., Bauman, M. L., & Bucci, J. P. (1997). Sertraline treatment of transition-associated anxiety and agitation in children with autistic disorder. *Journal of Child and Adolescent Psychopharmacology, 7*(1), 9–15.

Stigler, K. A., Desmond, L. A., Posey, D. J., Wiegand, R. E., & McDougle, C. J. (2004a). A naturalistic retrospective analysis of psychostimulants in pervasive developmental disorders. *Journal of Child and Adolescent Psychopharmacology, 14*(1), 49–56.

Stigler, K. A., Posey, D. J., & McDougle, C. J. (2004b). Aripiprazole for maladaptive behavior in pervasive developmental disorders. *Journal of Child and Adolescent Psychopharmacology, 14*(3), 455–463.

Stigler, K. A., Mullett, J. E., Erickson, C. A., Posey, D. J., & McDougle, C. J. (2012). Paliperidone for irritability in adolescents and young adults with autistic disorder. *Psychopharmacology (Berl), 223*(2), 237–245.

Subcommittee on Attention-Deficit/Hyperactivity, D., Steering Committee on Quality, I., Management, Wolraich, M., Brown, L., Brown, R. T., … Visser, S. (2011). ADHD: clinical practice guideline for the diagnosis, evaluation, and treatment of attention-deficit/hyperactivity disorder in children and adolescents. *Pediatrics, 128*(5), 1007–1022.

Sugie, Y., Sugie, H., Fukuda, T., Ito, M., Sasada, Y., Nakabayashi, M., et al. (2005). Clinical efficacy of fluvoxamine and functional polymorphism in a serotonin transporter gene on childhood autism. *Journal of Autism and Developmental Disorders, 35*(3), 377–385.

Suren, P., Roth, C., Bresnahan, M., Haugen, M., Hornig, M., Hirtz, D., et al. (2013). Association between maternal use of folic acid supplements and risk of autism spectrum disorders in children. *JAMA, 309*(6), 570–577.

Symons, F. J., Thompson, A., & Rodriguez, M. C. (2004). Self-injurious behavior and the efficacy of naltrexone treatment: A quantitative synthesis. *Mental Retardation and Dvelopmental Disabilities Research Review, 10*(3), 193–200.

The Clomipramine Collaborative Study Group. (1991). Clomipramine in the treatment of patients with obsessive-compulsive disorder. *Archives of General Psychiatry, 48*(8), 730–738.

Toichi, M., & Kamio, Y. (2003). Paradoxical autonomic response to mental tasks in autism. *Journal of Autism and Developmental Disorders, 33*(4), 417–426.

Urbano, M., Okwara, L., Manser, P., Hartmann, K., Herndon, A., & Deutsch, S. I. (2014). A trial of D-cycloserine to treat stereotypies in older adolescents and young adults with autism spectrum disorder. *Clinical Neuropharmacology, 37*(3), 69–72.

Vahabzadeh, A., & McDougle, C. J. (2013). Maternal folic acid supplementation and risk of autism. *JAMA, 309*(21), 2208.

Valicenti-McDermott, M. R., & Demb, H. (2006). Clinical effects and adverse reactions of off-label use of aripiprazole in children and adolescents with developmental disabilities. *Journal of Child and Adolescent Psychopharmacology, 16*(5), 549–560.

Valicenti-McDermott, M., Lawson, K., Hottinger, K., Seijo, R., Schechtman, M., Shulman, L., et al. (2019). Sleep problems in children with autism and other developmental disabilities: A brief report. *Journal of Child Neurology, 34*(7), 387–393.

Wang, M., Ramos, B. P., Paspalas, C. D., Shu, Y., Simen, A., Duque, A., et al. (2007). Alpha2A-adrenoceptors strengthen working memory networks by inhibiting cAMP-HCN channel signaling in prefrontal cortex. *Cell, 129*(2), 397–410.

Wang, Y., Wang, M., Rong, Y., He, H., & Yang, C. (2019). Oxytocin therapy for core symptoms in autism spectrum disorder: An updated meta-analysis of randomized controlled trials. *Research in Autism Spectrum Disorders, 64*, 63–75.

Wasserman, S., Iyengar, R., Chaplin, W. F., Watner, D., Waldoks, S. E., Anagnostou, E., et al. (2006). Levetiracetam versus placebo in childhood and adolescent autism: A double-blind placebo-controlled study. *International Journal of Clinical Psychopharmacology, 21*(6), 363–367.

Watanabe, T., Abe, O., Kuwabara, H., Yahata, N., Takano, Y., Iwashiro, N., et al. (2014). Mitigation of sociocommunicational deficits of autism through oxytocin-induced recovery of medial prefrontal activity: A randomized trial. *JAMA Psychiatry, 71*(2), 166–175.

Watanabe, T., Otowa, T., Abe, O., Kuwabara, H., Aoki, Y., Natsubori, T., et al. (2017). Oxytocin receptor gene variations predict neural and behavioral response to oxytocin in autism. *Social Cognitive and Affective Neuroscience, 12*(3), 496–506.

Wilens, T. E., Adler, L. A., Adams, J., Sgambati, S., Rotrosen, J., Sawtelle, R., et al. (2008). Misuse and diversion of stimulants prescribed for ADHD: A systematic review of the literature. *Journal of the American Academy of Child and Adolescent Psychiatry, 47*(1), 21–31.

Wilens, T. E., Spencer, T. J., Biederman, J., Girard, K., Doyle, R., Prince, J., et al. (2001). A controlled clinical trial of bupropion for attention deficit hyperactivity disorder in adults. *American Journal of Psychiatry, 158*(2), 282–288.

Willemsen-Swinkels, S. H., Buitelaar, J. K., Nijhof, G. J., & van England, H. (1995a). Failure of naltrexone hydrochloride to reduce self-injurious and autistic behavior in mentally retarded adults. Double-blind placebo-controlled studies. *Archives of General Psychiatry, 52*(9), 766–773.

Willemsen-Swinkels, S. H., Buitelaar, J. K., Weijnen, F. G., & van Engeland, H. (1995b). Placebo-controlled acute dosage naltrexone study in young autistic children. *Psychiatry Research, 58*(3), 203–215.

Williams, K., Brignell, A., Randall, M., Silove, N., & Hazell, P. (2013). Selective serotonin reuptake inhibitors (SSRIs) for autism spectrum disorders (ASD). *Cochrane Database of Systematic Reviews,* (8), CD004677.

Williams, K. W., Wray, J. J., & Wheeler, D. M. (2005). Intravenous secretin for autism spectrum disorder. *Cochrane Database of Systematic Reviews,* (3), CD003495.

Yamasue, H., Okada, T., Munesue, T., Kuroda, M., Fujioka, T., Uno, Y., … Kosaka, H. (2018). Effect of intranasal oxytocin on the core social symptoms of autism spectrum disorder: A randomized clinical trial. *Molecular Psychiatry.*

Yatawara, C. J., Einfeld, S. L., Hickie, I. B., Davenport, T. A., & Guastella, A. J. (2016). The effect of oxytocin nasal spray on social interaction deficits observed in young children with autism: A randomized clinical crossover trial. *Molecular Psychiatry, 21*(9), 1225–1231.

Zingarelli, G., Ellman, G., Hom, A., Wymore, M., Heidorn, S., & Chicz-DeMet, A. (1992). Clinical effects of naltrexone on autistic behavior. *American Journal of Mental Retardation, 97*(1), 57–63.

Interprofessional Training in Developmental and Behavioral Health Within a Pediatric Residency Program: An Organizational Systems Case Study

Jeffrey D. Shahidullah, Paul W. Kettlewell, Kathryn A. DeHart, Sharon L. Larson, and Paul J. Bellino

Abstract A systemic issue in traditional health service delivery models to children and adolescents is the difficulty in accessing quality developmental/behavioral health (D/BH) care. Contributors to this problem include the lack of available specialty D/BH specialists (e.g., child and adolescent psychiatrists and psychologists, developmental-behavioral pediatricians), as well as issues with insurance coverage and reimbursement when these services are paneled through behavioral health "carve-outs." Given the difficulty in accessing these services, primary care physicians such as pediatricians and pediatric residents often become the de facto D/BH providers. However, a major barrier that these providers express in managing D/BH concerns is the lack of training they receive in medical school and residency. This chapter presents an organizational systems-level case study detailing how concerned stakeholders in a healthcare delivery system and training program have responded to problems pertaining to the need for improved care and resident training in D/BH. The case study intends to inform those who design, revise, and operate service delivery and training systems on a daily basis. To facilitate a more nuanced examination of implementation experiences, a simulated question and answer discussion is included at the end of this chapter.

Those involved in the provision of developmental/behavioral health (D/BH) services to children, adolescents, and their families who receive care in traditional health delivery systems are likely aware of two profound problems that call for attention and response. The first problem concerns the lack of access to care. While 20% of

J. D. Shahidullah (✉)
Department of Psychiatry, University of Texas at Austin Dell Medical School, Austin, TX, USA
e-mail: Jeff.Shahidullah@austin.utexas.edu

P. W. Kettlewell
Department of Psychiatry, Geisinger Health System, Danville, PA, USA

K. A. DeHart · P. J. Bellino
Department of Pediatrics, Geisinger Health System, Danville, PA, USA

S. L. Larson
Center for Population Health Research, Main Line Health System, Thomas Jefferson University, Philadelphia, PA, USA

M. B. McClain et al. (eds.), *Interprofessional Care Coordination for Pediatric Autism Spectrum Disorder*, https://doi.org/10.1007/978-3-030-46295-6_26

children suffer from a D/BH condition (Strine et al., 2008), 80% of them do not receive needed services (Kataoka, Zhang, & Wells, 2002). Reasons for the ineffectiveness in providing D/BH services in these health delivery systems are numerous; chief among them being a shortage of well-trained specialty D/BH providers (Kim, 2003), causing long wait times for care. Even when specialty providers are available, failure of follow-through by patients to these externally referred services occurs frequently (Cummings & O'Donohue, 2011).

Due to this difficulty in accessing services, pediatricians and pediatric residents practicing in primary care (i.e., primary care providers; PCPs) have long been expected to provide basic D/BH services and have become the "de facto" D/BH delivery system (Regier et al., 1993). This reality highlights the second problem in traditional health delivery systems—lack of training in D/BH delivery for PCPs who are expected to manage the 50–70% of their patients who present with D/BH concerns (Belar, 2008; Gatchel & Oordt, 2013).

Not only do pediatric residents report receiving inadequate training in managing D/BH problems (Hampton, Richardson, Bostwick, Ward, & Green, 2015; Shahidullah et al., 2018a, 2018b), but resident training in this area appears to have remained largely stagnant. This conclusion stems from surveys of residents' competencies in managing D/BH problems in 2004 and again in 2013 demonstrating no meaningful changes (Horwitz et al., 2015). In fact, training has remained so stagnant that the American Academy of Pediatrics (AAP) recently issued a policy statement (Foy, Green, Earls, & Committee on Psychosocial Aspects of Child and Family Health, Mental Health Leadership Work Group, 2019) and technical report (Green, Foy, Earls, & AAP Committee on Psychosocial Aspects of Child and Family Health, Mental Health Leadership Work Group, 2019) citing the need for pediatric residency programs to develop curricular innovations to improve residents' attitudes, knowledge, and skills in D/BH service delivery.

Over several years, members of the departments of pediatrics and psychiatry at Geisinger Health System in Danville, Pennsylvania, a large rural health system, held discussions related to these problems in their own delivery system. This process subsequently led to a call for action to address the poor access to D/BH services and shortcomings in pediatric resident training in primary care D/BH delivery. These stakeholders recognized the need to develop and implement an integrated delivery model whereby behavioral health clinicians (BHCs; pediatric psychologists) are embedded in primary care offices to offer greater access to D/BH services by positioning them where patients receive their general medical care.

Because of the advocacy efforts by these stakeholders, a D/BH pilot project was initiated in 2010, which integrated pediatric psychologists into primary care clinics to serve patients in conjunction with the PCP. Three pediatric primary care practice sites were selected for the initial pilot. The goals of the initiative were to improve access to and quality of D/BH care via insertion of evidence-based practices into primary care, while increasing continuity of care with PCPs.

1st Pilot: Integrating Developmental/Behavioral Health Within Primary Care

The results of the pilot were consistently positive with improved access to care, improved patient and PCP satisfaction, positive clinical outcomes for patients, improved quality of life and some cost reductions (see Novotney, 2014 for an overview of the integration of psychologists into primary care). These results were consistent with a recent outcome study of BH integration in pediatric primary care with a 5-year follow demonstrating improved access to quality BH services and averting some of the expected increased costs associated with providing more clinical services (Walter et al., 2019). Additionally, a meta-analysis evaluating data from similar integrated D/BH and primary care models demonstrated broad positive outcomes (Asarnow, Rozenman, Wiblin, & Zeltzer, 2015). This model has led to increased access to D/BH services for many children and their families that otherwise may not have been seen by a BHC. These families greatly benefited from the significantly shorter wait times to see a BHC, as typically they were seen on the same day or even same visit. Additionally, having the visit within the PCP office reduced the perceived stigma sometimes identified from obtaining services at a D/BH specialists' office.

Consistent feedback from the pediatric PCPs emphasized appreciation and enthusiasm for the integrated care model. Access to quality care improved in the integrated care sites as PCPs were doing a better job of identifying D/BH concerns and introducing these patients to the BHC during their clinic visit. However, the clinical model was not adequately addressing the D/BH training needs of pediatric residents so that residents could manage the BH concerns more independently (without simply using the on-site BHC as a readily available referral source). Stakeholders from psychiatry and pediatrics continued to meet to identify possible methods of improving direct training in D/BH for residents. Two major limitations to delivering training were identified: (1) lack of internal funding/compensation to dedicate additional time to teaching from BHCs and (2) lack of time in the pediatric residency training process that could be devoted to new educational elements given an already full curriculum. Realizing these limitations, the new model of enhanced residency training would need to be structured to be both time and cost-effective.

2nd Pilot: Improving Resident Education in Primary Care Developmental/Behavioral Health

The second wave of this new D/BH delivery system incorporated the same integration of care as the 1st wave, but expanded the model to include the pediatric residency training site (i.e., continuity clinic). In efforts to be systematic and responsive to AAP's call (Foy et al., 2019; Green et al., 2019) for addressing D/BH competencies for future pediatricians through pediatric residency training, stakeholders focused on frequently occurring clinical presentations (e.g., ADHD, anxiety, depression, suicidality) and learner variables (i.e., knowledge and skills) specifically highlighted in the policy statements. Residents receiving enhanced training in D/BH in a primary care delivery system were expected to not only improve their knowledge and skills in D/BH, but also develop competencies to work in similar interprofessional and team-based settings in the future.

The use of the integrated D/BH pediatric primary care model in community practice sites plus the expansion into the continuity clinic site, resulted in the ability to address both previously identified problems: (1) improving access to D/BH care and (2) improving D/BH training for resident PCPs. Details about how this was accomplished as well as the key components of both the integrated service delivery model and the enhanced training model are next described in this chapter. The synergy between these two parallel efforts was critical to the success in making both comprehensive and sustainable health system changes. This chapter also discusses the importance of including both of these system changes as vital steps for making sustainable advancement in the D/BH delivery approach. Both quantitative and qualitative data were collected pertaining to D/BH learning enhancement of pediatric residents. The reader is referred to other sources to review that data, as the focus of this article is to describe the process by which the organizational innovation occurred.

Systems Intervention

Development

Stakeholder feedback. Clinicians and leaders in the health delivery system uniformly recognized that inadequate access to care and provider training clearly existed. This resulted in informal discussion among stakeholders and, subsequently, a more refined response from system leaders based on these stakeholder frustrations. The following are the key stakeholders and those committed to system changes described in the case study.

1. ***Behavioral health clinicians***. These included primarily pediatric psychologists, but also child and adolescent psychiatrists who have provided services in specialty mental health clinics and other settings in the hospital including consults in the children's hospital, emergency department, and a mixed adult/adolescent inpatient psychiatric unit. These providers were acutely aware of the limited services for children and adolescents with D/BH problems available in their rural catchment area.
2. ***Those involved in training of pediatric residents in developmental/behavioral health***. These included pediatric psychologists, developmental-behavioral pediatricians, and the pediatric residency and assistant residency program directors. These stakeholders recognized the inherent difficulty in being expected to provide quality D/BH training during the required 4-week developmental-behavioral

pediatrics (DBP) rotation. This rotation lacked the longitudinal continuity that residents cited as most beneficial to developing and honing skills in this area. There was a push by faculty stakeholders to embed D/BH training across the 3 years of residency training, rather than relying too heavily on the DBP rotation by itself to address these needs.

3. ***Child and adolescent patients and their families***. Patients and families have frequently reported problems with access to D/BH care (appropriate care provided in a reasonable time period at a reasonable distance from their home).
4. ***Pediatric primary care clinicians in community practice settings***. These include general pediatricians, family physicians, and pediatric midlevel practitioners. They have reported longstanding difficulty in providing D/BH care due to time and training limitations as well as access to appropriate D/BH specialists for patient referrals.
5. ***Department leaders***. These include the Chairperson and Vice President/Administrative Lead for the Department of Psychiatry for Geisinger Health System. Although they were acutely aware of problems patients have had with access to D/BH services, they also articulated a clear need for implementing service delivery approaches that are financially sustainable.
6. ***Philanthropist***. This individual made a significant financial contribution for innovative D/BH services and challenged the system to expand services for children and adolescents.
7. ***System health plan leaders***. Psychologists and Department of Psychiatry leaders made requests to leaders of the systems' health plan (which covers approximately one-third of the patients served by the health system) to support changes in how D/BH services are delivered and paid for and how providers are trained in D/BH. They accepted the message and provided collaboration in developing service delivery innovations and provided financial support over three years for both an integrated care pilot project and a pilot project for enhanced D/BH training for pediatric residents.
8. ***Director of behavioral health research***. This individual embraced these innovations and offered support and expertise in adequately measuring the outcomes of these innovations.
9. ***Senior leadership of the health system***. These leaders were interested in the specific innovations implemented and the outcome data. Primarily because of their awareness of limitations with traditional service delivery models and the positive outcomes from prior pilot projects, they have supported expansion within the health system. In fact, this health delivery system at large has developed a reputation for encouraging innovation in healthcare delivery. Systems' leaders have had a history of being relatively flexible and supportive of innovation including implementation/evaluation of pilot projects to improve care.

The following sections describe the development of the two parallel innovations—D/BH integration in primary care and enhanced D/BH training for pediatric residents. Although these two processes enhance and impact the other, each will be described separately for clarity.

Steps taken to develop an integrated developmental/behavioral health service delivery system.

1. ***Awareness of limitations of the current developmental/behavioral health delivery model***. These innovations would not have occurred without an awareness of the limitations of the traditional D/BH delivery system. These include long wait times from initial referral for D/BH services to the first appointment, high no-show rates to specialty clinics, problems with insurance coverage (including lack of insurance, limited insurance for mental health services, inconsistency of D/BH clinicians participating with some BH carve-out insurance companies), and D/BH outpatient specialty clinics being located at significant distances from patient's homes and PCP clinics.
2. ***Financial support***. A local philanthropist challenged decision-makers in the system to provide quality D/BH care that is timely and sufficient to children and adolescents. A financial gift from this donor provided freedom for the stakeholders to consider many options and challenge the assumptions of traditional D/BH service delivery approaches with an aim to identify possible alternatives, such as an integrated primary care D/BH model.
3. ***Identify/adapt other successful integrated primary care behavioral health models***. Discussions with directors and providers from other successful systems located in rural and underserved areas across the United States were conducted and provided a more detailed understanding of their models and how specific aspects of it may be replicated. Additionally, a pediatric psychologist and a pediatric psychology postdoctoral trainee were recruited from an existing program, which had already successfully implemented integrated primary care D/BH models.
4. ***Garnering support from key departments (Psychiatry, Pediatrics)***. This occurred in a variety of ways including informal discussions, presentations at internal conferences such as pediatric and psychiatry grand rounds, and presentations/discussions at administrative meetings.
5. ***Presentation to leaders of the systems health plan***. Advocates from the departments of psychiatry and pediatrics made a request to leaders of the systems' health plan to present their concerns about the D/BH delivery system and the need for change. This request was received positively with an assigned task to design a pilot project and evaluate the consequences of that pilot project. Health plan leaders then provided financial support for the initial pilot project.
6. ***Needs assessment with pediatric PCPs***. Recognizing the importance of input from PCPs, an early step was to assess their views about problems with the current service model to identify their perceived areas of greatest need and suggestions for changes. Several specific problem areas were identified, although the PCP's overarching concern was the lack of access to quality D/BH care.
7. ***Pilot project in which psychologists were fully integrated in primary care sites***. Several potential sites were considered (site visits, staff interviews) and three sites were selected based on factors such as perceived need, enthusiasm

of PCPs for an integrated care model, projected volume of patients and practical issues such as space and administrative support. At the beginning of this pilot project, the PCP attendings and psychologists working collaboratively in the three pilot sites participated in a two-day training provided by *The Reach Institute* (www.thereachinstitute.org/)—a multi-disciplinary organization with a prominent history of training PCPs in interdisciplinary collaboration and in the dissemination of high-quality scientific findings into applied settings.

8. ***Development of a research design to evaluate outcomes***. Metrics assessed included access to care, patient satisfaction, provider satisfaction, patient outcomes such as target behavior and quality of life changes, degree of collaboration between PCPs and BHCs, and costs. This research design involved naturally occurring control methods that allowed comparison of the results from the three integrated care sites with (a) those same sites prior to implementation of the integrated care model and (b) non-integrated care primary care sites in the system (see Petts et al., 2018; Shahidullah et al., 2017, 2018a, 2018b for outcomes evaluations from this project).
9. ***Review of the results from the integrated primary care behavioral health implementation pilot project***. Data obtained from the pilot project demonstrated consistent positive findings: improved patient satisfaction with care, improved PCP satisfaction with care, three-fold improvement in access to care, improved quality of life, and cost changes such as reductions in prescriptions for all medication and emergency department use.
10. ***Presentations of details of the pilot project including data about outcomes to health system leaders***. Presentations were made to a group of the health systems' leaders and then at a quarterly meeting of the systems' board of directors. This led to support for expansion of this model to three more primary care sites (including the pediatric primary care training clinic for pediatric residents highlighted in this case study).

Steps taken to enhance developmental/behavioral health training for pediatric residents.

Once the integrated care delivery model was implemented successfully for several years and was demonstrated to improve access to D/BH services, an additional initiative was undertaken to address the issue of inadequate training for pediatric residents in primary care D/BH delivery and team-based care. To address this problem, the following steps were taken:

1. ***Awareness of the limits of the 1-month mandated developmental-behavioral pediatrics rotation for residents***. The health systems' pediatric residency program has an ACGME-mandated rotation in DBP. This rotation fulfills the national requirements for training in D/BH. Although providing some worthwhile training, the limitations of this model include (1) limited amount of days spent by residents in the rotation (actual time spent engaged in D/BH education is impacted by resident vacation, post-call duty hours restrictions, and required longitudinal continuity clinic participation one-half day per week); (2) unpredictable patient types (it is difficult to ensure that the most pertinent diagnostic categories are

consistently assessed or treated by residents during the rotation); (3) a skewed patient population from which to learn as developmental-behavioral pediatricians and pediatric psychologists often see more severe or atypical patient types that are less frequently managed by general pediatricians (e.g., complex patients with autism, genetic conditions, eating disorders versus problems like ADHD and adolescent depression); (4) patients in specialty clinics are usually already diagnosed and have progressed in their presentation so the initial diagnosis and triage are not part of the training; and (5) treatment in the specialty setting does not account for the limited time or resources residents will face in their eventual outpatient clinics.

2. ***Development of a developmental/behavioral health training task force***. This group was formed to consider ways to enhance D/BH training of pediatric residents in the context of an integrated care model. The task force was composed of those involved as supervisors of the mandated DBP training month as well as residency directors. Members included the pediatric residency director, assistant residency director, two developmental-behavioral pediatricians, two child psychiatrists, and four pediatric psychologists. This task force was charged with developing an enhanced training model consistent with the AAP's (2009; this Policy Statement was recently updated by the Foy et al., 2019 Policy Statement and Green et al., 2019 Technical Report) call for innovation. The task force recommended expanding the integrated care model to the pediatric resident continuity and acute care clinic and providing enhanced D/BH training to residents in that setting in addition to the DBP rotation.
3. ***Development of guiding principles of enhanced developmental/behavioral health training***. The D/BH Training Task Force developed three guiding principles for their approach. First, the training model should fit consistently with the integrated care delivery model, such that the BH providers in the primary care sites are the key staff members that participate in the D/BH training for the residents. Second, the training model should be financially feasible and sustainable. Although the enhanced model is expected to require more staff time and subsequently more expense, it should be developed in a way that can be cost and time-efficient. Third, the training model should be able to be replicated and evaluated. This would require clear descriptions of the model so that others could replicate and evaluate the program.
4. ***Request for internal funding***. Funding was obtained through an internal "Quality Fund" supported by the system's health plan, which partially supported two years of implementation of this training innovation. This internal funding source has supported other innovative approaches to health care delivery within the health system, including support for the development and evaluation of the initial integrated care pilot project.
5. ***Placement of behavioral health clinicians within the continuity and acute care training clinic***. In September 2015, a pediatric psychologist and postdoctoral fellow began working full time in the training clinic with the dual goal of facilitating the integrated care delivery model and providing enhanced D/BH training via integrated service delivery and didactic exposure components. This location

served as the site for both resident general pediatric continuity clinic as well as the training site for pediatric urgent care. Key elements of the service delivery model included two BHCs embedded on-site for 5 days a week. These clinicians shared office space with attending and resident PCPs where they were available during clinic hours to receive what have been termed "warm handoffs" and "curbside consults." Warm handoffs consist of brief, unscheduled encounters during which the PCP introduces the patient to the BHC for brief assessment and intervention for D/BH concerns. Curbside consults are defined as brief consultations regarding a specific patient issue or broad D/BH topic from the BHC to the PCP without bringing the BHC to the exam room to meet a patient.

The BHCs' schedules were split to ensure that one of the two was always available for unscheduled warm handoffs and consults while the other provider was with their scheduled visits. Resident PCPs would either send a page to the BHC or precept directly with the BHC in conjunction with the attending PCP after identifying a D/BH issue with their patient. The BHC and resident PCP would briefly meet to discuss the patient's history and reason for referral before the PCP would introduce the BHC to the patient in the exam room. Having a BHC always available for warm handoffs removed the need for PCPs to interrupt the BHC in their office/exam room while they were with scheduled patients.

6. ***Curriculum development***. A curriculum was subsequently developed collaboratively by members of the departments of pediatrics and psychiatry based on the needs assessment and other stakeholder feedback. The curriculum consisted of two major elements—a didactic exposure component and an integrated service delivery experiential component (see Table 1). The didactic exposure included presentations delivered by BHCs, readings/quizzes on specific BH topics, and facilitated vignettes and case discussion. The integrated service delivery exposure consisted of warm-hand-offs, curbside consults, and clinical observations with performance feedback delivered by BHPs. A standardized patient simulation training was initiated 2 years later in 2017. In addition to facilitating learning enhancement in the context of more realistic clinical scenarios, Standardized patients also offer a mechanism in which to assess D/BH competencies on actual patient interactions is compared to simply relying on trainee self-report of their attitudes, knowledge, and competence (Shahidullah & Kettlewell, 2017). See Petts, Shahidullah, Kettlewell, and DeHart (2018) and Petts, Shahidullah, Jaques, Kettlewell, and DeHart (2019) for outcomes in response to standardized patient trainings within this D/BH curriculum. Standardized patient training was also used successfully with other pediatric resident learners within Geisinger (see Whitehead, Shahidullah, Kettlewell, Quinlan, & Strony, 2017 for outcomes from Geisinger's emergency medicine residents).
7. ***Development of a research plan to evaluate outcomes of the enhanced training curriculum***. Rather than considering the broad outcomes of the integrated care pilot project (access to care, patient satisfaction, cost, patient outcomes), the quantitative outcomes selected were specific to measuring changes in pediatric residents. These included key learner variables suggested by AAP (2009) of

Table 1 Enhanced training curricula for pediatric residents

Didactic exposure	
Lectures on D/BH topics	• Consists of BHPs (psychologist and postdoctoral fellow) delivering lectures on common BH concerns in primary care • 12 total lecture hours throughout year; approximately one per month • Topics included: *The Art of the Behavioral Health Referral, Behavior Management I & II, ADHD I & II, Anxiety I & II, Depression I & II, Suicide/Crisis Response I & II, Sleep, Feeding, Toileting, Child Abuse, Medical Unexplained Physical Symptoms, Common Factors I & II, Collaborating with Schools*
Readings and quizzes	• Consists of assigning readings for residents to read before each lecture • Readings consisted of relevant practice parameters or standards of care for each topic; if formal practice parameters or standards of care did not exist, then relevant journal articles were selected for each topic; resources from the AAP's Mental Health Toolkit[a] • Pre-lecture quizzes were administered to residents for some topics (e.g., ADHD, anxiety, depression, suicidality); feedback and discussion of answers were embedded into the lectures
Case vignettes/discussions	• Consists of residents reading case vignettes corresponding to each lecture topic, then describing BH concerns and identifying appropriate evaluation steps, diagnosis, and treatment plans based on information presented in the lecture • Case discussions are built into lectures and discussed as a group • Time is allotted to discuss actual cases that residents see in continuity clinic
Standardized patient simulations[b]	• Consisted of trained and paid child/adult actors enacting commonly occurring behavioral health scenarios for training pediatric resident training purposes • Observation and performance feedback was provided individually by BHC and faculty preceptors as well as in a group format ("fishbowl" method)

(continued)

Table 1 (continued)

Integrated primary care exposure	
Warm handoffs	• Consists of on-site BHPs (pediatric psychologist and postdoctoral fellow) collaborating with residents on BH concerns through direct patient care • PCP directly introduces patient to BHP at the time of patient's medical visit • To facilitate enhanced learning, accommodations were made to residents schedules to allow them to remain in the room to observe BHPs interactions with the patient
Curbside consults	• Consists of on-site BHPs collaborating with residents through indirect (informal discussions in resident clinic workroom) patient care • The resident informally obtains information or advice from the BHP to assist in the management of a patient with BH concerns
In vivo observation/performance feedback	• Consists of BHPs being in the room to observe residents in their conducting evaluations for ADHD, anxiety, depression, and/or suicidality, and to provide performance feedback to the resident after the clinical encounter • Feedback sessions were standardized to include the joint completion of a checklist • Checklist components consisted of degree to which the resident adhered to evidence-based practice parameters for a given condition as well as their use of "common factors" in the patient interaction (asking open-ended questions, reflective listening, allowing the patient ample time to talk) • This discussion included time for residents to self-reflect and assess their performance as well as to identify action steps to improve future performance
Joint precepting	• Psychologist precepts residents and psychology fellows in shared space • Psychologist also precepts the resident in conjunction with medical preceptor

[a]https://www.aap.org/en-us/advocacy-and-policy/aap-health-initiatives/Mental-Health/Pages/Addressing-Mental-Health-Concerns-in-Primary-Care-A-Clinicians-Toolkit.aspx
[b]This training enhancement began in 2017 and was not part of the first 2 years of the D/BH curricula

knowledge and skills. Surveys and focus groups were administered at the beginning and end of the training year to measure growth over time in response to the curriculum. The Geisinger IRB provided approval for all data collection procedures. In an effort to demonstrate that learner variables improved over time in response to the curriculum (rather than other factors such as maturation or clinical experiences/opportunities within the residency program), a control group of pediatric residents from comparable pediatric residency programs in the region were included. Sites did not differ significantly in their baseline knowledge and skills scores. See Shahidullah et al. (2017 IJHSE; 2018 NJ Pediatrics) for a review of the survey instrument, data collection methodology, and quantitative outcomes. Preliminary results indicate greater improvement in skills scores for residents in this pilot project who worked within the integrated care model alongside pediatric psychologists, when compared to residents at comparison sites. Qualitative data was also collected via focus groups held with pediatric residents both prior to and after integration with pediatric psychologists in the primary care continuity clinic occurred to inquire about attitudes, comfort, and confidence in managing D/BH concerns. Focus groups with a comparison site's residents were also held as a control group. Discussion of these results is beyond the scope of this chapter. However, the reader is referred to Petts et al. (2018) for a comprehensive review of the focus group methodology and outcomes.

Curriculum Implementation Case Study

The following case study describes the curriculum implementation chronologically from the beginning (July 2015) to the end (June 2016) of the pediatric residency training year.

July

At the beginning of the residency training year, both quantitative and qualitative needs assessment data were collected and ongoing discussions were held with systems stakeholders and the residency program leadership and training faculty. The obtained data indicated a clear need for enhanced D/BH training. Two BHCs were assigned to provide integrated D/BH services to clinic patients as well as to develop a didactic curriculum to be delivered in conjunction with this service integration. In an effort to maximize BHC availability given their clinical responsibilities, the didactics occurred during the residents Morning Report time slot, prior to usual clinic hours. The utilization of an already recurring educational time slot for residents ensured that as many participants as possible would be present. The didactic curriculum was developed based on the feedback from the initial needs assessment and focus groups transcripts. Participants in the focus group were asked about specific D/BH conditions they felt uncomfortable handling and would like focused didactics to help improve their knowledge and skills. Residents largely identified depression and anxiety as areas with uncertainly for which they would rely on making a referral. A number of more common D/BH issues that regularly presented to the general pediatrician were also included although not specifically identified by the focus group data. These include topics such as somatic complaints/medically unexplained physical symptoms, trauma, suicidality, academic underachievement/learning disabilities, and procedural anxiety. The lack of identification of these issues by residents suggests either their lack of recognition of the prevalence of these conditions or lack of recognition of the potential role that BHCs can have in their management.

September

In September, two BHCs were embedded (shared space, office staff, and electronic health record [EHR]) in the continuity and acute care training clinic and began providing training via integrated service delivery. To be responsive to training needs, additional mechanisms to receive iterative feedback from residents and training stakeholders were implemented. Individual brief interviews with chief residents and select residents from each academic level were held within the first 2 months of training, and then periodically throughout the year. Additionally, the two BH training faculty attended all monthly primary care office management meetings for clinic staff which included the pediatric medical faculty. The agenda for these meetings included defined time to discuss progress, updates, and issues pertaining to both the integrated service delivery and didactic exposure for residents. Feedback was received from faculty that informed intervention/curriculum refinement throughout the training year. During the first meeting, two issues were raised by the BHCs. The first pertained to the lack of D/BH referrals received early on, compared to what was expected based on D/BH referral patterns at the other previously established primary care clinics in the hospital system. One hypothesis was that the academic school year had just begun and thus academic, developmental, behavioral, and emotional problems had not begun to be fully realized. However, another hypothesis, stemming from the needs assessment focus group data, suggested that the lack of referrals was due to a general lack of awareness on the part of residents as to the range of possible D/BH concerns that could potentially be addressed in primary care in general, and by BHCs specifically, or possibly the residents were not asking families about these issues.

Given the initial underutilization of the BHC in the clinic setting, an adaptation of the didactic curriculum was made. Rather than beginning as planned with the behavior management module, the BHCs and other training faculty determined that the initial lecture should provide a general overview to D/BH and the range of possible and appropriate referrals, with specific directions for the warm handoff and curbside consult process.

The second issue raised by the BHCs came from the recognition that residents had the potential to achieve a higher degree of learning through the referral. It was noted that residents would often make the handoff to the BHC and then leave the exam room to see their next scheduled patient. Although efficient from a patient throughput standpoint, it resulted in missed opportunities for training as residents did not remain in the room to observe the BHC delivering time-limited evaluation and intervention. While no solution materialized that would encompass all situations, it was agreed upon that both BHCs and medical preceptors would encourage residents who had available time to remain in the room and observe. Preceptors also agreed to provide as much flexibility as possible in order to facilitate this interaction such as reassigning waiting patients to other residents who had openings. After this meeting and discussion, BHCs noticed an improvement in the number of residents who were able to remain in the room to observe the BHCs clinical interaction. Moreover, many of these residents shared that they found the experience to be beneficial to their learning.

October

BHCs began delivering the bi-weekly didactic curriculum for the duration of the training year. The didactics were delivered from 7:30 to 8:00 am during the Morning Report. The short time slot forced BHCs to keep the talks focused and applicable. Typically, there was at least an 80% attendance rate for the 33 residents in the program. At least one of the two chief residents and usually one faculty member was in attendance. This provided another avenue of quality control by having feedback from faculty on the relevance of lectures to training needs and objectives, as well as general feedback on presentation delivery. Feedback from all participants largely indicated that the lectures were beneficial and few changes needed to be made. However, some suggestions included making the lectures align with the American Board of Pediatrics Certifying Exam content and saving time at the end of lecture to discuss actual cases seen in continuity clinic.

November

During the first 2 months of enhanced D/BH training, warm handoffs and curbside consults were the extent of the integrated service delivery training components. However, informal feedback from residents indicated that their optimal learning typically came through authentic exposure to clinical situations and subsequent performance feedback. They noted that this type of learning was commonly facilitated by using simulated patients in their medical school training, although they had never had similar experiences in which the focus was on D/BH concerns. It was suggested that the BHC may be well-positioned to accompany the residents into the exam room, not to provide care, but to simply observe the resident and provide feedback. Training faculty worked with the systems' research center to develop a clinical observation checklist rubric that aligned with practice parameters (see Shahidullah et al., 2017 IJHSE; Shahidullah et al., 2018a, 2018b NJ Pediatrics for descriptions) for several of the most commonly presenting concerns in clinic and identified as areas of focus in the AAP's (2009) policy statement. Collaboration with the research center ensured that the checklists were developed and scored in such a way that they could be used for systematic follow-up evaluation.

In mid-November, BHCs began observing residents during actual patient encounters when specific D/BH concerns were identified in an effort to evaluate the resident's patient interactions as well as provide management for these concerns. After the patient encounter, the resident would briefly meet with the BHC to review the clinical care checklist and discuss the components that they carried out in alignment with evidence-based practice parameters. Strengths were emphasized and areas for improvement were also generated. These conversations were confidential and information was not shared with the resident's attendings, medical preceptors, or residency program faculty. Scores were for resident education and self-monitoring only, not for research purposes.

December

Around the mid-point of the training year, additional feedback was received from residents and training faculty through individual interviews as well as the monthly clinic staff meetings. It was noted that residents found it suboptimal to pause an encounter when they identified a patient that had a D/BH concern in order to have a BHC observe the visit. This practice was deemed impractical and disruptive to patient flow and resident-patient rapport. A solution was alternatively developed to have the residents and the BHC meet in the morning before clinic to review and discuss patient lists and identify those scheduled appointments that clearly described the reason for appointment in the EHR as fitting a D/BH category. When identified in advance, the BHC would plan to be available to go into the exam room with the resident from the start of the appointment, after receiving verbal approval from patient, to observe and provide performance feedback.

This strategy was immediately implemented and improved communication and coordination of care. When BHCs sat down with each resident at the outset as they reviewed patients and pre-charted, they were not only able to identify which patients they could potentially have a BHC provide in vivo performance feedback, but also which patients had a high likelihood of eliciting a warm handoff. This coordination also facilitated opportunities curbside consultation from the BHC on specific patient concerns or D/BH topics in general.

January

January brought a noticeable increase in patients presenting with positive depression screens via clinic-wide use of the PHQ-9 for all adolescents. BHCs were available to manage these patient concerns via warm handoffs to conduct suicide risk assessments and provide intervention. Although at times, after making the handoff to the BHC, residents needed to see their next scheduled patient, it was strongly encouraged that residents remain in the room and continue with the patient interview, assessing level and nature of suicidal risk with the BHC available to provide real-time observation and feedback before the handoff was made. If able, after the formal handoff, the resident remained in the room in order to observe the BHC establish rapport, carry out a suicide risk assessment, and arrive at a disposition. After a plan was implemented, a time was arranged for the resident and BHC to discuss the case in more depth in conjunction with the medical preceptor or attending.

Despite the availability of BHCs to provide support for suicidal crises during continuity clinic hours (typically 8 am to 5 pm), residents did not have immediate access to BHCs during all Acute Care Clinic hours (weekend mornings and weeknight evenings). Without a BHC present during these times, resident and attending PCPs sent these patients immediately to the emergency room (ER). In some cases, this was an appropriate disposition. However, in many cases the ER transfer was not indicated, as the patient may not have had any plan or intent beyond ideation. In these cases, an appropriate alternative option may have been to send the patient home with a safety plan and communicate with the BHC requesting an urgent appointment for the next clinic day. In response to the increased demand and requests for more training on responding to suicidal crises, an extra lecture was added to the didactic schedule in the spring which addressed voluntary vs involuntary hospital admission, suicide risk assessments (including evaluation of risk/protective factors), and developing a safety plan with the patient and their family.

June

At the end of the training year, in addition to the quantitative (see Shahidullah et al., 2017 IJHSE; 2018 NJ Pediatrics) and qualitative (see Petts et al., 2018) data collection, feedback was again obtained from residents ($n = 13$) through a brief survey asking the following three questions (topics are then listed in parentheses based on frequency counts and followed by any descriptive comments):

1. *What lecture topic was most helpful to you?* ADHD ($n = 5$), toileting ($n = 4$), behavior management ($n = 2$), anxiety, depression, referral resources available, motivational interviewing, suicide, learning disabilities, child abuse/trauma/ACES ($n = 1$ each), left blank ($n = 2$)
2. *What lecture topic was least helpful to you?* ADHD: "because we talk about it a lot, but I still think it's worth going over, $n = 1$); school programs ($n = 1$), left blank ($n = 6$); (other comments: "sometimes material very repetitive")
3. *Is there a topic that was not covered that you believe would be helpful? Please list*: bullying ($n = 2$), eating disorders ($n = 2$); substance abuse ($n = 2$), diet/exercise/weight ($n = 1$), left blank or "none" response ($n = 4$)

Teaching faculty and pediatric residency program leadership provided feedback suggesting that residents needed more training in interpersonal communication skills, particularly working from a motivational interviewing framework. Possible next steps in curriculum development should include training specifically on interpersonal communication and patient engagement skills focused on fostering patient autonomy and shared decision-making (i.e., "Common Factors"; see Foy, 2014 article for description). This may likely come from expanding the motivational interviewing module and perhaps use of the institution's standardized patient committee.

Conclusion

This organizational systems-level case study described how enhanced D/BH training was delivered in conjunction with an integrated service delivery model. This integrated care model offered a platform that created synergy between these two parallel efforts that were developed to specifically address two major problems in traditional health service delivery models—lack of access that these systems afford to D/BH care and the lack of training that PCPs receive in D/BH and team-based care. As described in the case study, this effort occurred over the course of several years and with the fiscal and logistical support from numerous stakeholders. While some aspects of the innovation may be amenable for off-site adoption, other aspects may not be without substantial financial or personnel support. Future research should assess the feasibility of delivering the training components with a high degree of fidelity. As all elements of this program may not be feasible within other sites, future research should evaluate the implementation and individual validity of the specific components within the program (didactics, warm handoffs, curbside consults, observations with performance feedback, joint precepting, standardized patients). This may be accomplished with a future dismantling study or component analysis study. Finally, some programs may be capable of utilizing additional training modalities that were not included in the package such as the use of standardized patients, computer-based learning, or electronic health record audits with performance feedback. The "value-added" that these learning enhancement opportunities provide must be evaluated in the context of their inherent "costs" (e.g., patient flow disruptions in busy clinics as a result of having the resident observe the BHC or vice versa). Financial costs should also be explored in future research by including key cost metrics given the importance and desire for financially sustainable D/BH services and training support. Partnerships with healthcare economists to examine this data could serve as an additional advocacy tool for the D/BH training initiative. To facilitate a more nuanced examination of implementation experiences, a simulated question and answer discussion is included at the end of this chapter.

Authors Respond to Questions Concerning the Systems-Level Innovation: Dr. Paul Kettlewell (PK), Psychologist Involved in Training Curricula Implementation, Dr. Paul Bellino (PB), Pediatric Residency Program Director

Question 1. You described several possible options for enhanced D/BH training (didactics, shared care for patients, case conferences, simulated patients, etc.). How did you decide which training approaches to use in the training model and which approaches to exclude?

PB: Determining the method for training for me is more of a practical thing than any data driven decision. The truth is that time for any additional educational activity in residency is limited, so activities that overlay or enhance already developed and practiced curricular elements fit better into this already cramped timeframe. Also, I am a believer that one learns best from experience rather than a presentation or some on-line activity that requires no effort other than clicking a mouse. When a resident is engaged in the entire process of managing a real patient, taking responsibility for all elements of patient care as well as the risk associated with the outcome, they will not forget the lessons they learn. I personally prefer to expose residents to these situations in their training as I believe it will offer a lasting and deep understanding of the issues at hand. Since not all possible scenarios can be covered during the process of caring for patients, additional lectures or other formats should be used to supplement the needed medical knowledge, but these should still try to draw off the experiential learning process obtained during the actual care of patients.

Having said that, there are some times where a quick passage of medical knowledge is all that is needed. In those cases, an hour lecture or self-directed activity is adequate. It seems to me that you can pack in more information with a lecture, but younger physicians seem to like doing role-playing or case-based discussions. These are common processes in medical schools now. Personally, I think they are a waste of time, but I am from a different era than these guys. So, when I can, I ask presenters to at a minimum wrap their presentations around a case that can be used as an anchor for the material that they will be presenting.

Computer-based activities are interesting. They can be fun and look cool, however, in my experience, when a resident has to do something on their own time, it rarely gets done unless you spend a lot of time policing them. As such, I have found these not worth the effort it takes to develop and implement them. Some residents are quite keen to complete them and prefer this type of learning, so I do have them as supplemental activities or for special things that only involve selected residents (global health curriculum, etc.). Outside of that, if it something I want everyone to do, I rarely choose a computer-based activity.

Question 2. It appears that you have taken logical and progressive steps in the development of both the integrated care model and then enhanced D/BH training approach. You have and will continue to get some data and informal feedback from stakeholders (pediatric residents, pediatric attendings, business

leaders, and patients) you likely will need to make some modifications to your approach. How do you conduct applied outcome research when you have an intervention that is not "fully fixed" and that likely will change gradually even if modestly over the next few years?

PB: Residency education is a fluid thing. The ACGME puts out mandates that are general and do not specifically spell out exactly how a program is to accomplish a required element. This is to permit programs to best utilize the resources that they have in a matter that best suits their purposes. We have had many unique training activities over the years that cannot be replicated in most programs because of Geisinger's unique attributes. Identifying resources and using them in creative ways is commonplace in resident education.

Whenever you begin a new educational process, it is imperative to review the outcomes to determine if it is having the desired effect. I expect that we will be able to review several things pertaining to this activity to determine if additional changes are needed. It will probably be easiest to obtain general feedback from residents and faculty about the basic processes, looking specifically at their attitudes about the manner in which the integrated D/BH activity functions as well as how they feel it impacts their patients and the resident's education. Subjective evidence like this is always easiest to come by and it offers a good starting point to make changes. The changes made from this information from my standpoint are done to get additional buy-in and correct dissatisfaction with the new process. This is not hard scientific data that can be used to determine if the outcome of the program is as expected. That will need to be seen over time and more time-consuming efforts will be needed to determine this. Directly testing residents on D/BH issues, looking at ABP and ISE scores in D/BH domains, and potentially identifying changes in the handling of patients with D/BH issues by residents by utilizing the EHR are all potential ways of seeing this objective data.

Even when all of this is completed and it is felt that the system is running well, change will be inevitable. Alterations in facilities, patient expectations, social issues, ACGME educational requirements, etc., all will occur over time, making continued evaluation and alteration of the program necessary. It is anticipated that this process will need to be altered at some point to meet the changing needs of our learners, faculty, and their patients.

Question 3. Pediatric residents have numerous demands on them during their residency. What challenges did you face in getting them to commit to learning about behavioral health and doing the things you required such as attending didactic lectures or collaborating with psychologists in their continuity clinics?

PB and PK: Any primary care provider is, by definition, a generalist and is expected to handle a broad range of health problems. For a resident in training this is a daunting and at times an overwhelming task. It is one of the reasons that some residents choose to specialize, so that they have more sense of mastery over the areas of healthcare they are expected to be competent in managing. Because of that challenge for broad skills that pediatric residents must master and the limited time they have, we developed our training model to be especially efficient. Most specifically, the curriculum involves lectures/discussions on D/BH topics that are only 30 min long and emphasize bottom-line knowledge and skills, with each lecture labeled, “What every pediatrician should know about ....”. Additionally, by moving our D/BH training to their continuity clinic, and providing help to them with their own patients, they could acquire skills in managing D/BH problems at the time in which they are most in need. Rather than being another training experience they have to squeeze into a busy week, our training experience often helped them get their job done more adequately and efficiently, which improved their “buy-in” with our training and curricula.

We also introduced numerous mechanisms to ensure that we received direct feedback from residents so that our training curricula could be implemented in an iterative process. Examples included focus groups, individual meetings with residents and faculty, confidential rating systems during didactic lectures for feedback, as well as other informal mechanisms such as conversations with residents in their continuity clinic. As indicated in the case study, there were numerous changes that occurred throughout the training year that were adaptations/modifications from the original curricular design. I would add that residents are motivated by the fear that they will need to know how to do something when they get out of residency. They know full well that they will need to handle D/BH issues and quite frankly are anxious that they will not have the needed skills to do so adequately. In educating residents, feeding off of this anxiety is quite useful. Residents will be more likely to cooperate with processes that offer them the practical information and practice experience that they feel will be needed for their future work as a general pediatrician.

Question 4. Health care organizations change leadership and resulting areas of emphasis at times. How can the changes you have made in service delivery and in enhanced training be sustainable if your organization’s priorities change? How can you solidify your changes so they are more likely to “stick”?

PK: In some ways it is fortunate for any of us involved in D/BH service delivery and training that in almost all health care delivery systems, there is a shortage of adequate D/BH services and training. Therefore, if a health care organization changes leadership, when the new leadership team assesses service delivery and training needs, D/BH will be among key areas that require attention. More importantly, if the D/BH training is of value and helps pediatric residents become both more competent and comfortable handling D/BH problems, it will be valued by both resident and attending pediatricians. Additionally, by combining our D/BH training with the implementation of the integrated pediatric primary care model we attempted to help attending pediatricians’ and residents’ experience the added value that the integrated care model provided. At least some of the pediatric primary care providers have told us that they no longer are willing to practice in a primary care setting without a BHC as a central member of their team.

In our health system, we did experience a change of senior leadership (a new CEO) from the time that our initiative (to change our D/BH service delivery and training approaches) was developed and proposed until the time we actually implemented it. The changes in leadership involved a transition from an emphasis on sound business strategies to an emphasis on excellence in the patient experience. This involved some clear differences in emphasis, but frankly, both approaches required sound business approaches as well as genuine care for patients, so the changes were more complementary and a natural progression than a radical change. As a result, our initiative was not negatively impacted by system leadership changes.

Also, research shows that an element of organizational capacity that has been repeatedly found to be central to any type of systems innovation is strong leadership. We are fortunate that the key stakeholders behind this initiative—division heads and leaders from the systems health plan—were very supportive of the program and all the people who implemented it. This type of active support is critical, particularly when organizational turnover occurs—our health system's CEO in our case—as these stakeholders in leadership positions can often engage the new decision-makers for ongoing support.

References

American Academy of Pediatrics. (2009). Policy statement—The future of pediatrics: Mental health competencies for the care of children and adolescents in primary care settings. *Pediatrics, 124,* 410–421.

Asarnow, J. R., Rozenman, M., Wiblin, J., & Zeltzer, L. (2015). Integrated medical-behavioral care compared with usual primary care for child and adolescent behavioral health: A meta-analysis. *JAMA Pediatrics, 169,* 929–937.

Belar, C. D. (2008). Clinical health psychology: A health care specialty in professional psychology. *Professional Psychology: Research and Practice, 39,* 229–233.

Cummings, N. A., & O'Donohue, W. (2011). *Understanding the behavioral healthcare crisis: The promise of integrated care and diagnostic reform.* New York: Routledge.

Foy, J. M. (2014). Enhancing pediatric mental health care: Algorithms for primary care. *Pediatrics, 125,* S109–S125.

Foy, J. M., Green, C. M., Earls, M. F., & Committee on Psychosocial Aspects of Child and Family Health, Mental Health Leadership Work Group. (2019). Mental health competencies for pediatric practice. *Pediatrics, 144,* 1–16.

Gatchel, R. J., & Oordt, M. S. (2013). *Clinical health psychology and primary care: Practical advice and clinical guidance for successful collaboration.* Washington, DC: American Psychological Association.

Green C. M., Foy, J. M., Earls, M. F., & AAP Committee on Psychosocial Aspects of Child and Family Health, Mental Health Leadership Work Group. (2019). Achieving the pediatric mental health competencies. *Pediatrics, 144*(5), e20192758.

Hampton, E., Richardson, J. E., Bostwick, S., Ward, M. J., & Green, C. (2015). The current and ideal state of mental health training: Pediatric resident perspectives. *Teaching and Learning in Medicine, 27,* 147–154.

Horwitz, S. M., Storfer-Isser, A., Kerker, B. D., Szilagyi, M., Garner, A., O'Conner, K. D., ... Stein, R. E. K. (2015). Barriers to the identification and management of psychosocial problems: Changes from 2004 to 2013. *Academic Pediatrics, 15,* 613–620.

Kataoka, S., Zhang, L., & Wells, K. B. (2002). Unmet need for mental health care among U.S. children: Variation by ethnicity and insurance status. *American Journal of Psychiatry, 159,* 1548–1555.

Kim, W. J. (2003). Child and adolescent psychiatry workforce: A critical shortage and national challenge. *Academic Psychiatry, 27,* 277–282.

Novotney, A. (2014). Integrated care at work. *Monitor on Psychology, 45*(7). Retrieved November 14, 2018, from http://www.apa.org/monitor/2014/07-08/integrated-care.aspx.

Petts, R. A., Shahidullah, J. D., Kettlewell, P. W., DeHart, K. A., Rooney, K., Ladd, I. G., … Larson, S. L. (2018). As a pediatrician, I don't know the second, third, or fourth thing to do: A qualitative study of pediatric residents' training and experiences in behavioral health. *International Journal of Health Sciences Education, 5*, 1–11.

Petts, R. A., Shahidullah, J. D., Jaques, M., Kettlewell, P. W., & DeHart, K. A. (2019). Evaluation of a group-based standardized patient training. *New Jersey Pediatrics, 2,* 30–33.

Petts, R., Shahidullah, J. D., Kettlewell, P. W., & DeHart, K. A. (2018b). Trainee perceptions of a group-based standardized patient training for challenging behavioral health scenarios in the United States. *Journal of Educational Evaluation for Health Professionals, 15,* 15.

Regier, D. A., Narrow, W. E., Rae, D. S., Manderscheid, R. W., Locke, B. Z., & Goodwin, F. K. (1993). The de facto US mental and addictive disorder service system: Epidemiologic catchment area prospective 1-year prevalence rates of disorders and services. *Archives of General Psychiatry, 50,* 85–94.

Shahidullah, J. D., Kettlewell, P. W., Palejwala, M. H., Forman, S. G., Billups, A., Anismatta, S., & Madsen, B. (2018a). Behavioral health training in pediatric residency programs: A national survey of training directors. *Journal of Developmental and Behavioral Pediatrics, 39*, 292–302.

Shahidullah, J. D., Kettlewell, P. W., DeHart, K. A., Palejwala, M. H., Rooney, K., Diaz, L., … Carlson, J. M. (2018b). Pediatric residency training and behavioral health: Preliminary outcomes from an interprofessional education curriculum. *New Jersey Pediatrics, 1*, 32–38.

Shahidullah, J. D., Kettlewell, P. W., DeHart, K. A., Rooney, K., Signore, A., Ladd, I. G., … Larson, S. L. (2017). An empirical approach to assessing pediatric residents' attitudes, knowledge, and skills in primary care behavioral health. *International Journal of Health Sciences Education, 4,* 1–14.

Shahidullah, J. D., & Kettlewell, P. W. (2017). Using standardized patients for training and evaluating medical trainees in behavioral health. *International Journal of Health Sciences Education, 4,* 1–14.

Strine, T. W., Mokdad, A. H., Balluz, L. S., Gonzalez, O., Crider, R., Berry, J. T., & Kroenke, K. (2008). Depression and anxiety in the United States: Findings from the 2006 behavioral risk factor surveillance system. *Psychiatric Services, 59*, 1383–1390.

Walter, H. J., Vernacchio, L., Trudell, E. K., Bromberg, J., Goodman, E., Barton, J., … Focht, G. (2019). Five-year outcomes of behavioral health integration in pediatric primary care. *Pediatrics, 144*, e20183243.

Whitehead, M. R., Shahidullah, J. D., Kettlewell, P. W., Quinlan, N., & Strony, R. (2017). An empirical approach to assessing needs for emergency department management of intentional self-harm and related behaviors in the United States. *Journal of Educational Evaluation for Health Professionals, 14,* 1–30.

Conclusions and Future Directions in Interprofessional Care Coordination for Pediatric Autism Spectrum Disorder

Katherine R. Mezher, Jeffrey D. Shahidullah, and Maryellen Brunson McClain

Abstract In the concluding chapter of the book, a brief review of preceding chapters is provided. The purpose of this chapter is to reflect on common themes throughout the chapters, and to highlight some key areas for future work in interprofessional care coordination (ICC) for autism spectrum disorder. Specifically, some current and future priorities may include (1) person-centered and family-centered care coordination, (2) innovative assessment and service management approaches, and (3) teaming and telehealth models that reduce barriers to accessing coordinated services.

Review of Preceding Chapters

The preceding chapters provide a comprehensive review of interprofessional care coordination (ICC) for pediatric autism spectrum disorder (ASD). The chapters first introduce the need for and benefits of ICC for children with ASD and their families. Through examples, case studies, practical suggestions, and specific service models, the authors illustrate how families and professionals from a variety of disciplines can work together to improve outcomes for children with ASD. It is important to note that authors in this book also represent numerous disciplines (e.g., psychology, speech and language pathology, medicine, social work) and work in a variety of settings (e.g., schools, universities, hospitals, community clinics).

An aforementioned aim of this book is to provide professionals who have ICC experience with new and innovative ideas to strengthen current and develop new collaborative interprofessional relationships. For example, interprofessional school teams may identify new ways to collaborate and coordinate care with physicians prescribing medication (e.g., chapter "Interprofessional Roles to Support Psychotropic

K. R. Mezher (✉)
Department of Educational Psychology, Miami University, Oxford, OH, USA
e-mail: krohnkr@miamioh.edu

J. D. Shahidullah
Department of Psychiatry, University of Texas at Austin Dell Medical School, Austin, TX, USA

M. B. McClain
Department of Psychology, Utah State University, Logan, UT, USA

M. B. McClain et al. (eds.), *Interprofessional Care Coordination for Pediatric Autism Spectrum Disorder*, https://doi.org/10.1007/978-3-030-46295-6_27

Medication Prescribing for ASD)", to revisit interprofessional work within special or general education (e.g., chapters "Promoting Academic Success" and "Supporting Students with Autism Spectrum Disorder in Schools Through Multi-Tiered Systems of Support"), or to establish home-school partnerships (e.g., chapter "Partners in School: An Example of Care Coordination to Ensure Consistency of Evidence-Based Practices Across Home and School for Youth with Autism Spectrum Disorder (ASD)") and enhance treatment fidelity, effectiveness, and acceptability.

Another aim of this book is to encourage professionals who do not yet engage in ICC to consider developing such interprofessional relationships. Related to this, is a call for trainers to address pre-professionals' development of ICC competencies through interprofessional education (IPE). Please see chapter "Interprofessional Education and Training", which described types of IPE (e.g., semester-long coursework; the federally funded Leadership Education in Neurodevelopmental and Related Disabilities program) as well as instructional delivery methods (e.g., teleECHO case-based discussions, role-play, clinical experiences).

Future Directions for Interprofessional Care Coordination

Following reflection of the preceding chapters, some interprofessional care priorities may include but are not limited to (1) person-centered and family-centered planning, (2) innovative ICC to positively impact assessment and service management, and (3) overcoming barriers to allow for better access to services, including ICC and sustained partnerships.

Person- and Family-Centered Planning

Given the importance of person-centered and family-centered planning, additional steps should be taken to build teams of interprofessional professionals who prioritize the unique needs of each child and family. As a specific example, the "Screening and Surveillance" chapter introduced Family Navigation, which is a case management framework that has been applied for medical and mental health needs to facilitate access to needed services, and is more recently being applied to ASD (see Broder-Fingert et al., 2019). Many authors in the book describe this need for school or community providers to support an individual or family's ability to *efficiently* find assessment and treatment services, and in particular to meet health and mental health needs. Medical conditions commonly co-occur with ASD, such as epilepsy, gastrointestinal issues, sleep problems, feeding disorders, and immune dysfunction (Tye, Rinicles, Whitehouse, & Alvares, 2019). The chapter titled "Medical Comorbidities in Pediatric Autism Spectrum Disorder" provided more information on medical comorbidities, and included these noteworthy statistics: "A recent review found that 99.1% of their sample of 3,278 children with ASD had at least one co-occurring condition and that 58.2% had at least four co-occurring conditions (Vargason, Frye, McGuinness, & Hahn, 2019)." Thus, it is likely that treating medical and mental health co-occurring conditions will be prioritized by individuals and their families given the significant impact such conditions may have on daily functioning.

Innovative ICC in Assessment and Service Management

This book presents many innovative solutions related to screening, diagnostic evaluation, and timely service access and management. For example, screenings may occur in accessible settings (e.g., home, preschool, child care, other community programs) rather than solely relying on primary care clinicians for screening at well-child visits (see chapters "Screening and Surveillance" and "Developmental Screening in Community-Based Settings"). Also, as some authors highlighted, using an interprofessional team for ASD diagnostic evaluation is faster and more cost-effective than a typical evaluation by a psychologist (Ahlers et al., 2019; see chapters "Interdisciplinary Evaluation of Autism Spectrum Disorder" and "Dell Children's (S)TAAR Model of Early Autism Assessment" for an in-depth review of evaluation). Finally, timely access to services is described in the "Management" and "Transition to Early Schooling for Children with ASD" chapters, which is particularly relevant at this time given that the American Academy of Pediatrics recently shared new recommendations for identifying and supporting children with ASD (Hyman, Levy, Myers, & AAP Council on Children with Disabilities, 2020). Specifically, one noteworthy recommendation was for children to be able to access intervention even before receiving an ASD diagnosis.

Overcoming Barriers to Access and Sustain ICC

Given health professional shortages, including professionals trained in ASD, limited capacity at specialized ASD clinics, and disparities in access for rural and underserved urban populations, telehealth delivery to allow families to access care from their homes was highlighted as an important future direction (see the chapter "Telehealth Approaches to Care Coordination in Autism Spectrum Disorder"). Another future direction is the ECHO Autism program, which seeks to address some of these challenges by leveraging videoconferencing technology to provide interprofessional training and mentorship to community-based providers on ASD best practices.

Finally, interprofessional team involvement is needed not only in early childhood but also for adolescents in the transition to adulthood (see the chapter "Transition from Adolescence to Adulthood in Those Without a Comorbid Intellectual Disability"), particularly as it relates to life skills and their development of independence and autonomy. Sustained collaboration between multiple providers may require team members who have received ICC-specific training (see chapters "Interprofessional Education and Training" and "Interprofessional Training in Developmental and Behavioral Health Within a Pediatric Residency Program An Organizational Systems Case Study") and who understand the philosophical underpinnings, scope of practice, and training of the other professionals (see LaFrance, Weiss, Kazemi, Gerenser, & Dobres, 2019, as astutely highlighted in the chapter "Coordinating ABA Services").

References

Ahlers, K., Gabrielsen, T. P., Ellzey, A., Brady, A., Litchford, A., Fox, J., … Carbone, P. S. (2019). A pilot project using pediatricians as initial diagnosticians in multidisciplinary autism evaluations for young children. *Journal of Developmental and Behavioral Pediatrics, 40*, 1–11.

Broder-Fingert, S., Stadnick, N. A., Hickey, E., Goupil, J., Diaz Lindhart, Y., & Feinberg, E. (2019). Defining the core components of Family Navigation for autism spectrum disorder. *Autism, 24*(2), 526–530.

Hyman, S. L., Levy, S. E., Myers, S. M., & AAP Council on Children with Disabilities, Section on Developmental and Behavioral Pediatrics (2020). Identification, evaluation, and management of children with autism spectrum disorder. *Pediatrics, 145*(1), e20193447.

LaFrance, D. L., Weiss, M. J., Kazemi, E., Gerenser, J., & Dobres, J. (2019). Multidisciplinary teaming: Enhancing collaboration through increased understanding. *Behavior Analysis in Practice, 12*, 709–726.

Tye, C., Rinicles, A. K., Whitehouse, A. J. O., & Alvares, G. A. (2019). Characterizing the interplay between autism spectrum disorder and comorbid medical conditions: An integrative review. *Frontiers in Psychology, 9*.

Vargason, T., Frye, R. E., McGuinness, D. L., & Hahn, J. (2019). Clustering of co-occurring conditions in autism spectrum disorder during early childhood: A retrospective analysis of medical claims data. *Autism Research*.

Index

M. B. McClain et al. (eds.), *Interprofessional Care Coordination for Pediatric Autism Spectrum Disorder*, https://doi.org/10.1007/978-3-030-46295-6

9783030462949